.V.Sc., FRCVS.

C0001S3333

Handbook of Histology Methods
for Bone and Cartilage

D. P. ATTENBURROW B.V.Sc., FRCVS.

Handbook of Histology Methods for Bone and Cartilage

Edited by

Yuehuei H. An, MD

Department of Orthopaedic Surgery,
Medical University of South Carolina, Charleston, SC;
and Department of Bioengineering, Clemson University, Clemson, SC

and

Kylie L. Martin, BSc

Department of Orthopaedic Surgery,
Medical University of South Carolina, Charleston, SC

Humana Press ✳ Totowa, New Jersey

© 2003 Humana Press Inc.
999 Riverview Drive, Suite 208
Totowa, New Jersey 07512

www.humanapress.com

All rights reserved. No part of this book may be reproduced, stored in a retrieval system, or transmitted in any form or by any means, electronic, mechanical, photocopying, microfilming, recording, or otherwise without written permission from the Publisher.

Due diligence has been taken by the publishers, editors, and authors of this book to assure the accuracy of the information published and to describe generally accepted practices. The contributors herein have carefully checked to ensure that the drug selections and dosages set forth in this text are accurate and in accord with the standards accepted at the time of publication. Notwithstanding, as new research, changes in government regulations, and knowledge from clinical experience relating to drug therapy and drug reactions constantly occurs, the reader is advised to check the product information provided by the manufacturer of each drug for any change in dosages or for additional warnings and contraindications. This is of utmost importance when the recommended drug herein is a new or infrequently used drug. It is the responsibility of the treating physician to determine dosages and treatment strategies for individual patients. Further it is the responsibility of the health care provider to ascertain the Food and Drug Administration status of each drug or device used in their clinical practice. The publisher, editors, and authors are not responsible for errors or omissions or for any consequences from the application of the information presented in this book and make no warranty, express or implied, with respect to the contents in this publication. All authored papers, comments, opinions, conclusions, or recommendations are those of the author(s), and do not necessarily reflect the views of the publisher.

This publication is printed on acid-free paper. ⧜
ANSI Z39.48-1984 (American Standards Institute) Permanence of Paper for Printed Library Materials.

Production Editor: Kim Hoather-Potter.

Cover design by Yuehuei H. An and Patricia F. Cleary.

Cover art: Background image: multiple fluorochrome labeling of bone (*see* Chapter 5). From left to right: root with periodontal ligament, alveolar bone, fatty bone marrow of the mandible (*see* Chapter 16); micrograph of a pediatric distal femoral physis (*see* Chapter 21); osteoblasts and woven bone areas stained with toluidine blue and acid fuchsin (*see* Chapter 23); scanning electron micrograph of a bone specimen following removal of marrow and bone cells (*see* Chapter 34); and growth plate cartilage and bone of rat distal femur (contributed by Dr. Q. Kay Kang).

For additional copies, pricing for bulk purchases, and/or information about other Humana titles, contact Humana at the above address or at any of the following numbers: Tel: 973-256-1699; Fax: 973-256-8341; E-mail: humana@ humanapr.com, or visit our Website at www.humanapress.com

Photocopy Authorization Policy:
Authorization to photocopy items for internal or personal use, or the internal or personal use of specific clients, is granted by Humana Press Inc., provided that the base fee of US $20.00 per copy is paid directly to the Copyright Clearance Center at 222 Rosewood Drive, Danvers, MA 01923. For those organizations that have been granted a photocopy license from the CCC, a separate system of payment has been arranged and is acceptable to Humana Press Inc. The fee code for users of the Transactional Reporting Service is: [0-89603-960-9/03 $20.00].

Printed in the United States of America. 10 9 8 7 6 5 4 3 2 1

Library of Congress Cataloging in Publication Data

Handbook of histology methods for bone and cartilage/edited by Yuehuei H. An and
Kylie L. Martin.
     p.;cm
  Includes bibliographical references and index.
  ISBN 0-89603-960-9 (alk. paper)   E-ISBN 1-59259-417-4
   1. Bones--Histology--Handbooks, manuals, etc. 2. Cartilage--Histology--Handbooks,
manuals, etc. I. An, Yuehuei H. II. Martin, Kylie L.
   [DNLM: 1. Bone and Bones--anatomy & histology--Handbooks. 2. Bone and
Bones--physiology--Handbooks. 3. Cartilage--anatomy & histology--Handbooks. 4.
Cartilage--physiology--Handbooks. 5. Histological Techniques--Handbooks. 6. Tissue
Harvesting--Handbooks. WE 39 H23613 2003]
QM101.H33 2003
611'.0184--dc21
                                                           2002035286

To Q. Kay Kang, MD
Without her love, inspiration, and support,
this book would not have been possible.

Yuehuei H. An, MD

To my husband Charles, and my daughters Lisa and Heather,
for their patience, understanding, love, and support.

Kylie L. Martin, BSc

PREFACE

Histotechnology and histomorphometry are the major methodologies in bone and cartilage-related research. *Handbook of Histology Methods for Bone and Cartilage* is an outgrowth of the editors' own quest for information on bone and cartilage histology and histomorphometry. It is designed to be an experimental guide for personnel who work in the areas of basic and clinical bone and cartilage, orthopedic, or dental research. It is the first inclusive and organized reference book on histological and histomorphometrical techniques on bone and cartilage specimens. The topic has not previously been covered adequately by any existing books in the field.

Handbook of Histology Methods for Bone and Cartilage has six major parts and is designed to be concise as well as inclusive, and more practical than theoretical. The text is simple and straightforward. Large numbers of tables, line drawings, and micro- or macro-photographs, are used to help readers better understand the content. Full bibliographies at the end of each chapter guide readers to more detailed information. A book of this length cannot discuss every method for bone and cartilage histology that has been used over the years, but it is hoped that major methods and their applications have been included.

Yuehuei H. An, MD
Kylie L. Martin, BSc

TABLE OF CONTENTS

ABOUT THE EDITORS

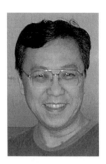

Yuehuei H. (Huey) An, MD, graduated from the Harbin Medical University, Harbin, China in 1983 and was trained in orthopedic surgery at the Beijing Ji Shui Tan Hospital, and in hand surgery at Sydney Hospital, Sydney, Australia. In 1991, Dr. An joined Dr. Richard J. Friedman in the Department of Orthopaedic Surgery at the Medical University of South Carolina to establish the Orthopaedic Research Laboratory, which is now a multifunctional orthopedic research center. Dr. An has published more than 100 scientific papers and book chapters, more than 100 research abstracts, and has also edited 5 books, including *Animal Models in Orthopaedic Research* (CRC Press, 1999), *Mechanical Testing of Bone and the Bone-Implant Interface* (CRC Press, 2000), *Handbook of Bacterial Adhesion* (Humana Press, 2000), *Internal Fixation in Osteoporotic Bone* (Thieme, 2002), and *Orthopaedic Issues in Osteoporosis* (CRC Press, 2002). He is an active member of eight academic societies in the fields of orthopedic surgery, biomaterials, biomechanics, and tissue engineering.

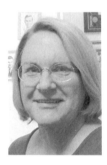

Kylie L. Martin, BSc, is an histological technician and laboratory manager of the Orthopaedic Research Laboratory for the Department of Orthopaedic Surgery, Medical University of South Carolina, Charleston, SC, USA. Ms. Martin received her baccalaureate degree from the Western Australian Institute of Technology (now Curtin University of Technology). She has been at the Medical University of South Carolina since 1979, working in a number of research laboratories, and has extensive experience in experimental histology and cell biology. Ms. Martin has published several journal articles and book chapters.

CONTRIBUTORS

Jean E. Aaron, PhD, *Lecturer, School of Biomedical Sciences, University of Leeds, Leeds, UK*

Yuehuei H. An, MD, *Associate Professor, Director of Orthopaedic Research Laboratory, Department of Orthopaedic Surgery, Medical University of South Carolina, Charleston, SC; and Assistant Professor of Bioengineering, Department of Bioengineering, Clemson University, Clemson, SC, USA*

Troels T. Andreassen, MD, *Associate Professor, Department of Connective Tissue Biology, Institute of Anatomy, University of Aarhus, Aarhus, Denmark*

Kyriacos A. Athanasiou, PhD, PE, *Professor, Department of Bioengineering, Rice University, Houston, TX, USA*

Thomas W. Bauer, MD, PhD, *Professor, Departments of Pathology and Orthopaedic Surgery, The Cleveland Clinic Foundation, Cleveland, OH, USA*

Robert B. Bourne, MD, FRCSC, *Division of Orthopaedic Surgery, London Health Sciences Center, University of Western Ontario, London, Ontario, Canada*

Warwick Bruce, *Department of Orthopaedic Surgery, Concord Hospital, Concord, New South Wales, Australia*

Karen J. L. Burg, PhD, *Assistant Professor, Tissue Engineering Laboratory, Department of Bioengineering, Clemson University, Clemson, SC, USA*

Cathy S. Carlson, DVM, PhD, *Department of Veterinary Diagnostic Medicine, University of Minnesota, Minneapolis, MN, USA*

Ada A. Cole, PhD, *Department of Biochemistry, Rush Medical College, Chicago, IL, USA*

Karl Donath, MD, DDS, MDhc, PhD, *Head and Professor of the Department of Oral Pathology, University of Hamburg, Hamburg, Germany*

Michael J. Dunbar, MD, FRCSC, PhD, *Division of Orthopaedics, QE II Health Sciences Centre, Dalhousie University, Halifax, Nova Scotia, Canada*

John L. Eady, MD, *Professor and Chairman, Department of Orthopaedic Surgery, University of South Carolina School of Medicine, Columbia, SC, USA*

Ryland B. Edwards, III, DVM, MS, *Department of Surgical Sciences, Comparative Orthopaedic Research Laboratory, School of Veterinary Medicine, University of Wisconsin-Madison, Madison, WI, USA*

Reinhold G. Erben, MD, DVM, *Associate Professor, Institute of Animal Physiology, Ludwig Maximilians University, Munich, Germany*

Gian Antonio Favero, MD, DDS, *Professor, Dental School, University of Padua, Padua, Italy*

Elisabetta Fiera, DDS, *Research Fellow, Dental School, University of Chieti, Chieti, Italy*

Victor Fornasier, MD, FRCPC, *Professor, Department of Laboratory Medicine and Pathobiology, Director of Laboratory of Bone and Joint Pathology, St. Michael's Hospital, University of Toronto, Toronto, Ontario, Canada*

Ronald M. Gillies, *Orthopaedic Research Laboratory, Department of Orthopaedic Surgery, University of New South Wales, Prince of Wales Hospital, Sydney, New South Wales, Australia*

Helen E. Gruber, PhD, *Senior Scientist and Director of Research Histology, Orthopaedic Research Biology, Carolinas Medical Center, Charlotte, NC, USA*

Ellen M. Hauge, MD, PhD, *Institute of Pathology, University of Aarhus, Aarhus, Denmark*

Joseph Hemmerlé, PhD, *Institut National de la Santé et de la Recherche Médicale U424, Fédération de Recherche Odontologie, Strasbourg, France*

Seiichi Hirota, MD, *Associate Professor, Department of Pathology, Osaka University Medical School, Suita Osaka, Japan*

Charles L. Ho, RT, HTC (HKU), *Laboratory of Bone and Joint Pathology, St. Michael's Hospital, University of Toronto, Toronto, Canada*

Jerry C. Y. Hu, BSc, *Department of Bioengineering, Rice University, Houston, TX, USA*

Giovanna Iezzi, DDS, *Research Fellow, Dental School, University of Chieti, Chieti, Italy*

Jane A. Ingram, BS, HT, *Orthopaedic Research Laboratory, Carolinas Medical Center, Charlotte, NC, USA*

John A. Jansen, DDS, PhD, *Professor and Head, Department of Biomaterials, University Medical Center Nijmegen, Nijmegen, The Netherlands*

Linda L. Jenkins, HT (ASCP), *Histology Supervisor, Department of Bioengineering, Clemson University, Clemson, SC, USA*

Yebin Jiang, MD, PhD, *Associate Professor of Radiology, Osteoporosis and Arthritis Research Group and Section of Musculoskeletal Radiology, Department of Radiology, University of California San Francisco, San Francisco, CA, USA*

Qian K. Kang, MD, *Senior Research Fellow, Orthopaedic Research Laboratory, Department of Orthopaedic Surgery, Medical University of South Carolina, Charleston, SC, USA*

Jasvir S. Khurana, MD, *Department of Pathology, Temple University Hospital, Philadelphia, PA, USA*

Christel P. A. T. Klein, DVM, PhD, *Head, Central Animal Facility, University Groningen, Groningen, The Netherlands*

Jackie C. LaBreck, HT (ASCP), *Former Research Administrator, Department of Orthopaedic Surgery, Medical University of South Carolina, Charleston, SC, USA*

Lars Lidgren, MD, PhD, *Professor of Department of Orthopaedics, Lund University Hospital, Lund, Sweden*

Mandi J. Lopez, DVM, MS, PhD, *Department of Medical Sciences, Comparative Orthopaedic Research Laboratory, School of Veterinary Medicine, University of Wisconsin-Madison, Madison, WI, USA*

Suzanne Maher, PhD, *Department of Biomedical Mechanics and Materials, The Hospital for Special Surgery, New York, NY, USA*

Diane Mahovlic, HT (ASCP), *Departments of Pathology and Orthopaedic Surgery, The Cleveland Clinic Foundation, Cleveland, OH, USA*

Mark D. Markel, DVM, PhD, *Professor and Chair, Department of Medical Sciences, Associate Dean for Advancement, Comparative Orthopaedic Research Laboratory, School of Veterinary Medicine, University of Wisconsin-Madison, Madison, WI, USA*

Kylie L. Martin, BSc, *Histological Technician and Laboratory Manager, Orthopaedic Research Laboratory, Department of Orthopaedic Surgery, Medical University of South Carolina, Charleston, SC*

Patricia L. Moreira, PhD, *Orthopaedic Research Laboratory, Department of Orthopaedic Surgery, Medical University of South Carolina, Charleston, SC, USA*

Takashi Nakamura, *Department of Orthopaedic Surgery, Kyoto University, Kyoto, Japan*

Stefan Nehrer, MD, *Department of Orthopaedic Surgery, University of Vienna, Vienna, Austria*

Masashi Neo, *Department of Orthopaedic Surgery, Kyoto University, Kyoto, Japan*

Andreas G. Nerlich, MD, *Professor and Chief of Department of Pathology, University of Munich, Munich, Germany*

Shintaro Nomura, MD, *Associate Professor of Department of Pathology, Osaka University Medical School, Suita Osaka, Japan*

Theodore R. Oegema, Jr., PhD, *Professor, Departments of Orthopaedic Surgery and Biochemistry, University of Minnesota, Minneapolis, MN, USA*

Giovanna Orsini, DDS, MS, *Research Fellow, Dental School, University of Chieti, Chieti, Italy*

Giovanna Petrone, DDS, PhD, *Research Fellow, Dental School, University of Chieti, Chieti, Italy*

Adriano Piattelli, MD, DDS, *Professor of Oral Pathology and Medicine, Dean and Director of Studies and Research, Dental School, University of Chieti, Chieti, Italy*

Manlio Quaranta, MD, DDS, *Professor of Prosthetic Dentistry, University of Rome "La Sapienza," Rome, Italy*

William L. Ries, DDS, PhD, *Professor, Departments of Stromatology and Pediatrics, College of Medicine, Medical University of South Carolina, Charleston, SC, USA*

Michael D. Rohrer, DDS, MS, *Director, Division of Oral and Maxillofacial Pathology, University of Minnesota School of Dentistry, Minneapolis, MN, USA*

Cecil H. Rorabeck, MD, FRCSC, *Division of Orthopaedic Surgery, London Health Sciences Centre, University of Western Ontario, London, Ontario, Canada*

Antonio Scarano, DDS, *Research Fellow, Dental School, University of Chieti, Chieti, Italy*

Patricia A. Shore, MSc, *Bone Structural Biology Laboratory, School of Biomedical Sciences, University of Leeds, Leeds, UK*

Robert A. Skinner, HTL (ASCP), *Center for Orthopaedic Research, University of Arkansas for Medical Sciences, Little Rock, AR, USA*

Myron Spector, PhD, *Professor, Department of Orthopaedic Surgery, Brigham and Women's Hospital, Harvard Medical School, Boston, MA, USA*

Torben Steiniche, MD, DMSci, *Associate Professor, Institute of Pathology, Aarhus University Hospital, Aarhus, Denmark*

Martin Svehla, *Orthopaedic Research Laboratory, Department of Orthopaedic Surgery, University of New South Wales, Prince of Wales Hospital, Sydney, New South Wales, Australia*

Krishan K. Unni, MB, MS, *Professor, Department of Pathology, Mayo Clinic, Rochester, MN, USA*

Gonzalo G. Valdivia, MD, FRCSC, *Division of Orthopaedic Surgery, London Health Sciences Centre, University of Western Ontario, London, Ontario, Canada*

Jan-Paul C. M. van der Waerden, BSc, *Department of Biomaterials, University Medical Center Nijmegen, Nijmegen, The Netherlands*

William R. Walsh, PhD, *Associate Professor, University of New South Wales, Director of Orthopaedic Research Laboratory, Department of Orthopaedic Surgery, Prince of Wales Hospital, Sydney, New South Wales, Australia*

Mark Walton, *Department of Orthopaedic Surgery, University of Otago School of Medicine, Dunedin, New Zealand*

Jian-Sheng Wang, MD, PhD, *Department of Orthopedics, Lund University Hospital, Lund, Sweden*

Yunzhao Wang, MD, *Professor, Department of Radiologic Pathology, Beijing Institute of Traumatology and Orthopaedics, Beijing Ji Shui Tan Hospital, Beijing, P.R. China*

Robert S. Weinstein, MD, *Professor, Division of Endocrinology and Metabolism, Center for Osteoporosis and Metabolic Bone Diseases, Department of Internal Medicine, and the Arkansas Veterans Healthcare System, University of Arkansas for Medical Sciences, Little Rock, AR, USA*

Winston W. Wiggins, BA, *Supervisor, Cannon Electron Microscopy Laboratory, Carolinas Medical Center, Charlotte, NC, USA*

Joop G. C. Wolke, PhD, *Department of Biomaterials, University Medical Center Nijmegen, Nijmegen, The Netherlands*

Dianmin Xue, *Department of Radiologic Pathology, Beijing Institute of Traumatology and Orthopaedics, Beijing Ji Shui Tan Hospital, Beijing, P.R. China*

Yuming Yin, MD, *Radiology Resident, Washington University School of Medicine, St. Louis, MO, USA*

Yan Yu, *Orthopaedic Research Laboratory, Department of Orthopaedic Surgery, University of New South Wales, Prince of Wales Hospital, Sydney, New South Wales, Australia*

COLOR PLATES

Color plates 1–24 appear as an insert following p. 270.

I   Introduction

1

Introduction to Experimental Bone and Cartilage Histology

Yuehuei H. An[1] and Helen E. Gruber[2]

[1]*Orthopaedic Research Laboratory, Medical University of South Carolina, Charleston, SC, USA*
[2]*Orthopaedic Research Biology, Carolinas Medical Center, Charlotte, NC, USA*

I. INTRODUCTION

Experimental and diagnostic histotechnology and histomorphometry are two consecutive steps that are essential for clinical work and research in bone or cartilage. Unlike routine histological or pathological laboratories, a laboratory for bone-tissue processing has unique characteristics, such as more demanding fixation, the challenging process of decalcification, media infiltration and embedding, the need for heavy-duty microtomes, diamond circular or wire saws for tissue sectioning, and grinders or grinding machines for section thinning and grinding. The existence of metal or other implants adds further complexity to the process. In addition to the routine microscopic evaluation of cellular and structural features, histomorphometry is a unique facet of bone and cartilage histology. A laboratory engaged in experimental bone and cartilage histology should have both basic and specialized equipment for its unique needs. Histotechnology and histomorphometry are both techniques and arts. They require patience and skilled hands as well as basic biological and anatomical knowledge at the level of organs, tissues, cells, and even molecules. Pre-employment and continuing education are necessary for maintaining adequate knowledge of biological tissues, basic and specific histological techniques, good laboratory practice, and laboratory safety issues.

II. BASIC FACILITY AND EQUIPMENT

A. General Surgical Dissecting Instruments

Ideally, an operating table should be available in the laboratory or in a nearby location. Some basic surgical instruments (such as scalpel, forceps, and scissors), as well as a supply of surgical towels, gloves, plastic bags, and saline should also be readily available in or near the laboratory for proper specimen preparation.

B. X-Ray Machine

A compact cabinet X-ray machine is ideal for a hard-tissue histology laboratory. Common models include Faxitron or Torrex Cabinet X-Ray Systems made by Faxitron X-Ray Corpo-

From: *Handbook of Histology Methods for Bone and Cartilage*
Edited by: Y. H. An and K. L. Martin © Humana Press Inc., Totowa, NJ

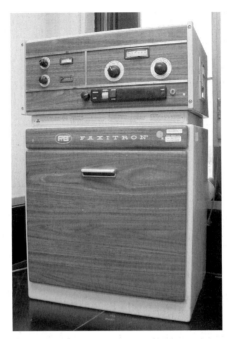

Figure 1. Easy-to-operate Faxitron 43855A cabinet X-ray System (Courtesy of Faxitron X-Ray Co., Wheeling, IL).

ration (Wheeling, IL). High-resolution radiographs can be obtained using these machines. An easy-to-operate model is the Faxitron 43855A cabinet X-ray System (Fig. 1). The Faxitron® Specimen Radiography System Model MX-20 is available for extremely high-resolution and high-magnification specimen radiography. The system's X-ray tube has a thin beryllium window and 20-μm focal spot size which, combined with its low kV capability can create extremely high-resolution specimen radiographs at up to 5 times radiographic magnification. The use of specialized mammography film improves image resolution.

C. Diamond Saws and Grinders

1. Saws for Specimen Harvesting and Rough Cutting

Handsaws with small or fine cutting teeth, hand-held wire saws, trephines, or surgical oscillating saws can be used to harvest bone specimens at necropsy or in the operating room. Further preparation (rough cutting) of specimens for histological processing requires several key tools. A band saw with a 1/4-inch or 1/2-inch fine-toothed blade is an invaluable general resource for cutting and resizing of bone specimens (Fig. 2). A Dremel rotary tool (Dremel, Racine, WI), with its wide variety of grinding and cutting attachments, is also a useful tool.

2. Diamond Circular Saws

Diamond circular saws are used for cutting plastic- or resin-embedded specimens to obtain thin sections before being ground to the desired thickness. There are several major manufacturers of diamond circular saws. The Isomet™ low-speed saw made by Buehler Ltd. (Lake Bluff, IL) is a popular one (Fig. 3). However, in the authors' laboratory an old high-speed dia-

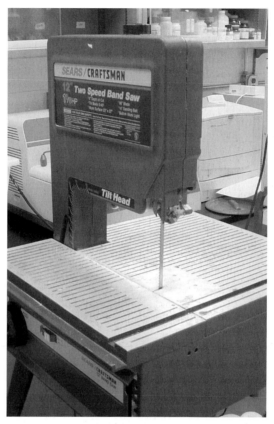

Figure 2. A band saw with a 1/4-inch fine-toothed blade is an invaluable general resource for cutting and resizing of bone specimens. It requires careful degreasing and cleaning after each use.

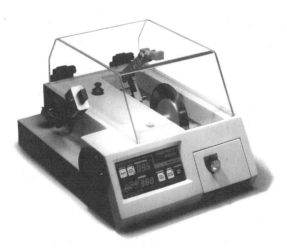

Figure 3. Isomet™ low-speed saw made by Buehler Ltd. (Courtesy of Buehler Ltd., Lake Bluff, IL) is a popular cut-off saw for trimming and sectioning plastic or resin-embedded specimens.

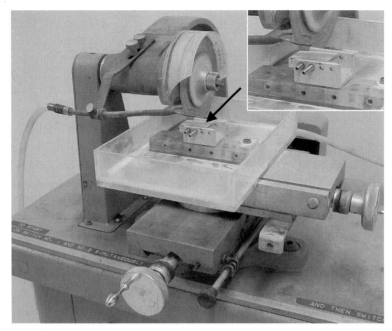

Figure 4. An old high-speed diamond circular saw with a motor-driven specimen stage is used to cut bone specimens containing hard metal implants, such as stainless steel or cobalt chromium alloy.

mond circular saw with a motor-driven specimen stage is used to cut bone specimens containing hard metal implants, such as stainless steel or cobalt chromium alloy (Fig. 4).

3. Diamond Wire Saws

Diamond wire saws are also used for cutting plastic or resin-embedded specimens to obtain thin sections before being ground to the desired thickness. There is only one major manufacturer of fine diamond wire saws that fit the needs of hard-tissue sectioning, Well Diamond Wire Saws, Inc. (Norcross, GA and Mannheim, Germany). In the author's laboratory, a Well model 3241 Precision Wire Saw (Fig. 5) has been successfully used for cutting plastic-embedded specimens. A more advanced version, Well model 4240 (Fig. 6), which has recently been tested in the authors' laboratory, creates a smoother cutting surface and can accommodate large tissue blocks.

4. Grinders or Grinding Systems

A wheel grinder/polisher (Fig. 7) is a basic tool for thinning and polishing bone sections before and after gluing to glass or Plexiglas slides. This machine is a major part of the basic sawing-grinding procedure, which is the routine method for hard-tissue histology in the majority of bone histology laboratories throughout the world. Several manufacturers make automated grinding systems, including Buehler, Struers, and Leco.

5. Specialized Sectioning/Grinding Equipment

A sawing/grinding system, the Exakt System (Exakt Apparatebau, Germany and Exakt Technologies, Inc., Oklahoma City, OK), is available but it is costly.[20] It consists of a

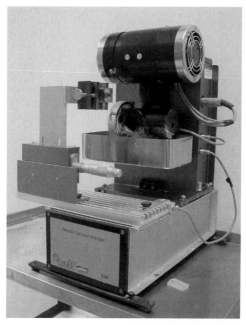

Figure 5. Well model 3241 Precision diamond wire saw (Courtesy of Well Diamond Wire Saws, Inc., Norcross GA, USA and Mannheim, Germany).

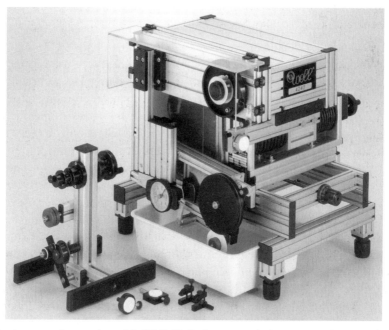

Figure 6. A more advanced model, Well 4240, has recently been tested in the authors' laboratory. It can create a smoother cutting surface and can accommodate large tissue blocks (Courtesy of Well Diamond Wire Saws, Inc., Norcross GA, USA and Mannheim, Germany).

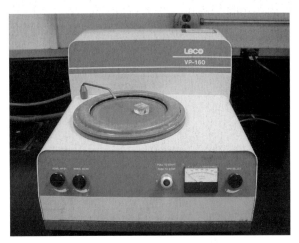

Figure 7. A basic wheel grinder/polisher (Leco Corp., St. Joseph, MI).

diamond-coated band-saw and an automated grinding unit (*see* Chapter 16). This system is frequently used in sectioning implants.

A modified inner circular "sawing" system (Fijnmetaal Techniek, Amsterdam, The Netherlands), reported by van der Lubbe and Klein (*see* Chapter 17), is available in Europe.[50,104] This system can cut thin sections (according to original users, as thin as 10 μm) directly, without grinding.

D. Microtomes

The majority of rotary microtomes have a protective metal casing to guard the mechanism against dust and accidental damage. They have stationary knife holders and a ball-joint block holder clamp. Rotary microtomes are the basic microtomes used in most histology laboratories for routine paraffin-embedded soft-tissue sectioning and sectioning of decalcified hard tissue (Fig. 8). They can also be used for cutting small celloidin-embedded tissues.

Leica has recently developed a new type of microtome, the rotating disc microtome (Fig. 9). This design offers a different approach to histological applications. In these microtomes, the specimen block sits on a vertical disc that rotates over the cutting knife in a circular motion, advancing toward the knife with each rotation, whereas with conventional microtomes, the knife advances toward the specimen. The specimen-changing position in this new design is located a safe distance from the knife, outside the sectioning zone. According to the manufacturer's web site, this system offers a number of advantages over rotary microtomes, including improved section quality, enhanced ergonomics, and greater user safety.

Sliding microtomes are commonly used for direct cutting of celloidin-embedded large tissues or small, hard tissues embedded in plastic or resin. The Leica SM2500 (Fig. 10) is a heavy-duty sliding microtome recommended for applications such as sectioning of hard tissues or materials embedded in plastic or resin, large specimens embedded in paraffin, and hard industrial materials. It may also be used for large, soft specimens (e.g., elastomers) with the addition of a liquid nitrogen-freezing attachment.

The Leica SP1600 microtome (Fig. 11) has a diamond-coated inner-hole saw blade at the center. Slices of very hard materials can be prepared without destroying their mor-

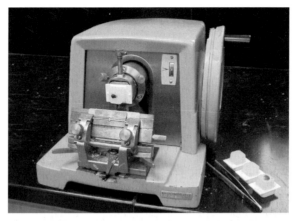

Figure 8. An old rotary microtome manufactured by American Optical Corp.

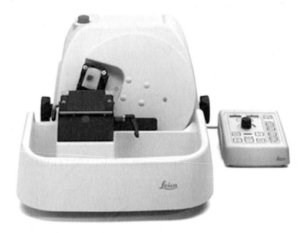

Figure 9. Leica's new rotating disc microtome (Courtesy of Meyer Instruments, Inc., Langham Creek, Houston, TX).

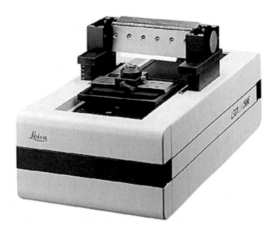

Figure 10. The Leica SM2500 heavy-duty sliding microtome (Courtesy of Meyer Instruments, Inc., Langham Creek, Houston, TX).

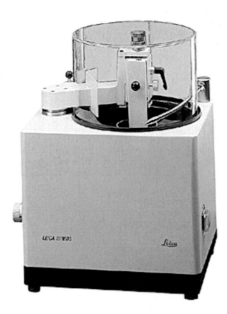

Figure 11. The Leica SP1600 microtome uses a diamond-coated inner-hole saw blade (Courtesy of Meyer Instruments, Inc., Langham Creek, Houston, TX).

phology for investigation using light microscopy. Under optimal conditions, sections with a thickness of 30 μm can be achieved. To prepare a section, the object holder is guided slowly toward the rotating cutting edge of the saw blade. With this sectioning technique, serial sections can be produced, unlike the conventional sawing technique in which the user must calculate the loss of material caused by the "thick" diamond-coated saw blade. The speed of the rotating blade is approx 600 rpm. A built-in water-cooling device prevents the objects from overheating and removes cutting debris from the blade's edge.

E. Other Useful Equipment and Tools

Many small items are necessary or useful for a bone histology lab. These include: adhesive for binding large specimens to molds and rings prior to sectioning (Technovit 3040 glue; Heraeus Kulzer GmbH, Germany and Energy Beam Sciences, Inc., Agawam, MA); "super glue" for gluing sections to glass or Plexiglas slides; electronic calipers or micrometers for measuring section thickness; vacuum pumps and desiccators for proper infiltration; small plastic molds for embedding specimens ("Peel-Away," Electron Microscopy Sciences, Fort Washington, PA) (Fig. 12); megacassettes for embedding large specimens (Surgipath Medical Instruments, Richmond, IL); bone histomorphometry software (OsteoMeasureTM: OsteoMetrics, Inc., Atlanta, GA); and microtome knives (Delaware Diamond Knives, Wilmington, DE).

III. BASIC PROCEDURES AND PRECAUTIONS

The basic procedures for tissue containing bone, teeth, or hard materials (such as metal implants) include fixation, decalcification (used only for paraffin or celloidin embedding), dehydration, infiltration and embedding, sectioning, and staining.

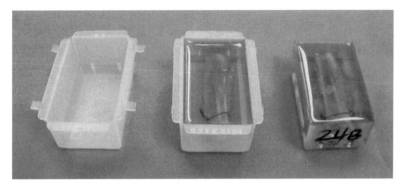

Figure 12. Tissue block embedded in Spurr's resin using a "Peel-A-Way" plastic mold ("Peel-A-Way", Electron Microscopy Sciences, Fort Washington, PA).

A. Tissue Fixation

Fixation is used for preventing tissue decomposition and preservation of cell and matrix structure, and to intensify subsequent staining. The specimen must be fixed immediately after harvesting to avoid artifacts. Specimens should be rough-cut into small pieces. Large specimens may require perfusion fixation or vacuum-assisted infiltration of fixative solutions for thorough fixation (*see* Chapter 8). There may be several undesirable effects of fixation, including shrinkage and hardening of tissue.

Ideally, the choice of a fixative should be governed by the tissue type and by enzyme or histochemical needs. A pilot study to test fixation procedures in unique experiments is always advisable. Although many fixatives are available, 10% neutral buffered formalin (NBF) remains the most popular fixative for fixation of bone and cartilage tissues. It is basically a general-purpose fixative for most biological tissues. It penetrates tissues continuously, rapidly (or slowly), and evenly. It permits the use of most staining and impregnation techniques. Tissues should be switched to 70% ethanol for long-term storage.

Other commonly used fixatives include 70% or 75% ethanol, glutaraldehyde, mercuric chloride, picric acid, Bouin's solution, and Carnoy's fluid. For enzyme studies of bone, alkaline phosphatase and acid phosphatase have specialized fixation needs.

Proper fixation is the first key step in bone histological processing (*see* Chapter 8). If possible, every effort should be made to reduce the specimen size before fixation, which dramatically helps the specimen to be properly fixed. Make sure the volume ratio between the fixative and specimen is large enough (>10:1). For most small bone specimens (less than 5 mm in thickness) 24–48 h fixation is enough. For large specimens or small dense bone, at least 48–72 h fixation is needed. For large bone specimens, perfusion fixation is recommended.

B. Dehydration and Clearing

The water in the tissue to be embedded is removed by bathing successively in a graded series of alcohols (usually 70%, 95%, 100% ethanol, two changes for each concentration). For both decalcified and undecalcified bone tissues, serial ethanol changes are the most commonly used method, but the times required for undecalcified tissue are much longer. Other reagents can be used for tissue dehydration, including acetone, butyl alcohol, and isopropyl alcohol. Acetone causes more shrinkage and hardening of tissue com-

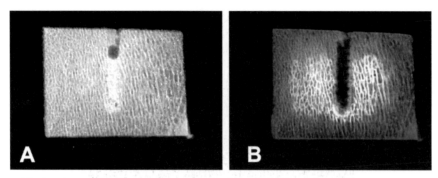

Figure 13. Radiographs show (A) a thin bone slice from bovine femoral condyles (3 mm in thickness) and (B) partial decalcification after 6 h immersion in Cal-Ex decalcifying solution (Fisher Scientific).

pared to alcohol. Automatic tissue processors allow variable infiltration schedules to be selected.

Before embedding in paraffin or other embedding media, the ethanol in the tissue is replaced by a lipid solvent such as xylene. As the tissues become impregnated with the solvent, they usually become transparent; this step is called "clearing." However, not all clearing agents can create this transparency; thus, so a more general term is "dealcoholization." For plastic embedding of undecalcified tissues, clearing is not often used. Xylene substitutes that offer convenience and safety advantages are now available, such as Clear-Rite (a blend of isoparaffinic aliphatic hydrocarbons) (Richard-Allan Scientific, Kalamazoo, MI).[89] Other clearing agents include toluene, benzene, carbon bisulphide, cedarwood oil, and methyl salicylate. Brain[9] and Skinner[95,96] suggested the use of cedar wood and methyl salicylate, which does not make tissue brittle, even after prolonged clearing time.

C. Decalcification, Paraffin Embedding, and Sectioning

Paraffin-embedding and sectioning remains the most common method for histological study of soft tissues (subcutaneous tissue, muscle, tendon, ligament), cartilage, and decalcified bone specimens. When using celloidin embedding, decalcification is also needed. In decalcifying bone specimens, the goal is to achieve sufficient decalcification (Fig. 13) to allow successful sectioning but to avoid over-decalcification so that cellular details remain intact. Commonly used solutions for decalcification include hydrochloric acid, formic acid, and ethylene diamine tetraacetic acid (EDTA) (*see* Chapters 10, 13, and the review by Brain[9] and Skinner et al.)[96] for the details of decalcification, embedding, and sectioning methods.

D. Plastic Embedding and Sectioning

Undecalcified embedding and sectioning are specialized procedures used for the evaluation of osseous tissues (bone, teeth, or calcified tissues), dental tissues, and especially specimens containing metal implants (*see* reviews by Sheehan and Hrapchak,[93] Baron et al.,[4] Sanderson,[89] Gruber and Starky,[34] and Parts III and IV of this book for details). With this technique, specimens are embedded in plastics or resins such as glycol methacrylate, methyl methacrylate (MMA) or Spurr's resin (Fig. 12).[89,97,110] In choosing a plastic-embedding medium, the goal is to match the hardness of the embedding medium to the

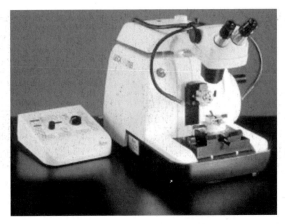

Figure 14. Automatic rotary microtome, Leica RM2165 (Courtesy of Meyer Instruments, Inc., Langham Creek, Houston, TX).

hardness of the bone or cartilage in order to produce successful sections. Embedding in plastic offers many advantages in hard-tissue histology. Generally, there is no need for decalcification. Using a sliding or heavy-duty rotary microtome, thin sections can be made because of the better support given by the media to cellular components.

There are some differences between plastic embedding and paraffin embedding in terms of tissue processing and sectioning. The time required for each step is much longer for plastic embedding; no decalcification is needed; clearing is not always used; and more choices of sectioning methods exist for plastic-embedded specimens. There are three major sectioning methods for plastic-embedded specimens: direct sectioning using a heavy-duty microtome, "sawing-grinding," and sawing only.

1. Sectioning with Microtomes

Small undecalcified bone specimens embedded in glycol methacrylate or MMA can be cut using automatic rotary microtomes such as the Leica RM2165 (Fig. 14) with a tungsten carbide blade (for MMA or glycol methacrylate) or with a large glass blade (for glycol methacrylate). Larger undecalcified specimens can be cut using a sliding microtome, such as the Leica SM2500 (Fig. 10).

2. Sawing-Grinding Methods

"Sawing-grinding" is the traditional method used for plastic-embedded specimens. The specimen is sectioned with a diamond-coated wafering saw (e.g., Buehler Isomet 2000, Struers Accutome-5, or Leco VC-50) into 0.2–1.0-mm-thick slices. The slices are then glued onto a Plexiglas slide and ground on a grinding machine (such as the Buehler Ecomet 3, Struers Dap-V, or Leco VP-160) to produce 30–100-μm-thick sections. In patient and skilled hands, the thickness of the ground sections can be less than 50 μm.[80] The process is tedious and time-consuming. Because the slices cut are relatively thick, in small specimens it is important that all cuts are successful to avoid excess tissue loss.

Well-controlled systems with automatic grinding capacity, such as the Exakt sawing-grinding system (Exakt Apparatebau, Germany and Exakt Technology, Inc., Oklahoma City, OK,)[20,87] are efficient, useful, and precise, but fairly expensive (*see* Chapter 16).

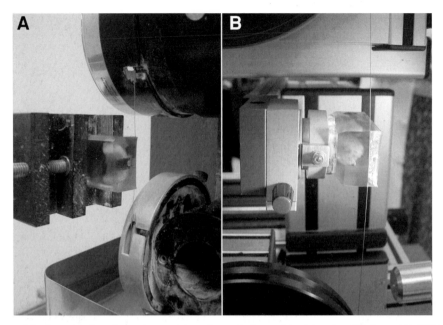

Figure 15. Images showing wires cutting through tissue blocks using Well model 3241 (A) and model 4240 (B) diamond wire saws. They can cut sections as thin as 75 μm (from small tissue blocks), and can cut specimen blocks as large as 10 cm in diameter.

3. Sawing Methods

Two systems are available for sawing hard tissues embedded in plastics and resins. One is the modified inner circular sawing technique (Fijnmetaal Techniek Amsterdam, The Netherlands) originally reported by van der Lubbe and Klein (*see* Chapter 17).[50,104] This technique can create 12 ± 5-μm sections without grinding.

Another sawing system is a diamond-coated wire saw unit, Well model 3241 or 4240 Precision Wire Saw (Well Diamond Wire Saws, Inc., Norcross GA). According to our experience and that of others,[12] small sections as thin as 75 μm can be cut using this method, in a matter of minutes (Fig. 15). The sections are then glued onto slides, stained, and coverslipped. Because of their simplicity, efficiency, and relatively lower cost compared to the Exakt system, these saws are becoming more popular for the sectioning of undecalcified or implant-containing specimens.

The advantage of these two techniques is that they are capable of sectioning hard tissues or implant-containing specimens without grinding.

4. Thickness of Section and Effects of Overlapping

The thickness at which sections are cut influences the usefulness of the sections. In general, thin sections are required for observing cellular detail and thick sections for lower-magnification histomorphometric analysis. For general applications, sections of 4–5 μm are cut from decalcified bone specimens. Direct cutting of plastic-embedded tissues using a heavy-duty rotary microtome can create sections as thin as 3 μm, although 5–7 μm are more realistic. The inner circular diamond saw described in Chapter 17 can cut as thin as 10 μm from MMA-embedded undecalcified hard tissues or tissues

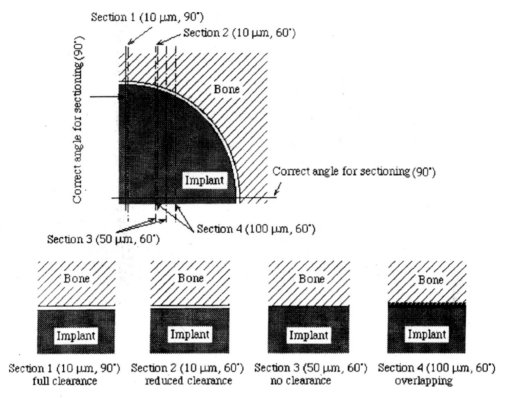

Section 1 (10 μm, 90°)

Section 2 (10 μm, 60°)

Correct angle for sectioning (90°)

Bone

Implant

Correct angle for sectioning (90°)

Section 4 (100 μm, 60°)

Section 3 (50 μm, 60°)

Bone	Bone	Bone	Bone
Implant	Implant	Implant	Implant

Section 1 (10 μm, 90°)   Section 2 (10 μm, 60°)   Section 3 (50 μm, 60°)   Section 4 (100 μm, 60°)

full clearance   reduced clearance   no clearance   overlapping

Figure 16. Schematic diagram showing the effects of section thickness and the angle of sectioning plane on the appearance of the implant-bone interface (a clearance at the interface is assumed).

containing metal implants. However, for most sawing-grinding methods, either manual or automatic, an appropriate range of thickness is 50–150 μm.

Overlapping between the boundaries of implant and tissue may occur as a result of the porosity of some implant surfaces or because of an imperfect angle between the interface and the sectioning plane (the correct angle is 90 degrees).[79,80] This can be overcome by making the thinnest sections possible and orienting the angle between the interface and sectioning plane at 90 degrees. If a cylindrical implant is used, the plane of the cut should be perpendicular to the long axis of the implant. This allows multiple, correctly angled cuts to be made without repositioning the implant. If the cut is made parallel to the long axis of the implant, wrong-angle phenomenon may occur because theoretically, no right-angle sections can be made in this orientation (since the thickness of the section cannot be zero) (Fig. 16). Parr et al.[79] demonstrated that interlabel distances were not significantly affected by section thickness. They suggested that the use of microradiographs for histomorphometric analysis of the implant-bone interface is superior to bright-field analysis because of the low variability of microradiographic data and the added ability to obtain bone-mineral-density measurements. However, the correct sectioning angle (90°) and the thinnest possible sections should always obtained in order to utilize the advantages of bright-field observation (visibility of cellular detail and the composition of tissues around the implant).

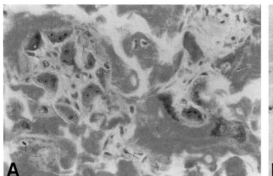 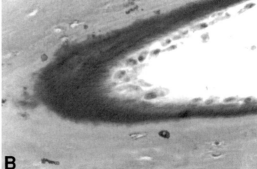

Figure 17. Goldner's trichrome stain of a cutting cone and a filling cone during the process of bone remodeling. (A) A histologic section taken from a nondecalcified bone biopsy core from a child being treated for osteopetrosis. The cutting cone of a forming osteon is shown, and its the circumference is lined with multinucleated osteoclasts (brown). Note the streaks of unstained mineralized cartilage (white) that course through the bone (green), a pattern pathognomonic of osteopetrosis. Goldner's trichrome stain. Original magnification ×400. (B) A section from nondecalcified cortical bone (green) of an iliac crest biopsy. A portion of the filling cone of a forming osteon is shown, and its wall is lined with osteoblasts. The osteoid seam (magenta) next to the osteoblastic cellular layer varies in width because of the plane of the section. Goldner's trichrome stain. Original magnification ×400. (*See* color plate 1 appearing in the insert following p. 270.)

E. Staining Procedures

1. Basic and Special Staining Methods

Many staining methods are available. Hematoxylin & eosin (H&E) staining remains the basic and most common procedure for most tissues. It can be used for both decalcified and undecalcified specimens. Both Goldner's trichrome stain and the von Kossa stain allow differentiation of osteoid from mineralized bone matrix, although von Kossa provides little other information. Other common stains for bone sections include Giemsa, toluidine blue (often used for ground sections),[21] methylene blue/basic fuchsin, and Stains-All.[33] Safranin O (for glycosaminoglycans)/fast green,[103] Alcian blue (for proteoglycans), and periodic acid-Schiff (for chondroitin sulfate and glycoproteins)[49] are commonly used in the evaluation of articular cartilage. Goldner's or Masson's trichrome are useful for both bone and cartilage staining in paraffin-embedded and plastic-embedded sections.[31]

Tetracycline labeling is a bone label that is administered during the experiment and before animals are sacrificed (*see* Chapter 5). It is based on the fact that most tetracycline antibiotics form stable tetracycline-calcium chelates, which fluoresce at wavelengths used with standard ultraviolet microscopy. Different tetracyclines fluoresce with different colors, and thus multiple time-spaced labels can be individually identified in the bone-forming sites. Tetracycline labeling is used for examining bone growth and remodeling, and requires undecalcified bone embedding. Tetracycline evaluation is *not* staining as the word is used in histology.

Intravascular injections of India ink or other dyes prior to tissue fixation are used for studying the vascularity of various tissues, such as bone or callus, meniscus, ligament, or tendon (*see* Chapter 38). Enzyme staining procedures have been developed for localization of alkaline phosphatase (ALP) and acid phosphatase (ACP) in bone,[38] cartilage,[32] and the tissues surrounding an implant.[81]

2. H&E or a Single Stain?

The Cole's hematoxylin[17]-only staining method has been used routinely in the author's laboratory for staining ground sections of bone and bone containing implants to be evaluated histomorphometrically. The areas of bone are stained in bluish purple. The marrow spaces are not stained. Similar results can be obtained by using toluidine blue, a single color stain that is very easy to use. If eosin is used on the same section with hematoxylin, marrow space and background resin will be stained red. As a result, there is reduced contrast between bone, soft tissues, and marrow space. This is not a problem when performing manual evaluation, but can create a large error if bone areas are digitized automatically using a computer program.

3. Goldner's Masson Trichrome Stain

Specialized adaptations have been developed for the application of Goldner's Masson trichrome stain to plastic-embedded undecalcified bone specimens.[31] This stain can be used successfully on bones embedded in methyl methacrylate, glycol methacrylate, and Spurr's resin.[31] The stain affords the advantage of good cellular staining because of the hematoxylin component with concomitant sharp discrimination of mature bone matrix (which stains green), immature new bone matrix (also known as osteoid tissue, which stains red), and calcified cartilage (which stains very pale green) (Fig. 17). Use of red filters during photomicrography aids in bone-osteoid discrimination in black-and-white photographs.

4. Immunohistochemical Staining

Immunohistochemical staining techniques have been further developed in recent years (*see* Chapter 22). These techniques are used for examining biochemicals in cartilage, bone, ligament, tendon, and other tissues. Immunostaining can be used to identify types I, II, and IV collagen, glycoproteins, laminin, tenasin, and fibronectin in plastic-embedded bone specimens.[57] Common macromolecules such as cartilage matrix protein,[72] types I, II, and III collagen,[14,63,66] and proteoglycans[106] have also been successfully localized in cartilage specimens. Other cartilage biochemicals for which immunohistochemical staining methods have been developed include types V, VI, X and XI collagen,[6,63] chondroitin sulfate, keratan sulfate,[27] stromelysin, tumor necrosis factor-α (TNF-α), TNF receptors,[18] and fibronectin.[59] Immunohistochemical techniques have been used to demonstrate the distribution of types I, II, and III collagen at the soft-tissue-implant interface,[107] the healing tendon-bone interface,[56] and the ligament-to-bone attachment.[27] Immunohistochemical staining procedures for substance P, tyrosine hydroxylase, and neurofilament have been used to evaluate nerve regeneration[26] (*see* Part V of this book for additional immunohistochemical staining techniques). Successful antibody localization may be fixative-sensitive; often ethanol fixation or non-fixed frozen sections may be needed for successful immunohistochemistry.

5. Vital Staining

Vital fluorescent staining can be used to determine chondrocyte viability in the cartilage layer. After it has been cut away from the underlying bone, the cartilage is stained

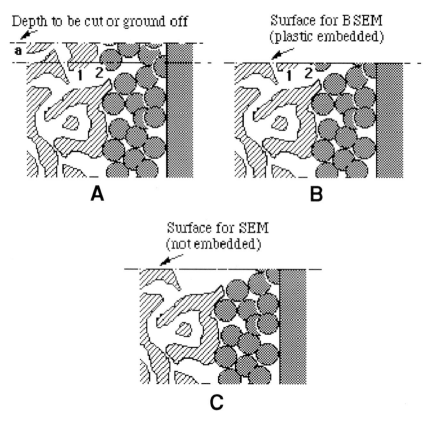

Figure 18. Schematic diagram showing the effects of SEM sample preparation on the trabecular bone volume. The upper surface of the tissue block containing implant-bone interface is cut or ground off to create a surface for SEM or BSEM evaluation (A). If the specimen is embedded in plastic media, the end of trabeculae "1" and the lower part of bead "2" will be preserved on the surface (B). If the specimen is not embedded, the end of trabeculae "1" and the lower part of bead "2" may fall off the surface, assuming there are no continuities or connections on the sagittal plane (C).

with either fluorescein diacetate/propidium iodide or calcein/ethidium homodimer in phosphate-buffered saline (PBS).[71] After staining, the cartilage slice is mounted on a slide (kept moist with PBS), and optical regional sectioning performed using a confocal laser-scanning microscope to determine cell viability and cell distribution within the cartilage tissue. The method of determining the distribution of live cells is based on the principle that viable and nonviable cells differ in their ability to exclude specific dyes. The cell membranes of damaged, dead, or dying cells are penetrated by propidium iodide or ethidium homodimer, and their nuclei will fluoresce red. Viable cells with intact membranes and active cytoplasm metabolize either fluorescein diacetate or calcein, and will fluoresce green.[71]

IV. GENERAL CONSIDERATIONS OF HISTOLOGICAL EVALUATION OF BONE AND CARTILAGE

A. *Histological Evaluation*

Histological evaluation and characterization of bone and cartilage tissues are normally done with light microscopy. Descriptive histology and histomorphometry are the two main types of histological study. Depending on the particular situation, either or both methods may be used. Descriptive histology is used to provide a general evaluation of the tissue of interest, including the morphology, structure, and arrangement of cells, matrix, implant, or tissue-implant interface. Scoring systems are often designed in order to semi-quantify the components of interest. An example of this is the estimation of the quantity of new bone formation in a bone defect.[54] Full bone formation in a defect is scored as 3, moderate bone formation as 2, mild bone formation as 1, and no new bone formation as 0. The data are analyzed using nonparametric analysis of variance. Examples of other similar scoring systems can be found in the literature for evaluation of fracture healing,[54] articular cartilage repair,[69,83] and biocompatibility of implants in soft tissues.[42]

B. *Histomorphometry*

Histomorphometric analysis has been performed using histological sections, micro-radiographs,[79] and backscattered electron microscopic (BSEM) images (on plastic-embedded surfaces).[74,101,117] Standard scanning electron microscopy (SEM) images of a specimen's surface are less desirable for histomorphometric analysis because overlying components from adjacent areas are not well-demonstrated (Fig. 18).

Histomorphometry is a methodology for quantitatively analyzing i) length (perimeter or boundary), such as the surface perimeter of an implant, ii) distance between points, such as the clearance at the implant-tissue interface or the distance between the central lines of two trabeculae, iii) area, such as trabecular bone area or repair tissue area, and iv) the number of components of interest, such as trabecular number, vessel number, or cell number.[78,86] These parameters are the four primary measurements that can be made based on two-dimensional (2D) images. Three-dimensional (3D) parameters or structures can be calculated or reconstructed from 2D measurements according to carefully considered assumptions. Although accurate 3D data is necessary for proper comparison between different specimens (such as treated and control bone structure), it is impossible to reconstruct a 3D structure based on a single 2D image because the structures of most biological tissues (such as bone tissue) are anisotropic. This problem has been partially conquered by the introduction of quantitative CT (QCT),[48,64,70] MRI,[70] and confocal laser-scanning microscopy, all of which section and reconstruct the specimen.

Despite its limitations, 2D histomorphometric analysis remains a common and useful method for analyzing the structural changes in trabecular bone,[45,78] the callus composition in healing fracture sites, the repair tissues of bone or cartilage defects, the pathological changes in arthritis, the bone apposition and ingrowth into implant surfaces (*see* Chapter 26 and 27), and the soft-tissue-implant interface (*see* Chapter 32).

Standard nomenclature, symbols, and units for bone histomorphometry can be found in Chapter 25 and in the review by Parfitt et al.[78] The more commonly used terms for trabecular bone structures include BV (bone volume or TBA, trabecular bone area, which is the trabecular surface area divided by the total area in mm^2); Tb.Th (trabecular thickness, the average thickness of trabeculae in μm); and Tb.Sp (trabecular separation, the average distance between trabeculae, representing the amount of marrow space in μm). Common parameters for trabecular bone spatial connectivity include Tb.N (trabecular number, the average number of continuous trabecular elements encountered per unit area), Ho.N (hole number, the average number of holes per unit area), N.Nd (trabecular node number, nodes: trabecular branch points), N.Tm (trabecular terminus number, termini: trabecular end points), and Nd/Tm ratio. Most of the parameters can be measured using specialized imaging software.

Quantifiable paramenters can be used for histomorphometric analysis of fracture callus,[111,112] repair tissues of bone defects,[19,114] cartilage defects,[10] ectopic bone formation (soft-tissue ossicles),[41,61] mineralized bone, non-mineralized bone, new bone, old bone, chondral tissue, fibrocartilage, hyaline cartilage, and fibrous vascular tissue. Parameters for cartilage repair, cartilage thickness and area, degree of attachment, and surface roughness have also been developed.[35]

Parameters that are used in the evaluation of experimental arthritis include articular cartilage thickness and area, synovial-cell-layer thickness, subchondral bone-plate thickness, periarticular bone structure, and spatial connectivity.[1,7,40,45] Other measurements of synovial or cartilage morphology include synovial-cell density, chondrocyte- and necrotic-cell density, the concentration of lipid-containing cells, and mean surface-destruction grade.[58]

In the histomorphometric analysis of the implant-bone interface, the useful parameters are: i) bone apposition (or ongrowth), which is the fractional linear extent of bone apposed to implant surface divided by the total surface perimeter of the implant (i.e., the surface potentially available for apposition)[1,25] and ii) bone ingrowth, which represents the amount of ingrown bone per unit of available surface area, porous space and ingrowth depth.[1,23,62,105] In the case of bone ingrowth within an osteopenic bone bed, the structure of the bone, represented by TBA, Tb.Th, Tb.N, and Tb.Sp, should be also analyzed.[1,23] Characterization of the soft-tissue-implant interfaces produced in percutaneous and sc implantation may include quantification of epidermal downgrowth, sulcus width, capsule thickness, macrophage density, or fibroblast density.[77,102]

In examining the scar tissue within a ligament defect, areas of interest that have been analyzed include blood vessels, fat cells, loosely arranged collagen, disorganized collagen, dense cellular infiltrates, and the combination of these elements.[94]

For vascular repair, Karim et al.[46] reported a histomorphometric analysis of the number of vascular smooth-muscle cells, actin-stain-positive cells, total cells, and the neointimal collagen area.

Like macro-measurements of bone dimensions, there may be significant intermethod or interobserver variability in histomorphometric analysis. When necessary, several observers may need to perform the same procedure independently, or more than one method may be employed for comparison.[116]

V. OTHER METHODS FOR MORPHOLOGICAL EVALUATION OF BONE AND CARTILAGE

A. Scanning Electron Microscopy

Scanning electron microscopy (SEM) and back-scatter scanning electron microscopy (BSEM) are important methods for evaluation of the structure and morphology of bone structures,[45,113] trabecular bone surfaces,[43] the osteoclast-bone interfaces,[120] cartilaginous surfaces or structures,[51] implant surfaces,[25,65] wear debris,[109] implant beds,[100] and implant-tissue interfaces.[60,73,74] SEM is also a popular method for examining the vascular structure of various corrosion-casted tissues (using Mercox injection), including bone,[76,108] muscle,[75] joint,[36] ligament, and tendon.[52]

The limitations of SEM are that the specimen must be dried before observation, causing distortion of the original spatial structure and morphology,[51] and the limited specimen size in some instruments. The first problem seems to have been solved by the new low-temperature or cryo-SEM system.[51,85]

B. Transmission Electron Microscopy

Transmission electron microscopy (TEM) is the most powerful method for evaluating the ultrastructure and morphology of large molecules (such as proteoglycans or collagens), subcellular components, cells, and even the implant-tissue interface. Immuno-labeled electron microscopy makes it possible to locate biochemicals of interest such as proteoglycans within cartilage,[84] collagens within cartilage cells and matrix,[15,119] and osteopontin, fibronectin, and osteocalcin within the cells or matrix adjacent to implant surfaces.[73] A relatively new, high-voltage electron microscopic tomography method can be used to view the structural relationships between collagen and mineral in bone.[53] The system also has direct 3D imaging capability.

Specially fixed and dehydrated tissues are embedded in Epon or Spurr's resin,[97] and ultrathin sections (50 nm to 2 μm) are cut.[13,16,53] Section preparation of metal implant-tissue interface has been a challenge for some time. In many cases, the implants are removed for easier preparation of ultrathin sections.[39,98] However, implant removal inevitably damages the implant-tissue interface. Therefore, several methods for preparing ultrathin tissue sections containing the intact implant-tissue interface have been explored. These include: using a soft-cored implant coated with a thin layer of metal,[13,55] removing bulk metal with electrochemical dissolution before embedding,[5,39] and removing bulk metal by sawing-grinding techniques.[37,47] Also, 10–20-μm sections created by the inner circular "sawing" technique can be used directly for TEM examination (*see* Chapter 17).[50]

C. Radiography and CT

1. Plain Radiography

Radiography is the basic method for evaluating fracture healing and bone-defect repair. Preoperative radiographs confirm normal anatomy and demonstrate the size of the bone, which is very helpful for designing or choosing fixation devices and implants of appropriate size or shape. In the operating room, roentgenograms using a C-arm unit are useful in determining the quality of internal fixation and the placement of implants. Radiographs should be taken immediately after surgery to examine the position of the fracture or defect and the quality of fixation. Periodic radiographs of the fracture or defect site are essential for monitoring the process of repair. In addition, angiography has been used to examine the revascularization of a healing fracture or a vascularized bone graft.[30]

2. High-Resolution Radiography and Microradiography

Bone specimens can be radiographed using a high-resolution X-ray machine, such as a Faxitron (Faxitron X-Ray Co., Wheeling, IL). Microradiography (also using a high-reso-

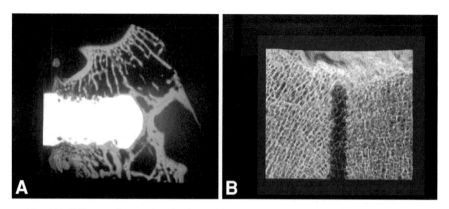

Figure 19. (A). Microradiographs shows a thin bone slice from rabbit distal femur (0.8 mm in thickness) containing a porous titanium implant. (B) Microradiograph shows a thin bone slice from bovine femoral condyles (2 mm in thickness). The structure of trabeculae and a screw hole are visualized.

lution X-ray machine) based on thin bone sections (about 0.5–1.0 mm) provides detailed images of bone structures. It can be used in the quantification of bone apposition and ingrowth into an implant (Fig. 19).[44,117,118] The quality of the bone structure around an implant can also be assessed using this method. A variation called microradiographic videodensitometry is also useful for analyzing bone structures and bone density.[44] The vascularity of repaired bone tissues can be evaluated using microradiography (or microangiography). In this technique, radio-opaque substances such as Micropaque, barium sulfate, or lead oxide are injected into the arterial vasculature prior to specimen processing. This allows visualization of the cross-sectioned vessels on thin sections. Vascular trees can also be demonstrated using larger sections.[11,90,92]

3. Computerized Tomography

Computerized tomography (CT) has been used for examining bone structure, bone destruction, new bone formation during fracture healing, and bone lengthening in animal models.[3,91] Quantitative CT (QCT) is capable of analyzing bone structure, even in small rat bones, and is believed to be more sensitive than dual-energy X-ray absorptiometry (DEXA).[28] The spatial resolution of CT on cancellous specimens can reach 8–80 μm.[8,29] Based on a 2D array, Feldkamp developed what has become known as the micro-CT (μ-CT) scanner for the 3D reconstruction of bone.[22] The recent development of compact desktop μ-CT scanners (SCANCO USA, Inc., Wayne, PA) has resulted in 3D images with high resolution, which can be used for studying 3D morphology of cancellous bone (Fig. 20).[88] Another CT method for 3D reconstruction is the X-ray tomographic microscope (XTM), which allows in vivo evaluation of cancellous bone.[48]

D. Confocal Microscopy

Developed less than 20 years ago, confocal laser scanning microscopy (CLSM) has become a star among the numerous imaging methods used in biomedical research. It has a wide variety of applications, and its use has become widespread in orthopedic research. The technique utilizes a laser beam, which penetrates tissue to a depth of 300–500 μm

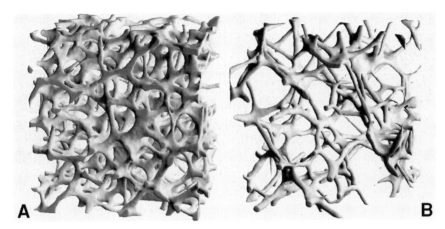

Figure 20. Three-dimensional µCT reconstruction of cancellous bone structure. (A) Normal cancellous bone structure. (B) Osteoporotic bone. (The images were kindly provided by Prof. Ralph Mueller, Institute for Biomedical Engineering, University of Zurich, Zurich, Switzerland and Harvard Medical School, Boston, MA, USA.)

and thus reflects images beneath the surface of a specimen. Stored multilayer 2D images can then be reorganized to show 3D or cross-sectional pictures. The advantages of CLSM over conventional SEM are its ability to view the structures within a specimen or cell and the fact that it can be used with unfixed, wet specimens.

CLSM has been used for viewing the structures at the implant-tissue interface, such as unmineralized bone matrix or mineralized bone.[82,99] Using CLSM, Piattelli et al.[82] found that in a rabbit tibial model a layer of unmineralized bone matrix lies at the interface of mineralized bone and titanium-screw surface. Their study revealed that although 40% of the titanium surface contained bone apposition, only 10% of the bone was in direct contact with the screw surface, and the other 30% was separated from the surface by an unmineralized tissue layer. Confocal microscopy has also been employed to determine the location of viable chondrocytes in frozen and thawed osteochondral articular cartilage.[71] CLSM has also been used for examining cell location and population in cell-seeded porous constructs[24] or explants and to detect the location of type IX collagen in cartilage[115] and type X and XI collagen in the bovine collateral ligament-bone junction.[67,68]

VI. GOOD LABORATORY PRACTICE

A. Why?

Medical devices, drugs, and biological products intended for human and animal use are regulated by the Food and Drug Administration (FDA), and must undergo preclinical testing prior to clinical testing. Standards exist for testing such FDA-regulated products. Research studies that support applications for such products must follow strict criteria that are delineated in the document entitled Good Laboratory Practice (GLP) for Nonclinical Laboratory Studies.[2] Adherence to the practices described in the document are intended to ensure the quality and integrity of the safety data filed in accordance with applicable sections of the Food, Drug, and Cosmetic Act and the Public Health Service

Act. The regulations concerning GLP studies are comprehensive, and include standards for all personnel, facilities, equipment, test articles, and records. GLP studies are essential but extremely time-consuming endeavors.

B. Elements of the GLP Study

Standard operating procedures must be in place to ensure the quality and integrity of the data collected during the course of a study, and any deviation from the written proto-col must be documented as part of the raw data. Standard operating procedures should include minimum animal care requirements; animal facility procedures; methods used to receive, identify, store, handle, mix, and sample control and test articles; animal observa-tions; laboratory tests; procedures for handling animals found moribund or dead during a study; necropsy procedures, collection and identification of specimens; histology proto-cols; data handling, storage, and retrieval; maintenance and calibration of equipment; and animal transfer, placement, and identification. Special emphasis is given to having procedures in place that could affect the outcome of the study, such as inadvertent ani-mal misidentification or exposures to test or control articles. Food and water provided to animals must be analyzed periodically during the course of the study for contaminants that may reasonably be expected to be present and affect study results. Histology proto-cols must be written and carefully observed with specific detailed methods prepared for all aspects of specimen procurement, preparation, and analysis. Records and report details are also carefully regulated in GLP studies.

The entire GLP study must be conducted in written accordance with the study protocol, appropriately documented by the individuals involved, and all deviations must be recorded. While the study is in progress, all GLP documents are periodically reviewed by a quality assurance unit. At the conclusion of a study, a comprehensive final report signed by the principal investigator must be prepared, which includes the objectives of the study, all methodologies involved in data collection and analysis, a description of the animals used, identification of all personnel involved in the study, and a description of where all raw data and specimens will be stored.

VII. LABORATORY SAFETY

A. Personnel

General laboratory safety principles should be applied when working in a histological laboratory. One of the most important aspects is ensuring that all laboratory personnel have been adequately trained in the handling of potentially biohazardous materials as well as general laboratory safety procedures. The laboratory director is responsible for ensur-ing adequate training of personnel.

Safety precautions must be established, posted, and observed to ensure protection from physical, chemical, biochemical, and electrical hazards and biohazardous materials.

Everyone who works in the laboratory should wear a lab coat and gloves (perhaps not for some sectioning procedures). These may be supplemented by such items as shoe cov-ers, face shields, and safety glasses as required for specific procedures.

All personnel should be aware that eating, drinking, smoking, and applying makeup are hazardous in the laboratory setting.

Laboratory personnel must practice safe disposal methods for any biological and chemical waste generated, and must follow the established procedures for their particular institution.

B. Facility and Equipment

The laboratory must be constructed, arranged, and maintained to ensure adequate space and ventilation for conducting all phases of testing, including the pre-analytic (pre-testing), analytic (testing), and post-analytic (post-testing).

A fume hood is essential for a histology laboratory for handling toxic or hazardous chemicals, such as xylene. Staining and cover slipping should be done in a well-ventilated area preferably using a fume hood. Handling of fixatives (e.g., formalin) should also be done under the fume hood.

Chemical storage should follow product and institutional regulations. Use an explosion-proof cabinet for storing small quantities of volatile solvents in the laboratory, and ensure that the solvents stored together are compatible. Acids and other corrosive agents should be stored separately.

An eyewash station and emergency "deluge" type shower should be installed in the laboratory to be used in the event of chemical accidents. A fire extinguisher rated for use on both chemical and electrical fires should also be in close proximity to the laboratory, and all personnel should be made aware of its location and mode of operation. All safety equipment should be tested monthly to ensure its readiness for use.

REFERENCES

1. An YH, Friedman RJ, Jiang M, et al: Bone ingrowth to implant surfaces in an inflammatory arthritis model. *J Orthop Res* 16:576–584, 1998.
2. Anonymous: *Good Laboratory Practice (GLP) for Nonclinical Laboratory Studies.* Department of Health and Human Services, Washington, DC, 1992.
3. Augat P, Merk J, Genant HK, et al: Quantitative assessment of experimental fracture repair by peripheral computed tomography. *Calcif Tissue Int* 60:194–199, 1997.
4. Baron R, Vignery A, Neff L, et al: Processing of undecalcified bone specimens for bone histomorphometry. In: Recker RR, ed: *Bone Histomorphometry: Techniques and Interpretation.* CRC Press, Boca Raton, FL, 1983, 13.
5. Bjursten LM, Emanuelsson L, Ericson LE, et al: Method for ultrastructural studies of the intact tissue-metal interface. *Biomaterials* 11:596–601, 1990.
6. Bland YS, Ashhurst DE: Development and ageing of the articular cartilage of the rabbit knee joint: distribution of the fibrillar collagens. *Anat Embryol (Berl)* 194:607–619, 1996.
7. Bogoch E, Gschwend N, Bogoch B, et al: Juxtaarticular bone loss in experimental inflammatory arthritis. *J Orthop Res* 6:648–656, 1988.
8. Bonse U, Busch F, Gunnewig O, et al: 3D computed X-ray tomography of human cancellous bone at 8 microns spatial and 10(–4) energy resolution. *Bone Miner* 25:25–38, 1994.
9. Brain EB: *The Preparation of Decalcified Sections.* Charles C. Thomas, Springfield, IL, 1966.
10. Breinan HA, Minas T, Hsu HP, et al: Effect of cultured autologous chondrocytes on repair of chondral defects in a canine model. *J Bone Joint Surg [Am]* 79:1439–1451, 1997.
11. Brueton RN, Brookes M, Heatley FW: The vascular repair of an experimental osteotomy held in an external fixator. *Clin Orthop* 257:286–304, 1990.
12. Burr DB, Milgrom C, Boyd RD, et al: Experimental stress fractures of the tibia. Biological and mechanical aetiology in rabbits. *J Bone Joint Surg [Br]* 72:370–375, 1990.

13. Chehroudi B, Ratkay J, Brunette DM: The role of implant surface geometry on mineralization in vivo and in vitro: A transmission and scanning electron microscopic study. *Cells Mater* 2:89–104, 1992.

14. Claassen H, Kirsch T: Temporal and spatial localization of type I and II collagens in human thyroid cartilage. *Anat Embryol (Berl)* 189:237–242, 1994.

15. Clark JM, Norman A, Notzli H: Postnatal development of the collagen matrix in rabbit tibial plateau articular cartilage. *J Anat* 191:215–221, 1997.

16. Clokie CM, Warshawsky H: Morphologic and radioautographic studies of bone formation in relation to titanium implants using the rat tibia as a model. *Int J Oral Maxillofac Implants* 10:155–165, 1995.

17. Cole EC: Studies of hematoxyin stains. *Stain Technol* 18:125–152, 1943.

18. Comer JS, Kincaid SA, Baird AN, et al: Immunolocalization of stromelysin, tumor necrosis factor (TNF) alpha, and TNF receptors in atrophied canine articular cartilage treated with hyaluronic acid and transforming growth factor beta. *Am J Vet Res* 57:1488–1496, 1996.

19. DeVries WJ, Runyon CL, Martinez SA, et al: Effect of volume variations on osteogenic capabilities of autogenous cancellous bone graft in dogs. *Am J Vet Res* 57:1501–1505, 1996.

20. Donath K, Breuner G: A method for the study of undecalcified bones and teeth with attached soft tissues. The Sage-Schliff (sawing and grinding) technique. *J Oral Pathol* 11:318–326, 1982.

21. Eurell JA, Sterchi DL: Microwaveable toluidine blue stain for surface staining of undecalcified bone sections. *J Histotechnol* 17:357–359, 1994.

22. Feldkamp LA, Goldstein SA, Parfitt AM, et al: The direct examination of three-dimensional bone architecture in vitro by computed tomography. *J Bone Miner Res* 4:3–11, 1989.

23. Fini M, Nicoli Aldini N, Gandolfi MG, et al: Biomaterials for orthopedic surgery in osteoporotic bone: a comparative study in osteopenic rats. *Int J Artif Organs* 20:291–297, 1997.

24. Freed LE, Grande DA, Lingbin Z, et al: Joint resurfacing using allograft chondrocytes and synthetic biodegradable polymer scaffolds. *J Biomed Mater Res* 28:891–899, 1994.

25. Friedman RJ, An YH, Jiang M, et al: Influence of biomaterial surface texture on bone ingrowth in the rabbit femur. *J Orthop Res* 14:455–464, 1996.

26. Fromm B, Schafer B, Parsch D, et al: Reconstruction of the anterior cruciate ligament with a cyropreserved ACL allograft. A microangiographic and immunohistochemical study in rabbits. *Int Orthop* 20:378–382, 1996.

27. Gao J, Messner K, Ralphs JR, et al: An immunohistochemical study of enthesis development in the medial collateral ligament of the rat knee joint. *Anat Embryol (Berl)* 194:399–406, 1996.

28. Gasser JA: Assessing bone quantity by pQCT. *Bone* 17:145S–1454S, 1995.

29. Gluer CC, Wu CY, Jergas M, et al: Three quantitative ultrasound parameters reflect bone structure. *Calcif Tissue Int* 55:46–52, 1994.

30. Gonzalez del Pino J, Knapp K, Gomez Castresana F, et al: Revascularization of femoral head ischemic necrosis with vascularized bone graft: a CT scan experimental study. *Skeletal Radiol* 19:197–202, 1990.

31. Gruber HE: Adaptations of Goldner's Masson trichrome stain for the study of undecalcified plastic embedded bone. *Biotech Histochem* 67:30–34, 1992.

32. Gruber HE, Marshall GJ, Nolasco LM, et al: Alkaline and acid phosphatase demonstration in human bone and cartilage: effects of fixation interval and methacrylate embedments. *Stain Technol* 63:299–306, 1988.

33. Gruber HE, Mekikian P: Application of Stains-All for demarcation of cement lines in methacrylate embedded bone. *Biotech Histochem* 66:181–184, 1991.

34. Gruber HE, Stasky AA: Histological study in orthopaedic animal research. In: An YH, Friedman RJ, eds. *Animal Models in Orthopaedic Research.* CRC Press, Boca Raton, FL, 1999, 115–138.

35. Hacker SA, Healey RM, Yoshioka M, et al: A methodology for the quantitative assessment of articular cartilage histomorphometry. *Osteoarthritis Cartilage* 5:343–355, 1997.
36. He SZ, Xiu ZH, Hansen ES, et al: Microvascular morphology of bone in arthrosis. Scanning electron microscopy in rabbits. *Acta Orthop Scand* 61:195–200, 1990.
37. Hemmerle J, Voegel JC: Ultrastructural aspects of the intact titanium implant-bone interface from undecalcified ultrathin sections. *Biomaterials* 17:1913–1920, 1996.
38. Hillmann G, Hillman B, Donath K: Enzyme, lectin and immunohistochemistry of plastic embedded undecalcified bone and other hard tissues for light microscopic investigations. *Biotech Histochem* 66:185–193, 1991.
39. Holgers KM, Thomsen P, Tjellstrom A, et al: Electron microscopic observations on the soft tissue around clinical long-term percutaneous titanium implants. *Biomaterials* 16:83–90, 1995.
40. Holm IE, Bunger C, Melsen F: A histomorphometric analysis of subchondral bone in juvenile arthropathy of the dog knee. *Acta Pathol Microbiol Immunol Scand [A]* 93:299–304, 1985.
41. Ishaug-Riley SL, Crane GM, Gurlek A, et al: Ectopic bone formation by marrow stromal osteoblast transplantation using poly(DL-lactic-co-glycolic acid) foams implanted into the rat mesentery. *J Biomed Mater Res* 36:1–8, 1997.
42. Jansen JA, Dhert WJ, van der Waerden JP, et al: Semi-quantitative and qualitative histologic analysis method for the evaluation of implant biocompatibility. *J Invest Surg* 7:123–134, 1994.
43. Jayasinghe JA, Jones SJ, Boyde A: Scanning electron microscopy of human lumbar vertebral trabecular bone surfaces. *Virchows Arch A Pathol Anat Histopathol* 422:25–34, 1993.
44. Kalebo P, Jacobsson M: Recurrent bone regeneration in titanium implants. Experimental model for determining the healing capacity of bone using quantitative microradiography. *Biomaterials* 9:295–301, 1988.
45. Kang Q, An YH, Butehorn HF, et al: Morphological and mechanical study of the effects of experimentally induced inflammatory knee arthritis on rabbit long bones. *J Mater Sci Mater Med* 9:463–473, 1998.
46. Karim MA, Miller DD, Farrar MA, et al: Histomorphometric and biochemical correlates of arterial procollagen gene expression during vascular repair after experimental angioplasty. *Circulation* 91:2049–2057, 1995.
47. Kayser MV, Downes S, Ali SY: An electron microscopy study of intact interfaces between bone and biomaterials used in orthopaedics. *Cells Mater* 4:353–358, 1991.
48. Kinney JH, Lane NE, Haupt DL: In vivo, three-dimensional microscopy of trabecular bone. *J Bone Miner Res* 10:264–270, 1995.
49. Kiviranta I, Tammi M, Jurvelin J, et al: Demonstration of chondroitin sulphate and glycoproteins in articular cartilage matrix using periodic acid-Schiff (PAS) method. *Histochemistry* 83:303–306, 1985.
50. Klein CP, Sauren YM, Modderman WE, et al: A new saw technique improves preparation of bone sections for light and electorn microscopy. *J Appl Biomater* 5:369–373, 1994.
51. Kobayashi S, Yonekubo S, Kurogouchi Y: Cryoscanning electron microscopy of loaded articular cartilage with special reference to the surface amorphous layer. *J Anat* 188:311–322, 1996.
52. Kraus BL, Kirker-Head CA, Kraus KH, et al: Vascular supply of the tendon of the equine deep digital flexor muscle within the digital sheath. *Vet Surg* 24:102–111, 1995.
53. Landis WJ, Hodgens KJ, Arena J, et al: Structural relations between collagen and mineral in bone as determined by high voltage electron microscopic tomography. *Microsc Res Tech* 33:192, 1996.
54. Lane JM, Sandhu HS: Current approaches to experimental bone grafting. *Orthop Clin North Am* 18:213–225, 1987.
55. Linder L: Ultrastructure of the bone-cement and the bone-metal interface. *Clin Orthop* 276:147–156, 1992.

56. Liu SH, Panossian V, al-Shaikh R, et al: Morphology and matrix composition during early tendon to bone healing. *Clin Orthop* 339:253–260, 1997.

57. Lucena SB, Duarte MEL, Fonseca EC: Plastic embedded undecalcified bone biopsies: an immunohistochemical method for routine study of bone marrow extracellular matrix. *J Histotechnol* 20:253, 1997.

58. Lukoschek M, Schaffler MB, Burr DB, et al: Synovial membrane and cartilage changes in experimental osteoarthrosis. *J Orthop Res* 6:475–492, 1988.

59. Lust G, Burton-Wurster N, Leipold H: Fibronectin as a marker for osteoarthritis. *J Rheumatol* 14 Spec No: 28–29, 1987.

60. McNamara A, Williams DF: Scanning electron microscopy of the metal-tissue interface. II. Observations with lead, copper, nickel, aluminium, and cobalt. *Biomaterials* 3:165–176, 1982.

61. Mohr H, Kragstrup J: Morphostereometry of heterotopic ossicles in the rat. *Acta Orthop Scand* 62:257–260, 1991.

62. Moroni A, Caja VL, Egger EL, et al: Histomorphometry of hydroxyapatite coated and uncoated porous titanium bone implants. *Biomaterials* 15:926–930, 1994.

63. Morrison EH, Ferguson MW, Bayliss MT, et al: The development of articular cartilage: I. The spatial and temporal patterns of collagen types. *J Anat* 189:9–22, 1996.

64. Muller R, Hildebrand T, Hauselmann HJ, et al: In vivo reproducibility of three-dimensional structural properties of noninvasive bone biopsies using 3D-pQCT. *J Bone Miner Res* 11:1745–1750, 1996.

65. Nakashima Y, Hayashi K, Inadome T, et al: Hydroxyapatite-coating on titanium arc sprayed titanium implants. *J Biomed Mater Res* 35:287–298, 1997.

66. Nerlich AG, Wiest I, von der Mark K: Immunohistochemical analysis of interstitial collagens in cartilage of different stages of osteoarthrosis. *Virchows Arch B Cell Pathol Incl Mol Pathol* 63:249–255, 1993.

67. Niyibizi C, Sagarrigo Visconti C, Gibson G, et al: Identification and immunolocalization of type X collagen at the ligament-bone interface. *Biochem Biophys Res Commun* 222:584–589, 1996.

68. Niyibizi C, Visconti CS, Kavalkovich K, et al: Collagens in an adult bovine medial collateral ligament: immunofluorescence localization by confocal microscopy reveals that type XIV collagen predominates at the ligament-bone junction. *Matrix Biol* 14:743–751, 1995.

69. O'Driscoll SW, Keeley FW, Salter RB: Durability of regenerated articular cartilage produced by free autogenous periosteal grafts in major full-thickness defects in joint surfaces under the influence of continuous passive motion. A follow-up report at one year. *J Bone Joint Surg [Am]* 70:595–606, 1988.

70. Odgaard A: Three-dimensional methods for quantification of cancellous bone architecture. *Bone* 20:315–328, 1997.

71. Ohlendorf C, Tomford WW, Mankin HJ: Chondrocyte survival in cryopreserved osteochondral articular cartilage. *J Orthop Res* 14:413–416, 1996.

72. Okimura A, Okada Y, Makihira S, et al: Enhancement of cartilage matrix protein synthesis in arthritic cartilage. *Arthritis Rheum* 40:1029–1036, 1997.

73. Orr RD, de Bruijn JD, Davies JE: Scanning electron microscopy of the bone interface with titanium, titanium alloy and hydroxyapatite. *Cells Mater* 2:241–251, 1992.

74. Overgaard S, Soballe K, Josephsen K, et al: Role of different loading conditions on resorption of hydroxyapatite coating evaluated by histomorphometric and stereological methods. *J Orthop Res* 14:888–894, 1996.

75. Pannarale L, Gaudio E, Marinozzi G: Microcorrosion casts in the microcirculation of skeletal muscle. *Scanning Electron Microsc* (Pt 3):1103–1108, 1986.

76. Pannarale L, Morini S, D'Ubaldo E, et al: SEM corrosion-casts study of the microcirculation of the flat bones in the rat. *Anat Rec* 247:462–471, 1997.

77. Paquay YC, De Ruijter AE, van der Waerden JP, et al: A one stage versus two stage surgical technique. Tissue reaction to a percutaneous device provided with titanium fiber mesh applicable for peritoneal dialysis. *Asaio J* 42:961–967, 1996.

78. Parfitt AM, Drezner MK, Glorieux FH, et al: Bone histomorphometry: standardization of nomenclature, symbols, and units. Report of the ASBMR Histomorphometry Nomenclature Committee. *J Bone Miner Res* 2:595–610, 1987.

79. Parr JA, Young T, Dunn-Jena P, et al: Histomorphometrical analysis of the bone-implant interface: comparison of microradiography and brightfield microscopy. *Biomaterials* 17:1921–1926, 1996.

80. Pazzaglia UE, Bernini F, Zatti G, et al: Histology of the metal-bone interface: interpretation of plastic embedded slides. *Biomaterials* 15:273–277, 1994.

81. Piattelli A, Scarano A, Piattelli M: Detection of alkaline and acid phosphatases around titanium implants: a light microscopical and histochemical study in rabbits. *Biomaterials* 16:1333–1338, 1995.

82. Piattelli A, Trisi P, Passi P, et al: Histochemical and confocal laser scanning microscopy study of the bone-titanium interface: an experimental study in rabbits. *Biomaterials* 15:194–200, 1994.

83. Pineda S, Pollack A, Stevenson S, et al: A semiquantitative scale for histologic grading of articular cartilage repair. *Acta Anat* 143:335–340, 1992.

84. Ratcliffe A, Fryer PR, Hardingham TE: The distribution of aggregating proteoglycans in articular cartilage: comparison of quantitative immunoelectron microscopy with radioimmunoassay and biochemical analysis. *J Histochem Cytochem* 32:193–201, 1984.

85. Read ND, Jeffree CE: Low-temperature scanning electron microscopy in biology. *J Microsc* 161:59–72, 1991.

86. Recker RR: *Bone Histomorphometry: Techniques and Interpretation.* CRC Press, Boca Raton, FL, 1983.

87. Rohrer MD, Schubert CC: The cutting-grinding technique for histologic preparation of undecalcified bone and bone-anchored implants. Improvements in instrumentation and procedures. *Oral Surg Oral Med Oral Pathol* 74:73–78, 1992.

88. Ruegsegger P, Koller B, Muller R: A microtomographic system for the nondestructive evaluation of bone architecture. *Calcif Tissue Int* 58:24–29, 1996.

89. Sanderson C: Entering the realm of mineralized bone processing: a review of the literature and techniques. *J Histotechnol* 20:259, 1997.

90. Schliephake H, Neukam FW, Hutmacher D, et al: Experimental transplantation of hydroxylapatite-bone composite grafts. *J Oral Maxillofac Surg* 53:46–51, 1995.

91. Schumacher B, Albrechtsen J, Keller J, et al: Periosteal insulin-like growth factor I and bone formation. Changes during tibial lengthening in rabbits. *Acta Orthop Scand* 67:237–241, 1996.

92. Seitz H, Hausner T, Schlenz I, et al: Vascular anatomy of the ovine anterior cruciate ligament. A macroscopic, histological and radiographic study. *Arch Orthop Trauma Surg* 116:19–21, 1997.

93. Sheehan DC, Hrapchak BB, eds: *Theory and Practice of Histotechnology.* Battelle Press, Columbus, OH and Richland, WA, 1980:89–117.

94. Shrive N, Chimich D, Marchuk L, et al: Soft-tissue "flaws" are associated with the material properties of the healing rabbit medial collateral ligament. *J Orthop Res* 13:923–929, 1995.

95. Skinner RA: The value of methyl salicylate as a clearing agent. *J Histotechnology* 9:27–28, 1986.

96. Skinner RA, Hickmon SG, Lumpkin CK, et al: Decalcified bone: twenty years of successful specimen management. *J Histotechnol* 20:267–277, 1997.

97. Spurr AR: A low-viscosity epoxy resin embedding medium for electron microscopy. *J Ultrastruct Res* 26:31–43, 1969.

 98. Takeshita F, Ayukawa Y, Iyama S, et al: Long-term evaluation of bone-titanium interface in rat tibiae using light microscopy, transmission electron microscopy, and image processing. *J Biomed Mater Res* 37:235–242, 1997.

 99. Takeshita F, Iyama S, Ayukawa Y, et al: Study of bone formation around dense hydroxyapatite implants using light microscopy, image processing and confocal laser scanning microscopy. *Biomaterials* 18:317–322, 1997.

100. Takeshita F, Murai K, Ayukawa Y, et al: Effects of aging on titanium implants inserted into the tibiae of female rats using light microscopy, SEM, and image processing. *J Biomed Mater Res* 34:1–8, 1997.

101. Tanzer M, Harvey E, Kay A, et al: Effect of noninvasive low intensity ultrasound on bone growth into porous-coated implants. *J Orthop Res* 14:901–906, 1996.

102. Therin M, Christel P, Meunier A: Analysis of the general features of the soft tissue response to some metals and ceramics using quantitative histomorphometry. *J Biomed Mater Res* 28:1267–1276, 1994.

103. Thompson Jr., RC, Oegema Jr., TR, Lewis JL, et al: Osteoarthrotic changes after acute transarticular load. An animal model. *J Bone Joint Surg [Am]* 73:990–1001, 1991.

104. van der Lubbe HB, Klein CP, de Groot K: A simple method for preparing thin (10 μm) histological sections of undecalcified plastic embedded bone with implants. *Stain Technol* 63:171–176, 1988.

105. Vigorita VJ, Minkowitz B, Dichiara JF, et al: A histomorphometric and histologic analysis of the implant interface in five successful, autopsy-retrieved, noncemented porous-coated knee arthroplasties. *Clin Orthop* 293:211–218, 1993.

106. Visco DM, Johnstone B, Hill MA, et al: Immunohistochemical analysis of 3-B-(-) and 7-D-4 epitope expression in canine osteoarthritis. *Arthritis Rheum* 36:1718–1725, 1993.

107. von Recum AF, Opitz H, Wu E: Collagen types I and III at the implant/tissue interface. *J Biomed Mater Res* 27:757–761, 1993.

108. Wallace CD, Amiel D: Vascular assessment of the periarticular ligaments of the rabbit knee. *J Orthop Res* 9:787–791, 1991.

109. Wang A, Essner A, Stark C, et al: Comparison of the size and morphology of UHMWPE wear debris produced by a hip joint simulator under serum and water lubricated conditions. *Biomaterials* 17:865–871, 1996.

110. Weaker FJ, Richardson L: A modified processing and sectioning technique for hard tissues. *Am J Med Technol* 44: 1030–1032, 1978.

111. West PG, Rowland GR, Budsberg SC, et al: Histomorphometric and angiographic analysis of bone healing in the humerus of pigeons. *Am J Vet Res* 57:1010–1015, 1996.

112. West PG, Rowland GR, Budsberg SC, et al: Histomorphometric and angiographic analysis of the humerus in pigeons. *Am J Vet Res* 57:982–986, 1996.

113. Whitehouse WJ, Dyson ED, Jackson CK: The scanning electron microscope in studies of trabecular bone from a human vertebral body. *J Anat* 108:481–496, 1971.

114. Wolff D, Goldberg VM, Stevenson S: Histomorphometric analysis of the repair of a segmental diaphyseal defect with ceramic and titanium fibermetal implants: effects of bone marrow. *J Orthop Res* 12:439–446, 1994.

115. Wotton SF, Jeacocke RE, Maciewicz RA, et al: The application of scanning confocal microscopy in cartilage research. *Histochem J* 23:328–335, 1991.

116. Wright CD, Vedi S, Garrahan NJ, et al: Combined inter-observer and inter-method variation in bone histomorphometry. *Bone* 13:205–208, 1992.

117. Yan WQ, Nakamura T, Kobayashi M, et al: Bonding of chemically treated titanium implants to bone. *J Biomed Mater Res* 37:267–275, 1997.

118. Young FA, Spector M, Kresch CH: Porous titanium endosseous dental implants in Rhesus monkeys: microradiography and histological evaluation. *J Biomed Mater Res* 13:843–856, 1979.

119. Young RD, Lawrence PA, Duance VC, et al: Immunolocalization of type III collagen in human articular cartilage prepared by high-pressure cryofixation, freeze-substitution, and low-temperature embedding. *J Histochem Cytochem* 43:421–427, 1995.
120. Zhou H, Cherncky R, Davies JE: Scanning electron microscopy of the osteoclast-bone interface in vivo. *Cells Mater* 3:141–150, 1993.

II Structure and Function of Bone and Cartilage

Cell Structure and Biology of Bone and Cartilage

**William R. Walsh,[1] Mark Walton,[2] Warwick Bruce,[3] Yan Yu,[1]
Ronald M. Gillies,[1] and Martin Svehla[1]**

*[1]Orthopaedic Research Laboratories, University of New South Wales,
Prince of Wales Hospital, Sydney, New South Wales, Australia
[2]Department of Orthopaedic Surgery, University of Otago School of Medicine,
Dunedin, New Zealand
[3]Department of Orthopaedic Surgery, Concord Hospital, Concord, New South Wales, Australia*

I. INTRODUCTION

Bone and cartilage are highly specialized connective tissues that are engineered by nature to perform a variety of specialized tasks. As a result, these tissues have unique cellular constituents and ultrastructural organization that help optimize the biochemical demands and biomechanical loads in vivo. Our understanding of these connective tissues has increased over the past few centuries, and progress continues as techniques are defined and improved or new ones are developed. The understanding of the ultrastructural and mechanical properties of bone and cartilage is a dynamic area that is constantly evolving with new understanding. This chapter departs from traditional overviews of bone and cartilage, and presents an examination of cellular constituents and ultrastructural organization of these tissues in the context of recent experimental and theoretical studies. It is the hope of the authors to bring to light many new and exciting findings.

II. BONE

Bone is a complex calcified, living, biological composite that exists on many levels. It is this hierarchical organization, from the macroscopic to the ultrastructural level of the organic and inorganic constituents, that makes this tissue so exciting. The spatial relationships and distribution of the cellular and structural aspects reflect the complex nature of this tissue. On a gross scale, bone can be broken down to three phases or compartments: the cellular components; the hydrated extracellular organic matrix; and the extracellular mineral phase.[151]

A. Cellular Components: Osteoblasts, Osteocytes, and Osteoclasts

There are four different cell types found in bone that reside in different locations, which in part reflect their biological function or role. The bone-forming activity rests with the osteoblasts[116] and osteocytes, which reside along with bone-lining cells and osteoclasts on

From: *Handbook of Histology Methods for Bone and Cartilage*
Edited by: Y. H. An and K. L. Martin © Humana Press Inc., Totowa, NJ

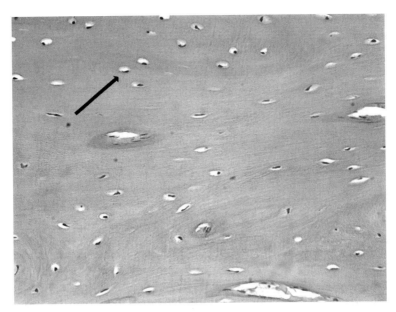

Figure 1. Hematoxylin and eosin (H&E) staining (20× objective) of adult rabbit bone viewed in the circumferential axis. Osteocytes (arrow) are surrounded by the mineralized bone matrix.

the bone surface. *Bone-lining cells* are considered the immediate precursors of the osteoblast, and lie within close proximity to the osteoblasts lining the bone-forming surface. Bone-lining cells are flat, elongated, inactive cells that cover bone surfaces that are not undergoing bone formation or resorption. Bone-lining cells have also been identified adjacent to the Haversian canal wall,[93] and may create a "bone surface-cell barrier"[92] and control fluxes of ions between compartments.[111] *Osteoblasts* are derived from local osteoprogenitor cells that are pluripotential.[38] They are considered *osteocytes* (Fig. 1) as soon as they are surrounded by a mineralized matrix or lacunae.[116] Osteoblasts are fully differentiated cells that synthesize membrane-associated alkaline phosphatase and regulate the deposition of the bone matrix molecules, including type I collagen and a variety of non-collagenous proteins. Osteoblast morphology at the light and electron microscopic level has been summarized by Holtrop.[59] A microscopic view of adult cancellous bone from the distal femur of sheep, which demonstrates a layer of osteoblasts on the surface, is shown in Fig. 2.

Cells derived from primary cultures of bone tissue (bone-derived cells) are commonly used to explore how osteoblast-like cells attach, proliferate, and differentiate in cell culture on a variety of different materials. Osteoblasts are nearly indistinguishable from fibroblasts in cell culture in the absence of a mineralized matrix.[38] The attachment of osteoblasts to surfaces plays a vital role in the clinical success of implant metals and polymers in craniofacial, dental, and orthopedic surgery. Many studies have examined the attachment, proliferation, and differentiation of osteoblasts to materials.[32,133,134] Interest in spatial control of osteoblast attachment to materials has extended the understanding of how these cells attach and spread on a material. Different attachment factors such as fibronectin and vitronectin have been shown to play vital roles in the interaction of osteoblast-like cells with materials (Fig. 3).[34,87,88,146]

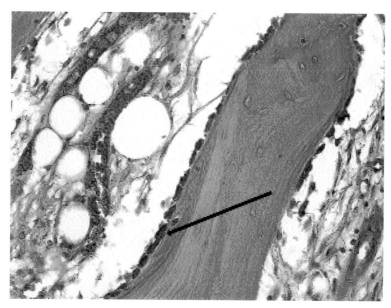

Figure 2. Hematoxylin and eosin (H&E) staining (40× objective) of adult cancellous bone from the distal femur of sheep demonstrating a layer of osteoblasts on the surface (arrow).

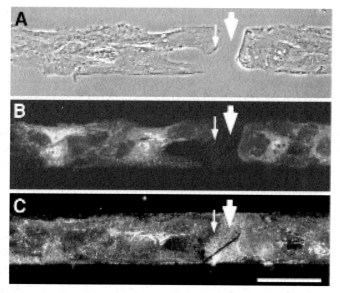

Figure 3. Initial HBD cell attachment and protein profile on EDS/DMS patterned surfaces. HBD cells in medium containing 10% (v/v) serum were seeded onto patterned surfaces. After 2 h incubation, non-adherent cells were removed and adherent cells fixed (A) and immunostained for fibronectin (Fn) (B) and vitronectin (Vn) (C). Note high levels of Vn staining on the EDS region (large arrowhead), and low levels at cellular focal adhesion sites (small arrows). In contrast, Fn is primarily cell-associated, suggesting that initial cell adhesion to the EDS regions is mediated by the localized adsorption of Vn from serum. Bar represents 50 μm. (*See* color plate 2 appearing in the insert following p. 270.)

The isolated location of the osteocytes within the mineralized bone matrix is by no means a life of solitary confinement, considering the compartmental nature and communication of the bone fluid spaces.[61] They remain in contact with each other and with cells on the bone surface through gap-junction-coupled cell processes passing through the matrix via the canaliculi that connect the cell-body-containing lacunae with each other. Various theories on osteocyte function have been proposed related to their role in bone remodeling, mechanotransduction, and functional adaptation of bone.[1,29,80,90,114,149]

Osteoblasts that have been recently incorporated into the bone matrix but are yet to mineralize represent a transitory stage referred to as the osteocytic-osteoblast[113,161] or osteoid-osteocyte.[118] Palumbo[118] has presented an elegant piece of work on the morphology and ultrastructure of osteoid-osteocytes in serial transmission electron microscopy (TEM). This work demonstrated the active nature of these cells, which seems to be polarized toward the mineralization front.[118]

Osteoclasts are multinucleated giant cells responsible for resorbing the mineralized bone matrix. Osteoclasts were recognized and described as early as 1873.[72] They are hematopoietic in origin,[140] and are formed by the fusion of mononuclear progenitors of the monocyte/macrophage family.[24,81,128,143,144]

Bone resorption by osteoclasts occurs through a multi-step complex pathway that involves proliferation of immature osteoclast precursors, close contact with the bone surface, secretion of protons, and hydrolases that can degrade the organic and inorganic constituents of bone tissue. The formation of the so-called "ruffled membrane" is a classic feature of the osteoclast during bone resorption. Macrophage colony-stimulating factor (M-CSF) and receptor for activation of nuclear factor kappa B (NF-κB) (RANK) ligand (RANKL) (also referred to as osteoclast differentiation factor), and osteoprotegerin (OPGL or TRANCE) are essential and sufficient to promote osteoclastogenesis.[24,81,128,143,144] The role of M-CSF in osteoclast development has been demonstrated in studies with a mouse point mutation in the M-CSF gene.[166] This mutation results in severe osteopetrosis because of an absence of osteoclasts. Injection of M-CSF into these animals has improved skeletal sclerosis, and has implicated M-CSF for early osteoclast development. RANK ligand is a member of the tumor necrosis factor (TNF) family,[166] binds to the RANK receptor on osteoclast precursors, and induces osteoclast formation. A variety of other factors influence osteoclast development and activity, including interleukin 1, 6, and 11 (IL-1, -6, -11) as well as TGF-α and the TNFs.[51,128] Duong and colleagues have also recently reviewed the role of integrins—heterodimeric adhesion receptors that mediate cell-matrix and cell-cell interactions—as they relate to osteoclasts.[39]

Wear-particle-induced osteolysis, following replacement of a natural joint by a metal and/or plastic prosthetic component, presents an interesting model for the study of osteoclast biology.[33,65,66,89,109,110,126] The mechanisms and possibility for control of the osteoclast development and resorption of bone has sparked great interest in total joint replacement. Hirashima et al.[58] suggested that osteolysis induced via wear particles from the joint articulation (e.g., ultrahigh molecular-weight polyethylene, UHMWPE) may not need direct contact with the debris. Activation of macrophages triggered by the presence of wear particles causes the release of humoral factors (inflammatory cytokines) (Fig. 4). These cytokines may be transported to the bone marrow tissues around the implants where they stimulate the differentiation of the bone marrow cells into osteoclasts.[58]

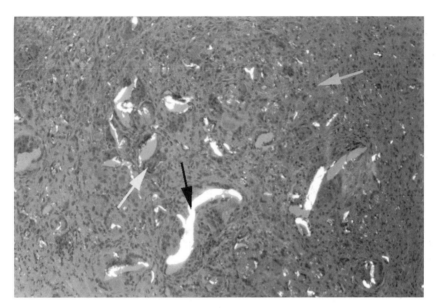

Figure 4. Pseudocapsule tissue from a revision total shoulder arthroplasty stained with IL-1β cDNA probe and viewed under polarizing light (10× objective) demonstrating PE wear debris (black arrow) as well as giant cells (yellow arrow) and niacrophages (green arrow) and macrophages (red). A positive signal for IL-1β mRNA in macrophages is seen throughout the section. (*See* color plate 3 appearing in the insert following p. 270.)

B. Organization and Constituents of Bone

The hierarchical structure of bone reveals a number of interesting features that can be identified. The complexity of bone is such that there is no level of organization at which one can say they are looking at "bone."[31] Bone is a porous viscoelastic anisotropic composite material with three types of constituents; water, a variety of organic constituents (protein and cellular), and an inorganic mineral phase. On a weight percentage, the cellular constituents, matrix, and mineral phase are approx 8%, 25% and 67%, respectively.[151] The mineral and organic phase of bone comprise about 40–45% and 35–40% of the bone volume, and the porosity makes up the remainder.[49] The relative proportions of these constituents and their orientation or organization as well as their individual properties play a role in determining the mechanical properties of bone tissue.

On a macroscopic level, bones can be classified based on their function (weight-bearing, articulating, or protecting), shape (long, short, or flat) or mechanism of formation (endochondral or intramembraneous ossification).[9] Using the femur as our "model" bone, it is considered to be a nonhomogenous anisotropic material (Fig. 5). The two major types of bone apparent at this level are cortical (or compact) bone, which resides primarily in the diaphyses, and cancellous (or trabecular) bone present at the metaphyses and epiphyses as well as in cuboid bones (vertebrae). Cortical bone is much more dense than cancellous bone. The density of both types of bone can vary with position, as illustrated in the dual energy X-ray absorptiometry (DEXA) scan of the proximal femur (Fig. 6). The nonhomogenous nature of bone and the variations in the density (and therefore

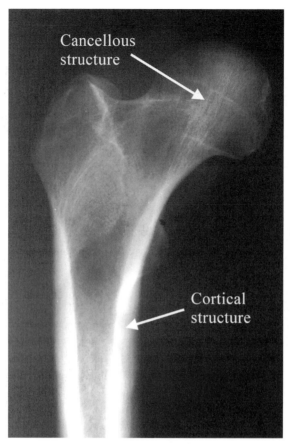

Figure 5. Anteroposterior radiographic view of a human femur demonstrating cancellous bone and cortical bone.

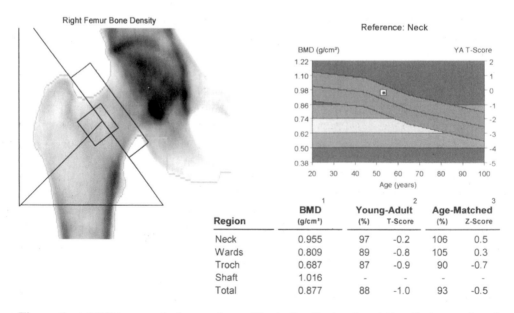

Region	BMD¹ (g/cm³)	Young-Adult² (%)	T-Score	Age-Matched³ (%)	Z-Score
Neck	0.955	97	-0.2	106	0.5
Wards	0.809	89	-0.8	105	0.3
Troch	0.687	87	-0.9	90	-0.7
Shaft	1.016	-	-	-	-
Total	0.877	88	-1.0	93	-0.5

Figure 6. A DEXA scan of a human femur illustrating the local variations in bone mineral density in the cortical as well as cancellous bone.

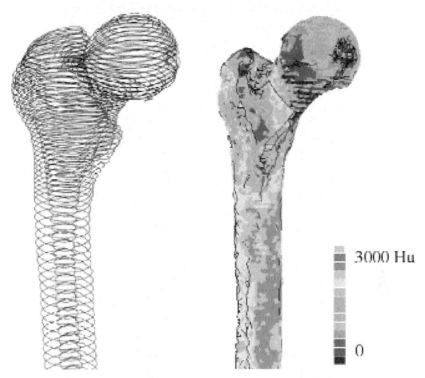

Figure 7. Extracted computed tomography (CT) contours and the CT data (Houndsfield units, Hu) applied to a finite element (FE) model of the femur. (*See* color plate 4 appearing in the insert following p. 270.)

mechanical properties as well) can also be demonstrated with quantitative computed tomography (QCT). CTs are often used to generate finite element models for engineering analyses. An example of a finite element model of the femur developed in our laboratory is shown in Fig. 7.

The most striking difference between cortical and cancellous bone relates to differences in porosity, which is known to change with age as well as various disease conditions. The cellular structure of cancellous bone consists of an interconnected network of rods or plates[47] and has a complex mechanical behavior.[45,95,96] The mechanical properties of cancellous bone, a cellular solid, are greatly influenced by density[23] and vary with position,[95] age,[23] and disease conditions.[47]

The porosity of bone and bone fluid has recently been reviewed by Cowin.[28] Cowin presents bone porosity in a hierarchical manner, with the porosity at the level of cancellous bone (on the order of 1 mm) being the largest. This is followed by the vascular porosity (on the order of 20 μm), which encompasses the osteonal canals as well as the smaller Volkmann canals. The spaces in the lacunae and the canaliculi (lacunar-canalicular porosity) (on the order of 0.1 μm) are identified as the most important porosity related to mechanotransduction effects and the osteocytes.[28] Bone porosity at the next level is associated with the spaces between the collagen and mineral crystals (on the order of 10 nm). Fluid movement at this level is considered negligible because of the bound water layer with the inorganic mineral.[112]

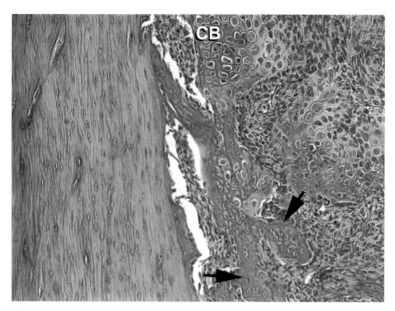

Figure 8. Hematoxylin and eosin (H&E) staining (20× objective) at 2 wk in a rat femoral fresh fracture. New woven bone (arrows) as well as the presence of chondroblastic cells "CB" can be seen in the section.

Bone consists of two forms at the microscopic level: woven and lamellar. Woven bone, an immature disorganized form of bone, is found during embryonic development, in metaphyseal regions during growth or in fracture repair (Fig. 8). Woven bone is characterized by a nonuniform collagen distribution and a random distribution of cells,[8] which imparts a more isotropic behavior. Lamellar bone, however, actively replaces woven bone (Fig. 9) over time and is found in a several structural and functional units with greater organization. The structure-function relationship in lamellar bone has been reviewed by Weiner and colleagues.[160] A lamellar unit is composed of five sublayers made up of mineralized collagen fibers oriented in complex rotated plywood-like structure.[160] Layers of lamellar bone and woven bone can be found together and comprise plexiform bone, often found in larger animals that experience rapid growth. Haversian bone represents the most complex form of cortical bone, and is often referred to as secondary bone. The osteon (or Haversian system) is a characteristic feature of Haversian bone (Fig. 10), with a central channel containing blood vessels, lining cells, and occasionally nerves and continues to be an area of intense research.[3] Cement lines are present at the boundaries of an osteon and represent the limit of a structural remodeling between the osteoblast and osteoclast.

III. EXTRACELLULAR MATRIX

Examination of the extracellular matrix (ECM) of bone finds the structural organic phase of bone composed primarily of type I collagen (90%) with a variety of non-collagenous proteins (NCPs)[145,151] glycoproteins, and proteoglycans in relatively small proportions.[48] The structure and chemistry of type I collagen has been extensively reported.[91,121] The tropocollagen molecule consists of two different subunits that are arranged into a

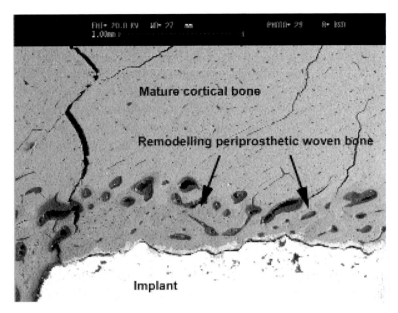

Figure 9. Backscatter SEM depicting periprosthetic bone formation at 8 wk around a HA-coated titanium alloy implant in a skeletally mature ovine model. Note that the region of darker bone is woven bone that is undergoing remodeling.

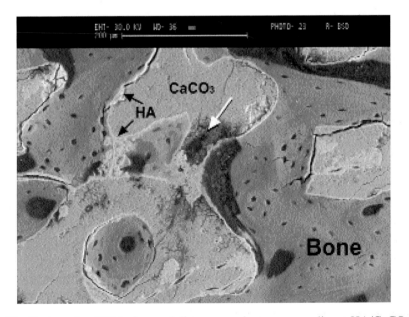

Figure 10. Backscatter SEM of remodeling woven bone surrounding a $HA/CaCO_3$ bone-graft substitute (ProOsteon 500R, Interpore-Cross, Irvine, CA) in an adult rabbit tibia at 6 wk. Evidence of bone remodeling and the formation of a Haversian system are noted (dark arrows). Degradation of the calcium carbonate bone graft substitute is also evident (white arrow).

water bond, stabilized left-handed superhelix. The collagen molecules are considered to be arranged in axial fashion with a "1/4" stagger arrangement.[121]

Boskey et al. recently revisited collagen and bone strength.[10] Suarez and colleagues have also revealed the differences between type I collagen in bone vs soft tissue, as well as between cortical and cancellous bone.[139] The content of hydroxylysine, glycosylated hydroxylysine, and pyridinium crosslinks of collagen from cortical and trabecular bone was determined in 100-d-old rats. Cortical bone was found to contain a higher amount of hydroxylysine residues, and in trabecular bone glycosylation of hydroxylysine was found to be higher and pyridinium crosslink concentration to be lower.[139] Tzaphlidou et al. reported structural alterations of bone collagen fibrils induced following ovariectomy as well as the influence of nutritional factors.[67,150] The architecture of bone collagen was disturbed in the estrogen-deficient state, and increasing dietary levels of calcium resulted in an improvement in the fibril packing as compared to controls.[67,150] Thus, although the ultrastructure of the type I collagen in bone and soft tissue or even between cortical and cancellous bone is similar, there are differences, and their significance is not yet completely understood.

Although the NCPs of bone make up only a small percentage, their role in regulating or controlling mineralization has received a great deal of attention.[9,62,108,145] The complexity of the NCP pool of bone has been demonstrated through a variety of extraction protocols.[108,145,151] Nanci reported the content and distribution of some of the non-collagenous proteins in bone using immunocytochemistry[108] and the importance of NCPs in bone and the mineralization process. Bone sialoprotein and osteopontin were found to co-distribute and accumulate in the cement lines and spaces among mineralized collagen fibers.[62] It was suggested that one of the major roles of NCPs is to fill spaces created during collagen assembly, and impart cohesion by allowing mineral deposition across the entire collagen meshwork.[108] An additional hypothesis for the role of NCPs has been offered by Ingram and colleagues, who suggested that they represent a regulatory mechanism by which the extracellular matrix (ECM) influences cell dynamics and remodeling.[62] Further understanding of the role of some of these proteins, such as the bone morphogenetic proteins (BMPs) in bone formation and fracture healing has provided new therapeutic possibilities for the future.[131]

IV. BONE MINERAL

Mineralization of bone is a complex event.[2] The mineral phase of bone is a calcium-deficient, carbonate-containing, poorly crystalline analog of the naturally occurring calcium phosphate mineral species known as hydroxyapatite $[Ca_{10}(PO_4)_6(OH)_2]$,[122] and has been the source of many reviews.[9,13,94,123,124] Bone mineral is also known as dahllite.[127] The surface chemistry of bone mineral provides a variety of attachment sites for anionic and cationic domains of proteins.[94] Bundy hypothesized that the effectiveness of bonding between the mineral and organic phases could be an important influence on the behavior of bone with respect to its mechanical properties,[20] which have been demonstrated to play an important role in the biomechanical behavior of bone.[74,153–155]

The shape, size, location, and interaction(s) between the mineral and organic constituents of bone tissue has motivated a variety of composite models.[20,21,30,31,70,73] Examination at the ultrastructural level provides insight into the location and relationship between the collagen and mineral.[46,78,79,148,157–159] As early as 1973, Katz and Li suggested that the position of the mineral was located within the collagen fibril and associated with the collagen surface.[68,69] Weiner and Traub reported the bone mineral crystals to be extremely small plate-shaped crystals of carbonate apatite, just hundreds of angstroms in length and width and some 20–30 angstroms thick, arranged in parallel layers within the collagenous framework. The mineral-filled collagen fibrils are ordered into arrays in which the fibril axes and the crystal layers are organized into a three-dimensional (3D) structure that makes up a lamella of bone a few microns thick. Using a calcifying turkey tendon model, Landis and colleagues confirmed the platelet-shaped hydroxyapatite crystals in association with the surface of collagen fibrils. Mineral was also observed in closely parallel arrays within the collagen holes and overlap zones.[79] In another study using high-voltage electron microscopic tomography, Landis et al.[78] reported the size of the mineral crystals to be variable, and found that they measured up to $80 \times 30 \times 8$ nm in length, width, and thickness, respectively. The longest crystal dimension, corresponding to the c-axis crystallographically, was generally parallel to the collagen fibril long axis. Individual crystals were oriented parallel to one another in each fibril examined. Bone mineral crystals were periodically (approx 67 nm repeat distance) arranged along the fibrils and their location appeared to correspond to collagen hole and overlap zones. Landis and colleagues suggest that platelet-shaped crystals are arranged in channels or grooves, which are formed by collagen hole zones in register, and that crystal sizes may exceed the dimensions of whole zones.[78,79]

V. COMPOSITE MODELING

Information concerning the structural biology of bone may help to provide more realistic composite models of this complex interaction. Pidaparti and colleagues[120] proposed that the elastic properties of osteonal bone could be modeled a simple fiber-reinforced composite. Their model assumes that bone mineral crystals act as short fibers reinforcing the collagen matrix, and suggests that collagen is aligned 30 degrees from the long axis of the bone and that 75% of the mineral phase resides outside of the collagen fibers with their c-axis in the longitudinal direction.[120] Braidotti and colleagues[11] suggest a laminated composite material for bone with a matrix composed of extracellular non-collagenous calcified proteins, and that the reinforcement is the calcified collagen fiber system. Kotha and Guzelsu[73] recently offered a simple shear lag model to analyze stress transfer between the organic and mineral constituents of bone tissue in the presence of an interface and changes in bonding. An analytical model was developed that assumed interactions between overlapped bone-mineral platelets. The platelets were believed to carry the axial stresses, while the organic matrix transfers the stresses from one platelet to another by shear. A decrease in the interface mechanical properties decreases the elastic modulus as a result of increased shear between the overlapped platelets. They suggested the aspect ratio and volume fraction of the mineral in the remaining bone tissue would increase because of a reduction in the density of the bone.[73]

VI. CARTILAGE

Cartilage is a porous, viscoelastic composite that relies on a complex interaction and organization of its constituents to provide the resilient load-bearing, energy-dissipating

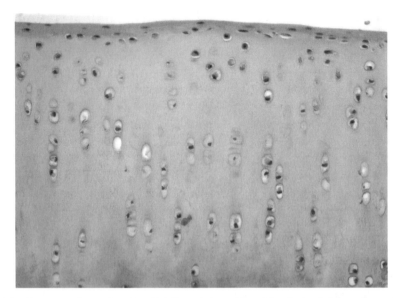

Figure 11. Hematoxylin and eosin (H&E) staining (40× objective) of the surface of articular cartilage from an adult rabbit demonstrating the presence of chondrocytes in the matrix as well as overall organization.

lubrication and frictional properties.[103] Articular cartilage is a form of hyaline cartilage that covers the articulating surfaces of long bones and sesamoid bones within synovial joints. The impressive load-bearing capacity of this tissue reflects in part the intrinsic matrix toughness and turgidity, as the ability of the tissue to swell is opposed by the internal structure. The degradation, loss, or breakdown of this unique relationship between the collagenous matrix and heavily hydrated charge-carrying proteoglycans caused by trauma or chronic and progressive degenerative joint disease (e.g., osteoarthrosis or rheumatoid arthritis) has great functional, biomechanical, clinical, and social implications. This section explores the cellular components, matrix constituents, and ultrastructural organization of articular cartilage.

A. Cellular Components: Chondrocytes

Chondrocytes are specialized cells, which produce and maintain the ECM of cartilage (Fig. 11).[106] Chondrocytes occupy only 5% of the volume and are isolated within the matrix.[71] These cells exist in a unique physiological and mechanical environment[56] in the ECM and exhibit different sizes, shapes, and possibly metabolic activity in the various zones of cartilage. The development of chondrocytes during embryogenesis has been recently reviewed.[35,117]

Interactions between chondrocytes and the ECM regulate many biological processes important to cartilage homeostasis and repair including cell attachment, growth, differentiation, and survival.[82] The integrin family of cell-surface receptors appears to play a major role in mediating cell-matrix interactions that are important in regulating these processes. Chondrocytes have been found to express several members of the integrin family (cell-surface receptors), which can serve as receptors for fibronectin (alpha5beta1), types II and VI collagen (alpha1beta1, alpha2beta1, alpha10beta1), laminin (alpha6beta1), and vitronectin and osteopontin (alpha5beta3). Integrin binding stimulates intracellular signaling that can affect gene expression and regulate chondrocyte function. The chondrocyte mechanical environment is another important factor in the cellular response.[54]

Chondrocyte apoptosis (cell death) has recently received attention because of its role in osteoarthrosis.[84,129] Controlling chondrocyte apoptosis may be of therapeutic value after cartilage injury and in arthrosis. Lotz and colleagues[84] have shown that chondrocyte apoptosis can be induced in vitro by nitric oxide donors, but not by pro-inflammatory cytokines, such as IL-1 or TNF. A subset of chondrocytes, located in the superficial zone of cartilage, expresses the Fas antigen. Activation of the Fas receptor triggers apoptosis in these cells.[84] Sandell and colleagues have recently reported that apoptosis probably occurs primarily in the calcified cartilage,[129] which has great implications for the local bony response in osteoarthrosis.

B. Constituents and Organization of Cartilage

The major constituents of articular cartilage in the hydrated state fall into three main classes: water (68–85%); collagens (10–20%), and proteoglycans (5–10%).[102] The interstitial water is the most abundant component of articular cartilage.[102,147] The amount of water in the tissue partly reflects the proteoglycan concentration[86] and the amount of dissolved ions in solution as the organization of the collagenous matrix.[102,103]

The type and relationship of collagens in normal and degenerative articular cartilage has been extensively well studied.[12,16,25–27,36,40–44,75,103,163–165] Of the 18 different types of collagen identified to date,[102] articular cartilage contains at least five types.[40,83] Types II, IX, and XI are cartilage-specific, crosslinked fashion that forms the cartilage extracellular framework. Type II collagen provides the basic architecture[16,42,43,75] and type XI is probably copolymerized with type II collagen in the matrix.[40,42,164] Type VI collagen is found in the normal articular cartilage.[57] In osteoarthrosis, type VI collagen is increased in the pericellular region in the middle and deep zones of articular cartilage, but is reduced in the superficial layer relative to normal cartilage.[57] Type IX collagen (1% of total collagen in cartilage) is covalently linked to the surface of type II collagen fibrils.[36,41,163,165] Collagen type X is restricted to the underlying calcified zone of articular cartilage.

Proteoglycans consist of a protein core and many glycosaminoglycan chains (long unbranched polysaccharide chains consisting of repeating disaccharides that contain an amino sugar) (Fig. 12).[71,106] The charge-carrying capacity of proteoglycans combined with the interstitial ion-carrying water phase makes for an ideal environment for interactions. A variety of glycosaminoglycans (GAGs) are found in cartilage, including hyaluronic acid, chondroitin sulfate, keratan sulfate, and dermatan sulfate.[15,71] Two major classes of proteoglycans reside in articular cartilage: large aggregating proteoglycan monomers or aggrecans,[132,156] and small proteoglycans including decorin, biglycan, and fibromodulin.[71] The tissue may also contain other small proteoglycans that have not yet been identified.[15,71] Proteoglycans are key molecules in the mechanical behavior of articular cartilage.[4,15,55,85;86,97,98] They also play a cellular role, and mediate cell interactions.[119]

Proteoglycan aggregates form as a result of the noncovalent interactions between hyaluronic acid and other small NCPs.[17–19,142] The formation of these aggregates provides, in part, the spatial relationship between the constituents reflected in the mechanical properties.[60] Verbruggen and colleagues reported a decline in aggrecan synthesis rates and

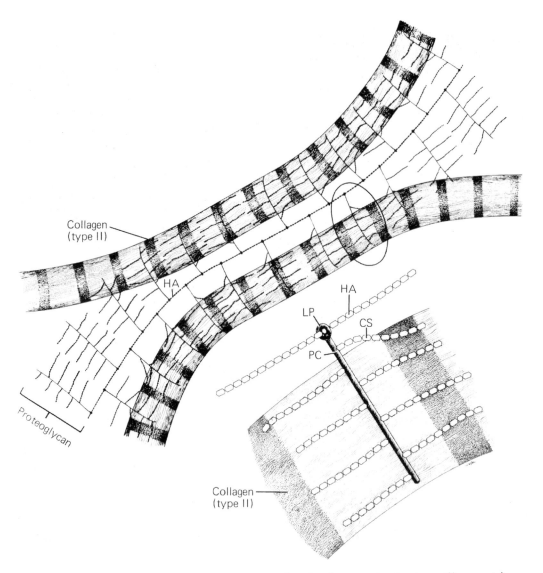

Figure 12. Schematic representation of proposed molecular organization in cartilage matrix. Linking proteins (LP) covalently bind the protein core (PC) of proteoglycans to the linear hyaluronic acid (HA) molecules. The chondroitin sulfate (CS) side chains of the proteoglycan electrostatically bind to the collagen fibrils, forming a crosslinked rigid matrix (reproduced with permission from Junqueira, L.C. and Carneiro, J., Basic Histology, 4th ed. LANGE Medical, Los Altos, CA).

decreased capability in macromolecular assembly with age in humans, and confirmed the progressive failure in the repair function of chondrocytes.[152] This has led to a wide range of treatment options for cartilage injuries, repair, and regeneration.[115]

At the histological level, articular cartilage, like all biological tissues, is fascinating to examine (Fig. 13). The structure and composition at the microscopic levels varies significantly with depth and can be separated into four poorly defined zones; superficial,

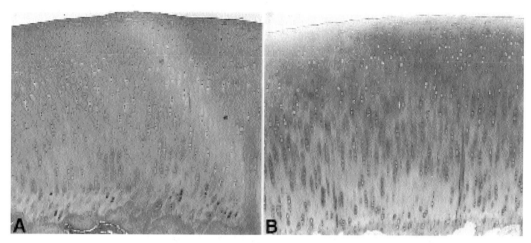

Figure 13. Hematoxylin and eosin (H&E) staining (A) and Safranin O staining (B) of the surface of articular cartilage in an adult sheep distal femur. These sections demonstrate the multi-zones of articular cartilage as well as the variation in proteoglycan concentration with depth (B). (*See* color plate 5 appearing in the insert following p. 270.)

transitional, a middle (radial), or deep zone and a zone of calcified cartilage.[14,15] The superficial zone consists of two layers. Layer 1 is composed of fine fibrils with little polysaccharide and no cells that cover the joint surface and is often referred to as the lamina splendens, which can be peeled from the articular surface in some regions. The scanning electron micrograph (Fig. 14) displays this highly specialized zone of articular cartilage. The mechanical behavior of this zone plays an important role in resisting tensile forces generated during surface deformation under load. Damage to the superficial zone is one of the first detectable structural changes in the experimentally induced degeneration of articular cartilage,[55] may contribute to the development of osteoarthrosis by changing the mechanical behavior, and may possibly release molecules that stimulate an immune or inflammatory response.[15]

The transitional zone is larger than the superficial zone, and demonstrates a difference in cellularity and organization. Cells in the transitional zone are more spheroidal in shape, and synthesize a matrix that has larger-diameter collagen fibrils, a higher concentration of proteoglycan, and lower concentrations of water and collagen that does the matrix of the superficial zone.[15] Speer and Dahners,[136] using scanning electron microscopy (SEM) and light microscopy, reported that within the transitional zone there is a narrow band with no vertical or horizontal collagen fibers, and in which collagen fibers intersect predominantly at angles ranging between 45 and 135 degrees. The chondrocytes in the middle (radial) zone are spheroidal in shape, and tend to align themselves in columns perpendicular to the joint surface. The largest diameter collagen fibrils, the highest concentration of proteoglycans, and the lowest concentration of water are found in the middle zone.[15] The deepest, calcified zone forms a mechanical transition between the relatively deformable cartilage above and the hard bone below. A so-called "tidemark" delineates the extent of mineralization, yet collagen fibers continue across this line. No such continuum exists in the zone

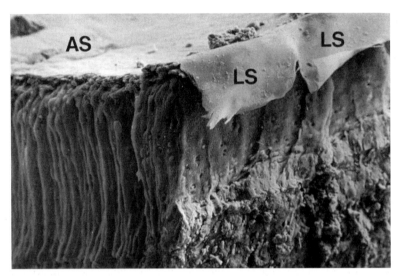

Figure 14. Freeze-fracture SEM view of the mouse femoral condyle. The hierarchical organization of the articular cartilage can been seen. The articular surface (AS) is a smooth, thin layer often referred to as the lamina splendens (LS).

4-bone interface that instead is convoluted, thus distributing the compressive loads over a larger surface area. The calcified cartilage layer makes up the final zone that separates the middle zone from the underlying subchondral bone.

Cartilage permeability has been shown to be related to the depth into the tissue. Gonsalves and colleagues[50] recently reported the use of scanning electrochemical microscopy, a high-resolution chemical imaging technique, to probe the distribution and mobility of solutes in articular cartilage. Areas of high permeability were observed in the cellular and pericellular regions of articular cartilage.[50] Oxygen tension modulates the abundance of mRNAs encoding structural molecules, several cytokines, beta-1 integrin, and integrin-linked kinase in articular chondrocytes, and may be important during disease progression.[52]

Although the structure of cartilage has been well-reported,[136] two recent studies continue to provide insight into this unique tissue. Jurvelin and colleagues examined bovine humeral head articular cartilage using atomic force microscopy as well as TEM.[64] Local discontinuities in the superficial zone were observed, through which the underlying network of collagen fibrils—oriented parallel to the surface and displaying the staggering banding pattern—could be seen.[64] Camacho and colleagues reported the first results using Fourier transform infrared (FTIR) spectroscopy to assess articular cartilage.[22] Comparison of polarized FTIR microscopy from the superficial and deep zones of cartilage showed changes in intensities of the collagen absorbance, suggesting differences in spatial organization.

Ultrastructural interconnected organization[42] reflects a complex relationship in which the collagen fibrils are loaded in tension when the hydrophilic proteoglycans interact with water.[86] Broom and Silyn-Roberts[12] used TEM to demonstrate a complex 3D meshwork of type II collagen fibers in a radial arrangement that repeatedly defect laterally as short oblique segments. Fibrils were noted to associate at "nodal" points in a transient manner that may have important implications for interfibrillar interactions.[12] Collagen-proteoglycan and proteoglycan-proteoglycan interactions are very important in the mechanical behavior of cartilage.[100,102–105] These interactions are in part dictated by the fixed-charged density of these constituents in ionic solution.[86,100] Applying a compressive force to cartilage would bring these charged groups closer together, increase the Donnan osmotic pressure, and increase charge-to-charge repulsive forces.

VII. MODELING

Improvements in the understanding of the ultrastructure, constituents, and their interactions in cartilage have resulted in improvements in modeling this tissue. Much of our understanding regarding the mechanical properties of articular cartilage is reflected in the work of Professor V. C. Mow and his colleagues over the past 25 years.[4–7,53,76,77,85,97–104,107,125,130,135,137,138,141] Linear elasticity theory (single phase) has been used for analysis of a number of connective tissues including articular cartilage. The well-accepted biphasic model has been used to examine a range of cartilages, confirming the complex nature as well as nonhomogenity of this tissue.[99] The biphasic theory assumes the solid matrix to be intrinsically incompressible. The interstitial fluid phase can move through the tissue by a pressure gradient. The viscous component of the tissue results from the frictional drag of the interstitial fluid flow through the "porous" permeable collagenous meshwork.[100] The mechanical properties and modeling of articular cartilage continue to be the topic of a number of investigations.[37,63,64,162]

The current composite model for articular cartilage biomechanics is the triphasic theory. Originally proposed in 1991 by Lai et al.,[77] the triphasic model accounts for two fluid-solid phases (biphasic), and an ion phase, representing cation and anion of a single salt, to describe the deformation and stress fields for cartilage under chemical and/or mechanical loads. This triphasic theory combines the physico-chemical theory for ionic and polyionic (proteoglycan) solutions with the biphasic theory for cartilage.

VIII. CONCLUDING REMARKS

Bone and cartilage are fascinating tissues to explore, in the native, diseased, and healing/regenerative states. Our understanding of constituent interactions from a biomechanical as well as biochemical point of view continues to progress for both of these tissues. Many of the "classical" studies on the ultrastructure and biochemistry of cartilage have been advanced with new and exciting techniques. Advances in molecular biology and cross-fertilization of a number of scientific disciplines will certainly see a number of advances in our understanding of these complex biological composites.

REFERENCES

1. Aarden EM, Burger EH, Nijweide PJ: Function of osteocytes in bone. *J Cell Biochem* 55:287–299, 1994.
2. Anderson HC: Mechanism of mineral formation in bone. *Lab Invest* 60:320–330, 1989.
3. Ardizzoni A: Osteocyte lacunar size-lamellar thickness relationships in human secondary osteons. *Bone* 28:215–219, 2001.
4. Armstrong CG, Lai WM, Mow VC: An analysis of the unconfined compression of articular cartilage. *J Biomech Eng* 106:165–173, 1984.

5. Ateshian GA, Lai WM, Zhu WB, et al: An asymptotic solution for the contact of two biphasic cartilage layers. *J Biomech* 27:1347–1360, 1994.
6. Ateshian GA, Warden WH, Kim JJ, et al: Finite deformation biphasic material properties of bovine articular cartilage from confined compression experiments. *J Biomech* 30:1157–1164, 1997.
7. Athanasiou KA, Rosenwasser MP, Buckwalter JA, et al: Interspecies comparisons of in situ intrinsic mechanical properties of distal femoral cartilage. *J Orthop Res* 9:330–340, 1991.
8. Bianco P: Structure and mineralization of bone. In: Bonucci E, ed: *Calcification in Biological Systems.* CRC Press, Boca Raton, FL, 1992:243–268.
9. Boskey AL, Posner AS: Bone structure, composition, and mineralization. *Orthop Clin North Am* 15:597–612, 1984.
10. Boskey AL, Wright TM, Blank RD: Collagen and bone strength. *J Bone Miner Res* 14:330–335, 1999.
11. Braidotti P, Branca FP, Stagni L: Scanning electron microscopy of human cortical bone failure surfaces. *J Biomech* 30:155–162, 1997.
12. Broom ND, Silyn-Roberts H: The three-dimensional "knit" of collagen fibrils in articular cartilage. *Connect Tissue Res* 23:261–277, 1989.
13. Buckwalter JA, Cooper RR: Bone structure and function. *Instr Course Lect* 36:27–48, 1987.
14. Buckwalter JA, Hunziker EB, Rozenberg LC, et al: Articular cartilage. Composition and structure. In: Woo SL-Y, Buckwalter JA, eds: *Injury and Repair of the Musculoskeletal Soft Tissues.* American Academy of Orthopaedic Surgeons, Park Ridge, IL, 1988:405–425.
15. Buckwalter JA, Mankin HJ: Articular cartilage. Part 1: Tissue design and chondrocyte-matrix interactions. *J Bone Joint Surg [Am]* 79:600–611, 1997.
16. Buckwalter JA, Mankin HJ: Articular cartilage: tissue design and chondrocyte-matrix interactions. *Instr Course Lect* 47:477–486, 1998.
17. Buckwalter JA, Rosenberg LC: Electron microscopic studies of cartilage proteoglycans. Direct evidence for the variable length of the chondroitin sulfate-rich region of proteoglycan subunit core protein. *J Biol Chem* 257:9830–9839, 1982.
18. Buckwalter JA, Rosenberg LC, Tang LH: The effect of link protein on proteoglycan aggregate structure. An electron microscopic study of the molecular architecture and dimensions of proteoglycan aggregates reassembled from the proteoglycan monomers and link proteins of bovine fetal epiphyseal cartilage. *J Biol Chem* 259:5361–5363, 1984.
19. Buckwalter JA, Roughley PJ, Rosenberg LC: Age-related changes in cartilage proteoglycans: quantitative electron microscopic studies. *Microsc Res Tech* 28:398–408, 1994.
20. Bundy KJ: Determination of mineral-organic bonding effectiveness in bone—theoretical considerations. *Ann Biomed Eng* 13:119–135, 1985.
21. Burstein AH, Zika JM, Heiple KG, et al: Contribution of collagen and mineral to the elastic-plastic properties of bone. *J Bone Joint Surg [Am]* 57:956–961, 1975.
22. Camacho NP, West P, Torzilli PA, et al: FTIR microscopic imaging of collagen and proteoglycan in bovine cartilage. *Biopolymers* 62:1–8, 2001.
23. Carter DR, Hayes WC: The compressive behavior of bone as a two-phase porous structure. *J Bone Joint Surg [Am]* 59:954–962, 1977.
24. Chambers TJ: Regulation of the differentiation and function of osteoclasts. *J Pathol* 192:4–13, 2000.
25. Chen MH, N Broom: On the ultrastructure of softened cartilage: a possible model for structural transformation. *J Anat* 192:329–341, 1998.
26. Clarke IC: Articular cartilage: a review and scanning electron microscope study. 1. The interterritorial fibrillar architecture. *J Bone Joint Surg [Br]* 53:732–750, 1971.
27. Clarke IC: Surface characteristics of human articular cartilage—a scanning electron microscope study. *J Anat* 108:23–30, 1971.
28. Cowin SC: Bone poroelasticity. *J Biomech* 32:217–238, 1999.

29. Cowin SC, Weinbaum S: Strain amplification in the bone mechanosensory system. *Am J Med Sci* 316:184–188, 1998.

30. Currey JD: The relationship between the stiffness and mineral content of bone. *J Biomechanics* 2:477–480, 1969.

31. Currey JD: *The Mechanical Adaptation of Bones.* Princeton University Press, Princeton, NJ, 1984.

32. Davies JE: *The Bone-Biomaterial Interface.* University of Toronto Press, Toronto, Canada, 1991.

33. Dean DD, Schwartz Z, Liu Y, et al: The effect of ultra-high molecular weight polyethylene wear debris on MG63 osteosarcoma cells in vitro. *J Bone Joint Surg [Am]* 81:452–461, 1999.

34. Degasne I, Basle MF, Demais V, et al: Effects of roughness, fibronectin and vitronectin on attachment, spreading, and proliferation of human osteoblast-like cells (Saos-2) on titanium surfaces. *Calcif Tissue Int* 64:499–507, 1999.

35. DeLise AM, Fischer L, Tuan RS: Cellular interactions and signaling in cartilage development. *Osteoarthritis Cartilage* 8:309–334, 2000.

36. Diab M, Wu JJ, Eyre DR: Collagen type IX from human cartilage: a structural profile of intermolecular cross-linking sites. *Biochem J* 314:327–332, 1996.

37. DiSilvestro MR, Zhu Q, Wong M, et al: Biphasic poroviscoelastic simulation of the unconfined compression of articular cartilage: I—Simultaneous prediction of reaction force and lateral displacement. *J Biomech Eng* 123:191–197, 2001.

38. Ducy P, Schinke T, Karsenty G: The osteoblast: a sophisticated fibroblast under central surveillance. *Science* 289:1501–1504, 2000.

39. Duong LT, Lakkakorpi P, Nakamura I, et al: Integrins and signaling in osteoclast function. *Matrix Biol* 19:97–105, 2000.

40. Eyre DR: The collagens of articular cartilage. *Semin Arthritis Rheum* 21:2–11, 1991.

41. Eyre DR, Apon S, Wu JJ, et al: Collagen type IX: evidence for covalent linkages to type II collagen in cartilage. *FEBS Lett* 220:337–341, 1987.

42. Eyre DR, Wu JJ: Collagen structure and cartilage matrix integrity. *J Rheumatol Suppl* 43:82–85, 1995.

43. Eyre DR, Wu JJ, Woods PE: The cartilage collagens: structural and metabolic studies. *J Rheumatol Suppl* 27:49–51, 1991.

44. Eyre DR, Wu JJ, Woods PE, et al: The cartilage collagens and joint degeneration. *Br J Rheumatol* 30:10–15, 1991.

45. Fenech CM, Keaveny TM: A cellular solid criterion for predicting the axial-shear failure properties of bovine trabecular bone. *J Biomech Eng* 121:414–422, 1999.

46. Gadaleta SJ, Camacho NP, Mendelsohn R, et al: Fourier transform infrared microscopy of calcified turkey leg tendon. *Calcif Tissue Int* 58:17–23, 1996.

47. Gibson LJ, Ashby MF: *Cellular Solids.* Pergamon Press, Oxford, UK 1988.

48. Goldberg HA, Domenicucci C, Pringle GA, et al: Mineral-binding proteoglycans of fetal porcine calvarial bone. *J Biol Chem* 263:12,092–12,101, 1988.

49. Gong JK, Arnold JS, Cohn SH: Composition of trabecular and cortical bone. *Anat Rec* 149:325–332, 1964.

50. Gonsalves M, Barker AL, Macpherson JV, et al: Scanning electrochemical microscopy as a local probe of oxygen permeability in cartilage. *Biophys J* 78:1578–1588, 2000.

51. Greenfield EM, Bi Y, Miyauchi A: Regulation of osteoclast activity. *Life Sci* 65:1087–1102, 1999.

52. Grimshaw MJ, Mason RM: Modulation of bovine articular chondrocyte gene expression in vitro by oxygen tension. *Osteoarthritis Cartilage* 9:357–364, 2001.

53. Gu WY, Lai WM, Mow VC: A triphasic analysis of negative osmotic flows through charged hydrated soft tissues. *J Biomech* 30:71–78, 1997.

54. Guilak F, Jones WR, Ting-Beall HP, et al: The deformation behaviour and mechanical properties of chondrocytes in articular cartilage. *Osteoarthritis Cartilage* 7:59–70, 1999.

55. Guilak F, Ratcliffe A, Lane N, et al: Mechanical and biochemical changes in the superficial zone of articular cartilage in canine experimental osteoarthritis. *J Orthop Res* 12:474–484, 1994.

56. Hall AC, Horwitz ER, Wilkins RJ: The cellular physiology of articular cartilage. *Exp Physiol* 81:535–545, 1996.

57. Hambach L, Neureiter D, Zeiler G, et al: Severe disturbance of the distribution and expression of type VI collagen chains in osteoarthritic articular cartilage. *Arthritis Rheum* 41:986–996, 1998.

58. Hirashima Y, Ishiguro N, Kondo S, et al: Osteoclast induction from bone marrow cells is due to pro-inflammatory mediators from macrophages exposed to polyethylene particles: a possible mechanism of osteolysis in failed THA. *J Biomed Mater Res* 56:177–183, 2001.

59. Holtrop ME: Light and electron microscopic structure of bone-forming cells. In: Hall BK, ed: *Bone: The Osteoblast and Osteocyte.* Telford Press, Caldwell, NJ, 1990:1–41.

60. Huber M, Trattnig S, Lintner F: Anatomy, biochemistry, and physiology of articular cartilage. *Invest Radiol* 35:573–580, 2000.

61. Hughes S, Davies R, Khan R, et al: Fluid space in bone. *Clin Orthop* 134:332–341, 1978.

62. Ingram RT, Clarke BL, Fisher LW, et al: Distribution of noncollagenous proteins in the matrix of adult human bone: evidence of anatomic and functional heterogeneity. *J Bone Miner Res* 8:1019–1029, 1993.

63. Jurvelin JS, Arokoski JP, Hunziker EB, et al: Topographical variation of the elastic properties of articular cartilage in the canine knee. *J Biomech* 33:669–675, 2000.

64. Jurvelin JS, Muller DJ, Wong M, et al: Surface and subsurface morphology of bovine humeral articular cartilage as assessed by atomic force and transmission electron microscopy. *J Struct Biol* 117:45–54, 1996.

65. Kadoya Y, Kobayashi A, Ohashi H: Wear and osteolysis in total joint replacements. *Acta Orthop Scand Suppl* 278:1–16, 1998.

66. Kadoya Y, Revell PA, Kobayashi A, et al: Wear particulate species and bone loss in failed total joint arthroplasties. *Clin Orthop* 340:118–129, 1997.

67. Kafantari H, Kounadi E, Fatouros M, et al: Structural alterations in rat skin and bone collagen fibrils induced by ovariectomy. *Bone* 26:349–353, 2000.

68. Katz EP, Li ST: The intermolecular space of reconstituted collagen fibrils. *J Mol Biol* 73:351–369, 1973.

69. Katz EP, Li ST: Structure and function of bone collagen fibrils. *J Mol Biol* 80:1–15, 1973.

70. Katz JL: The structure and biomechanics of bone. *Symp Soc Exp Biol* 34:137–168, 1980.

71. Knudson CB, Knudson W: Cartilage proteoglycans. *Semin Cell Dev Biol* 12:69–78, 2001.

72. Kolliker A: *Die normale resorption des knochengewebes in ihre bedeutung fur die entstehung der typischen knochenformen.* FC Vogel, Leipzig, 1873:86.

73. Kotha SP, Guzelsu N: The effects of interphase and bonding on the elastic modulus of bone: changes with age-related osteoporosis. *Med Eng Phys* 22:575–585, 2000.

74. Kotha SP, Walsh WR, Pan Y: Varying the mechanical properties of bone tissue by changing the amount of its structurally effective bone mineral content. *Biomed Mater Eng* 8:321–334, 1998.

75. Kuettner KE: Biochemistry of articular cartilage in health and disease. *Clin Biochem* 25:155–163, 1992.

76. Kwan MK, Lai WM, Mow VC: A finite deformation theory for cartilage and other soft hydrated connective tissues. I. Equilibrium results. *J Biomech* 23:145–155, 1990.

77. Lai WM, Hou JS, Mow VC: A triphasic theory for the swelling and deformation behaviors of articular cartilage. *J Biomech Eng* 113:245–258, 1991.

78. Landis WJ, Hodgens KJ, Arena J, et al: Structural relations between collagen and mineral in bone as determined by high voltage electron microscopic tomography. *Microsc Res Tech* 33:192–202, 1996.

79. Landis WJ, Hodgens KJ, Song MJ, et al: Mineralization of collagen may occur on fibril surfaces: evidence from conventional and high-voltage electron microscopy and three-dimensional imaging. *J Struct Biol* 117:24–35, 1996.

80. Lanyon LE: Osteocytes, strain detection, bone modeling and remodeling. *Calcif Tissue Int* 53:S102–6; discussion S106–7, 1993.

81. Lerner UH: Osteoclast formation and resorption. *Matrix Biol* 19:107–120, 2000.

82. Loeser RF: Chondrocyte integrin expression and function. *Biorheology* 37:109–116, 2000.

83. Loeser RF, Sadiev S, Tan L, et al: Integrin expression by primary and immortalized human chondrocytes: evidence of a differential role for alphalbeta1 and alpha2beta1 integrins in mediating chondrocyte adhesion to types II and VI collagen. *Osteoarthritis Cartilage* 8:96–105, 2000.

84. Lotz M, Hashimoto S, Kuhn K: Mechanisms of chondrocyte apoptosis. *Osteoarthritis Cartilage* 7:389–391, 1999.

85. Mak AF, Lai WM, Mow VC: Biphasic indentation of articular cartilage—I. Theoretical analysis. *J Biomech* 20:703–714, 1987.

86. Maroudas AI: Balance between swelling pressure and collagen tension in normal and degenerate cartilage. *Nature* 260:808–809, 1976.

87. McFarland CD, Mayer S, Scotchford C, et al: Attachment of cultured human bone cells to novel polymers. *J Biomed Mater Res* 44:1–11, 1999.

88. McFarland CD, Thomas CH, DeFilippis C, et al: Protein adsorption and cell attachment to patterned surfaces. *J Biomed Mater Res* 49:200–210, 2000.

89. Merkel KD, Erdmann JM, McHugh KP, et al: Tumor necrosis factor-alpha mediates orthopedic implant osteolysis. *Am J Pathol* 154:203–210, 1999.

90. Mikuni-Takagaki Y: Mechanical responses and signal transduction pathways in stretched osteocytes. *J Bone Miner Metab* 17:57–60, 1999.

91. Miller EJ. Chemistry of the collagens and their distribution. In Reddi KA, Piez AH, eds: *Extracellular Matrix Biochemistry.* Elsevier, New York, NY, 1984:41–78.

92. Miller SC, Bowman BM, Smith JM, et al: Characterization of endosteal/bone-lining cells from fatty marrow bone sites in adult beagles. *Anat Rec* 198:163–173.

93. Miller SC, WS Jee. The bone lining cell: a distinct phenotype? *Calcif Tissue Int* 41:1–5, 1987.

94. Misra DN: Surface chemistry of bone and tooth mineral. In: Dickson GR, ed: *Methods of Calcified Tissue Preparation.* Elsevier, Amsterdam, 1984, 435–460.

95. Morgan EF, Keaveny TM: Dependence of yield strain of human trabecular bone on anatomic site. *J Biomech* 34:569–577, 2001.

96. Morgan EF, Yeh OC, Chang WC, et al: Nonlinear behavior of trabecular bone at small strains. *J Biomech Eng* 123:1–9, 2001.

97. Mow VC. Biphasic rheological properties of cartilage. *Bull Hosp Joint Dis* 38:121–124, 1977.

98. Mow VC, Ateshian GA, Spilker RL. Biomechanics of diarthrodial joints: a review of twenty years of progress. *J Biomech Eng* 115:460–467, 1993.

99. Mow VC, Gibbs MC, Lai WM, et al: Biphasic indentation of articular cartilage–II. A numerical algorithm and an experimental study. *J Biomech* 22:853–861, 1989.

100. Mow VC, Hou JS, Owens JM, et al: Biphasic and quasilinear viscoelastic theories for hydrated soft tissues. In: Mow VC, Woo SL, Ratcliffe A, eds: *Biomechanics Of Diarthrodial Joints.* Springer-Verlag, New York, NY, 1990:215–260.

101. Mow VC, Kuei SC, Lai WM, et al: Biphasic creep and stress relaxation of articular cartilage in compression? Theory and experiments. *J Biomech Eng* 102:3–84, 1980.

102. Mow VC, Ratcliffe A: Structure and function of articular cartilage and meniscus. In: Mow VC, Hayes WC, eds. *Basic Orthopaedic Biomechanics,* Lippincott-Raven, Philadelphia, PA, 1997:113–177.

103. Mow VC, Ratcliffe A, Poole AR: Cartilage and diarthrodial joints as paradigms for hierarchical materials and structures. *Biomaterials* 13:67–97, 1992.

104. Mow VC, Wang CC: Some bioengineering considerations for tissue engineering of articular cartilage. *Clin Orthop* 367:S204–S223, 1999.

105. Mow VC, Wang CC, Hung CT: The extracellular matrix, interstitial fluid and ions as a mechanical signal transducer in articular cartilage. *Osteoarthritis Cartilage* 7:41–58, 1999.

106. Muir H: The chondrocyte, architect of cartilage. Biomechanics, structure, function and molecular biology of cartilage matrix macromolecules. *Bioessays* 17:1039–1048, 1995.

107. Myers ER, Lai WM, Mow VC: A continuum theory and an experiment for the ion-induced swelling behavior of articular cartilage. *J Biomech Eng* 106:151–158, 1984.

108. Nanci A: Content and distribution of noncollagenous matrix proteins in bone and cementum: relationship to speed of formation and collagen packing density. *J Struct Biol* 126:256–269, 1999.

109. Neale SD, Athanasou NA: Cytokine receptor profile of arthroplasty macrophages, foreign body giant cells and mature osteoclasts. *Acta Orthop Scand* 70:452–458, 1999.

110. Neale, SD, Haynes DR, Howie DW, et al: The effect of particle phagocytosis and metallic wear particles on osteoclast formation and bone resorption in vitro. *J Arthroplasty* 15:654–662, 2000.

111. Neuman WF, Neuman MW: On the measurement of water compartments, pH, and gradients in calvaria. *Calcif Tissue Int* 31:135–145, 1980.

112. Neuman WF, Neuman MW: *The Chemical Dynamics of Bone.* Chicago University Press, Chicago, IL, 1958.

113. Nijweide PJ, van der Plas A, Scherft JP: Biochemical and histological studies on various bone cell preparations. *Calcif Tissue Int* 33:529–540, 1981.

114. Noble BS, Reeve J: Osteocyte function, osteocyte death and bone fracture resistance. *Mol Cell Endocrinol* 159:7–13, 2000.

115. O'Driscoll SW: The healing and regeneration of articular cartilage. *J Bone Joint Surg [Am]* 80:1795–1812, 1998.

116. Owen M: Histogenesis of bone cells. *Calcif Tissue Res* 25:205–207, 1978.

117. Pacifici M, Koyama E, Iwamoto M, et al: Development of articular cartilage: what do we know about it and how may it occur? *Connect Tissue Res* 41:175–184, 2000.

118. Palumbo C: A three-dimensional ultrastructural study of osteoid-osteocytes in the tibia of chick embryos. *Cell Tissue Res* 246:125–134, 1986.

119. Perrimon N, Bernfield M: Cellular functions of proteoglycans—an overview. *Semin Cell Dev Biol* 12:65–67, 2001.

120. Pidaparti RM, Chandran A, Takano Y, et al: Bone mineral lies mainly outside collagen fibrils: predictions of a composite model for osteonal bone. *J Biomech* 29:909–916, 1996.

121. Piez KA: Molecular aggregate structures of the collagens. In: Reddi KA, Piez AH, eds: *Extracellular Matrix Biochemistry.* Elsevier, New York, NY, pp 1–35, 1984.

122. Posner AS: Crystal chemistry of bone mineral. *Physiol Rev* 49:760–792, 1969.

123. Posner AS: The mineral of bone. *Clin Orthop* 200:87–99, 1985.

124. Posner AS: The structure of bone apatite surfaces. *J Biomed Mater Res* 19:241–250, 1985.

125. Prendergast PJ, van Driel WD, Kuiper JH: A comparison of finite element codes for the solution of biphasic poroelastic problems. *Proc Inst Mech Eng [H]* 210:131–136, 1996.

126. Revell PA, al-Saffar N, Kobayashi A: Biological reaction to debris in relation to joint prostheses. *Proc Inst Mech Eng [H]* 211:187–197, 1997.

127. Robinson RA: An electron microscopy study of cartilage and bone and its relationship to the organic matrix. *J Bone Joint Surg [Am]* 34:389–434, 1952.

128. Roodman GD: Cell biology of the osteoclast. *Exp Hematol* 27:1229–124, 1999.

129. Sandell LJ, Aigner T: Articular cartilage and changes in arthritis. An introduction: cell biology of osteoarthritis. *Arthritis Res* 3:107–113, 2001.

130. Schmidt MB, Mow VC, Chun LE, et al: Effects of proteoglycan extraction on the tensile behavior of articular cartilage. *J Orthop Res* 8:353–363, 1990.

131. Schmitt JM, Hwang K, Winn SR, et al. Bone morphogenetic proteins: an update on basic biology and clinical relevance. *J Orthop Res* 17:269–278, 1999.

132. Schwartz NB, Pirok 3rd, EW, Mensch Jr., JR, et al: Domain organization, genomic structure, evolution, and regulation of expression of the aggrecan gene family. *Prog Nucleic Acid Res Mol Biol* 62:177–225, 1999.

133. Schwartz Z, Boyan BD: Underlying mechanisms at the bone-biomaterial interface. *J Cell Biochem* 56:340–347, 1994.
134. Schwartz Z, Lohmann CH, Oefinger J, et al: Implant surface characteristics modulate differentiation behavior of cells in the osteoblastic lineage. *Adv Dent Res* 13:38–48, 1999.
135. Setton LA, Zhu W, Mow VC: The biphasic poroviscoelastic behavior of articular cartilage: role of the surface zone in governing the compressive behavior. *J Biomech* 26:581–92, 1993.
136. Speer DP, Dahners L: The collagenous architecture of articular cartilage. Correlation of scanning electron microscopy and polarized light microscopy observations. *Clin Orthop* 139:267–275, 1979.
137. Spilker RL, Donzelli PS, Mow VC: A transversely isotropic biphasic finite element model of the meniscus. *J Biomech* 25:1027–1045, 1992.
138. Spilker RL, Suh JK, Mow VC: A finite element analysis of the indentation stress-relaxation response of linear biphasic articular cartilage. *J Biomech Eng* 114:191–201, 1992.
139. Suarez KN, Romanello M, Bettica P, et al: Collagen type I of rat cortical and trabecular bone differs in the extent of posttranslational modifications. *Calcif Tissue Int* 58:65–69, 1996.
140. Suda T, Takahashi N, Martin TJ: Modulation of osteoclast differentiation. *Endocr Rev* 13:66–80, 1992.
141. Suh JK, Li Z, Woo SL: Dynamic behavior of a biphasic cartilage model under cyclic compressive loading. *J Biomech* 28:357–364, 1995.
142. Tang LH, Buckwalter JA, Rosenberg LC: Effect of link protein concentration on articular cartilage proteoglycan aggregation. *J Orthop Res* 14:334–339, 1996.
143. Teitelbaum SL: Bone resorption by osteoclasts. *Science* 289:1504–1508, 2000.
144. Teitelbaum SL: Osteoclasts, integrins, and osteoporosis. *J Bone Miner Metab* 18:344–349, 2000.
145. Termine JD: Non-collagenous proteins in bone. In: Rodan GA, ed: *Cell and Molecular Biology of Vertebrate Hard Tissues.* John Wiley and Sons, Chichester, UK, 1988:178–206.
146. Thomas CH, McFarland CD, Jenkins ML, et al: The role of vitronectin in the attachment and spatial distribution of bone-derived cells on materials vitronectin in the attachment and spatial distribution of bone-derived cells on materials with patterned surface chemistry. *J Biomed Mater Res* 37:81–93, 1997.
147. Torzilli PA: Water content and equilibrium water partition in immature cartilage. *J Orthop Res* 6:766–769, 1988.
148. Traub W, Arad T, Weiner S: Origin of mineral crystal growth in collagen fibrils. *Matrix* 12:251–255, 1992.
149. Turner CH, Pavalko FM: Mechanotransduction and functional response of the skeleton to physical stress: the mechanisms and mechanics of bone adaptation. *J Orthop Sci* 3:346–355, 1998.
150. Tzaphlidou M, Kafantari H: Influence of nutritional factors on bone collagen fibrils in ovariectomized rats. *Bone* 27:635–638, 2000.
151. Veis A: Bones and teeth. In: Reddi KA, Piez AH, eds: *Extracellular Matrix Biochemistry.* Elsevier, New York, NY, 1984:329–372.
152. Verbruggen G, Cornelissen M, Almqvist KF, et al: Influence of aging on the synthesis and morphology of the aggrecans synthesized by differentiated human articular chondrocytes. *Osteoarthritis Cartilage* 8:170–179, 2000.
153. Walsh WR, Guzelsu N: The role of ions and mineral-organic interfacial bonding on the compressive properties of cortical bone. *Biomed Mater Eng* 3:75–84, 1993.
154. Walsh WR, Guzelsu N: Compressive properties of cortical bone: mineral-organic interfacial bonding. *Biomaterials* 15:137–145, 1994.
155. Walsh WR, Labrador DP, Kim HD, et al: The effect of in vitro fluoride ion treatment on the ultrasonic properties of cortical bone. *Ann Biomed Eng* 22:404–415, 1994.
156. Watanabe H, Yamada Y, Kimata K: Roles of aggrecan, a large chondroitin sulfate proteoglycan, in cartilage structure and function. *J Biochem (Tokyo)* 124:687–693, 1998.

157. Weiner S, Traub W: Organization of hydroxyapatite crystals within collagen fibrils. *FEBS Lett* 206:262–266, 1986.
158. Weiner S, Traub W: Crystal size and organization in bone. *Connect Tissue Res* 21:259–265, 1989.
159. Weiner S, Traub W: Bone structure: from angstroms to microns. *Faseb J* 6:879–885, 1992.
160. Weiner S, Traub W, Wagner HD: Lamellar bone: structure-function relations. *J Struct Biol* 126:241–255, 1999.
161. Wetterwald A, Hoffstetter W, Cecchini MG, et al: Characterization and cloning of the E11 antigen, a marker expressed by rat osteoblasts and osteocytes. *Bone* 18:125–132, 1996.
162. Wong M, Ponticiello M, Kovanen V, et al: S. Volumetric changes of articular cartilage during stress relaxation in unconfined compression. *J Biomech* 33:1049–1054, 2000.
163. Wu JJ, Eyre DR: Covalent interactions of type IX collagen in cartilage. *Connect Tissue Res* 20:241–246, 1989.
164. Wu JJ, Eyre DR: Structural analysis of cross-linking domains in cartilage type XI collagen. Insights on polymeric assembly. *J Biol Chem* 270:18,865–18,870, 1995.
165. Wu JJ, Woods PE, Eyre DR: Identification of cross-linking sites in bovine cartilage type IX collagen reveals an antiparallel type II-type IX molecular relationship and type IX to type IX bonding. *J Biol Chem* 267:23,007–23,014, 1992.
166. Yoshida H, Hayashi S, Kunisada T, et al: The murine mutation osteopetrosis is in the coding region of the macrophage colony stimulating factor gene. *Nature* 345:442–444, 1990.

3

Normal Structure and Function of Bone

Torben Steiniche[1] and Ellen M. Hauge[2]

[1]*Institute of Pathology, Aarhus University Hospital AKH, Aarhus, Denmark*
[2]*Institute of Pathology, Aarhus University Hospital AAS, Aarhus, Denmark*

I. INTRODUCTION

Bones are the 206 individual organs that comprise the human skeletal system. Like other connective tissues, bone consists of cells, fibers, and ground substance, but unlike the others, its extracellular components are calcified, making it a hard and firm substance that is ideally suited for its supportive and protective function in the skeleton.[2]

Bone provides the foundation for the internal support of the body and for the attachment of muscles and tendons. It serves as rigid levers for muscles to act against as they hold the body upright in defiance of gravity, and thus it is essential for locomotion. It protects the vital organs of the cranial and thoracic cavities from injuries, and within its cavities it houses and protects the blood-forming marrow. Finally, bone has an important metabolic role as a storage area for ions—especially calcium and phosphate, which can be drawn upon in situations with increased demands, thus maintaining serum homeostasis.

The regulation of bone mass and structure is to a great extent governed by the mechanical demands placed upon the bone tissue. The apparent biological goal is the maintenance of a minimum adequate structure, in which the margin of safety between normal mechanical demands and fracture is balanced by the cost of excessive bone mass on mobility.[44]

A. Macroscopic Structure of Bone

The skeleton is divided into two regions: the axial skeleton, including the skull, vertebrae, ribs, sternum, and hyoid, and the peripheral skeleton, including the limbs and pelvis.[34] Bones can be classified according to shape into long, short, flat, and irregular bones. However, this traditional classification has no great merit. Bones must be studied individually, and considered in relation to the functional demands placed upon them.[39]

In the individual bone, two types of bone tissue are distinguishable—compact bone, which is usually limited to the cortices of mature bone (cortical bone), and spongy bone (cancellous bone), which forms the central regions of the bones. Cortical bone appears as a solid continuous mass, in which spaces can be visualized only with the aid of the microscope. Cancellous bone consists of thin trabeculae (bony spicules) arranged in a three-dimensional (3D) lattice. The size and thickness of the cortex and the architecture of the

From: *Handbook of Histology Methods for Bone and Cartilage*
Edited by: Y. H. An and K. L. Martin © Humana Press Inc., Totowa, NJ

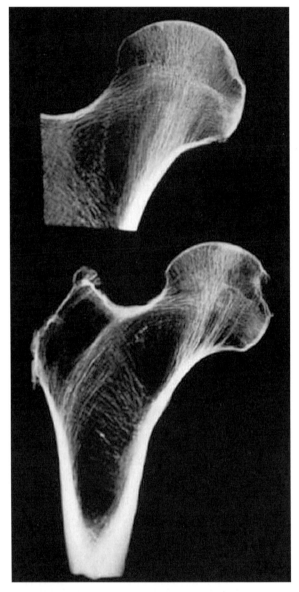

Figure 1. A section through the proximal end of the femur reveals that the cancellous bone is organized according to prevailing mechanical stress.

cancellous lattice are designed to match the type and direction of the forces that the individual bone must resist (Fig. 1). Thus, bone cannot be considered an isotropic tissue, a factor that must be taken into account when histomorphometric measurements are performed.[17] In order to obtain correct and unbiased measurements of highly anisotropic tissues such as cancellous bone, specially designed procedures are required to obtain and cut the specimens, combined with the use of specially designed grid systems.[17,45]

The diaphysis (tubular shaft) of a long bone such as the tibia or femur consists of a thick-walled cylinder of cortical bone with a central marrow cavity (Fig. 2). The tubular

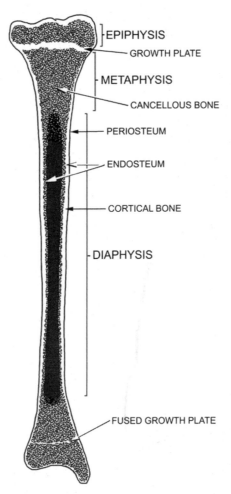

Figure 2. Schematic view of a longitudinal section through the growing tibia (long bone).

shape is ideal for withstanding the bending and torsional loads imposed on the bone shaft, since a hollow cylinder, weight for weight, is stronger than a solid one.[5] Toward the metaphysis and the epiphysis, the compact bone becomes progressively thinner and the internal space is filled with cancellous bone. Here, the bone is designed to support and distribute mostly compression forces created during joint movements.[39] Cortical bone constitutes approx 80% of the skeletal mass, and cancellous bone approx 20%. The relative proportions of cortical and cancellous bone differ considerably in various parts of the skeleton.[24] The vertebral and iliac bones, which are often studied in human as well as in experimental animal models, are mainly composed of cancellous bone with a rather thin shell of cortical bone. This cortical shell still has a major influence upon bone strength.[46] Decreasing cortical thickness with age is observed in both sexes in the axial and in the appendicular skeleton.[3] The diameter of the cortical bone increases throughout life,[16] but an even greater enlargement of the marrow cavity simultaneously occurs, leading to the cortical thinning.[3] Resistance of tubular bones to bending and torsion is influenced by the bone geometry, and the most effectual shape of the bone is that in which the osseous tissue is distributed far from the neutral axis (center of the medullary cavity).[7] The increase in bone diameter may thus to a certain degree compensate for the bone loss because of the cortical thinning. The amount of cancellous bone also decreases with age,[36] but the loss of bone volume is accompanied by structural changes that may reduce the strength of the bone to a greater extent than the reduction in the amount of bone itself would suggest.[31] In the vertebrae, the bone mass, expressed as the ash-density, decreases from the age of 20 yr to 50–55%, whereas the vertical cancellous bone compressive stress decreases to 20–25% and the horizontal compressive stress to only 5–10% of the value at the age of 20 yr.[23] Men and women may lose cancellous bone tissue in different ways. Women appear to lose cancellous bone predominantly by trabecular perforations with loss of the whole structural element, whereas men appear to lose cancellous bone predominantly by trabecular thinning.[6] This loss of cancellous bone architecture with age, and the potential for a different loss pattern in men and women, may explain the observed increase in fractures with age that are expecially in common in women in skeletal regions dominated by cancellous bone.

B. Microscopic Structure of Bone

At the microscopic level, bone can be divided into two distinct types: woven and lamellar bone. In woven or immature bone, the collagen fibers are arranged randomly in a meshwork pattern. In lamellar bone, the collagen fibers are arranged in parallel sheets and bundles, and the orientation of collagen fibers alternates between successive lamellae. This explains the shifting light and dark bands seen in polarized light (Figs. 3, 4). The number of osteocytes per unit volume in woven bone is higher than in lamellar bone, and they are unevenly distributed.[22] Woven bone is formed during rapid bone formation, as during development and fracture healing, or in tumors and some metabolic bone diseases. The disorientation of the collagen fibers gives woven bone tissue its isotropic mechanical characteristics. When woven bone tissue is tested, the mechanical behavior is similar— regardless of the orientation of the applied forces—in contrast to lamellar bone, which shows the greatest resistance to load when the forces are directed in a parallel fashion to the longitudinal axis of the collagen fibers.[7] After the age of 4 yr, the majority of bone tissue is lamellar,[7] either arranged in osteons or as interstitial bone tissue.

The cornerstone of cortical as well as cancellous bone is the osteon (Fig. 3, 4). The correct name is the secondary osteon, used in order to distinguish it from the primary osteon formed during the initial generation of bone. Approximately two-thirds of cortical volume is formed by intact secondary osteons. The remainder is made up of interstitial bone, which represents the remnants of previous generations of secondary osteons, and a continuous layer of a few lamellae at the surfaces, termed the subperiosteal and subendosteal circumferential lamellae. The 3D architecture of a secondary cortical osteon is that of branching cylindrical columns[41] with a mean of 2.5 mm between the branch points.[1] This distance is conveniently taken as the mean length of the secondary cortical osteon. The diameter of the secondary osteon in the iliac crest is approx 150 μm, with a central vascular canal of about 40 μm in diameter (the Haversian canal).[3]

The Haversian canals are connected to one another, and communicate with the periosteum and with the marrow cavity via transverse and oblique channels known as the Volkmann's canals. The blood vessels of the Volkmann's canals are often larger than those of

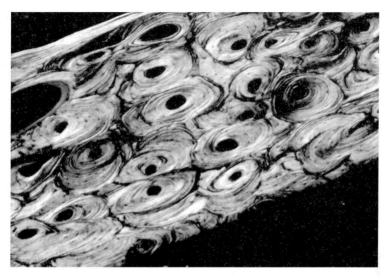

Figure 3. Cross-section of cortical osteons with concentric lamellae surrounding vascular canals (polarized light).

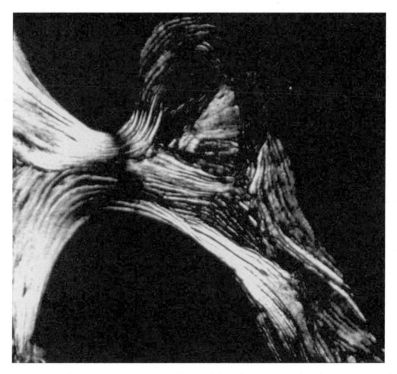

Figure 4. Crescent-shaped cancellous osteons (packets) with lamellae running parallel to the bone-marrow interface (polarized light).

the Haversian canals.[2] The secondary cortical osteons are usually oriented in the long axis of tubular bone.[41] In the center of the secondary cortical osteon is the Haversian canal, with one or two capillaries lined by fenestrated endothelium surrounded by a basal lamina. Usually there are also some unmyelinated and occasional myelinated nerve fibers.[39] Concentric lamellae of bone are centered around this canal. At the periphery, the secondary osteon is sharply demarcated from the surrounding bone by a cement line, which is a region of reduced mineralization containing sulfated mucosubstances,[4] and probably little or no collagen. The cement line can also be interpreted as the reversal line marking the extension of bone resorption that precedes bone formation. Osteocytes are regularly dispersed within the osteon with the long axes of the cells parallel to the lamellae. The osteocytes are located in lacunae that are interconnected by canaliculi.[22,25] The osteocyte is considered the most mature or terminally differentiated cell of the osteoblast lineage. By means of cytoplasmic projections within the canaliculi, the cells get nutrition and maintain contact with cell processes from the osteocytes or with processes from the cells lining the bone surface.[19,22]

The secondary cancellous osteons have the same basic construction as the secondary cortical osteons, but with a different shape (Fig. 4). The osteons resemble broad bands, which are made up of parallel lamellae, bounded on one side by the bone marrow and on the other side by an irregular cement line. The mean thickness is much less than the mean extent in the other dimensions (the ratio is less than 0.2). A single 3D osteon can therefore give rise to a varying number of profiles in a single random two-dimensional (2D) section.[20] As in cortical bone, interstitial bone is seen between the secondary osteons, representing remnants of previous generations of secondary cancellous osteons.

C. Ultrastructure of Bone

The fundamental constituents of bone are the cells and the mineralized extracellular matrix (ECM). Only 10–20% of the bone matrix mass is water. Sixty-seven percent of the dry weight is made up of inorganic mineral salts (mainly hydroxyapatite), 30–40% is collagen, and the remainder (about 5%) is non-collagenous protein (NCP) and carbohydrates.[21] The ratio of collagen to NCP is quite unique for bone, with collagenous protein comprising 90% of the organic matrix compared with 10–20% in other tissues.[38]

Bone salts form the inorganic constituents of the bone matrix and convert the soft organic matrix into a rigid structure, giving the bone tissue mechanical strength. Hydroxyapatite is the main component, but bone mineral contains numerous impurities.[21] The fluoride ion F^- may substitute OH^-, and the amount depends mainly on the fluoride content of the drinking water. Other impurities may be citrate, carbonate, magnesium, and sodium. The hydroxyapatite forms small slender rod-like crystals about 40 nm in length and 1.5–3 nm in thickness. The crystals are aligned along the collagen fiber axis at regular intervals of 60–70 nm.[2,38]

The predominant collagen of bone is type I, as in skin and tendons, and only minute amounts are of type III, V, and IX.[38] As in all connective tissues, the collagen fibrils serve mechanical functions in providing strength and elasticity. The tensile strength of the bone thus depends to a large extent upon the fibers. Collagen type I is a triple-helical molecule synthesized by the osteoblasts as a procollagen molecule, and characterized by strong covalent crosslinks holding the molecules together.[35]

The NCPs of bone are a complex set of molecules that arise from exogenous (mainly serum-derived proteins) or local sources (synthesized by osteoblasts).[42,43] Bone mineral has excellent adsorbent properties, and therefore binds many circulating proteins such as alpha 2-HS-glycoprotein from the blood and potent growth factors.[42] Osteoblasts produce a large number of proteins such as alkaline phosphatase, osteonectin, and osteocalcin. The exact role of all these NCPs is not well-defined, but they probably play a central role in matrix mineralization and in the control of osteoblastic and osteoclastic metabolism.[21]

D. Histogenesis of Bone

Replacement of pre-existing connective tissue is always the basis for bone formation. Two different modes of osteogenesis are observed: intramembranous ossification, in which bone formation occurs directly in primitive highly vascular connective tissue, and endochondral ossification, in which bone formation takes place in pre-existing cartilage.

1. Intramembranous Ossification

Certain flat bones of the skull—the frontal, parietal, occipital, and temporal bones—form by intramembranous ossification. In condensed vascular connective tissue, mesenchymal cells proliferate and differentiate directly into preosteoblasts and then into osteoblasts, which begin to synthesize bone matrix. This bone matrix will first appear as thin strands, or trabeculae, of eosinophilic material. The bone matrix will soon mineralize, and osteoblasts will be trapped in the growing bone as osteocytes. At the periphery, mesenchymal cells continue to differentiate to osteoblasts. The osteoblasts proceed with bone formation on the surface of trabeculae, creating the primary spongiosa (consisting of woven bone). If the trabeculae continue to thicken at the expense of the connective tissue, primitive cortical bone is formed. The bone is deposited in irregularly concentric layers, and has some similarity to the Haversian system, but is composed of woven bone (the primary osteons). In other areas, the trabecular thickening stops and the vascular connective tissue space is gradually transformed into hematopoietic tissue, creating the primitive cancellous bone. Later, this primary or primitive bone will be remodeled, and thereby progressively replaced by mature lamellar bone.[2,39]

2. Endochondral Ossification

Bones of the vertebral column, pelvis, and the extremities are first formed as cartilage models, which are subsequently replaced by bone in a process called endochondral ossification.[2,39] In contrast to bone, where apposition of new bone only can occur on the surface, cartilage can grow interstitially. In cartilage, new cells can be added within its volume, and it can increase its volume by elaborating ECM, thus expanding both its length and its diameter.[34] This is an advantage when rapid growth is required during prenatal life and childhood, as in the longitudinal growth of long bones. In early fetal life, condensed mesenchyme is replaced by an avascular cartilaginous model, which has the crude shape of the adult bone. In a long bone, the primary center of ossification is seen in the middle of the shaft of this cartilage model. Three events occur at almost the same time: i) around the mid-portion of the shaft (diaphysis), under the perichondrium, mesenchymal cells modulate to form osteoblasts, which lay down bone just outside the cartilage core, initially as a layer of type I collagen-rich osteoid that later becomes mineralized,[32] creating a periosteal collar; ii) the chondrocytes in the center of the cartilage core undergo hypertrophy, and as their lacunae enlarge, the intervening matrix is compressed to thin septa, which calcify; iii) blood vessels form the periosteum and penetrate the cartilage core accompanied by pericytes, hematopoietic and osteoprogenitor cells and osteoclasts.

In the interior of the cartilage model, the osteoprogenitor cells differentiate to osteoblasts, which begin to deposit bone on the septa of calcified cartilage. The earliest bony trabeculae thus have a core of calcified cartilage. These primary trabeculae soon become remodeled and replaced by secondary trabeculae of lamellar bone, or are replaced by marrow. After creation of the periosteal collar, no further interstitial growth of the diaphysis can occur, and the further expansion in diameter and shape is the result of subperiosteal appositional growth (intramembranous ossification).[34] Primary centers of ossification have developed in the diaphysis of the long bone by the third month of fetal life. Much later, usually after birth, secondary centers of ossification occur in the epiphyses of the long bones. In the secondary centers of ossification, the same sequence of events occurs as in the primary center of ossification, except that there is no associated subperichondral deposition of bone.[2] When the endochondral ossification originating from the primary center of ossification has reached the level of the diaphyseal-epiphysial junction, the rapid continuous longitudinal growth of the long bones depends on endochondral growth at the epiphyseal growth plate. Here, an ordered sequence of cartilage-cell cytomorphosis occurs, which is actually identical to the processes previously described in the primary center of ossification. Four different zones representing four different stages in cartilage cell cytomorphosis can be recognized: i) the resting zone; ii) the proliferative zone (chondrocyte proliferation); iii) the hypertrophic zone (the chondrocytes hypertrophy and line up in columns, and additional matrix is deposited); iv) the degenerative zone (the cartilage matrix calcifies and metaphyseal vascular ingrowth and collagen breakdown occur).[37] During this process of cartilage proliferation and mineralization, the bone continues to grow until it reaches its final length.

3. Modeling and Remodeling

Three basic mechanisms are involved in the development and turnover of bone: longitudinal growth, modeling, and remodeling. Longitudinal growth ceases with closure of the growth plates at the end of the growing period.

During the growth phase, a continuous adaption of the macroscopic shape of the bone takes place. Some surfaces are under continuous resorption and others are under continuous formation, a process known as modeling. Bone modeling thus sculpts the shape and sizes of bone by adding bone in some places and removing it in others.[13] Modeling plays its major role during growth, and becomes relatively ineffective around and after skeletal maturity.

Remodeling is the process by which the skeleton is continuously renewed. The process starts with fetal osteogenesis and continues throughout life. It results in turnover of lamellar bone without causing large changes in bone quantity, geometry, or size.[11] The purpose of remodeling is to adjust the skeleton to changes in mechanical demands, to prevent accumulation of fatigue damage, to repair micro fractures, to ensure the viability of the osteocytes, and to allow the skeleton to participate in the calcium homeostasis. Bone remodeling displays substantial regional variations between different skeletal sites.[33] Bone remodeling is a surface phenomenon and occurs at all bone surfaces. In bone, four different surfaces or envelopes can be identified—the periosteal (periost), Haversian canal (intracortical), endocortical (endosteal), and the trabecular surface(s). Besides a variation in remodeling activity between different skeletal sites, there is also a variation in the remodeling activity and bone balance between the different envelopes in the individual bone. In general, cancellous bone remodeling activity is 5–10 times greater than in cortical bone. The remodeling process turns bone over by localized osteoclastic resorption followed by osteoblastic formation, (i.e., the coupled process of bone remodeling). Bone remodeling, which in adults accounts for more than 90% of the normal bone turnover, occurs as a sequence of events performed by a committed team of cells called the bone multicellular unit (BMU).[18] After activation, osteoclasts start to erode and resorb bone. When a certain resorption depth is reached, the osteoclasts are apparently replaced by mononuclear cells that complete the resorption.[10] Following completion of resorption, preosteoblasts invade the area, differentiate into osteoblasts, and begin bone matrix formation. After a time period (the osteoid maturation time[30]), bone matrix is subsequently mineralized to lamellar bone. Osteoblasts continue to form bone matrix that subsequently mineralizes, thereby in essence repairing the resorption-mediated "defect" (the quantum concept of bone remodeling[27]). During this process, some osteoblasts are incorporated into the matrix.[22] As described here, resorption and formation are closely associated with each other both temporally (time) and spatially (location).[9–11] In the normal remodeling process, resorption will always be followed by formation, and formation will always be preceded by resorption (coupling).[18] The frequency with which a given site on the bone surface undergoes remodeling is known as the activation frequency.[30]

In cortical bone, the basic multicellular unit forms a complex and unique structure, which bores holes through the hard and compact cortical bone like a drill, creating a longitudinal tunnel, which appears as an enclosed cavity in cross section. In front is the cutting cone, where osteoclasts resorb bone. Closely following the osteoclasts comes a capillary loop with endothelial cells and perivascular mesenchymal cells, which are osteoblast progenitors. This initiates the closing cone, in which the longitudinal tunnel is refilled by new bone, and a new secondary cortical osteon is formed (Fig. 5).

In cancellous bone, the sequence of events is the same as in cortical bone[8] (Fig. 6). The duration of the total remodeling sequence in cancellous bone is approx 4 mo, with a resorption period of 1 mo and a formation period of 3 mo. In cancellous bone of the iliac crest, the sequence of events is recapitulated every second year (an activation frequency of 0.50 per yr) in normal young adults.[40]

The activation frequency in cortical bone (at the surface of the Haversian canals) is also around 0.50 per yr.[3] Thus, the surface-based activity appears to be nearly identical in cortical and cancellous bone. Since the extent of bone surface to bone volume is much lower in cortical than in cancellous bone, however, the volume-based turnover is much lower in cortical bone as compared to cancellous bone.

Bone balance is the difference between the amount of bone resorbed and reformed during the remodeling cycle. The bone balance may differ between the different bone envelopes, and is influenced by many local and systemic factors. To explain the observed changes in bone architecture with age, the bone balance must in general be positive at the periosteal surface (increased bone diameter with age), zero or slightly negative at the surface of the Haversian canals and negative at the endocortical surface (increased diameter of bone marrow cavity with age) and cancellous surface (decrease in the trabecular width with age).

Finally, this leads to considerations about how bone can be lost or gained by the remodeling process. Three different mechanisms seem to be involved (Fig. 7):

Cortical Bone Remodeling Sequence

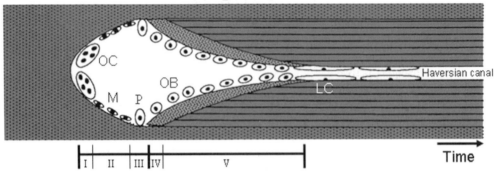

Figure 5. The bone remodeling unit (BRU) of cortical bone constitutes a cylinder with a cone-shaped top (cutting cone), in which osteoblastic resorption proceeds. The resorption is later followed by formation of new bone in the area of the closing cone, which results in refilling of the cavity. In cancellous bone, the BRU can be viewed as a cortical BRU cut through the middle. The structure is pancake-shaped. The remodeling sequence can be divided into different phases: I = osteoclastic phase; II = mononuclear phase; III = pre-osteoblastic phase; IV = initial mineralization lag time; V = mineralization period. Phase I–III = resorptive period. Phases IV–V = formative period. OC = osteoclasts, M = mononuclear resorptive cells, P = preosteoblasts, OB = osteoblasts, LC = lining cells.

Cancellous Bone Remodeling Sequence

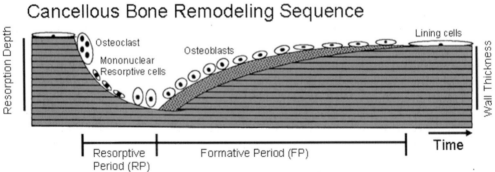

Figure 6. Throughout life, lamellar bone is renewed through internal reorganization known as remodeling. After activation, osteoclasts start to erode and form a resorption cavity. When a certain depth is reached, the osteoclasts are replaced by mononuclear cells that complete the resorption. Osteoblasts subsequently differentiate and form new bone at the same site. At first, the new bone is not as heavily mineralized as the old.

1. Reversible Bone Loss/Gain by Changes in Bone Turnover

The remodeling space is the amount of bone that has been removed by osteoclasts and not yet reformed by the osteoblasts during the remodeling sequence.[26] The total remodeling space within the skeleton depends on the number of ongoing remodeling cycles, the duration of the resorptive and formative periods, and the depth of the resorption lacunae. In normal individuals, the remodeling space is 6–8% of the skeletal volume.[26] An increase

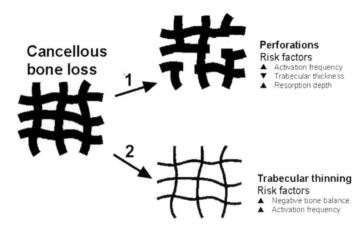

Figure 7. The remodeling process may cause bone to be lost irreversibly by two different mechanisms: (1) by perforations leadings to disintegration of the trabecular network and (2) by a negative bone balance at the remodeling site, leading to a thinning of the trabeculae.

in activation frequency leads to an increase in the number of ongoing remodeling cycles. This will increase the remodeling space and proportionally decrease the amount of bone. Obviously, the opposite effect is seen if the activation frequency is decreased. The process is reversible because the remodeling space, and thereby the bone volume, returns to normal when the metabolic challenge to the bone is removed, and the activation frequency returns to normal.

2. Irreversible Bone Loss/Gain by Changes in Bone Balance

In normal young adults, the amount of bone formed by the osteoblasts at the remodeling site is equal to the amount of bone previously resorbed. However, a negative balance may occur, leading to cortical and trabecular thinning and thereby to osteopenia. Obviously, an increase in cortical and trabecular thickness will occur if the bone balance per remodeling site is positive.

3. Irreversible Loss of Whole Trabecular Elements and Trabecularization of the Endocortical Surface

A very deep resorption lacuna may perforate a trabecular plate, removing the basis for the subsequent bone formation and thus causing the loss of a structural element adding to the disintegration of the trabecular network.[28] The risk of trabecular plate perforations depends on the activation frequency, resorption depth, and trabecular thickness. Although the loss of bone volume by this mechanism may be limited, the effect on the biomechanical competence (strength) may be very pronounced.[29]

After cessation of longitudinal growth, modeling and remodeling are the only biological mechanisms that can change a bone's size and shape, and the content and distribution of its bony tissue, thus determining the mechanical strength of the bone. Therefore, there must be biological mechanisms that are able to adjust the bone to the mechanical demands put upon it. These demands can range from complete disuse to maximal vigor. The mechanostat is a hypothesis presented by Harold M. Frost, which creates a link between mechanical use and bone modeling and remodeling.[14],[15] This hypothesis operates with four mechanical usage windows.[13]

- The disuse window: When the mechanical load normally put on the bone suddenly falls, such as during prolonged bedrest or space flight, for example, bone remodeling will increase dramatically. Under these circumstances, the bone balance per remodeling cycle will be negative, and rapid bone loss occurs. The modeling process is turned off.
- The adapted window: The mechanical load on the bone stays within a normal range. The bone remodeling process occurs at a normal speed, in order to carry out its role in preventing accumulation of fatigue damage, repairing micro fractures, and ensuring the viability of the osteocytes. The bone balance per remodeling cycle will be close to zero, and bone mass and architecture will be preserved. The modeling process is turned off. Healthy, normally active adult individuals function in this window.
- The mild overload window: The skeleton senses a mild mechanical overload. The remodeling process occurs with a normal speed, carrying out its many roles, but modeling is turned on in order to begin strengthening and changing the bone architecture to adapt the bone to the new mechanical challenge. Healthy, normally active growing individuals should function in this window.
- The pathologic overload window: The skeleton senses a severe mechanical overload. At first, the remodeling process occurs at normal speed, but bone remodeling subsequently increases because of an increase in micro fractures. Bone modeling will be turned on, but with woven bone formation. This process may be involved in loosening endoprostheses or implants that are poorly designed, or do not fit properly.

The mechanical loads that function as set points for these different windows may be under the influence of genetic factors and circulating agents. Endocrine and other changes accompanying menopause may thus raise the normal set point for the disuse window, and may be one of the mechanisms behind the increase in bone remodeling that occurs at menopause.[12]

REFERENCES

1. Beddoe AH: Measurements of the microscopic structure of cortical bone. *Phys Med Biol* 22:298–308, 1977.
2. Bloom W, Fawcett DW: Bone. In: Bloom W, Fawcett DW, eds: *A Textbook of Histology, 12th ed.* Chapman & Hall, New York, NY, 1994:194–233.
3. Brockstedt H, Kassem M, Eriksen EF, et al: Age- and sex-related changes in iliac cortical bone mass and remodeling. *Bone* 14:681–691, 1993.
4. Burr DB, Schaffler MB, Frederickson RG: Composition of the cement line and its possible mechanical role as a local interface in human compact bone. *J Biomech* 21:939–945, 1988.
5. Carter DR, Spengler DM: Mechanical properties and composition of cortical bone. *Clin Orthop* 135:192–217, 1978.
6. Compston JE, Mellish RW, Garrahan NJ: Age-related changes in iliac crest trabecular microanatomic bone structure in man. *Bone* 8:289–292, 1987.
7. Einhorn TA: The bone organ system: form and function. In: Marcus R, Feldman D, Kelsey J, eds: *Osteoporosis.* Academic Press, San Diego, CA, 1996:3–22.
8. Eriksen EF: Normal and pathological remodeling of human trabecular bone: three dimensional reconstruction of the remodeling sequence in normals and in metabolic bone disease. *Endocr Rev* 7:379–408, 1986.
9. Eriksen EF, Gundersen HJ, Melsen F, et al: Reconstruction of the formative site in iliac trabecular bone in 20 normal individuals employing a kinetic model for matrix and mineral apposition. *Metab Bone Dis Relat Res* 5:243–252, 1984.

10. Eriksen EF, Melsen F, Mosekilde L: Reconstruction of the resorptive site in iliac trabecular bone: a kinetic model for bone resorption of 20 normal individuals. *Metab Bone Dis Relat Res* 5:235–242, 1984.

11. Frost HM: Tetracycline-based histological analysis of bone remodeling. *Calcif Tissue Res* 3:211–237, 1969.

12. Frost HM: The mechanostat: a proposed pathogenic mechanism of osteoporosis and the bone mass effects of mechanical and nonmechanical agents. *Bone Miner* 2:73–85, 1987.

13. Frost HM: Perspectives: bone's mechanical usage windows. *Bone Miner* 19:257–271, 1992.

14. Frost HM: Suggested fundamental concepts in skeletal physiology [editorial]. *Calcif Tissue Int* 52:1–4, 1993.

15. Frost HM: Wolff's Law and bone's structural adaptations to mechanical usage: an overview for clinicians. *Angle Orthod* 64:175–188, 1994.

16. Garn SM, Rohmann CG, Wagner B, et al: Continuing bone growth throughout life: a general phenomenon. *Am J Phys Anthropol* 26:313–317, 1967.

17. Gundersen HJ, Bendtsen TF, Korbo L, et al: Some new, simple and efficient stereological methods and their use in pathological research and diagnosis. *APMIS* 96:379–394, 1988.

18. Hattner R, Epker BN, Frost HM: Suggested sequential mode of control of changes in cell behaviour in adult bone remodelling. *Nature* 206:489–490, 1965.

19. Holtrop ME: The ultrastructure of bone. *Ann Clin Lab Sci* 5:264–271, 1975.

20. Kragstrup J, Melsen F: Three-dimensional morphology of trabecular bone osteons reconstructed from serial sections. *Metab Bone Dis Relat Res* 5:127–130, 1983.

21. Lian JB, Stein GS, Canalis E, et al: Bone formation: osteoblast lineage cells, growth factors, matrix proteins, and the mineralization process. In: Favus MJ, *ed: Primer on the Metabolic Bone Diseases and the Disorders of Mineral Metabolism, 4th ed.* Lippincott Williams and Wilkins, Philadelphia, PA, 1999:14–29.

22. Marotti G: The structure of bone tissues and the cellular control of their deposition. *Ital J Anat Embryol* 101:25–79, 1996.

23. Mosekilde L: Normal age-related changes in bone mass, structure, and strength—consequences of the remodelling process. *Dan Med Bull* 40:65–83, 1993.

24. Mundy GR: Bone remodeling. In: Favus MJ, *ed: Primer on the Metabolic Bone Diseases and Disorders of Mineral Metabolism, 4th ed.* Lippincott Williams and Wilkins, Philadelphia, PA, 1999:30–38.

25. Parfitt AM: The actions of parathyroid hormone on bone: relation to bone remodeling and turnover, calcium homeostasis, and metabolic bone disease. Part III of IV parts; PTH and osteoblasts, the relationship between bone turnover and bone loss, and the state of the bones in primary hyperparathyroidism. *Metabolism* 25:1033–1069, 1976.

26. Parfitt AM: Bone histomorphometry: techniques and interpretation. In: Recker RR, ed: *The Physiologic and Clinical Significance of Bone Histomorphometric Data.* CRC Press Inc., Boca Raton, FL, 1983:143–224.

27. Parfitt AM: The cellular basis of bone remodeling: the quantum concept reexamined in light of recent advances in the cell biology of bone. *Calcif Tissue Int* 36:S37–S45, 1984.

28. Parfitt AM: Age-related structural changes in trabecular and cortical bone: cellular mechanisms and biomechanical consequences. *Calcif Tissue Int* 36:S123–S128, 1984.

29. Parfitt AM: Trabecular bone architecture in the pathogenesis and prevention of fracture. *Am J Med* 82:68–72, 1987.

30. Parfitt AM, Drezner MK, Glorieux FH, et al: Bone histomorphometry: standardization of nomenclature, symbols, and units. Reports of the ASBMR Histomorphometry Nomenclature Committee. *J Bone Miner Res* 2:595–610, 1987.

31. Parfitt AM, Mathews CH, Villanueva AR, et al: Relationships between surface, volume, and thickness of iliac trabecular bone in aging and in osteoporosis. Implications for the microanatomic and cellular mechanisms of bone loss. *J Clin Invest* 72:1396–1409, 1983.

32. Pechak DG, Kujawa MJ, Caplan AI: Morphological and histochemical events during first bone formation in embryonic chick limbs. *Bone* 7:441–458, 1986.

33. Podenphant J, Engel U: Regional variations in histomorphometric bone dynamics from the skeleton of an osteoporotic woman. *Calcif Tissue Int* 40:184–188, 1987.

34. Porter GA, Gurley M, Roth SI: Bone. In: Sternberg SS, ed: *Histology for Pathologists, 2nd* ed. Lippincott Raven, Philadelphia, PA, 1997:85–105.

35 Prockop DJ, Kivirikko KI, Tuderman L, et al: The biosynthesis of collagen and its disorders (first of two parts). *N Engl J Med* 301:13–23, 1979.

36. Riggs BL, Wahner HW, Melton LJ, III, et al: Rates of bone loss in the appenducular and axial skeletons of women. Evidence of substantial vertebral bone loss before menopause. *J Clin Invest* 77:1487–1491, 1986.

37. Robertson WW, Jr: Newest knowledge of the growth plate. *Clin Orthop* 253:270–278, 1990.

38. Robey PG, Boskey AL: The biochemistry of bone. In: Marcus R, Feldman D, Kelsey J, eds: *Osteoporosis.* Academic Press, San Diego, CA, 1996:95–183.

39. Soames RW: Skeletal system. In: Williams PL, Bannister LH, Berry MM, et al: *Gray's Anatomy, 38th ed.* Churchill Livingstone, New York, Edinburgh, London, Tokyo, Madrid, Melbourne, 1995:425–736.

40. Steiniche T: Bone histomorphometry in the pathophysiological evaluation of primary and secondary osteoporosis and various treatment modalities. *APMIS Suppl* 51:1–44, 1995.

41. Stout SD, Brunsden BS, Hildebolt CF, et al: Computer-assisted 3D reconstruction of serial sections of cortical bone to determine the 3D structure of osteons. *Calcif Tissue Int* 65:280–4, 1999.

42. Termine JD: Non-collagen proteins in bone. *Ciba Found Symp* 136:178–202, 1988.

43. Termine JD: Cellular activity, matrix proteins, and aging bone. *Exp Gerontol* 25:217–221, 1990.

44. Turner CH: Homeostatic control of bone structure: an application of feedback theory. *Bone* 12:203–217, 1991.

45. Vesterby A, Kragstrup J, Gundersen HJ, et al: Unbiased stereologic estimation of surface density in bone using vertical sections. *Bone* 8:13–17, 1987.

46. Vesterby A, Mosekilde L, Gundersen HJ, et al: Biologically meaningful determinants of the in vitro strength of lumbar vertebrae. *Bone* 12:219–224, 1991.

4

Structure and Function of Articular Cartilage

Jerry C. Y. Hu and Kyriacos A. Athanasiou

Department of Bioengineering, Rice University, Houston, TX, USA

I. INTRODUCTION

Cartilage is an aneural, avascular, alymphatic connective tissue. Like other tissues, chondrocytes arise from mesenchymal stem cells.[93] During skeletal development, cartilage grows rapidly and mineralizes to form bone. During the early process of bone fracture repair, cartilage is formed before mineralizing to bone. In the human adult, cartilage may be classified as hyaline, elastic, or fibrous.[74] Hyaline cartilage is glassy and forms the costal cartilages, articular cartilages of joints, and cartilages of the nose, larynx, trachea, and bronchi.[74] Elastic cartilage may be found in the epiglottic cartilage, the cartilage of the external ear and the auditory tube, and some of the smaller laryngeal cartilages. Histologically, elastic cartilage resembles hyaline cartilage, with a dense network of finely branched elastic fibers.[74] Fibrous cartilage, unlike other types of cartilage, contains mainly type I collagen. It may be found in the intra-articular lips, disks, menisci, and intervertebral discs, and it serves as a transitional tissue between dense connective tissue (tendon) and hyaline cartilage.[93] This chapter will focus on articular cartilage, which is a specialized form of hyaline cartilage. Articular cartilage covers the articulating ends of bones and serves as a lubricated, wear-resistant, friction-reducing surface that is slightly compressible to evenly distribute forces onto the bone. After injury, articular cartilage is unable to naturally restore itself back to a functional tissue, and, because of this, current efforts have been directed toward tissue engineering. Since articular cartilage contains zones that are specific in their functions, the replication of these zones may be important in obtaining a functional tissue-engineered construct, and histology will serve as the first tool in discerning these zonal variations.

II. COMPOSITION OF ARTICULAR CARTILAGE

Articular cartilage is composed of a fluid phase and a solid phase. The fluid phase is water with physiological concentrations of ionic and non-ionic solutes, and makes up 75–80% of the wet wt (ww) of cartilage.[81] By wet wt, the solid phase is composed of ~10% chondrocytes, 10–30% collagen, 3–10% proteoglycans, ~10% lipids, and minor amounts of glycoproteins.[94] The mechanical properties, and thus the function of cartilage, are dictated by the interactions of its matrix components. Since the organization and composition of cartilage varies with depth, its mechanical properties also vary accordingly.

From: *Handbook of Histology Methods for Bone and Cartilage*
Edited by: Y. H. An and K. L. Martin © Humana Press Inc., Totowa, NJ

A. Chondrocytes

Chondrocytes comprise only about 1–5% of the volume of the matrix. Chondrocytes differentiate from mesenchymal stem cells of the bone marrow and are responsible for matrix remodeling, secreting both the components that make up the matrix and the enzymes that degrade it.[93] Since articular cartilage is avascular, chondrocytes obtain nutrients from diffusion.[63] During movement, articulation of the joint results in mass transfer through the tissue by the compression and relaxation of cartilage that results in fluid exudation and absorption. A pericellular region that attaches the chondrocyte to the surrondings extracellular matrix (ECM) acts as a fluid-filled "bladder" to absorb mechanical loads and to provide hydrodynamic protection for the chondrocyte.[25,70] The formation of this chondrocytic pericellular matrix may be directed by hyaluronan receptors.[72] The territorial region comes next, containing collagen fibrils that follow the pericellular outlines close to the cell, but becoming less organized further away. The territorial region may enclose more than one chondrocyte. Outermost from the chondrocyte, and also the largest region that takes up the spaces between chondrocytes, is the interterritorial region. It is mainly responsible for the mechanical properties of cartilage.[106]

B. Cartilage Collagen

Collagen is a protein of approx 1000 amino acids, with a glycine at every third amino acid. Each collagen molecule is coiled into a left-handed helix, and three alpha helices coil around each other into a right-handed helix called a tropocollagen molecule. Collagen contains hydroxyproline, which stabilizes the triple helix, and hydroxylysine, which allows collagen to bind convalently to carbohydrates.[45] The types of collagen found in articular cartilage can be divided into fibril-forming and non-fibril-forming; types II and XI form fibrils, although types VI, IX, and X do not, but are also found to contribute to the ECM structure. Type II collagen fibrils contribute to the tensile strength of cartilage.[68] Its fibril thickness is affected by the other collagen types and varies through the depth of cartilage. Type II collagen is the most abundant type of collagen in hyaline articular cartilage, accounting for 90–95% of the collagen in the matrix. It is associated with type XI collagen to form a mesh. Type XI collagen may act to control fibril diameter. Type VI collagen is a microfibrillar collagen that forms elastic fibers and is preferentially located in the pericellular region of chondrocytes.[19] Type IX collagen is classified as a fibril-associated collagen with interrupted triple helices, and may function to act as a bridge between collagen fibrils and aggrecan.[125,145] Type X collagen is classified as a network-forming collagen and, although its function is not entirely clear, it is found mineralized in the calcified zone of cartilage. The collagen fibrils are stabilized by cartilage oligomeric matrix protein (COMP), a 100,000-kDa protein that is present in cartilage and tendons,[58] with multiple binding sites.

C. Cartilage Glycosaminoglycans

Glycosaminoglycans (GAG) are long chains of non-branching polysaccharides, consisting of repeating disaccharide units.[48] There is usually a sulfated group (SO_4^{2-}) per disaccharide. Less often, there are non-sulfated or disulfated disaccharides. This high occurrence of sulfated disaccharides and the presence of COO^- ionic groups give an overall negative charge to the GAG, which is crucial in controlling the hydration of cartilage, and ultimately, the mechanical properties of the tissue.

D. P. ATTENBURROW B.V.Sc., FRCVS.

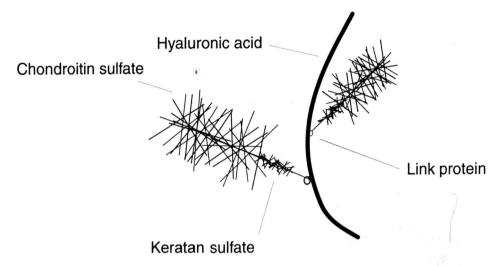

Figure 1. Aggrecan is formed with chondroitin sulfate and keratan sulfate attached to a core protein. This core protein is then stabilized to hyaluronic acid with a link protein.

The two main types of GAG in articular cartilage are keratan sulfate and chondroitin sulfate. Both chondroitin and keratan sulfate contain variations within their own group, such as differences in disaccharide units, sulfation, and amino acid epimerization. Thus, as an example, chondroitin may be divided into chondroitin A, B, and C, each molecule with different properties from each other. Chondroitin sulfate is also larger, at ~20 kDa, while keratan sulfate chains are ~5–15 kDa. The biosynthesis and control of both GAGs are not well-understood. It has been shown that the amount of keratan sulfate in cartilage increases with age.[93,151] The ratio of the two GAGs also varies with the depth of cartilage. Other GAGs present in cartilage include dermatan sulfate—which is chondroitin sulfate with epimerized amino acids—and heparan sulfate.[151]

D. Cartilage Proteoglycans

Proteoglycans are a special class of glycoproteins with long, unbranched, and highly charged GAG chains.[48] The major type of proteoglycan found in cartilage is aggrecan, which provides the compressive strength of cartilage.[68] Other proteoglycans include decorin, biglycan, and fibromodulin.

Aggrecan is formed by a core protein of high mol wt (~250,000), with attached GAG side chains, mostly chondroitin sulfate and keratan sulfate. Each aggrecan contains ~100 chondroitin sulfate chains and up to 60 keratan sulfate chains (Fig. 1). Aggrecan resembles a tube brush, since the GAG chains, with their high concentration of SO_4^{2-} and COO^- groups spaced 1–1.5 nm apart, repel each other. Expressed mostly in cartilaginous tissues, aggrecan aggregates with hyaluronan, an unbranched polysaccharide with mol wt up to several million, and a noncovalently bonded link protein stabilizes this aggregation.

The overall negative charge of aggrecan, called the fixed-change density (FCD), attracts cations from the fluid phase. The Donnan ion distribution law states that there are always more charged particles in the tissue than the bathing solution.[75] As a result, this

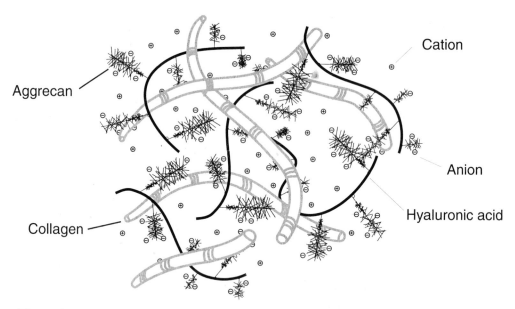

Figure 2. The anions on the proteoglycans of aggrecan attract cations. This causes the ion concentration within the tissue to be greater than that in the surrounding fluid, causing an osmotic pressure difference. Fluid is thus imbibed into cartilage, placing the collagen fibrils in tension.

difference in the concentration of ions creates a positive osmotic pressure, known as Donnan osmotic pressure, which causes the matrix to swell.[28,75,82] This swelling force is balanced by crosslinked collagen fibrils that contain the aggrecan (Fig. 2). The collagen is thus placed in tension,[28,82,83] giving cartilage the tendency to curl up when removed from the subchondral bone.[29] When cartilage is compressed, the interstitial water initially becomes pressurized and supports a significant portion of the load.[129] The water is then forced out of the matrix, and friction between the water and the matrix dissipates the applied force.[7,80] The cartilage equilibrates as the load balances out the osmotic pressure. When the load is removed, fluid is imbibed back into the aggrecan network. Thus, the biomechanical roles of aggrecan in cartilage are to provide the compressive stiffness of cartilage, to provide the Donnan osmotic pressure effect, to determine the premeability of cartilage to water, and to regulate the amount of water in the matrix.[7]

In articular cartilage, decorin and biglycan are synthesized with chondroitin sulfate or dermatan sulfate. Decorin exists mostly in the matrix and binds with fibronectin[115] and TGF-β.[61] It appears to delay collagen fibril formation in vitro.[115,146] Biglycan does not appear to interact with the fibrillar collagens,[30] and it is found around the pericellular matrix.[27] Fibromodulin binds specifically to collagen II, and may play a role in the formation and maintenance of fibrils.[59]

E. Zonal Arrangement of Cartilage

Articular cartilage can be divided into four distinct zones that vary both in material composition and in mechanical properties. Beginning with the articulating surface, cartilage can be separated into the superficial, middle, deep, and calcified zones (Fig. 3).

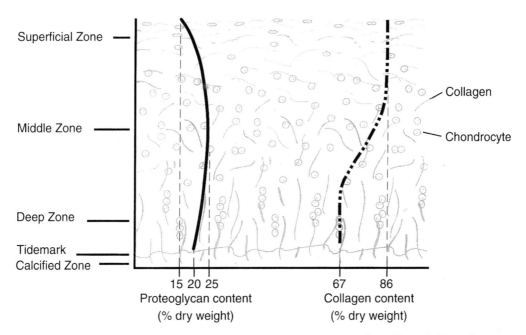

Superficial Zone —

Middle Zone —

Deep Zone —

Tidemark —
Calcified Zone —

Collagen

Chondrocyte

15 20 25
Proteoglycan content
(% dry weight)

67   86
Collagen content
(% dry weight)

Figure 3. The zonal arrangement of cartilage is characterized by flat cells and thin collagen fibrils aligned in the direction of shear in the superficial zone, a more random organization of both cells and thicker collagen fibrils in the middle zone, and cells in the deep zone that are arranged in columns, along thick radial collagen fibrils that extend into the calcified cartilage. From the superficial zone, the proteoglycan content starts off at 15% dry weight (dw) in the superficial zone (SZ), reaches a maximum of 25% dw in the middle zone (MZ), and is at 20% dw in the deep zone (DZ). Collagen content decreases steadily from around 87% in the superficial zone to around 67% in the deep zone. To show the orientation, the chondrocytes and collagen fibers have not been drawn to scale.

The proteoglycan content increases from around 15% dry weight (dw) in the superficial zone to a peak of 25% dw in the middle zone then falls to 20% in the deep zone. The collagen content falls from 86% dw in the superficial zone to 67% dw in the deep zone. The water content also falls linearly with respect to depth, from approx 84% to 40–60%.[81] Because of the compositional and organizational differences of these zones, the mechanical properties of these zones are also different, and efforts to replicate the function of cartilage using tissue-engineering approaches should also replicate the functions of these zones.

Covering the superficial zone is the lamina splendens, an acellular cover of type II collagen aligned in the direction of shear stress that serves as a gliding surface. The lamina splendens also allows the diffusion of small molecules, such as glucose, while retaining the ECM components of cartilage inside. Like the lamina splendens, the superficial zone contains densely packed collagen II fibrils, but it also contains a low density of flattened, elongated cells. Both the cells and collagen fibrils are oriented in the direction of shear stress. The superficial zone, along with the lamina splendens, makes up 10–20% of the full thickness of articular cartilage, and its collagens and proteoglycans are strongly interconnected, possibly to resist tension caused by shearing the cartilage during articulation.[32] Collagen in the superficial zone also plays a role in the fluid permeability of cartilage. It has been shown that permeability increases when the uppermost articualr cartilage surface is removed[140] or when collagen fibrils are removed.[55] The middle zone contains collagen fibers that are randomly oriented, although this randomness can also be seen as a transition from a tangential orientation to a radial orientation of collagen fibers. Because it has the highest proteoglycan content of all other layers, and is the thickest (40–60% of full thickness), the middle zone may contribute the most to compressive strength.[114] Cells in this zone are rounded.[81] In the deep zone, radial collagen fibers extend into the calcified zone to reinforce the bond between cartilage and bone. The deep zone is separated from the calcified zone by a distinct tidemark. The cells in the deep zone are aligned into radial columns and are ellipsoid in shape.[81] The calcified zone is the only cartilage zone that contains collagen X, which is associated with mineralization. The chondrocytes in this layer are believed to be inert, since they are trapped within the calcified matrix.[4] However, successful attempts to create calcified cartilage in vitro have been made using these cells.[67,153]

Although chondrocytes have been categorized as all belonging to the same phenotype, transient metabolic differences between the chondrocytes of different size[141] and zonal affiliation[5,20,21,121,154] have been observed in vitro. The chondrocytes in the superficial zone are flatter than chondrocytes from other zones, have few organelles and resemble fibroblasts,[4] and synthesize a specific proteoglycan of ~345 kDa.[116] This superficial zone protein had been shown to impart lubricating properties.[46] Superficial-zone chondrocytes were found to attach to tissue-culture plastic more slowly than chondrocytes from the deeper zones.[121] Deep-zone cells displayed a higher label for vimentin,[44,52] which has been hypothesized to resist compression of the cell.[104] Keratan sulfate synthesis has been observed to gradually increase through cartilage depth.[5,20,21,121,154] Just as many cells lose their phenotypes in vitro, these zonal differences in cell morphology and metabolic product decreased in time as cells were cultured in monolayers.[121] However, chondrocytes cultured in agarose retained morphological and proteoglycan synthesis differences.[5,20,21]

Aside from orientation, collagen fibers also differ in density and diameter through their depth. The fiber diameter is the finest on the surface, and gradually becomes coarser in the deep zone. This difference indicates a variation in ECM synthesis, since collagen fibril assembly is directed and affected by ECM components such as type XI and IX collagens and decorin. These variations also indicate a difference in mechanical property though the zones. The production rates of type II, IX, and XI mRNA in different zones of epiphyseal cartilage have been found to be different.[24] However, production rates of decorin, biglycan, and fibromodulin—all of which play a role in collagen fibril assembly—by chondrocytes of different zones have not yet been investigated.

III. FUNCTIONAL ASPECTS OF ARTICULAR CARTILAGE

Articular cartilage may experience loads up to 18 MPa in the hip when rising from a chair, as demonstrated by Hodge and associates[62] using an instrumented hip endoprosthesis. The typical cartilage thickness is 0.5–5 mm, so when comparing the amount of shock that can be absorbed by muscles and the energy absorbed by the much thicker bone, the energy cartilage can absorb from impact is comparably infinitesimal. Cartilage therefore serves only to provide a self-renewing, articulating surface that redistributes forces. The ability of cartilage to function is determined by its mechanical properties. The mechanical properties of cartilage are also important because they may modulate the forces transmitted to the chondrocytes, which respond by altering biosynthesis.

A. Mechanical Properties of Articular Cartilage

From a mechanics point of view, cartilage can be modeled as a porous solid phase that contains and interacts with a fluid phase that fills the pores. This biphasic theory models cartilage as consisting of an incompressible, porous-permeable solid and an incompressible viscous fluid.[92] The viscoelastic behavior of cartilage results from a viscoelastic dissipation within the collagen-proteoglycan matrix and a frictional resistance of the interstitial fluid to flow from the permeable solid matrix.[93] Thus, when cartilage is loaded, the force imposed on the cartilage is counterbalanced by the fluid-flow drag of the interstitial fluid with the solid matrix.

Modeling with biphasic theory yields three independent variables from an indentation test, the equilibrium compressive modulus, the Poisson's ratio, and the permeability. Human articular cartilage has thus been shown to have an aggregate modulus that ranges from 0.53 MPa to 1.34 MPa, a Poisson's ratio from 0.00–0.14, and a permeability from 0.90×10^{-15} m^4/Ns to 4.56×10^{-15} m^4/Ns.[8,9,16] The size of the "pores" in the solid matrix has been estimated to range from 30 to 60 Å.[71] Recently, a light-scattering technique has been used to measure the compressive modulus of cartilage by correlating the scattering of collagen.[73]

Cartilage also serves to lower the friction of articular joints, and a mathematical analysis of squeeze film lubrication yields the conclusion that loaded cartilage deforms to enlarge the load-bearing area and to also slow down the movement of the lubricating fluid film.[64] The calculations also show that a tensile hoop stress exists at the cartilage surface as a result of the radial flow of the interstitial fluid in the cartilage layer.[64] A surfactant known as lubricating glycoprotein-I has been shown to adsorb onto the cartilage surface to reduce friction.[135] As cartilage experiences a plowing motion, fluid is exuded at the leading edge of the motion, and imbibed at the trailing end.[80] In a model known as weeping lubrication, the exuded fluid during loading of articular cartilage forms a boundary lubricant that keeps the two articulating surfaces apart.[86] In another model known as boosted lubrication, the ability of cartilage to imbibe fluids because of its porosity is believed to leave concentrated puddles of lubricants at the articulating surfaces during loading.[79]

B. Variations in the Mechanical Properties of Articular Cartilage

Articular cartilage displays various mechanical properties in joints that serve different functions. Recently, the presence and absence of certain steroids and hormones have also been shown to affect the mechanical properties. Because of the different structure and composition of zones of articular cartilage, the mechanical properties of these zones are also different.

1. Variations From Joint to Joint

The mechanical properties of cartilage are a direct result of its function, and thus vary from anatomical location to location. A comparison of the mechanical properties of artic-

Table 1. Comparison of Material Properties of Cartilage from the Ankle, Elbow, Hip, Knee, and First Metatarsophalangeal Joint

Joint	H_A (MPa)	v_s	$k \times 10^{-15}$ (m⁴/Ns)	h (mm)	μ_s (MPa)
Elbow (n = 6, 132 test sites)[123]	0.80 ± 0.25	0.07 ± 0.08	1.29 ± 1.04	1.13 ± 0.31	0.37 ± 0.13
Hip (n = 5, 140 test sites)[8]	1.21 ± 0.61	0.05 ± 0.06	0.90 ± 0.54	1.34 ± 0.38	0.57 ± 0.30
Knee (n = 6, 196 test sites)[16]	0.60 ± 0.15	0.06 ± 0.07	1.45 ± 0.61	2.63 ± 1.04	0.28 ± 0.07
Ankle (n = 7, 196 test sites)[15]	1.11 ± 0.40	0.03 ± 0.05	1.23 ± 1.47	1.18 ± 0.29	0.54 ± 0.21
First metatarsophalangeal (n = 7, 108 test sites)[13]	0.98 ± 0.50	0.07 ± 0.07	2.02 ± 1.47	0.75 ± 0.21	0.45 ± 0.23

H_A = aggregate modulus; v_s = Poisson's ratio; k = permeability; h= thickness; μ_s = shear modulus.

Table 2. Comparison of the Mechanical Properties of Hip Cartilage at the Anterior Acetabulum from Different Animal Models[9]

Species	H_A (MPa)	v_s	$k \times 10^{-15}$ (m⁴/Ns)	h (mm)
Bovine (n = 12)	0.29 ± 0.2	0.25 ± 0.12	3.84 ± 1.49	1.40 ± 0.58
Canine (n = 12)	0.89 ± 0.33	0.31 ± 0.07	4.08 ± 1.02	0.47 ± 0.16
Papio (n = 12)	0.95 ± 0.26	0.26 ± 0.09	4.19 ± 2.11	0.70 ± 0.12
Human (n = 10)	1.24 ± 0.61	0.04 ± 0.04	0.91 ± 0.44	1.24 ± 0.15

H_A = aggregate modulus; v_s = Poisson's ratio; k = permeability; h= thickness; μ_s = shear modulus.

ular cartilage in various joints is provided in Table 1. Each of the joints has different functional requirements and different physiological loads. Even within a joint, high and low weight-bearing regions exist, and the compressive moduli, permeability, Poisson's ratio, and thickness may be different. The tissues from high weight-bearing areas are generally stiffer than low weight-bearing areas, as shown through a series of experiments on the ankle,[15] hip,[8] knee,[16] and first metatarsophalangeal joint.[13] Continuing with the functional development of cartilage, the thickness of articular cartilage may be indicative of the congruence of the joint surfaces. For instance, thicker cartilage may be required to distribute high local stresses in incongruent joints.[16]

Similarly, the same joint in different animals may be loaded differently and thus contain articular cartilage of different mechanical properties, a notable point when selecting animal models. An animal model comparison of hip cartilage is presented in Table 2. Athanasiou and associates[9] have shown that the aggregate moduli of the baboon acetabulum and femoral head are most similar to that of humans, and the bovine model is the least similar.

2. Zonal Variations in Mechanical Properties

The structure-function relationship of cartilage means that material heterogeneity is directly translated into mechanical differences. Variations in collagen fibril diameter, density, and orientation, and variation in the type and amount of GAGs with respect to depth also mean that the mechanical properties of cartilage vary over depth. Early compressive testing has mainly modeled cartilage as a homogenous tissue, but it has been shown recently that the compressive modulus increased from 0.079 ± 0.039 MPa in the superficial zone to 2.10 ± 2.69 MPa in the deepest zone.[114] Recently, a microindentation device also showed zonal differences in mechanical properties.[120]

It has also been shown that the tensile properties of cartilage vary with depth, with superficial zone samples that are cut parallel to the fibrils displaying strengths as high as 25 MPa, and deep-zone samples displaying a much reduced strength of 15 MPa.[68] Narmoneva and associates,[96] by measuring swelling induced strains in the absence of applied loading in articular cartilage, have provided further evidence of differences in the stress-strain state of the deep zone as compared to the middle and superficial zones.

Permeability also differs from zone to zone. The permeability of the middle zone is 35% higher than that of the superficial zone.[91] Considered together, the compressive and tensile moduli and permeability of ECM around chondrocytes vary from zone to zone. Since chondrocytes respond to mechanical signals, these differences may be responsible for the synthetic differences of chondrocytes from zone to zone.

The deformation of chondrocytes in a homogenous cartilage matrix has been modeled on a microscopic scale.[152] Guilak[53] used confocal laser-scanning microscopy (CLSM) to determine chondrocyte deformation in cartilage explants and showed that chondrocytes in the superficial zone deformed anisotropically, unlike those cells from other zones. Buschmann and colleagues[33] studied the effect of static and dynamic mechanical compression on the biosynthetic activity of chondrocytes cultured within agarose gel, and noted that the presence of matrix had a significant effect on the biosynthesis of these chondrocytes. Guilak and colleagues[54] also evaluated chondrocyte deformation using micropipet aspiration, and showed that the Young's moduli of the chondrocyte and its pericellular region is three orders of magnitude smaller than the ECM. The mechanical properties of chondrocytes without a pericellular matrix have also been measured using a cytoindenter[119] and cytodetacher,[18] and these instruments may be used to directly evaluate zonal variations in the mechanical properties of cells.

3. Variations Caused by Hormonal Changes

Recently, the effects of hormones—namely estrogen and methylprednisolone—have been studied in sheep and horses, respectively. In the first study, estrogen production was stopped in sheep by ovariectomy.[142] Ovariectomized sheep developed cartilage with lower aggregate and shear moduli as compared to control (sham) sheep and sheep that underwent estrogen replacement therapy. The compressive modulus of cartilage from sheep lacking estrogen decreased by approx 20%, and the shear modulus also decreased by approx 15%. Estrogen replacement helped to maintain the mechanical integrity of the cartilage (Fig. 4, 5).[142] Athanasiou and colleagues[95] did a comparison of cartilage from horses injected with methylprednisolone acetate (MPA), an anti-inflammatory steroid, or a diluent solution (Fig. 6). Compared to diluent-treated horses, MPA-treated cartilage had a compressive modulus that was 49% lower, was 55% more permeable, had a shear modulus that was 47% lower, and was 20% thinner than diluent-treated horses.[95] These results could have significant implications in ovariectomized women who undergo such procedures because of cervical or ovarian cancer. Similarly, anti-inflammatory steriod drugs prescribed to athletes may compromise the mechanical property of their joints.

4. Variations Due to Diabetes

It has been shown that patients with diabetes mellitus have an increased number of musculoskeletal injuries and experience more morbidity from treatment and injury than

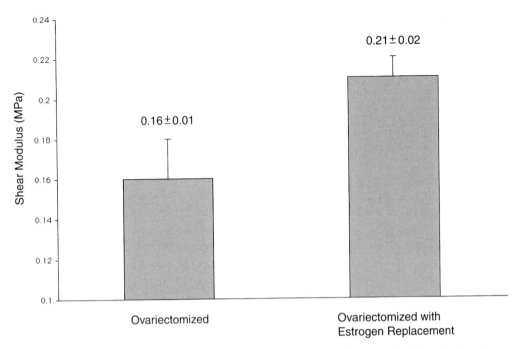

Figure 4. The shear modulus of cartilage in ovariectomized sheep is significantly less than that of ovariectomized sheep that have undergone estrogen replacement. Mean ± S.D.; $p = 0.05$.[142]

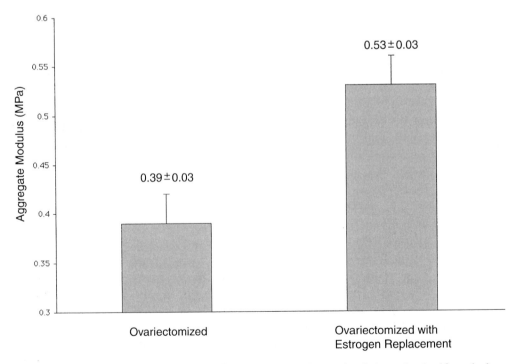

Figure 5. The aggregate modulus of cartilage in ovariectomized sheep is significantly less than that of ovariectomized sheep that have undergone estrogen replacement. Mean ± S.D.; $p = 0.01$.[142]

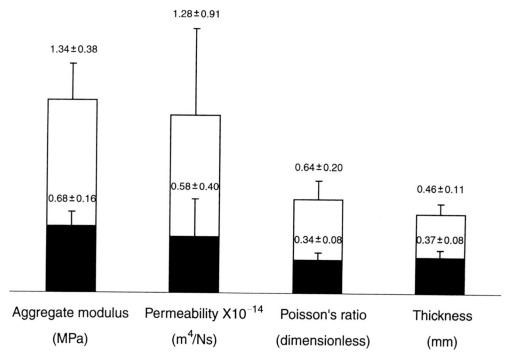

Figure 6. The cartilage from the middle carpal articular joint from steroid-treated horses (filled boxes) contained intrinsic material properties that are less than half of control horses (unfilled boxes). Mean ± S.D.; $p = 0.0001$.[95]

those without diabetes.[6,65,90] This may be the result of an accelerated degeneration of articular cartilage in these patients, and it has been shown that ankle cartilage from these patients has a lower stiffness and is more permeable than normal tissue (Fig. 7).[11] Although the decrease in aggregate modulus seems to support the idea that the cartilage proteoglycan content of diabetic patients is somehow changed, further studies must be done to correlate the biomechanical properties and the biochemical composition of cartilage from diabetic patients, and this may yield insight into the mechanisms of how diabetes may cause cartilage deterioration.

IV. ARTICULAR CARTILAGE AND INJURY

A. Types of Injuries and Natural Response

The response of articular cartilage to injury depends on the type of injury.[66] Articular cartilage injury may be imperceptible, such as a loss of the proteoglycans and the other matrix components that give strength to the tissue and allow it to function. In this case, the cells recognize this injury and upregulate the production of ECM. As long as the matrix that is lost or disrupted is less than or equal to that which the chondrocytes can synthesize, the tissue can recover. Otherwise, the chondrocytes will be exposed to excessive loading without the protection of the matrix, and the tissue eventually degenerates.[66] Chondral flaps, tears, and fissures are chondral injuries that result from focal mechanical disruptions. Shortly after this form of injury, chondrocytes proliferate and begin to synthesize

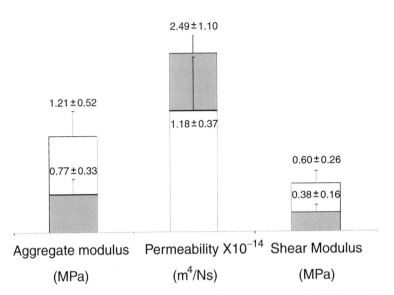

Figure 7. The mechanical properties of cartilage from patients with diabetes (filled boxes) and of normal tissue (empty boxes). Note that the permeability of cartilage from patients with diabetes is greater than that of normal tissue, possibly caused by disruption of the proteoglycan content. Mean ± S.D.; $p = 0.01$ for aggregate modulus; $p = 0.0002$ for permeability; $p = 0.009$ for shear modulus.[47]

more matrix. However, this burst of activity ceases after a few days, before the defect has been repaired, which results in the observation that chondral injuries are generally permanent. Further degeneration of the tissue may spread from the injury site.[66] Osteochondral injuries penetrate down to the subchondral bone. In chondral injuries, the chondrocytes are mainly responsible for proliferating and remodeling, but stem cells from the bone marrow can migrate to the defect site in an osteochondral injury to fill the site with fibrocartilage. However, fibrocartilage lacks the mechanical resilience of articular cartilage, and the repair tissue is bound to break down with usage.[31]

B. Clinical Approaches

Since partial thickness defects fail to heal because of inadequate chondrocyte response, various clinical approaches have been employed to provide more metabolically active cells to the articular surface. Efforts include cleaning and deepening the defect to perforate the subchondral bone, resurfacing the articular surface, transplants, and tissue engineering. Deepening a chondral defect allows bone-marrow stem cells to populate the defect, but this often leads to the formation of fibrous cartilage, which is mechanically ill-suited for articulation.[87,143] Resurfacing the articular surface has been attempted with various methodologies, but evaluation of these techniques does not usually include biomechanical analyses.[23,51,88] Transplantation includes perichondrial transplants, which are rich in osteochondral progenitor cells,[99] osteochondral plugs, and autologous chondrocyte transplantation,[36,89,104] These techniques have had variable levels of success, but limited donor site, lack of integration, fibrocartilage formation around or above the transplant, and the realization that the function is not immediately restored are problems with transplants. Because of the lack of long-term functional stability of current surgical approaches, much of the current effort in treating chondral/osteochondral defects has been directed toward tissue engineering.

C. Tissue Engineering of Articular Cartilage

The goal of fabricating a mechanically functional tissue engineered articular cartilage has been approached by manipulating four main variables, the cell type, the scaffold, chemical factors (growth factors), and mechanical forces.

1. Cell Type

The most obvious choice for a cell type to implant into an articular defect would be differentiated articular chondrocytes, since they already produce cartilage ECM. Because subpopulations of chondrocytes have different morphology and synthetic activities[20,21] it may be important to retain the zonal distribution of cells when harvesting. For instance, chondrocytes from the deep zone have been employed to regenerate cartilage with mineralized and non-mineralized zones.[153] Subpopulations of chondrocytes may also require different forces to induce them into forming a functional tissue, since proliferation and GAG synthesis rates of superficial and deep zone cells have been shown to differ under the same mechanical loading regimens.[77] However, an observed decrease in cellularity with age from the superficial zone[131] may make this difficult. Mesenchymal stem cells (MSC) from bone marrow,[3,107,148] muscle,[60] and the periosteum,[100,105] which may be present in repair cartilage in full-thickness defects, have also been attempted with some success. MSCs decrease in number with age, and their pluripotent nature may result in differentiation into cell types other than the desired chondrogenic lineage. Doherty and associates[43] have shown that an adenoviral vector successfully infected chondrocytes both before and after transplantation into cartilage, thus opening the door for the possibility of gene therapy in articular cartilage engineering.

2. Scaffold

The most widely studied natural polymer for articular cartilage engineering is collagen. Chondrocytes proliferate on collagen gels,[117] and it has been shown that chondrocytes maintain their phenotype longer on collagen type II than type I.[97,98] In full-thickness defects, the formation of a tidemark was absent in the use of type I collagen,[149] showing lack of integration, but indentation tests showed that the reformed cartilage had mechanical properties similar to native cartilage. On the other hand, when the subchondral bone is reformed by seeding MSCs, also in collagen I, regenerated cartilage is softer and still does not integrate with the native cartilage.[35] Lack of integration eventually led to degeneration. Other natural scaffolds include agarose, which has the advantage of maintaining the chondrogenic phenotype for 8 mo,[57] or allowing dedifferentiated chondrocytes to re-express their phenotype.[26] Other natural materials include fibrin glue,[122,138,144] hyaluronic acid,[128] and chitosan.[84]

Poly(DL-lactic acid) (PLA) and poly(glycolic acid) (PGA) are polymers whose biocompatibility has been studied extensively,[49,124] and are FDA approved. PLA is less crystalline and more stable than PGA, and has long been used as an orthopedic material. However, efforts to generate cartilage with PLA, have been unsuccessful because of the lower synthesis of sulfated GAGs than on PGA,[50] and presence of type I collagen when cultured with perichondral cells.[40,41] The copolymer of PLA and PGA, poly(DL-lactic-co-glycolic acid) (PLGA) is a polymer whose mechanical properties, biocompatibility, and sterilization and storage techniques has been studied extensively.[1,2,10,12,14] The degradation and release rate of bioactive agents from PLGA have also been studied both without and with dynamic loading.[17,137] Although the degradation products of PLGA are acidic, a technique has been developed to control the pH in and around it.[1] In addition, Spain and associates[130] have devised a copolymer prepared in a blend of three copolymers of 50:50 PLGA that has been shown to result in a slow degradation rate of up to 6 wk.

Other synthetic polymers include polyethylene and propylene oxide (P[EO-co-PO]), which is injectable, but studies thus far have not employed articular chondrocytes,[34] and poly(propylene fumarate) (PPF), which is currently being studied in conjunction with linked peptide sequences.[132–134]

3. Growth Factors

Depending on the cell type selected, various growth factors have been tested to evaluate their role in regulating cell growth and matrix production. One of the most commonly used growth factors is TGF-β. TGF-β has been shown to promote proliferation of immature cells and to promote the differentiation of committed cells, but conflicting views exist on its effects on chondrocytes. TGF-β has been observed to decrease PG production and switch the expression of collagen from type II to type I, both signs of chondrocyte de-differentiation.[111] However, it has also been shown that TGF-β stimulates the production of both collagen and GAG.[109,110] This elevation of ECM production has been employed in a goat model, where osteochondral defects were filled with 50:50 PLG with 180 ng and 1800 ng of TGF-β. Repair cartilage formed on the implant with 1800 ng of TGF-β showed statistically higher aggregate and shear moduli than cartilage formed in empty defects, defects filled with PLG only, and defects filled with PLG and 180 ng of TGF-β.[12] However, TGF-β also promotes the growth of fibroblasts, thus creating type I collagen in hyaline cartilage.[139] Bone morphogenetic proteins, which belong to the TGF-β superfamily, have been observed to maintain the articular cartilage phenotype,[113] and thus have been used in full-thickness defects to show accelerated formation of subchondral bone and improved histological appearance of the articular cartilage formed.[118] Insulin-like growth factors (ILGFs), which are believed to be necessary in leading osteoarthritic chondrocytes to produce matrix,[42] are another class of growth factors that may be used in tissue engineering of articular cartilage. The effect of platelet-derived growth factor (PDGF) has also been investigated in collagen gels, and although chondrocyte proliferation rate increased, the amount of proteoglycans synthesized on a per-cell basis decreased with PDGF stimulation.[150] When selecting a growth factor, it is important to note the effects of the chosen growth factor not only on the target cells of interest, but also on surrounding cells.

4. Mechanical Forces

Considering that cartilage is a highly mechanical tissue, and considering that cartilage development is subject to mechanical stimuli, mechanical forces contribute to maintain phenotype, up-regulate biosynthesis, and organize the ECM into a mechanically functional form. The usual forces experienced include shear, direct and hydrostatic compression, and tension.

Hydrostatic pressure on chondrocytes is one of the most heavily investigated types of forces, and has been employed in bioreactors to cultivate tissue-engineered constructs.

Hydrostatic pressure has been shown to alter the organization of the cytoskeleton,[102] to induce the expression of interleukin[5] and tumor necrosis factor (TNF) α mRNAs in a chondrocyte-like cell line,[136] and to alter the Golgi apparatus.[103] Regulation of proteoglycan synthesis using cyclic hydrostatic pressure[101] and upregulation of matrix synthesis by static hydrostatic pressure[56,78] have also been demonstrated. Smith and associates[127] have shown that an intermittent loading regimen of 4 h per d for 4 d showed a ninefold increase for type II collagen mRNA levels and a 20-fold increase for aggrecan mRNA levels. A semi-perfusion system has been designed to deliver intermittent physiological pressure in tissue-engineering cartilage.[36-38] In this case, chondrocytes were seeded on PGA and cultured for 5 wk under a hydrostatic pressure of 3.4 MPa and fed semi-continuously. The pressurized constructs were twice as high in proteoglycan content as the control, and also demonstrated a correlation in the compressive modulus with respect to proteoglycan content.[36-38]

Shear has been investigated by Vunjak-Novakovic and colleagues[147] to demonstrate that cells cultured in turbulent flow formed a tough capsule on the outside of the construct, although those that were cultured in laminar conditions (in a rotating bioreactor) displayed significantly higher matrix synthesis and better mechanical properties than constructs cultured in static conditions. However, shear has also been shown to increase GAG chain length and to increase the production of prostaglandin E_2, which are related to inflammatory degeneration of cartilage in osteoarthritis.[126]

Compression has been shown to affect chondrocyte biosynthesis in both cartilage explants,[22,69,112] and in scaffolds.[33,85] It has been found that the matrix around the cell affects biosynthesis during compression, and that dynamic compression stimulates biosynthesis, yet graded levels of compression resulted in decreases in biosynthesis.[33] Amplitudes around 10% and a frequency of 1 Hz have been found to be optimal for chondrocyte biosynthesis.[33,69,76,85,112] Recently, Lee and colleagues[77] have shown that subpopulations of chondrocytes from various zones of cartilage respond to compression with different proliferation rates and biosyntheses.

D. Current Challenges

Challenges in the tissue engineering of articular cartilage involve optimizing the parameters of tissue engineering. This includes finding the proper cell type(s), the selection of a scaffold that is both chemically and mechanically fitting, the selection and application of various growth factors, and the determination of how mechanical forces may be applied to optimize biosynthesis. All these variables must work together to produce a tissue that will be functionally stable. Histological processing often dissolves synthetic polymers, leaving the degradation rates and degraded structure of the polymer in question when evaluating tissue-engineered products. Thus, methods must be developed to visualize both the tissue components and the carrier scaffold. Currently, integration of the tissue-engineered tissue with the surrounding native tissue is poor, and boundaries may be easily discerned with staining alone. Eventually, the assessment of integration would require finer observations down to the level of collagen diameters and organization, and although electron microscopy has been widely applied to assess tissue-engineered constructs, its application to the implant/native tissue interface has not been widely used. A possibility for enhancing integration may be to implant incompletely formed tissues into defects. In this case, histological methods must be developed to distinguish between the implanted cells, with their newly synthe-sized ECM, from the cells of the native tissue. Finally, histology may serve to observe the zonal variations in the tissue-engineered construct to ensure the replication of the structure-function relationship.

V. CONCLUSION

The zonal arrangement of articular cartilage is indicative of different functional capa-bilities in these zones. The superficial zone, which is strong in tension because of the col-lagen fibers, resists the shear applied to cartilage during articulation. High amounts of proteoglycan in the middle and deep zones impart compressive strength to the tissue, which suggests that these zones bear and redistribute the majority of the applied load with their viscoelastic behavior. Finally, the deep zone contains collagen fibers that are contin-uous through the tidemark to mechanically integrate the cartilage with the subchondral bone. The fact that the structure-function relationships of these zones are distinctly unique and different from each other suggests that to tissue-engineer articular cartilage, it may be necessary to replicate the zonal arrangement of articular cartilage. If the tissue-engineered construct exhibits sufficient compressive strength, imparted by the middle and deep zones, but its superficial zone lacks the collagen fibers to resist tension, shear on the artic-ulating surface during physiological usage may soon damage the implanted tissue and thus result in destruction of the implant. Replication of zonal functions may be attempted by manipulating any of the tissue-engineering principles. For instance, culturing the superficial, middle, and deep zone cells separately may allow one to find different chemi-cal and mechanical stimuli that optimize cellular biosynthesis for each subpopulation of chondrocytes. To understand the mechanisms behind this process, the application of mechanical forces must be quantifiable at the cellular level to accurately model how mechanotransduction affects biosynthesis. This determination of the type of mechanical forces required may then be applied through the design of bioreactors that can deliver dif-ferent forces to various cell populations.

With a construct that performs well mechanically, one may also wish to integrate it into native cartilage, in order to have a continuity of mechanical properties that will prevent the formation of stress concentrations that can damage both the implanted and native tis-sues. Histological assessment techniques are central in our efforts to understand articular cartilage in terms of its state of health or disease, its healing potential, or the outcome of tissue-engineering approaches to enhance regeneration. Histology, in conjunction with gross morphology, remains the first convincing tool of tissue evaluation. It should cer-tainly be an integral part of our armamentarium for the cogent assessment of cartilage, which also includes gross morphology and quantitative tests such as biomechanical and biochemical evaluations. Our next challenge in this regard should be the establishment of correlations—assuming that they exist—between histology and quantitative tests.

REFERENCES

1. Agrawal CM, Athanasiou KA: Technique to control pH in vicinity of biodegrading PLA-PGA implants. *J Biomed Mater Res* 38:105–114, 1997.
2. Agrawal CM, Athanasiou KA, Heckman JD: Biodegradable PLA-PGA polymers for tissue engineering in orthopaedics. *Mater Sci Forum* 250:115–128, 1997.

3. Angele P, Kujat R, Nerlich M, Yoo J, et al: Engineering of osteochondral tissue with bone marrow mesenchymal progenitor cells in a derivatized hyaluronan-gelatin composite sponge. *Tissue Eng* 5:545–554, 1999.

4. Annefeld M: The chondrocyte—the living element of articular cartilage. In: *Articular Cartilage and Osteoarthrosis.* Hans Huber Publishers, Bern, Switzerland, 1983:30–41.

5. Archer CW, McDowell J, Bayliss MT, et al: Phenotypic modulation in sub-populations of human articular chondrocytes in vitro. *J Cell Sci* 97:361–371, 1990.

6. Arkkila PE, Kantola IM, Viikari JS: Limited joint mobility in type 1 diabetic patients: correlation to other diabetic complications. *J Intern Med* 236:215–223, 1994.

7. Ateshian GA, Warden WH, Kim JJ, et al: Finite deformation biphasic material properties of bovine articular cartilage from confined compression experiments. *J Biomech* 30:1157–1164, 1997.

8. Athanasiou KA, Agarwal A, Dzida FJ: Comparative study of the intrinsic mechanical properties of the human acetabular and femoral head cartilage. *J Orthop Res* 12:340–349, 1994.

9. Athanasiou KA, Agarwal A, Muffoletto A, et al: Biomechanical properties of hip cartilage in experimental animal models [published erratum appears in *Clin Orthop* 320:283,1995]. *Clin Orthop* 316:254–266, 1995.

10. Athanasiou KA, Agrawal CM, Barber FA, et al: Orthopaedic applications for PLA-PGA biodegradable polymers. *Arthroscopy* 14:726–737, 1998.

11. Athanasiou KA, Fleischli JG, Bosma J, et al: Effects of diabetes mellitus on the biomechanical properties of human ankle cartilage. *Clin Orthop* 368:182–189, 1999.

12. Athanasiou KA, Korvick D, Schenck RC: Biodegradable implants for the treatment of osteochondral defects in a goat model. *Tissue Eng* 3:363–373, 1997.

13. Athanasiou KA, Liu GT, Lavery LA, et al: Biomechanical topography of human articular cartilage in the first metatarsophalangeal joint. *Clin Orthop* 348:269–281, 1998.

14. Athanasiou KA, Niederauer GG, Agrawal CM: Sterilization, toxicity, biocompatibility and clinical applications of polylactic acid/polyglycolic acid copolymers. *Biomaterials* 17:93–102, 1996.

15. Athanasiou KA, Niederauer GG, Schenck Jr., RC: Biomechanical topography of human ankle cartilage. *Ann Biomed Eng* 23:697–704, 1995.

16. Athanasiou KA, Rosenwasser MP, Buckwalter JA, et al: Interspecies comparisons of in situ intrinsic mechanical properties of distal femoral cartilage. *J Orthop Res* 9:330–340, 1991.

17. Athanasiou KA, Singhal AR, Agrawal CM, et al: In vitro degradation and release characteristics of biodegradable implants containing trypsin inhibitor. *Clin Orthop* 315:272–281, 1995.

18. Athanasiou KA, Thoma BS, Lanctot DR, et al: Development of the cytodetachment technique to quantify mechanical adhesiveness of the single cell. *Biomaterials* 20:2405–2415, 1999.

19. Ayad S, Evans H, Weiss JB, et al: Type VI collagen but not type V collagen is present in cartilage [letter]. *Coll Relat Res* 4:165–168, 1984.

20. Aydelotte MB, Greenhill RR, Kuettner KE: Differences between sub-populations of cultured bovine articular chondrocytes. II. Proteoglycan metabolism. *Connect Tissue Res* 18:223–234, 1988.

21. Aydelotte MB, Kuettner KE: Differences between sub-populations of cultured bovine articular chondrocytes. I. Morphology and cartilage matrix production. *Connect Tissue Res* 18:205–222, 1988.

22. Bachrach NM, Valhmu WB, Stazzone E, et al: Changes in proteoglycan synthesis of chondrocytes in articular cartilage are associated with the time-dependent changes in their mechanical environment. *J Biomech* 28:1561–1569, 1995.

23. Bakay A, Csonge L, Papp G, et al: Osteochondral resurfacing of the knee joint with allograft. Clinical analysis of 33 cases. *Int Orthop* 22:277–281, 1998.

24. Balmain N, Leguellec D, Elkak A, et al: Zonal variations of types II, IX and XI collagen mRNAs in rat epiphyseal cartilage chondrocytes: quantitative evaluation of in situ hybridization by image analysis of radioautography. *Cell Mol Biol (Noisy-le-grand)* 41:197–212, 1995.

25. Benninghoff A: Form und Bau der Gelenkknorpel in ihren beziechungen zur funktion. I. Die modellierenden und formerhalterden Faktoren des Knorpelreliefs. *Z ges Anant* 76:43–63, 1925.

26. Benya PD, Shaffer JD: Dedifferentiated chondrocytes reexpress the differentiated collagen phenotype when cultured in agarose gels. *Cell* 30:215–224, 1982.

27. Bianco P, Fisher LW, Young MF, et al: Expression and localization of the two small proteoglycans biglycan and decorin in developing human skeletal and non-skeletal tissues. *J Histochem Cytochem* 38:1549–1563, 1990.

28. Broom ND: New experimental approaches to the understanding of structure-function relationships in articular cartilage. In: Maroudas A, Kuettner K, eds: *Methods in Cartilage Research.* Academic Press, San Diego, CA, 1990:70–73.

29. Broom ND, Poole CA: A functional-morphological study of the tidemark region of articular cartilage maintained in a non-viable physiological condition. *J Anat* 135:65–82, 1982.

30. Brown DC, Vogel KG: Characteristics of the in vitro interaction of a small proteoglycan (PG II) of bovine tendon with type I collagen. *Matrix* 9:468–478, 1989.

31. Buckwalter JA: Articular cartilage: injuries and potential for healing. *J Orthop Sports Phys Ther* 28:192–202, 1998.

32. Buckwalter JA, Hunziker EB, Rosenberg LC, et al: Articular cartilage: composition and structure. In: Woo SL, Buckwalter JA, eds: *Injury and Repair of the Musculoskeletal Soft Tissues, 2nd ed.* American Academy of Orthopaedic Surgeons, Park Ridge, IL, 1991:405–425.

33. Buschmann MD, Gluzband YA, Grodzinsky AJ, et al: Mechanical compression modulates matrix biosynthesis in chondrocyte/agarose culture. *J Cell Sci* 108:1497–1508, 1995.

34. Cao Y, Rodriguez A, Vacanti M, et al: Comparative study of the use of poly(glycolic acid), calcium alginate and pluronics in the engineering of autologous porcine cartilage. *J Biomater Sci Polym Ed* 9:475–487, 1998.

35. Caplan AI, Elyaderani M, Mochizuki Y, et al: Principles of cartilage repair and regeneration. *Clin Orthop* 342:254–269, 1997.

36. Carver SE, Heath CA: Increasing extracellular matrix production in regenerating cartilage with intermittent physiological pressure. *Biotechnol Bioeng* 62:166–174, 1999.

37. Carver SE, Heath CA: Influence of intermittent pressure, fluid flow, and mixing on the regenerative properties of articular chondrocytes. *Biotechnol Bioeng* 65:274–281, 1999.

38. Carver SE, Heath CA: Semi-continuous perfusion system for delivering intermittent physiological pressure to regenerating cartilage. *Tissue Eng* 5:1–11, 1999.

39. Chen FS, Frenkel SR, Di Cesare PE: Chondrocyte transplantation and experimental treatment options for articular cartilage defects. *Am J Orthop* 26:396–406, 1997.

40. Chu CR, Coutts RD, Yoshioka M, et al: Articular cartilage repair using allogeneic perichondrocyte-seeded biodegradable porous polylactic acid (PLA): a tissue-engineering study. *J Biomed Mater Res* 29:1147–1154, 1995.

41. Chu CR, Monosov AZ, Amiel D: In situ assessment of cell viability within biodegradable polylactic acid polymer matrices. *Biomaterials* 16:1381–1384, 1995.

42. Coutts RD, Sah RL, Amiel D: Effects of growth factors on cartilage repair. *Instr Course Lect* 46:487–494, 1997.

43. Doherty PJ, Zhang H, Tremblay L, et al: Resurfacing of articular cartilage explants with genetically-modified human chondrocytes in vitro. *Osteoarthritis Cartilage* 6:153–159, 1998.

44. Durrant LA, Archer CW, Benjamin M, et al: Organisation of the chondrocyte cytoskeleton and its response to changing mechanical conditions in organ culture. *J Anat* 194:343–353, 1999.

45. Eyre DR: Collagen: molecular diversity in the body's protein scaffold. *Science* 207:1315–1322, 1980.

46. Flannery CR, Hughes CE, Schumacher BL, et al: Articular cartilage superficial zone protein (SZP) is homologous to megakaryocyte stimulating factor precursor and is a multifunctional

proteoglycan with potential growth-promoting, cytoprotective, and lubricating properties in cartilage metabolism. *Biochem Biophys Res Commun* 254:535–541, 1999.

47. Fleischli JG, Laughlin TJ, Lavery LA, et al: The effects of diabetes mellitus on the material properties of human metatarsal bones. *J Foot Ankle Surg* 37:195–198, 1998.
48. Fosang AJ, Hardingham TE: Matrix proteoglycans. In: Comper WD, ed: *Extracellular Matrix.* Harwood Academic Publishers, Amsterdam, The Netherlands, 1996:200–229.
49. Freed LE, Grande DA, Lingbin Z, et al: Joint resurfacing using allograft chondrocytes and synthetic biodegradable polymer scaffolds. *J Biomed Mater Res* 28:891–899, 1994.
50. Freed LE, Marquis JC, Nohria A, et al: Neocartilage formation in vitro and in vivo using cells cultured on synthetic biodegradable polymers. *J Biomed Mater Res* 27:11–23, 1993.
51. Furukawa T, Eyre DR, Koide S, et al: Biochemical studies on repair cartilage resurfacing experimental defects in the rabbit knee. *J Bone Joint Surg [Am]* 62:679–689, 1980.
52. Ghadially FN: *Fine Structure of Synovial Joints: A Text and Atlas of the Ultrastructure of Normal and Pathological Articular Tissues.* Butterworths, London, 1983: 55.
53. Guilak F: Compression-induced changes in the shape and volume of the chondrocyte nucleus. *J Biomech* 28:1529–1541, 1995.
54. Guilak F, Jones WR, Ting-Beall HP, et al: The deformation behavior and mechanical properties of chondrocytes in articular cartilage. *Osteoarthritis Cartilage* 7:59–70, 1999.
55. Guilak F, Ratcliffe A, Lane N, et al: Mechanical and biochemical changes in the superficial zone of articular cartilage in canine experimental osteoarthritis. *J Orthop Res* 12:474–484, 1994.
56. Hall AC, Urban JP, Gehl KA: The effects of hydrostatic pressure on matrix synthesis in articular cartilage. *J Orthop Res* 9:1–10, 1991.
57. Hauselmann HJ, Fernandes RJ, Mok SS, et al: Phenotypic stability of bovine articular chondrocytes after long-term culture in alginate beads. *J Cell Sci* 107:17–27, 1994.
58. Hedbom E, Antonsson P, Hjerpe A, et al: Cartilage matrix proteins. An acidic oligomeric protein (COMP) detected only in cartilage. *J Biol Chem* 267:6132–6136, 1992.
59. Hedlund H, Mengarelli-Widholm S, Heinegard D, et al: Fibromodulin distribution and association with collagen. *Matrix Biol* 14:227–232, 1994.
60. Hendrickson DA, Nixon AJ, Grande DA, et al: Chondrocyte-fibrin matrix transplants for resurfacing extensive articular cartilage defects. *J Orthop Res* 12:485–497, 1994.
61. Hildebrand A, Romaris M, Rasmussen LM, et al: Interaction of the small interstitial proteoglycans biglycan, decorin and fibromodulin with transforming growth factor beta. *Biochem J* 302:527–534, 1994.
62. Hodge WA, Carlson KL, Fijan RS, et al: Contact pressures from an instrumented hip endoprosthesis. *J Bone Joint Surg [Am]* 71:1378–1386, 1989.
63. Honner R, Thompson RC: The nutritional pathways of articular cartilage. An autoradiographic study in rabbits using ^{35}S injected intravenously. *J Bone Joint Surg [Am]* 53:742–748, 1971.
64. Hou JS, Mow VC, Lai WM, et al: An analysis of the squeeze-film lubrication mechanism for articular cartilage. *J Biomech* 25:247–259, 1992.
65. Hough FS: Alterations of bone and mineral metabolism in diabetes mellitus. Part I. An overview. *S Afr Med J* 72:116–119, 1987.
66. Hunziker EB: Articular cartilage repair: are the intrinsic biological constraints undermining this process insuperable? *Osteoarthritis Cartilage* 7:15–28, 1999.
67. Kandel RA, Boyle J, Gibson G: In vitro formation of mineralized cartilagenous tissue by articular chondrocytes. *In Vitro Cell Dev Biol Anim* 33:174–181, 1997.
68. Kempson GE, Tuke MA, Dingle JT, et al: The effects of proteolytic enzymes on the mechanical properties of adult human articular cartilage. *Biochim Biophys Acta* 428:741–760, 1976.
69. Kim YJ, Sah RL, Grodzinsky AJ, et al: Mechanical regulation of cartilage biosynthetic behavior: physical stimuli. *Arch Biochem Biophys* 311:1–12, 1994.

70. Knight MM, Lee DA, Bader DL: The influence of elaborated pericellular matrix on the deformation of isolated articular chondrocytes cultured in agarose. *Biochim Biophys Acta* 1405:67–77, 1998.

71. Knudson CB: Hyaluronan receptor-directed assembly of chondrocyte pericellular matrix. *J Cell Biol* 120:825–834, 1993.

72. Knudson W, Knudson CB: Assembly of a chondrocyte-like pericellular matrix on non-chondrogenic cells. Role of the cell surface hyaluronan receptors in the assembly of a pericellular matrix. *J Cell Sci* 99:227–235, 1991.

73. Kovach IS, Athanasiou KA: Small-angle HeNe laser light scatter and the compressive modulus of articular cartilage. *J Orthop Res* 15:437–441, 1997.

74. Krause WJ, Cutts JH: Special connective tissue: cartilage, bone, and joints. In: Schnittman ER, Mastrodomenico A, eds: *Essentials of Histology: Text/Atlas/Review, 1st ed.* Little, Brown and Company, Boston, MA, 1994:105–140.

75. Lai WM, Mow VC, Zhu W: Constitutive modeling of articular cartilage and biomacromolecular solutions. *J Biomech Eng* 115:474–480, 1993.

76. Lee DA, Bader DL: Compressive strains at physiological frequencies influence the metabolism of chondrocytes seeded in agarose. *J Orthop Res* 15:181–188, 1997.

77. Lee DA, Noguchi T, Knight MM, et al: Response of chondrocyte subpopulations cultured within unloaded and loaded agarose. *J Orthop Res* 16:726–733, 1998.

78. Lippiello L, Kaye C, Neumata T, et al: In vitro metabolic response of articular cartilage segments to low levels of hydrostatic pressure. *Connect Tissue Res* 13:99–107, 1985.

79. Longfield MD, Dowson D, Walker PS, et al: "Boosted lubrication" of human joints by fluid enrichment and entrapment. *Biomed Eng* 4:517–522, 1969.

80. Mansour JM, Mow VC: The permeability of articular cartilage under compressive strain and at high pressures. *J Bone Joint Surg [Am]* 58:509–516, 1976.

81. Maroudas A: Physicochemical properties of articular cartilage. In: Freeman MAR, ed: *Adult Articular Cartilage, 2nd ed.* Pitman Medical, Kent, UK, 1979:215–290.

82. Maroudas A, Grushko G: Measurement of swelling pressure of cartilage. In: Maroudas A, Kuettner K, eds: *Methods in Cartilage Research.* Academic Press, New York, NY, 1990:298–301.

83. Maroudas AI: Balance between swelling pressure and collagen tension in normal and degenerate cartilage. *Nature* 260:808–809, 1976.

84. Mattioli-Belmonte M, Gigante A, Muzzarelli RA, et al: N,N-dicarboxymethyl chitosan as delivery agent for bone morphogenetic protein in the repair of articular cartilage. *Med Biol Eng Comput* 37:130–134, 1999.

85. Mauck RL, Soltz MA, Wang CC, et al: Functional tissue engineering of articular cartilage through dynamic loading of chondrocyte-seeded agarose gels. *J Biomech Eng* 122:252–260, 2000.

86. McCutchen CW: Joint lubrication. *Bull Hosp Joint Dis Orthop Inst* 43:118–129, 1983.

87. Menche DS, Frenkel SR, Blair B, et al: A comparison of abrasion burr arthroplasty and subchondral drilling in the treatment of full-thickness cartilage lesions in the rabbit. *Arthroscopy* 12:280–286, 1996.

88. Meyers MH, Akeson W, Convery FR: Resurfacing of the knee with fresh osteochondral allograft. *J Bone Joint Surg [Am]* 71:704–713, 1989.

89. Minas T, Peterson L: Advanced techniques in autologous chondrocyte transplantation. *Clin Sports Med* 18:13–44, 1999.

90. Moeckel B, Huo MH, Salvati EA, et al: Total hip arthroplasty in patients with diabetes mellitus. *J Arthroplasty* 8:279–284, 1993.

91. Mow VC, Holmes MH, Lai WM: Fluid transport and mechanical properties of articular cartilage: a review. *J Biomech* 17:377–394, 1984.

92. Mow VC, Kuei SC, Lai WM, et al: Biphasic creep and stress relaxation of articular cartilage in compression? Theory and experiments. *J Biomech Eng* 102:73–84, 1980.

93. Mow VC, Ratcliffe A, Poole AR: Cartilage and diarthrodial joints as paradigms for hierarchical materials and structures. *Biomaterials* 13:67–97, 1992.

94. Muir IHM: Biochemistry. In: Freeman MAR, ed: *Adult Articular Cartilage, 2nd ed.* Pitman Medical, Kent, UK, 1979: 145–214.

95. Murray RC, DeBowes RM, Gaughan EM, et al: The effects of intra-articular methylprednisolone and exercise on the mechanical properties of articular cartilage in the horse. *Osteoarthritis Cartilage* 6:106–114, 1998.

96. Narmoneva DA, Wang JY, Setton LA: Nonuniform swelling-induced residual strains in articular cartilage. *J Biomech* 32:401–408, 1999.

97. Nehrer S, Breinan HA, Ramappa A, et al: Chondrocyte-seeded collagen matrices implanted in a chondral defect in a canine model. *Biomaterials* 19:2313–2328, 1998.

98. Nehrer S, Breinan HA, Ramappa A, et al: Canine chondrocytes seeded in type I and type II collagen implants investigated in vitro [published erratum appears in *J Biomed Mater Res* 38:288, 1997]. *J Biomed Mater Res* 38:95–104, 1997.

99. O'Driscoll SW: Articular cartilage regeneration using periosteum. *Clin Orthop* 367:S186–S203, 1999.

100. O'Driscoll SW, Salter RB: The repair of major osteochondral defects in joint surfaces by neochondrogenesis with autogenous osteoperiosteal grafts stimulated by continuous passive motion. An experimental investigation in the rabbit. *Clin Orthop* 208:131–140, 1986.

101. Parkkinen JJ, Ikonen J, Lammi MJ, et al: Effects of cyclic hydrostatic pressure on proteoglycan synthesis in cultured chondrocytes and articular cartilage explants. *Arch Biochem Biophys* 300:458–465, 1993.

102. Parkkinen JJ, Lammi MJ, Inkinen R, et al: Influence of short-term hydrostatic pressure on organization of stress fibers in cultured chondrocytes. *J Orthop Res* 13:495–502, 1995.

103. Parkkinen JJ, Lammi MJ, Pelttari A, et al: Altered Golgi apparatus in hydrostatically loaded articular cartilage chondrocytes. *Ann Rheum Dis* 52:192–198, 1993.

104. Peterson L, Minas T, Brittberg M, et al: Two- to 9-year outcome after autologous chondrocyte transplantation of the knee. *Clin Orthop* 374:212–234, 2000.

105. Pitman MI, Menche D, Song EK, et al: The use of adhesives in chondrocyte transplantation surgery: in-vivo studies. *Bull Hosp Joint Dis Orthop Inst* 49:213–220, 1989.

106. Poole CA: Articular cartilage chondrons: from, function and failure. *J Anat* 191:1–13, 1997.

107. Radice M, Brun P, Cortivo R, et al: Hyaluronan-based biopolymers as delivery vehicles for bone-marrow-derived mesenchymal progenitors. *J Biomed Mater Res* 50:101–109, 2000.

108. Ralphs JR, Tyers RN, Benjamin M: Development of functionally distinct fibrocartilages at two sites in the quadriceps tendon of the rat: the suprapatella and the attachment to the patella. *Anat Embryol* 185:181–187, 1992.

109. Redini F, Lafuma C, Pujol JP, et al: Effect of cytokines and growth factors on the expression of elastase activity by human synoviocytes, dermal fibroblasts and rabbit articular chondrocytes. *Biochem Biophys Res Commun* 155:786–793, 1988.

110. Rosen DM, Stempien SA, Thompson AY, et al: Differentiation of rat mesenchymal cells by cartilage-inducing factor. Enhanced phenotypic expression by dihydrocytochalasin B. *Exp Cell Res* 165:127–138, 1986.

111. Rosen DM, Stempien SA, Thompson AY, et al: Transforming growth factor-beta modulates the expression of osteoblast and chondroblast phenotypes in vitro. *J Cell Physiol* 134:337–346, 1988.

112. Sah RL, Kim YJ, Doong JY, et al: Biosynthetic response of cartilage explants to dynamic compression. *J Orthop Res* 7:619–636, 1989.

113. Sailor LZ, Hewick RM, Morris EA: Recombinant human bone morphogenetic protein-2 maintains the articular chondrocyte phenotype in long-term culture. *J Orthop Res* 14:937–945, 1996.

114. Schinagl RM, Gurskis D, Chen AC, et al: Depth-dependent confined compression modulus of full-thickness bovine articular cartilage. *J Orthop Res* 15:499–506, 1997.

115. Schmidt G, Hausser H, Kresse H: Interaction of the small proteoglycan decorin with fibronection. Involvement of the sequence NKISK of the core protein. *Biochem J* 280:411–414, 1991.

116. Schumacher BL, Block JA, Schmid TM, et al: A novel proteoglycan synthesized and secreted by chondrocytes of the superficial zone of articular cartilage. *Arch Biochem Biophys* 311:144–152, 1994.

117. Schuman L, Buma P, Versleyen D, et al: Chondrocyte behaviour within different types of collagen gel in vitro. *Biomaterials* 16:809–814, 1995.

118. Sellers RS, Peluso D, Morris EA: The effect of recombinant human bone morphogenetic protein-2 (rhBMP-2) on the healing of full-thickness defects of articular cartilage. *J Bone Joint Surg [Am]* 79:1452–1463, 1997.

119. Shin D, Athanasiou K: Cytoindentation for obtaining cell biomechanical properties. *J Orthop Res* 17:880–890, 1999.

120. Shin D, Lin JH, Agrawal CM, et al: Zonal variations in microindentation properties of articular cartilage. 44th Annual Meeting of the Orthopaedic Reasearch Society, New Orleans, LA, March 16–19, 1998:903.

121. Siczkowski M, Watt FM: Subpopulations of chondrocytes from different zones of pig articular cartilage. Isolation, growth and proteoglycan synthesis in culture. *J Cell Sci* 97:349–360, 1990.

122. Silverman RP, Passaretti D, Huang W: Injectable tissue-engineered cartilage using a fibrin glue polymer. *Plast Reconstr Surg* 103:1809–1818, 1999.

123. Simon WH, Freidenberg S, Richardson S: A correlation of joint congruence and thickness of articular cartilage in dogs. *J Bone Joint Surg [Am]* 55:1614–1620, 1973.

124. Sittinger M, Reitzel D, Dauner M, et al: Resorbable polyesters in cartilage engineering: affinity and biocompatibility of polymer fiber structures to chondrocytes. *J Biomed Mater Res* 33:57–63, 1996.

125. Smith GN Jr, Brandt KD: Hypothesis: can type IX collagen "glue" together intersecting type II fibers in articular cartilage matrix? A proposed mechanism. *J Rheumatol* 19:14–17, 1992.

126. Smith RL, Donlon BS, Gupta MK, et al: Effects of fluid-induced shear on articular chondrocyte morphology and metabolism in vitro. *J Orthop Res* 13:824–831, 1995.

127. Smith RL, Lin J, Trindade MC, et al: Time-dependent effects of intermittent hydrostatic pressure on articular chondrocyte type II collagen and aggrecan mRNA expression. *J Rehabil Res Dev* 37:153–161, 2000.

128. Solchaga LA, Dennis JE, Goldberg VM, et al: Hyaluronic acid-based polymers as cell carriers for tissue-engineered repair of bone and cartilage. *J Orthop Res* 17:205–213, 1999.

129. Soltz MA, Ateshian GA: Experimental verification and theoretical prediction of cartilage interstitial fluid pressurization at an impermeable contact interface in confined compression. *J Biomech* 31:927–934, 1998.

130. Spain TL, Agrawal CM, Athanasiou KA: New technique to extend the useful life of a biodegradable cartilage implant. *Tissue Eng* 4:343–352, 1998.

131. Stockwell RA: The cell density of human articular and costal cartilage. *J Anat* 101:753–763, 1967.

132. Suggs LJ, Kao EY, Palombo LL, et al: Preparation and characterization of poly(propylene fumarate-co-ethylene glycol) hydrogels. *J Biomater Sci Polym Ed* 9:653–666, 1998.

133. Suggs LJ, Krishnan RS, Garcia CA, et al: In vitro and in vivo degradation of poly(propylene fumarate-co-ethylene glycol) hydrogels. *J Biomed Mater Res* 42:312–320, 1998.

134. Suggs LJ, Shive MS, Garcia CA, et al: In vitro cytotoxicity and in vivo biocompatibility of poly(propylene fumarate-co-ethylene glycol) hydrogels. *J Biomed Mater Res* 46:22–32, 1999.

135. Swann DA, Slayter HS, Silver FH: The molecular structure of lubricating glycoprotein-I, the boundary lubricant for articular cartilage. *J Biol Chem* 256:5921–5925, 1981.

136. Takahashi K, Kubo T, Arai Y, et al: Hydrostatic pressure induces expression of interleukin 6 and tumour necrosis factor alpha mRNAs in a chondrocyte-like cell line. *Ann Rheum Dis* 57:231–236, 1998.

137. Thompson D, Agrawal C, Athanasiou K: The effects of dynamic compressive loading on biodegradable implants of 50–50% polylactic acid-polyglycolic acid. *Tissue Eng* 2:61–74, 1996.
138. Ting V, Sims CD, Brecht LE, et al: In vitro prefabrication of human cartilage shapes using fibrin glue and human chondrocytes. *Ann Plast Surg* 40:413–420; discussion 420–421, 1998.
139. Tipton DA, Dabbous MK: Autocrine transforming growth factor beta stimulation of extracellular matrix production by fibroblasts from fibrotic human gingiva. *J Periodontol* 69:609–619, 1998.
140. Torzilli PA: Effects of temperature, concentration and articular surface removal on transient solute diffusion in articular cartilage. *Med Biol Eng Comput* 31:S93–S98, 1993.
141. Trippel SB, Ehrlich MG, Lippiello L, et al: Characterization of chondrocytes from bovine articular cartilage: I. Metabolic and morphological experimental studies. *J Bone Joint Surg [Am]* 62:816–820, 1980.
142. Turner AS, Athanasiou KA, Zhu CF, et al: Biochemical effects of estrogen on articular cartilage in ovariectomized sheep. *Osteoarthritis Cartilage* 5:63–69, 1997.
143. Vachon A, Bramlage LR, Gabel AA, et al: Evaluation of the repair process of cartilage defects of the equine third carpal bone with and without subchondral bone perforation. *Am J Vet Res* 47:2637–2645, 1986.
144. van Susante JL, Buma P, Schuman L, et al: Resurfacing potential of heterologous chondrocytes suspended in fibrin glue in large full-thickness defects of femoral articular cartilage: an experimental study in the goat. *Biomaterials* 20:1167–1175, 1999.
145. Vaughan L, Mendler M, Huber S, et al: D-periodic distribution of collagen type IX along cartilage fibrils. *J Cell Biol* 106:991–997, 1988.
146. Vogel K, Troter J: The effect of proteoglycans on the morphology of collagen fibrils in vitro. *Collagen Rel Res* 7:105–114, 1987.
147. Vunjak-Novakovic G, Martin I, Obradovic B, et al: Bioreactor cultivation conditions modulate the composition and mechanical properties of tissue-engineered cartilage. *J Orthop Res* 17:130–138, 1999.
148. Wakitani S, Goto T, Pineda SJ, et al: Mesenchymal cell-based repair of large, full-thickness defects of articular cartilage. *J Bone Joint Surg [Am]* 76:579–592, 1994.
149. Wakitani S, Goto T, Young RG, et al: Repair of large full-thickness articular cartilage defects with allograft articular chondrocytes embedded in a collagen gel. *Tissue Eng* 4:429–444, 1998.
150. Weiser L, Bhargava M, Attia E, et al: Effect of serum and platelet-derived growth factor on chondrocytes grown in collagen gels. *Tissue Eng* 5:533–544, 1999.
151. Woessner JFJ, Howell DS. *Joint Cartilage Degradation.* Marcel Dekker, New York, NY, 1993.
152. Wu JZ, Herzog W, Epstein M: Modelling of location- and time-dependent deformation of chondrocytes during cartilage loading. *J Biomech* 32:563–572, 1999.
153. Yu H, Grynpas M, Kandel RA: Composition of cartilagenous tissue with mineralized and non-mineralized zones formed in vitro. *Biomaterials* 18:1425–1431, 1997.
154. Zanetti M, Ratcliffe A, Watt FM: Two subpopulations of differentiated chondrocytes identified with a monoclonal antibody to keratan sulfate. *J Cell Biol* 101:53–59, 1985.

III | Tissue Harvesting, Fixation, and Preparation

5

Bone-Labeling Techniques

Reinhold G. Erben

Institute of Animal Physiology, Ludwig Maximillians University, Munich, Germany

I. INTRODUCTION

Labeling of the skeleton with intravital marker substances allows the quantitative measurement of bone formation and of bone remodeling dynamics. Therefore, in vivo bone labeling has become a standard technique in skeletal research.[15,16,68] It is the goal of this chapter to provide an overview of the substances used as bone labels, and to present the relevant information about how to employ these labeling substances in living organisms for specific purposes in a meaningful way. Another goal of this chapter is to describe how to avoid mistakes that are commonly made in the use of bone-labeling techniques.

In vivo bone-labeling methods that are rarely used today—such as the use of lead markers for the assessment of bone formation in decalcified bone histology—are not covered in this chapter. For further information about these methods, the reader is referred to older standard textbooks.[63] Also, this chapter does not describe techniques for radioactive labeling of skeletal tissues with ^{45}Ca or ^{3}H-tetracycline. These methods are useful for calcium kinetic studies and for the measurement of bone resorption at the organ or whole-body level, but are rarely used for autoradiography in bone sections.

II. FLUOROCHROMES

Fluorochromes used for bone labeling are calcium-seeking substances that are incorporated into the mineralization front of mineralizing surfaces, which can be visualized in histological specimens by their fluorescence under excitation with ultraviolet (UV) or blue light.

After oral or parenteral administration, fluorochromes enter the bloodstream and are preferentially bound at sites of new mineralized tissue formation in the skeleton and the teeth.[67] Fluorochromes bind to bone mineral through chelation of calcium ions at the surface of newly formed apatite crystals. The reason for selective binding of fluorochromes to newly mineralizing surfaces in bone, dentin, enamel, and cementum may be the smaller apatite crystal size formed during the initial stages of mineralization compared with older mineralizing sites.[1,2,67] Unlike radioactive calcium, fluorochromes are irreversibly deposited at sites of mineralized tissue formation.[64]

From: *Handbook of Histology Methods for Bone and Cartilage*
Edited by: Y. H. An and K. L. Martin © Humana Press Inc., Totowa, NJ

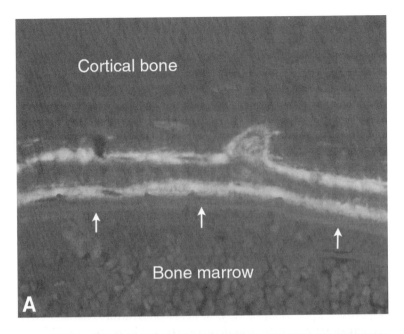

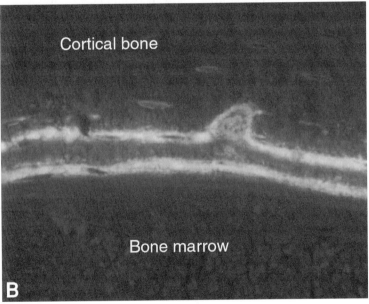

Figure 1. Calcein double-labeling of bone. (A) Shows the endocortical bone surface in the distal femur of a 3-mo-old female mouse, viewed under blue-violet excitation (395–440 nm). The mouse has been subcutaneously injected with calcein (20 mg/kg) 5 d and 2 d before sacrifice. The endocortical bone surface is intensely labeled with two green fluorescent bands. In the two days between administration of the second label and sacrifice of the animal, the second calcein label has been covered with new bone matrix. The bone surface is marked with arrows. (B) Shows the same site viewed under blue excitation (450–490 nm). Note the marked reduction of background fluorescence with blue excitation. Sections are 3 μm thick. Original magnification ×400. (*See* color plate 6 appearing in the insert following p.270.)

Fluorochrome labels are laid down in the form of bands in bone sections (Fig. 1). The width of the fluorochrome band depends on the velocity of mineralization progression and on the time the substance circulates in the extracellular fluid. In addition, because fluorochromes are able to diffuse into recently formed, low-density bone, the width of fluorochrome bands is increased when the accumulation of mineral during the initial phases of mineralization is delayed, such as in vitamin D deficiency.[1] In histological sections, the width of a fluorochrome band also depends on the angle at which a three-dimensional (3D) label plane has been sectioned.

Fluorochromes incorporated into bone formation sites stay there for very long periods of time, and are not released until the fluorochrome-containing bone matrix is resorbed by osteoclasts. Probably because of the resulting very low plasma concentrations, the fluorochromes released by osteoclastic bone resorption of labeled bone are not re-incorporated into new bone formation sites in a significant fashion.[26] Therefore, re-use of fluorochromes once bound to bone matrix and released through osteoclast activity is not a confounding factor for bone labeling.

A. Tetracyclines

Tetracyclines were originally developed as antibiotics. In addition to their antibacterial actions, tetracycline antibiotics form complexes with metal ions such as Ca^{2+}, Zn^{2+}, Mn^{2+}, or $Fe^{2+/3+}$, and show fluorescence under excitation with UV light. The optimal excitation wavelength for tetracyclines bound to bone mineral lies between 390 and 430 nm.[45] In the 1950s, tetracycline antibiotics were found to be incorporated into bone, which enables them to be used as markers of bone formation.[33] Of the tetracyclines currently in clinical use as antibiotics, tetracycline, chlortetracycline, oxytetracycline, and demeclocycline have also been used as bone-labeling substances. The color of the emitted fluorescent light varies slightly for the various tetracyclines. Tetracycline and oxytetracycline bound to apatite fluoresce yellowish-green, and demeclocycline reveals a golden-yellow fluorescence. Therefore, it is possible to distinguish tetracycline/oxytetracycline from demeclocycline in histological sections (Fig. 2).

Tetracyclines are orally available, and have low toxicity in humans. Thus, tetracyclines are the fluorochromes of choice in clinical studies. Daily oral doses given to humans for the purpose of bone labeling vary from 7–15 mg/kg for tetracycline or oxytetracycline and 4–8 mg/kg for demeclocycline.[3,29,44,51] Tetracyclines can result in staining of teeth and in dental enamel defects in children, and should therefore not be given to children, especially under the age of 8 years, or to pregnant or breastfeeding women.

It should be noted that although tetracyclines are an almost ideal bone-labeling substance in humans, they can be toxic to some animal species, especially at higher doses. For example, tetracyclines should be used with caution in horses because of the risk of life-threatening diarrhea.[52] In the author's experience, a single dose of demeclocycline can be hepatotoxic in rats at doses higher than 20 mg/kg. Demeclocycline should not be used in amphibians. In an experiment with toads, tetracycline at a dose of 100 mg/kg showed no signs of toxicity, but all animals died within a few weeks after a subcutaneous (sc) injection of 20 mg/kg demeclocycline.[6] With the exception of horses (10–15 mg/kg),[52,53] tetracycline and oxytetracycline can be given at the dose of 20–25 mg/kg to all animals. Demeclocycline is usually administered at a dose of 20 mg/kg. No undesirable side effects have been reported in rats,[9] mice,[57] amphibians,[14] rabbits,[62] guinea pigs,[60] dogs,[36,69] pigs,[23] sheep,[7,22] and monkeys[70] at these dose levels.

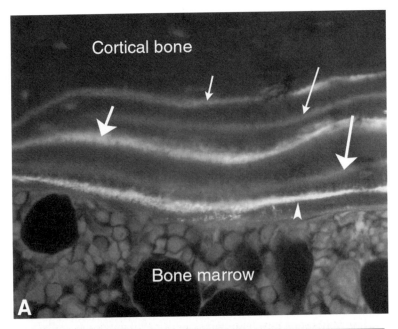

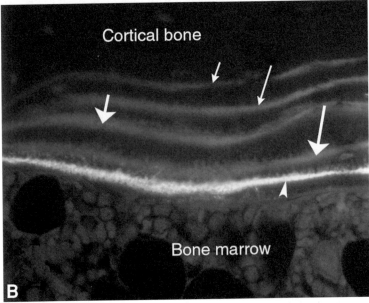

Figure 2. Multiple fluorochrome labeling of bone. (A) Shows the labeled endocortical bone surface in the proximal tibia of a 12-mo-old female rat, viewed under blue-violet excitation (395–440 nm). The rat has been intraperitoneally injected every 5 d with five different fluorochromes: oxytetracycline (25 mg/kg, short small arrow), xylenol orange (90 mg/kg, long arrow), demeclocycline (20 mg/kg, short large arrow), alizarin complexone (30 mg/kg, long large arrow), and calcein (20 mg/kg, arrowhead). Four days after the last label, the rat was sacrificed. The yellowish-green fluorescence of oxytetracycline can be clearly distinguished from the golden-yellow fluorescence of demeclocycline. (B) Shows the same site viewed under blue excitation (450–490 nm). Blue excitation improves the visualization of calcein, alizarin complexone, and xylenol orange, but decreases the brightness of the two tetracycline labels. Sections are 5 μm thick. Original magnification ×400. (*See* color plate 7 appearing in the insert following p. 270.)

1. Author's Preferred Method

For animal experimental studies, it is preferable to prepare the dosing solutions from a crystalline substance. Tetracyclines in powdered form can be dissolved in physiological saline at concentrations of 10–25 mg/mL. The pH of the solution should be controlled and adjusted to either pH 6.0–6.5 or pH 8.2–8.5. Solubility is often better in the acidic pH range. The solubility of tetracyclines in aqueous solution depends on pH, and consequently, on ionization of the molecule. Many tetracylines are insoluble in aqueous solution around pH 7. Aqueous solutions of tetracyclines are unstable and should not be stored. The dosing solutions should not be exposed to intense light.

Endotoxin-free water for injection purposes should be used for preparation of the solutions. Generally, sterile filtration of the solution should be performed before parenteral administration. However, this is not an absolute necessity for intraperitoneal or sc injection in rats and mice. The same applies for all the other fluorochromes.

B. Fluoresceins

Calcein is a calcium-chelating fluorescein that shows very intense green fluorescence when bound to bone mineral under UV, blue-violet, or blue excitation (Fig. 1). Optimal excitation of fluorescence is achieved with blue light.[45] Use of calcein as a bone label was explored in the 1960s and 1970s.[34,50] Because of its very bright fluorescence and its strong resistance to fading, calcein is the bone label of choice for animal studies. Calcein is administered at doses of 8–20 mg/kg. Doses of up to 20 mg/kg appear to be safe in all species studied (rats,[9] mice,[56] guinea pigs,[60] amphibians,[14] rabbits,[25] dogs,[39] pigs,[23] sheep,[22] horses,[59] and monkeys[30]). In aged rats (over 1 yr) and larger animals such as dogs, sheep, horses, or monkeys, a dose of 10 mg/kg is recommended. Undesirable side effects have not been reported at these dose levels. In the experience of the author, a dose of 10 mg/kg usually yields very good results in all animals.

Calcein blue is another fluorescein dye that shows blue fluorescence under UV illumination. It has been used at a dose of 30 mg/kg for bone labeling in some studies with rats, sheep, and rabbits.[46] However, an important disadvantage of calcein blue is its rapid fading, and therefore it cannot be classified as a recommended bone label.

1. Author's Preferred Method

Calcein is dissolved in 1.4% isotonic sodium bicarbonate ($NaHCO_3$) at a concentration of 10–20 mg/mL. The pH of the resulting solution lies between 7.7 (10 mg/mL) and 7.2 (20 mg/mL). Dissolution of calcein in solutions containing $NaHCO_3$ is associated with production of CO_2. Therefore, closed vials may be under pressure after dissolving the substance, and care should be taken when opening the vial. Repeated opening of the vial while dissolving the substance is recommended. The dosing solution can be stored at 4°C in the dark for several weeks.

C. Alizarins

Alizarins—natural plant dyes derived from madder—are fluorochromes that show a red fluorescence under UV or blue excitation (Fig. 2).[45] Although other alizarins, mainly alizarin red S,[32] were used initially, alizarin complexone is almost exclusively employed today for bone labeling because of its more intense red fluorescence and lower toxicity.[48] Optimal excitation of alizarin complexone is achieved with green light.[45] However, blue-violet or blue light can also be used for excitation with acceptable results. Alizarin complexone can be administered to rats,[9] mice,[10] guinea pigs,[60] dogs,[39] rabbits,[25] pigs,[55] sheep,[22] and monkeys[38] at a dose of 25–30 mg/kg. This dose appears to be well-tolerated in all species.

1. Author's Preferred Method

Alizarin complexone is dissolved in 1.4% isotonic $NaHCO_3$ at a concentration of 15–30 mg/mL. The pH of the resulting solution lies between 7.7 (15 mg/mL) and 7.1 (30 mg/mL). Similar to calcein, dissolution of alizarin complexone in solutions containing $NaHCO_3$ is associated with production of CO_2. Therefore, the same precautions apply as described previously for calcein. The dosing solution can be stored at 4°C in the dark for several weeks.

D. Other Fluorochromes

Xylenol orange is a useful bone label that is chemically different from tetracyclines, fluoresceins, and alizarins.[47] Xylenol orange bound to bone mineral exhibits an orange or red fluorescence under excitation with UV, blue-violet, or blue light (Fig. 2).[45] The dose of 90 mg/kg has been administered in most studies with good results, and appears to have no toxic side effects in rats,[9] amphibians,[14] rabbits,[25] dogs,[39] pigs,[37] sheep,[54] and monkeys.[5] However, if there is no specific need to use xylenol orange, preference should be given to alizarin complexone, which can be given at lower doses. Today, xylenol orange is almost exclusively used in multiple labeling regimens.

1. Author's Preferred Method

Xylenol orange is dissolved in physiological saline or in 1.4% isotonic $NaHCO_3$ at a concentration of up to 90 mg/mL. The dosing solution can be stored at 4°C in the dark for several weeks.

E. Route of Fluorochrome Administration

In humans, tetracyclines are usually administered orally. However, in animal experimental studies, fluorochromes are given intravenously, intraperitoneally, intramuscularly, or subcutaneously. Intravenous (iv) infusion of calcium-chelating substances is a potentially dangerous procedure because these compounds form complexes with blood-ionized calcium, resulting in the risk of severe and sometimes fatal hypocalcemia. Therefore, iv infusion of fluorochromes must be performed very slowly. In monkeys and horses, bone markers are usually given intravenously. In other animals, the author recommends sc administration of the substances. Intravenous injections in rodents are time-consuming and, therefore are not practical for many studies. Although fluorochromes have been given intraperitoneally in many studies with rats and mice, it is safer to administer the substances subcutaneously. With intraperitoneal (ip) injections there is always a risk of injecting the fluorochrome into the intestine, or sometimes into the seminal vesicles in male animals. This risk depends on the skill of the person performing the injections, and is especially high after major abdominal surgery with subsequent formation of adhesions. The sequelae of injecting the fluorochrome labels into the intestine or seminal vesicles are faint or absent bone labels. Therefore, sc administration of the fluorochromes greatly reduces the risk of absent bone labels. However, when animals receive daily sc injections of oily solutions, care must be taken that the aqueous fluorochrome solutions are not injected in close proximity to the oily solution injection sites, as the fluorochromes may not be properly absorbed. In this case, ip injection may be preferable.

As mentioned here, the width of a fluorochrome band in bone depends (among other factors) on the time the substance circulates in the blood. The time that a substance is present in the extracellular fluid depends on the route of administration, and on the pharmacokinetics of the drug (plasma half-life). Therefore, a single parenteral injection of a fluorochrome generally produces more distinct labels compared with oral administration, and substances with a short plasma half-life such as calcein or alizarin complexone result in more distinct labels compared with tetracyclines with a plasma half-life in the range of several hours or more.[27]

F. Histological Processing of Fluorochrome-Labeled Specimens

Because fluorochromes are bound in skeletal tissues as complexes with calcium, undecalcified bone histology is a prerequisite for their later microscopic study. Decalcification of the bone or dental specimens results in complete or almost complete loss of calcium-seeking fluorochromes. Therefore, acidic fixation media (such as Carnoy's, Bouin's, or unbuffered formalin) that may dissolve bone calcium should not be used for fluorochrome-labeled specimens. A good fixative for fluorochrome-labeled bone specimens is 40% ethanol at 4°C. Fixation with 40% ethanol at 4°C causes less shrinkage compared with 70% ethanol at room temperature. For optimal cell morphology, fixation in phosphate-buffered 4% paraformaldehyde at pH 7.4 is recommended.

Generally, the best preservation of fluorochrome labels is achieved when the fixed specimens are processed without interruption until they are embedded in plastic. However, if storage is necessary at earlier stages, specimens should be stored in 70% ethanol. Loss of fluorochrome labels in 70% ethanol is minimal when appropriate labeling regimens are used. Blocks and sections from fluorochrome-labeled tissue should be protected from intense light during processing, and stored in the dark. The labels are stable in blocks and sections for decades under appropriate storage conditions.

Sections prepared for analysis of fluorochrome labeling are left unstained, and the dry sections are mounted in a medium suitable for fluorescence microscopy (e.g., Fluoromount®, Boehringer Ingelheim). Using optimal microscopic equipment, it is not necessary to use thicker (e.g., 8–10-μm-thick) sections for analysis of fluorochrome labeling, compared with sections used for normal histology (3–5-μm-thick). The recommendation to use thicker sections stems from the fact that fluorescence is brighter in thicker sections. However, in thinner sections, double labels are better recognized.[4,31]

G. Visualization of Fluorochrome Labels by Epifluorescent Microscopy

Fluorochrome bands in bone or dental sections are visualized by UV, blue-violet, or blue excitation. The source of light for excitation is usually a super-pressure mercury vapor lamp, but can also be a laser in more sophisticated microscope systems. The spectrum produced by the mercury vapor lamp is filtered by an excitation filter (usually a band-pass filter) that transmits only the desired wavelengths. In an epifluorescent microscope, the short-waved length light used for excitation passes through the same objective that is used for the observation of the longer-waved length fluorescent light. The different wavelengths are separated by a beam splitter. In addition, a barrier filter (usually a low-pass filter) blocks the transmission of any light below a certain wavelength to the eyepiece.

Thus, filter systems used for epifluorescent microscopes consist of three components: an excitation filter, a beam splitter, and a barrier filter.

It is important to choose an appropriate fluorescence filter system for the analysis of fluorochrome labels in skeletal tissue. For optimal fluorescence, tetracyclines require blue-violet or UV excitation (Fig. 2). However, a disadvantage of UV and blue-violet illumination is that many cells and tissues show pronounced autofluorescence under these conditions. This is especially true for collagen fibers in unmineralized osteoid. Calcein, alizarin complexone, and xylenol orange are best visualized using a filter system developed for the observation of FITC (fluorescein isothiocyanate) fluorescence (Fig. 2). FITC filter systems use blue light for excitation. Blue excitation greatly reduces background fluorescence in skeletal and dental tissues compared with UV or blue-violet illumination (Fig. 1, 2). Moreover, *fading* (reduction in fluorescence intensity with time under constant exposure to the light used for excitation) is reduced under illumination with blue light relative to UV light.

The term *quenching* describes the reduction in fluorescence intensity through absorption of the emitted fluorescent light photons by the surrounding tissue. The use of any type of histological staining can result in considerable quenching of fluorescence in bone sections through absorption of fluorescent light by the dye. Therefore, the conditions for analysis of fluorochrome labels are optimal in unstained sections.

1. Author's Preferred Method

For visualization of tetracyclines, the author uses the Zeiss filter set No. 05, consisting of a 395–440-nm band-pass excitation filter, a 460-nm beam splitter, and a 470-nm low-pass barrier filter (Fig. 1, 2). For calcein, alizarin complexone, and xylenol orange, the author employs the Zeiss filter set No. 09, consisting of a 450–490 nm band-pass excitation filter, a 510-nm beam splitter, and a 520-nm low-pass barrier filter (Fig. 1, 2). When only alizarin complexone is studied, the most appropriate filter set is No. 14, consisting of a 510–560-nm band-pass excitation filter, a 580-nm beam splitter, and a 590-nm low-pass filter. In specimens that have been labeled with combinations of tetracyclines and other fluorochromes, we use the Zeiss filter set No. 05 (Fig. 2).

III. LABELING REGIMENS

In order to obtain the maximum amount of information from a specific study, it is important to determine the purpose of labeling bone in that study. Also, it can be very worthwhile to consider the possibility of further studies (beyond the major aim) on bones from a given experiment. For example, in a hypothetical study with rats, the primary goal may be to evaluate the effects of a certain drug on cancellous bone. However, after the experiment has been performed, there are also effects on periosteal bone envelopes that must be studied histologically. It saves time and money to consider this possibility in the planning phase of the study, and to make the necessary arrangements in the experimental design of the study.

With the exception of measuring longitudinal bone elongation and of assessing bone resorption, two labels given at different time-points are necessary for the calculation of mineral apposition rate, bone formation rate, or bone remodeling dynamics. Especially for studies in humans, a code is used for the labeling schedule. The code 2–10–2:4 means 2 d of labeling followed by 10 d without label, another 2 d of labeling, followed by 4 d of

**Table 1. Cancellous Bone Formation Periods and Appropriate
Marker Intervals in Different Species***

Species	Formation period	Optimal marker interval
Man[40,51]	60–250 d	12–50 d
Cynomolgus monkey[24,28]	20 (young)–75 d (mature)	4–15 d
Dog[36,58]	30–50 d	6–10 d
Sheep[7]	75 d	15 d
Minipig[35]	35–40 d	7–8 d
Rat[11]	15–25 d	3–5 d
Mouse>3 mo of age[10]	10–13 d	2–3 d
Mouse<2 mo of age[10]	5–10 d	1–2 d

*The marker intervals are based on a marker interval/formation period ratio of below 0.2. *See* text for details.

no label prior to bone biopsy.[18] The time interval between the bone labels is the marker interval. The marker interval is used for calculation of appositional rates. The labeling period is the duration of label administration.

It is very important to allow sufficient time between the last label and the biopsy or the sacrifice of the animal. During this time, the label stabilizes during further mineralization of the matrix, and is covered with new bone matrix (Fig. 1), so that it will not be lost by elution into solutions used for fixation or processing of the specimen later on.[49] Appropriate minimum time intervals after the last label are 4–5 d in humans, 2 d in rats, and 1 d in mice.

When choosing combinations of different fluorochromes for a study, later microscopic analysis can be made easier to if we consider that tetracyclines require UV or blue-violet excitation, and calcein, alizarin complexone, and xylenol orange are best visualized using blue excitation.

A. *Label Escape Error and Skewed Sampling Error*

When the purpose of fluorochrome labeling in a specific study is the measurement of bone formation and related parameters in cancellous or cortical bone remodeling units (BSU, bone structural units), it is very important to understand the nature of the label escape error and the skewed sampling error. For more detailed information about both errors, the reader is referred to the excellent description by Dr. Frost.[18,19] Remodeling is a cyclical renewal process in which bone resorption is followed by bone formation in the same bone site.[17,20,41] Remodeling activity in cancellous bone is not restricted to higher mammals, but is also the prevailing turnover activity in nongrowing or slowly growing bones of rats.[9] Therefore, the label escape and skewed sampling errors are relevant for all human and most animal studies. The length of the bone formation phase of the remodeling cycle is known as the formation period.[42] Typical formation periods for cancellous bone of different species are shown in Table 1.

It is important to note that the label escape error and the skewed sampling error do not apply to modeling drifts. In contrast to the remodeling activity, bone formation and bone resorption are independent and are not coupled during the modeling process. Bone formation can continue over extended periods of time in cancellous and cortical bone-modeling drifts.[21,41] Periosteal expansion is a typical modeling drift in cortical bone. Modeling is also the prevailing turnover activity for metaphyseal cancellous bone in the rapidly growing appendicular bones of young rats, and probably other species.[9]

Information about appositional rates can only be obtained when two bone labels are present in individual remodeling units. The mean distance between the labels divided by the marker interval corresponds to the mineral apposition rate (MAR).[42] When two bone labels are given at two different time-points, certain proportions of the remodeling units in their formation phase will take either two labels or one label. This is shown by a schematic graph in Fig. 3. It is evident that the proportion of remodeling units that take a double label depends on the ratio between the marker interval (MI) and the formation period (FP). The smaller the MI/FP ratio, the greater the proportion of double-labeled remodeling units. If the marker interval is longer than the formation period, no double labels will be found.

This phenomenon is known as label escape, and the resulting error is the label escape error. It is obvious that this error can result in severe underestimation of mineralizing surface and of all derived parameters, such as the bone-formation rate. The label escape error is especially important for animal studies in rats and mice in which the mineralizing surface is often calculated as the double-labeled surface. The magnitude of the label escape error is determined by the MI/FP ratio. It can be calculated that the MI/FP ratio should be below 0.2 in order to arrive at an acceptable label escape error of below 25%.[19] The marker intervals shown in Table 1 are based on a MI/FP ratio of approx 0.2.

The skewed sampling error affects the measurement of the MAR and all derived parameters such as formation period, remodeling period, or osteoid maturation time.[18] There are three physiological properties of the formation phase during the process of bone remodeling that can give rise to skewing in MAR measurements:

   i) The MAR is not uniform during the formation period. Rather, organic matrix formation and MAR are higher during the early phase of the formation period, and slow down considerably at the later stages of bone formation.[40]
  ii) Individual remodeling units have different appositional rates.
 iii) Osteoblastic activity may temporarily pause,[19] especially during the later stages of the formation phase. It is obvious that the value for an individual MAR measurement will be reduced when the first and second label span such an off period. It is not clear whether fluorochrome labels are taken up during off periods.

An increase in the marker interval statistically favors the longer phase of slow apposition in individual remodeling units, statistically favors remodeling units with slow apposition rates relative to units with higher rates, and increases the likelihood of inclusion of off periods. All these effects result in skewing of the measured MAR frequency distribution toward lower values with increasing marker intervals. Therefore, a marker interval that is too long will result in erroneously low mean MAR values. There is experimental proof for this theoretical concept. Using increasing marker intervals, Tam and Anderson[61] have shown that in cancellous bone of growing rats, marker intervals longer than 3 d result in underestimation of MAR.

Both the label escape and the skewed sampling error can be minimized by the reduction of the marker interval. However, double labels must still be separated sufficiently in the sections to allow for accurate microscopic measurement. Therefore, the marker interval used should be as short as possible, yet still allow accurate measurement of MAR. The accuracy of the MAR measurements can be improved by using an objective with higher

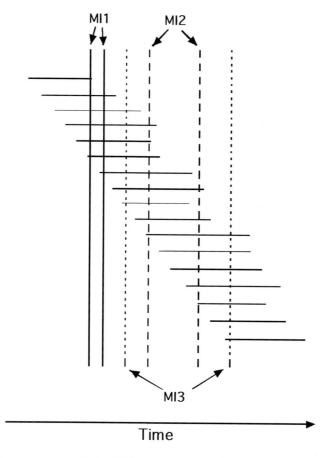

Figure 3. Label escape error. Each of the horizontal bars in this graph depicts the formation phase in an individual remodeling unit (BSU, bone structural unit). Bone formation in each unit proceeds along the time axis from left to right. New BSU are created with time, and are shown separately from each other on the dimensionless y-axis. The mean length of the horizontal bars represents the formation period (FP). In this example, three sets of fluorochrome double labels with different marker intervals (MI) are administered at specific time-points. A fluorochrome label given at a certain time-point labels all BSU that are actively mineralizing at that time. Therefore, every intersection of the vertical lines representing the markers with the horizontal bars representing the formation phases of individual BSU means that this remodeling unit takes the label. The marker set (solid line) with a short marker interval (MI1) labels 7 BSU; Five BSU took a double label (71%), and two BSU a single label (29%). The dashed-marker set has an about threefold longer marker interval (MI2) compared with MI1, and labels 11 BSU; three BSU took a double label (27%), and 8 BSU took a single label (73%). The dotted-marker set has a marker interval (MI3) that is longer than the formation period, and only single labels but no double labels are yielded. This schematic example clearly shows that the proportion of double-labeled BSU depends on the MI/FP ratio. The marker intervals MI1, MI2, and MI3 correspond to MI/FP ratios of about 0.2, 0.6, and 1.3, respectively. Adapted from Frost.[19]

power, such as ×40 or ×65 objectives. It is a bad strategy to take into account a large label escape and skewed sampling error simply because it is more convenient to measure MAR at lower magnification.

B. Clinical Studies in Humans

The purpose of fluorochrome labeling in human studies is usually the assessment of cancellous or endocortical bone turnover in iliac bone biopsies. It is necessary to administer two tetracycline labels. Other fluorochromes cannot be used in humans. Our studies have found that the use of two different tetracyclines for double labeling offers no significant advantage over using one fluorochrome for both labels. It has been shown that there are consistent differences in the amount of single-labeled surface for different tetracyclines.[43] Thus, the use of two different tetracyclines may introduce additional errors in the measurement. Tetracyclines are usually given orally in humans. Typical labeling schedules used in adult humans are 2–12–2:4,[3] 3–11–3:4,[44] or 3–14–3:5.[51]

C. Animal Studies

The range of possible applications for bone labeling in animal studies is wider than in clinical studies. In animal experiments, fluorochrome labeling can be used for the measurement of cancellous, endocortical, intracortical, and periosteal bone formation, for the evaluation of bone elongation, for multiple labeling regimens, and also for the assessment of bone resorption. When multiple doses of fluorochromes are administered to the same animal within a relatively short period of time, one should be aware that high cumulative doses of fluorochromes have the potential to inhibit bone mineralization.[8] However, this is mainly a concern for continuous labeling procedures or regimens using multiple labeling with very short marker intervals.

1. Assessment of Cancellous and Cortical Bone Formation and Bone Remodeling Dynamics

For this measurement, double labeling of bone is necessary. As mentioned in Section III.C., the use of two different fluorochromes for double labeling does not seem to offer any significant advantage over using one fluorochrome for both labels. The fluorochrome of choice is calcein. Calcein is nontoxic, can be administered at lower doses than all other fluorochromes, gives very distinct labels, fluoresces very brightly, and shows good resistance to fading. Typical optimal marker intervals for analysis of cancellous bone remodeling dynamics in different species are shown in Table 1.

Problems can arise when the same double-labeling schedule is planned for use for the measurement of both cancellous and periosteal bone formation. In young animals, periosteal bone apposition occurs at very high rates, so that usually the same marker interval can be used for cancellous and cortical bone. However, in aged animals, periosteal expansion slows down, and a marker interval optimized for cancellous bone remodeling can result in inseparable labels on periosteal envelopes.

To solve this problem, another label or another pair of labels must be introduced to allow accurate measurement of periosteal bone apposition with a longer marker interval. It is possible to administer three labels—for example, calcein on the 13th and third day and alizarin complexone on the eighth day before sacrificing the animals. The 10-d marker interval between the first calcein labels is then used for periosteal measurements, and the 5-d marker interval between the first calcein label and the alizarin label (or between the alizarin label and the second calcein label) for measurement of cancellous bone formation. When another pair of markers is used, it can be advantageous to use tetracyclines for the second pair of labels because different fluorescence filter systems can be employed to facilitate the separate analysis of the two pairs of labels. For example, give tetracycline on the 13th and third day, and calcein on the tenth and fifth day before sacrificing the animals. The 10-d marker interval between the tetracycline labels is then used for periosteal measurements, and the 5-d marker interval between the calcein labels for measurement of cancellous bone formation. It is important to note that three or more identical labels must not be administered when cancellous bone formation is also an end point. In this case, it will not be possible to make valid measurements because it is impossible to determine the correct marker interval unless all labels are present in a cancellous bone-forming site.

2. Assessment of Bone Elongation

The measurement of longitudinal bone elongation can be performed with a single label, and does not necessarily require a double fluorochrome label. Figure 4 shows how the measurement is performed using a single or a double label. In many cases, longitudinal bone elongation can be determined more easily, and also more accurately with the help of a single label of a different color (e.g., a tetracycline) compared with the pair of labels (e.g., calcein) used for measurement of cancellous bone formation.

There are some additional aspects to this method. In growing animals, a fluorochrome label given at baseline of a study can provide information about periosteal bone apposition or bone elongation over the entire study period.[65] Similarly, a baseline fluorochrome label in growing animals can help to distinguish between effects on pre-existent cancellous bone and on bone formed under the influence of some type of intervention. However, it must be taken into consideration that the time period that can be covered from baseline until the end of the trial is limited in long bones of the appendicular skeleton. Cancellous bone in the metaphyseal region of growing long bones is eventually resorbed toward the diaphyseal marrow cavity. Therefore, fluorochrome labels in metaphyseal cancellous bone will vanish after a certain period of time, depending on the growth rate of the animal. High bone turnover, such as that induced by estrogen deficiency in rats or mice, accelerates the loss of the metaphyseal label.[66]

3. Assessment of Bone Resorption

Fluorochrome-labeling of bone can also be used to estimate the activity of osteoclastic bone resorption.[66] When a single fluorochrome label is administered at the baseline of a study, the label is incorporated into active bone-formation sites. During the following weeks or months, osteoclastic bone resorption may be initiated at some sites carrying the label. Therefore, the label will disappear with time, and the rate of disappearance is an estimate of the activity of osteoclastic bone resorption. Any antiresorptive treatment results in increased preservation of a fluorochrome label administered at the baseline of the study.[12,66]

In metaphyseal bone of growing animals, such a label can be used to monitor bone resorption over a period of a few weeks because of the high rate of label disappearance,[66] yet in cancellous bone of the axial skeleton, the disappearance of the label can be followed over months.[12] The measurements can be expressed as a percentage of labeled cancellous bone perimeter or as labeled bone perimeter per bone area or per tissue area.[66] These values can be compared with baseline values and with those of control groups at the end of the experiment.

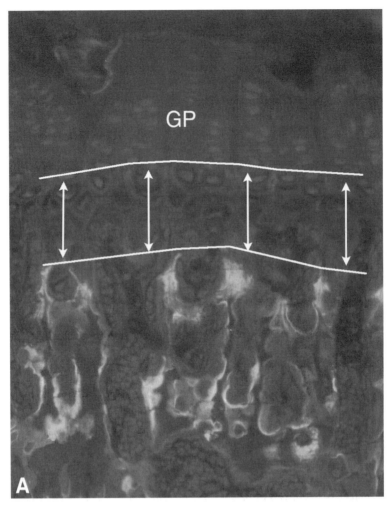

Figure 4. Measurement of longitudinal bone elongation. These fluorescence photomicrographs show the growth plate (GP) and the metaphysis of proximal tibias from growing rats. There are two ways to determine bone elongation. One method uses the fact that the earliest sites of fluorochrome incorporation into mineralized tissue are the calcifying cartilage septa in the growth plate. Some of the calcified cartilage septa are not resorbed, and form the template for osteoblastic bone formation in the primary spongiosa. With continuing bone elongation, the labeled calcified cartilage cores move distally toward the diaphysis. The 3-mo-old female rat in (A) has been labeled with calcein (20 mg/kg) 4 d prior to sacrifice. The distance between the most proximal traces of fluorochrome label in metaphyseal calcified cartilage cores (lower line) and the first calcified cartilage septa in the growth plate (upper line) is measured (arrows). This mean distance divided by the time interval between the administration of the label and the end of the experiment yields the bone elongation rate. The second method measures the mean distance between two fluorochrome labels in the metaphyseal cancellous bone. *(Figure continues)*

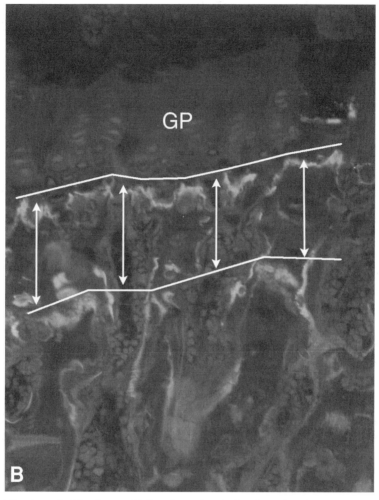

Figure 4. *(Continued)* The 6-mo-old female rat in (B) has been labeled with demeclocycline (20 mg/kg, golden-yellow fluorescence) and calcein (20 mg/kg, green fluorescence) with a marker interval of 10 d. The calcein label was administered 4 d before sacrificing the animal. The bone elongation rate is given by the mean distance (arrows) of the most proximal traces of the two labels (white lines) divided by the marker interval. For the measurement of the distance between the two fluorochrome bands, it is very helpful to use markers with different fluorescent colors. Blue-violet excitation. Original magnification ×200. (*See* color plate 8 appearing in the insert following p. 270.)

As mentioned here, it is advantageous to use a label of different fluorescent color for this purpose compared with the double label used to measure bone formation at the termination of the study. In order to increase the amount of labeled bone matrix, it is also possible to give the baseline label continuously over a certain period of time before initiation of the intervention.

4. Multiple Labeling

When used appropriately, multiple fluorochrome labeling makes it possible to quantitatively determine what happened to bone formation, for example in response to a pharmacological or surgical intervention, in the same animal over a certain period of time.[13] This technique is also commonly used to monitor the osseointegration of bone implants over time.[25,55,62] Therefore, multiple labeling can be a very powerful technique. The time period covered by the labeling regimen depends on the spacing of the individual fluorochrome labels in time. To fully exploit the possibilities of this technique, it is necessary that each label can be differentiated from the others by its specific fluorescence properties. Up to five different fluorochromes (e.g., oxytetracycline, xylenol orange, demeclocycline, alizarin complexone, and calcein) have been used successfully (Fig. 2).[9,13]

Acknowledgments: The writer is indebted to Stefanie Engert, Karin Begsteiger, and Claudia Bergow for their excellent technical assistance over many years.

REFERENCES

1. Baylink D, Stauffer M, Wergedal J, et al: Formation, mineralization, and resorption of bone in vitamin D-deficient rats. *J Clin Invest* 49:1122–1134, 1970.
2. Baylink D, Wergedal J, Stauffer M: Formation, mineralization, and resorption of bone in hypophosphatemic rats. *J Clin Invest* 50:2519–2530, 1971.
3. Bell KL, Loveridge N, Lindsay PC, et al: Cortical remodeling following suppression of endogenous estrogen with analogs of gonadotrophin releasing hormone. *J Bone Miner Res* 12:1231–1240, 1997.
4. Birkenhager-Frenkel DH, Birkenhager JC: Bone appositional rate and percentage of doubly and singly labeled surfaces: comparison of data from 5 and 20 micron sections. *Bone* 8:7–12, 1987.
5. Bosshardt D, Luder HU, Schroeder HE: Rate and growth pattern of cementum apposition as compared to dentine and root formation in a fluorochrome-labelled monkey (Macaca fascicularis). *J Biol Buccale* 17:3–13, 1989.
6. Böll S, Erben RG, Linsenmair E: Wie zuverlässig ist die skeletochronologische Altersbestimmung bei der Geburtshelferkröte *Alytes obstetricans?* In: Henle K, Vieth M, eds. *Naturschutzrelevante Methoden der Feldherpetologie—Mertensiella 7.* Deutsche Gesellschaft für Herpetologie und Terarrienkunde, Rheinbach, 1997:315–327.
7. Delmas PD, Vergnaud P, Arlot ME, et al: The anabolic effect of human PTH (1–34) on bone formation is blunted when bone resorption is inhibited by the bisphosphonate tiludronate—is activated resorption a prerequisite for the in vivo effect of PTH on formation in a remodeling system? *Bone* 16:603–610, 1995.
8. Engesaeter LB, Underdal T, Langeland N: Effects of oxytetracycline on mineralization of bone in young rats. *Acta Orthop Scand* 51:459–465, 1980.
9. Erben RG: Trabecular and endocortical bone surfaces in the rat: Modeling or remodeling? *Anat Rec* 246:39–46, 1996.
10. Erben RG: Unpublished results.
11. Erben RG, Eberle J, Stahr K, et al: Androgen deficiency induces high turnover osteopenia in aged male rats: a sequential histomorphometric study. *J Bone Miner Res* 15:1085–1098, 2000.
12. Erben RG, Mosekilde L, Thomsen JS, et al: Prevention of bone loss in ovariectomized rats by combined treatment with risedronate and $1\alpha,25$-dihydroxyvitamin D_3. *J Bone Miner Res* 17:1498–1511, 2002.
13. Erben RG, Scutt AM, Miao DS, et al: Short-term treatment of rats with high dose 1,25-dihydroxyvitamin D_3 stimulates bone formation and increases the number of osteoblast precursor cells in bone marrow. *Endocrinology* 138:4629–4635, 1997.
14. Francillon H, Castanet J: Experimental demonstration of the annual characteristic of the lines of arrest of skeletal growth in Rana esculenta (Amphibia, anura). *C R Acad Sci III* 300:327–332, 1985.

15. Frost HM: Relation between bone tissue and cell population dynamics, histology and tetracycline labeling. *Clin Orthop* 49:65–75, 1966.
16. Frost HM: Tetracycline-based histological analysis of bone remodeling. *Calcif Tissue Res* 3:211–237, 1969.
17. Frost HM: A method of analysis of trabecular bone dynamics. In: Meunier PJ, ed: *Bone Histomorphometry. Second International Workshop.* Armour Montagu, Paris, France, 1977:445–476.
18. Frost HM: Bone histomorphometry: choice of marking agent and labeling schedule. In: Recker RR, ed: *Bone Histomorphometry: Techniques and Interpretation.* CRC Press, Boca Raton, FL, 1983:37–52.
19. Frost HM: Bone histomorphometry: correction of labeling 'escape error.' In: Recker RR, ed: *Bone Histomorphometry: Techniques and Interpretation.* CRC Press, Boca Raton, FL, 1983:133–142.
20. Frost HM: *Intermediary Organization of the Skeleton.* CRC Press, Boca Raton, FL, 1986.
21. Frost HM: Skeletal structural adaptations to mechanical usage (SATMU): 1. Redefining Wolff's law: the bone modeling problem. *Anat Rec* 226:403–413, 1990.
22. Haas R, Donath K, Fodinger M, et al: Bovine hydroxyapatite for maxillary sinus grafting: comparative histomorphometric findings in sheep. *Clin Oral Implants Res* 9:107–116, 1998.
23. Iwaniec UT, Crenshaw TD: Distribution of mineralization indices of modeling and remodeling over eight months in middiaphyseal cross sections of femurs from adult swine. *Anat Rec* 250:136–145, 1998.
24. Jerome CP, Johnson CS, Vafai HAT, et al: Effect of treatment for 6 months with human parathyroid hormone (1–34) peptide in ovariectomized cynomolgus monkeys (*Macaca fascicularis*). *Bone* 25:301–309, 1999.
25. Jinno T, Goldberg VM, Davy D, et al: Osseointegration of surface-blasted implants made of titanium alloy and cobalt-chromium alloy in a rabbit intramedullary model. *J Biomed Mater Res* 42:20–29, 1998.
26. Klein L, Jackman KV: Assay of bone resorption in vivo with ^{3}H-tetracycline. *Calcif Tissue Res* 20:275–290, 1976.
27. Klein NC, Cunha BA: Tetracyclines. *Med Clin North Am* 79:789–801, 1995.
28. Lees CJ, Ramsay H: Histomorphometry and bone biomarkers in cynomolgus females: study in young, mature, and old monkeys. *Bone* 24:25–28, 1999.
29. Malluche HH, Faugere MC: *Atlas of Mineralized Bone Histology.* Karger, Basle, Switzerland, 1986.
30. Malouvier A, Martin F, Orus L, et al: Comparative use of calcein and oxytetracycline for the analysis of bone mineralisation in Rhesus monkeys. *Med Sci Res* 21:423–425, 1993.
31. Martin RB: Label escape theory revisited: the effects of resting periods and section thickness. *Bone* 10:255–264, 1989.
32. Miani A, Malossini L, Miani C: Alternate use of tetracycline and alizarin red S in the temporal study of osseous deposition. *Boll Soc Ital Biol Sper* 40:1260–1262, 1964.
33. Milch RA, Rall DP, Tobie JE: Fluorescence of tetracycline antibiotics in bone. *J Bone Joint Surg [Am]* 40:897–910, 1958.
34. Modis L, Petko M, Foldes I: Histochemical examination of supporting tissues by means of fluorescence. II. Fluorochromes as an indicator of lamellar bone mineralization. *Acta Morphol Acad Sci Hung* 17:157–166, 1969.
35. Mosekilde L, Weisbrode SE, Safron JA, et al: Evaluation of the skeletal effects of combined mild dietary calcium restriction and ovariectomy in Sinclair S-1 minipigs: A pilot study. *J Bone Miner Res* 8:1311–1321, 1993.
36. Nakamura T, Nagai Y, Yamato H, et al: Regulation of bone turnover and prevention of bone atrophy in ovariectomized beagle dogs by the administration of 24R,25(OH)$_2$D$_3$. *Calcif Tissue Int* 50:221–227, 1992.
37. Niederhagen B, Braumann B, Schmolke C, et al: Tooth-borne distraction of the mandible. An experimental study. *Int J Oral Maxillofac Surg* 28:475–479, 1999.

38. Ogura N, Mera T, Sato F, et al: Longitudinal observation of cementum regeneration through multiple fluorescent labeling. *J Periodontol* 62:284–291, 1991.

39. Paddock C, Youngs T, Eriksen E, et al: Validation of wall thickness estimates obtained with polarized light microscopy using multiple fluorochrome labels: correlation with erosion depth estimates obtained by lamellar counting. *Bone* 16:381–383, 1995.

40. Parfitt AM: The physiologic and clinical significance of bone histomorphometric data. In: Recker RR, ed: *Bone Histomorphometry: Techniques and Interpretation.* CRC Press, Boca Raton, FL, 1983:143–223.

41. Parfitt AM: The cellular basis of bone remodeling: the quantum concept reexamined in light of recent advances in the cell biology of bone. *Calcif Tissue Int* 36:S37–S45, 1984.

42. Parfitt AM, Drezner MK, Glorieux FH, et al: Bone histomorphometry: standardization of nomenclature, symbols, and units. Report of the ASBMR Histomorphometry Nomenclature Committee. *J Bone Miner Res* 2:595–610, 1987.

43. Parfitt AM, Foldes J, Villanueva AR, et al: Difference in label length between demethylchlortetracycline and oxytetracycline: implications for the interpretation of bone histomorphometric data. *Calcif Tissue Int* 48:74–77, 1991.

44. Parfitt AM, Villanueva AR, Foldes J, et al: Relations between histologic indices of bone formation: implications for the pathogenesis of spinal osteoporosis. *J Bone Miner Res* 10:466–473, 1995.

45. Rahn BA: Die polychrome Fluoreszenzmarkierung des Knochenanbaus—Instrumentelle Aspekte und experimentelle Anwendung. *Zeiss Informationen* 22/85:36–39, 1976.

46. Rahn BA, Perren SM: Calcein blue as a fluorescent label in bone. *Experientia* 26:519–520, 1970.

47. Rahn BA, Perren SM: Xylenol orange, a fluorochrome useful in polychrome sequential labeling of calcifying tissues. *Stain Technol* 46:125–129, 1971.

48. Rahn BA, Perren SM: Alizarin complexon-fluorochrome for bone and dentine labeling. *Experientia* 28:180–184, 1972.

49. Ramser JR, Villanueva AR, Frost HM: Cortical bone dynamics in osteomalacia, measured by tetracycline bone-labeling. *Clin Orthop* 49:89–102, 1966.

50. Rasmussen P: Effect of oxytetracycline and purified calcein (DCAF) on the apposition and mineralization of rat incisor dentin. *Scand J Dent Res* 83:233–237, 1975.

51. Recker RR, Kimmel DB, Parfitt AM, et al: Static and tetracycline-based bone histomorphometric data from 34 normal postmenopausal females. *J Bone Miner Res* 3:133–144, 1988.

52. Savage CJ, Jeffcott LB, Melsen F, et al: Bone biopsy in the horse. 1. Method using the wing of ilium. *Zentralbl Veterinarmed A* 38:776–783, 1991.

53. Savage CJ, Tidd LC, Melsen F, et al: Bone biopsy in the horse. 2. Evaluation of histomorphometric examination. *Zentralbl Veterinarmed A* 38:784–792, 1991.

54. Schemitsch EH, Turchin DC, Kowalski MJ, et al: Quantitative assessment of bone injury and repair after reamed and unreamed locked intramedullary nailing. *J Trauma* 45:250–255, 1988.

55. Schliephake H, Neukam FW, Hutmacher D, et al: Experimental transplantation of hydroxylapatite-bone composite grafts. *J Oral Maxillofac Surg* 53:46–51, 1995.

56. Schmidt J, Lumniczky K, Tzschaschel BD, et al: Onset and dynamics of osteosclerosis in mice induced by Reilly-Finkel-Biskis (RFB) murine leukemia virus—increase in bone mass precedes lymphomagenesis. *Am J Pathol* 155:557–570, 1999.

57. Sheng MH, Baylink DJ, Beamer WG, et al: Histomorphometric studies show that bone formation and bone mineral apposition rates are greater in C3H/HeJ (high-density) than C57BL/6J (low-density) mice during growth. *Bone* 25:421–429, 1999.

58. Snow GR, Anderson C: The effects of 17 beta-estradiol and progestagen on trabecular bone remodeling in oophorectomized dogs. *Calcif Tissue Int* 39:198–205, 1986.

59. Svalastoga E, Reimann I, Nielsen K: A method for quantitative assessment of bone formation using double labelling with tetracycline and calcein. An experimental study in the navicular bone of the horse. *Nord Vet Med* 35:180–183, 1983.

60. Takumida M, Zhang DM, Yajin K, et al: Polychromatic labeling of otoconia for the investigation of calcium turnover. *ORL J Otorhinolaryngol Relat Spec* 59:4–9, 1997.
61. Tam CS, Anderson W: Tetracycline labeling of bone in vivo. *Calcif Tissue Int* 30:121–125, 1980.
62. Tisdel CL, Goldberg VM, Parr JA, et al: The influence of a hydroxyapatite and tricalcium-phosphate coating on bone growth into titanium fiber-metal implants. *J Bone Joint Surg [Am]* 76:159–171, 1994.
63. Tonna EA, Singh IJ, Sandhu HS: Non-radioactive tracer techniques for calcified tissues. In: Dickson GR, ed. *Methods of Calcified Tissue Preparation.* Elsevier, Amsterdam, The Netherlands, 1984:333–367.
64. Treharne RW, Brighton CT: The use and possible misuse of tetracycline as a vital stain. *Clin Orthop* 140:240–246, 1979.
65. Turner RT: Cancellous bone turnover in growing rats: time-dependent changes in association between calcein label and osteoblasts. *J Bone Miner Res* 9:1419–1424, 1994.
66. Turner RT, Evans GL, Wakley GK: Mechanism of action of estrogen on cancellous bone balance in tibiae of ovariectomized growing rats: Inhibition of indices of formation and resorption. *J Bone Miner Res* 8:359–366, 1993.
67. Urist MR, Ibsen KH: Chemical reactivity of mineralized tissue with oxytetracycline. *Arch Pathol* 76:484–496, 1963.
68. Villanueva AR, Ilnicki L, Duncan H, et al: Bone and cell dynamics in the osteoporoses: a review of measurements by tetracycline bone labeling. *Clin Orthop* 49:135–150, 1966.
69. Wilson AK, Bhattacharyya MH, Miller S, et al: Ovariectomy-induced changes in aged beagles: Histomorphometry of rib cortical bone. *Calcif Tissue Int* 62:237–243, 1998.
70. Wronski TJ, Morey ER: Inhibition of cortical and trabecular bone formation in the long bones of immobilized monkeys. *Clin Orthop* 181:269–276, 1983.

6

Human Bone Biopsy

Robert S. Weinstein

Division of Endocrinology and Metabolism, Center for Osteoporosis and Metabolic Bone Diseases,
Department of Internal Medicine, and the Central Arkansas Veterans Healthcare System,
University of Arkansas for Medical Sciences, Little Rock, AR, USA

I. INTRODUCTION

During the last 15 years, the diagnostic approach to metabolic disorders of the skeleton has been considerably enhanced by new developments in bone densitometry and biochemical measurements of ionized calcium, parathyroid hormone, vitamin D metabolites, bone alkaline phosphatase, and urinary excretion of bone collagen fragments. Experience with these new tools now facilitates the detection and diagnosis of subtle abnormalities of bone metabolism that were previously unrecognized on routine radiographic images or with multi-channel chemistry panels.

However, bone loss in some patients remains unexplained even with these diagnostic advances, and therefore examination of bone biopsy specimens remains an indispensable part of the evaluation of disorders of bone and mineral metabolism. The analysis of bone specimens has rapidly evolved from the primordial studies of decalcified, rongeured bone fragments. Nordin and Bordier pioneered the use of unique trephines necessary to obtain an intact specimen of cortical and cancellous bone in an outpatient setting.[3] With the advent of plastic embedding and sledge microtomes, undecalcified bone sections that distinguish mineralized bone from osteoid became available.[5,8] Arguably, the most important advance was the pioneering work of Frost on the application of quantitative analysis to tetracycline-labeled bone.[2] The incorporation of tetracycline markers in newly mineralized bone allowed the first direct measurements of the rate of bone formation. Today, the use of microprocessor-operated, stereomicroscope-guided, heavy-duty rotary microtomes, computers with drawing tubes and digitizing tablets, and digital cameras with sophisticated image-analysis software contribute speed, precision, and accuracy to the histomorphometric examination of bone whether viewed by bright-field, epifluorescence, polarized light, phase-contrast, or differential interference contrast microscopy. A histomorphometric examination of bone is much more than a qualitative look at the overall structure and arrangement of bone tissue. Histomorphometry comprises a large repertoire of possible measurements including: cortical width and porosity; cancellous microarchitecture (trabecular width, separation, and number), osteoid area and width, wall width (the width of newly completed packets of bone); counts of osteoblasts, osteocytes,

From: *Handbook of Histology Methods for Bone and Cartilage*
Edited by: Y. H. An and K. L. Martin © Humana Press Inc., Totowa, NJ

and osteoclasts; the prevalence of bone-cell apoptosis; and kinetic measurements of bone formation. Selection of the best tissue specimens and subset of measurements to address a particular question is crucial. Correct interpretation of the results of the examination requires cooperation between clinician, biopsy operator, and histopathologist, and therefore to increase communication in this rapidly expanding field, the nomenclature, symbols, and units of bone histomorphometry have been standardized.[10]

II. REQUIREMENTS FOR BONE BIOPSY

A. When to Do a Bone Biopsy

- Unexplained bone loss.
- Borderline or inconclusive lab findings.
- Rapid progression *(Could this much bone loss have occurred since menopause?)*
- Unusually painful.
- Skeletal fragility with normal bone mineral density.
- Recognize subtle osteomalacia.
- Distinguish between the various forms of renal osteodystrophy.
- Chronic hypophosphatemia.

Bone biopsy is usually required to recognize subtle osteomalacia[1] and to distinguish between the various forms of renal osteodystrophy.[7] Bone biopsy may also be indispensable in the evaluation of a patient with unusually painful disease, rapidly progressive loss of bone density, or skeletal fragility with normal bone-mineral-density values, particularly when the results of the physical examination, radiographs, and biochemical findings are ambiguous. Biopsy is indicated in patients with unexplained chronic hypophosphatemia or long-term elevation of the bone alkaline phosphatase concentration. In osteoporosis, bone biopsy is the only method that reveals the trabecular architecture, so that the clinician can determine whether the bone loss is caused by trabecular atrophy, interruption of trabecular continuity, or both, and bone biopsy is the best way to reveal whether bone turnover is low, normal or elevated.[6,17] If treatment successfully increases bone mass, only biopsy can definitively show whether the new bone is of normal quality, the extent of restoration of the microarchitecture, and the treatment-induced changes in the rate of bone formation. For these reasons, the majority of bone biopsies performed today are done in pharmaceutical trials.

B. Limitations of Bone Biopsy

- Sample of only a single, relatively small skeletal site.
- Primary pathophysiology which caused bone loss may have abated but transient effects from medication may affect biopsy interpretation.
- Main usefulness is in renal osteodystrophy or suspected occult osteomalacia.
- The rate of bone resorption is difficult to estimate, except in diseases with extremely high bone turnover such as Paget's disease or severe renal hyperparathyroidism.

There are four limitations to the clinical utility of bone biopsy. The most restrictive of these is that bone biopsy samples only a single skeletal site. Clinicians are often concerned with the question of how representative the specimen is of the whole skeleton, because disorders such as postmenopausal osteoporosis and renal osteodystrophy are known to show considerable regional variation. However, the variation is usually in the severity of the findings; all bones show at least some recognizable involvement. Nevertheless, large regional variations in the rate of bone formation have been documented. In one

74-yr-old woman with osteoporosis who received two courses of oral tetracycline before she died, the bone formation rate was much lower in the spine than at the standard biopsy site, but this was caused by variation in the tetracycline-labeled cancellous perimeter rather than differences in the mineral appositional rate (MAR).[12]

The second limitation occurs when the primary pathophysiology that caused the loss of bone mass has abated or ceased and the current rate of bone remodeling is within normal limits. Even in this circumstance, bone histomorphometry based on the width of interstitial bone, contour of the cement lines, trabecular microarchitecture, and shape of the resorption cavities may reveal information about the original process.[9,11]

The third limitation is that convincing evidence of clinical benefit of bone biopsy in therapeutic decisions is primarily available in occult osteomalacia and renal osteodystrophy.[1,7] At present, subdivision of patients with osteoporosis into groups with normal, elevated, or low bone turnover based on bone biopsy has not facilitated choice of effective therapy.

The fourth limitation is the difficulty in estimating the rate of bone resorption by histomorphometry. However, because bone formation and bone resorption are closely coupled, the rate of bone formation is an index of skeletal turnover.[18] Under most circumstances, the error incurred by assuming that the rates of bone resorption and formation are equal is about 10%, less than the error of the measurements.[10] A unique phenomenon allowing direct measurement of the rate of bone resorption sometimes occurs in patients with greatly accelerated bone turnover. Aggressive osteoclasts in Paget's disease of bone or in recently postmenopausal women may be seen to pass through the tetracycline labels, which then act as temporal goalposts. From the depth of the erosion cavity through the double labels, the time of the last tetracycline administration and the date of the bone biopsy procedure, the minimum initial rate of bone resorption can be calculated in μm/d just as precisely as the MAR is measured from the distance between the double labels divided by the days between the courses of oral tetracycline administration.[16]

C. Bone Biopsy Arrangements

- First, learn as much as possible about the tetracycline labeling and bone biopsy procedure.
- Next, find an *experienced* bone biopsy operator.
- Locate a specialist in bone histomorphometry.
- Recruit someone to fix the core and do the paperwork.
- Let the subject read about the biopsy before you do the physical exam. After you complete the exam, tell her about the procedure. Give her a pictorial image of the tetracycline. Tell her to avoid dairy products, calcium, and antacids with the tetracycline. Highlight the steps taken to ensure her comfort: pre-biopsy analgesia, *Novocaine,* and suture removal.

Once it has been determined that a bone biopsy is needed, several arrangements must be carefully made. Foremost are the requirements to find a physician who understands and can explain the tetracycline regimen to the patient and an operator who is experienced in obtaining bone biopsy specimens with a large-diameter trephine.* Next, a pathologist must be recruited to help with proper fixation of the bone core and processing of the necessary paperwork. Most pathology laboratories cannot process undecalcified bone specimens or do histomorphometry, so unless the pathologist is familiar with plastic

---

* An excellent bone biopsy trephine is the Trocart de Bordier mod. Meunier in 8 mm, obtained from Lepine a Lyon, Instruments de Chirurge, Lyon, France.

Table 1. Instructions for Patients Scheduled For Bone Biopsy

1. Take the tetracycline capsules EXACTLY as ordered: one capsule three or four times a day for 3 days,_____, then 2 weeks without any tetracycline, and then one capsule three or four times a day for 3 more days,_____. Please notify Dr._____ if you have ever received any other tetracycline medications such as Achromycin, Tetracyn, Panmycin, Sumycin, Aureomycin, Terramycin, Declomycin, Rondomycin, Mysteclin, Vibramycin, or Minocin.
2. Mark the days on your calendar!
3. On the two 3-day periods that you take the tetracycline, you must avoid dairy products (especially milk), antacids (such as Tums, Maalox, Amphojel, Rolaids), calcium supplements, and iron-containing medications. During the 2-week interval without any tetracycline, you may take any food or medication that you used previously.
4. On the morning of the bone biopsy, have only a very light breakfast.
5. Come to the procedure room at 8:30 a.m. on_____.
6. You will be ready to return home before noon. Have someone ready to take you back home just in case the biopsy anesthetic medication has made you sleepy.
7. Call Dr. (_____) _____-_____, if you have any problems or questions or if you are sensitive or allergic to Demerol, Valium, Novacaine, Betadine, or adhesive gauze pads.
8. After the biopsy, the area must stay dry and covered with a gauze pad for 2 days. The sutures should be removed in 1 week. You may return to your normal daily activities as soon as you feel up to it. Results from the microscopic evaluation will be available in about 2 weeks. Dr._____will call you to discuss the findings as soon as they are available.

Adapted from Weinstein RS: The clinical use of bone biopsy. In: Coe FL, Favus MJ, eds: *Disorders of Bone and Mineral Metabolism.* Raven Press Ltd., New York, NY, 1992:455–474.

embedding and quantitative histological analysis, the specimen should be referred to a specialist in histomorphometry. Often the best solution is to refer the patient to the histomorphometry center for biopsy. This ensures satisfactory communication between the clinician, operator, and histopathologist, and is the best insurance against the incomplete, broken, or fragmented cores obtained by inexperienced operators.

Arrangements must begin as soon as possible, since the procedure must be delayed for 24 d while the patient receives two time-spaced courses of oral tetracycline (Table 1). The labeling regimen should be explained graphically to the patient to help ensure compliance with the instructions. A picture of the rings in a tree stump is a valuable visual aid (Fig. 1).

Several special situations may arise. Occasionally, the specimen may be obtained in the operating room at the time of an unrelated procedure, during an osteotomy, or in children under 12 or 13 years of age, in whom it is not reasonable to attempt the procedure with local anesthesia. In these cases, the clinician should go to the operating room to guarantee that an adequate specimen is obtained and properly fixed. Once obtained, a core for undecalcified quantitative histological analysis should remain in sight until it is brought or mailed to the histomorphometry laboratory. Remember that routine bone samples from the operating room are usually cut into small pieces and decalcified as soon as they are logged in at the surgical pathology receiving area. Surgical bone specimens are sometimes obtained from a fracture site, but these specimens are of little or no value in the evaluation of metabolic disorders.

Some patients refuse meperidine before the biopsy, and patients with epilepsy should not receive meperidine because it lowers the seizure threshold. In these situations, the procedure can be done comfortably with only diazepam and local lidocaine. Patients

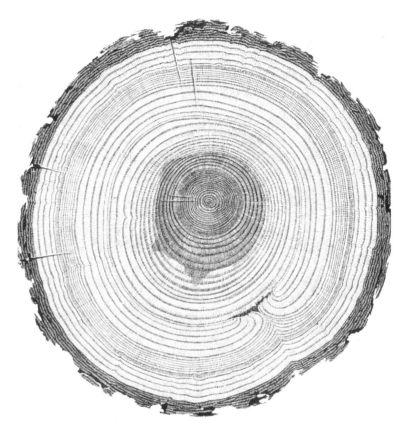

Figure 1. A picture of the rings visible on a smooth tree stump helps to explain the tetracycline regimen to the patient. A light and dark ring are made each year (xylem and phloem). Closely spaced rings indicate years of light rainfall or drought during which the tree had minimal growth. Widely spaced rings indicate abundant rainfall and luxuriant growth.

with severe diarrhea or malabsorption must receive 2 or 3 g of tetracycline each day of their labeling regimen to ensure that enough tetracycline is absorbed to make a clearly visible mark in bone. If there is a convincing history of allergy to tetracycline, doxycycline may be used, but the pale green fluorescent labels that result may require epifluorescence with a mercury light source for adequate visualization. When the patient has recently received previous tetracycline treatment for acne, prostatitis, bronchitis, or bacterial intestinal overgrowth, the bone-labeling regimen must use a different tetracycline that gives a contrasting fluorescence. Demeclocycline appears orange yellow, doxycycline pale green, oxytetracycline leaf green, and tetracycline golden yellow. Even with the use of different tetracyclines, the colors of the individual labels may be difficult to distinguish and multiple fluorescent rings in the specimen may complicate measurement of the rate of bone formation.

With the closed-needle transilial bone biopsy procedure described in Section IID below, it is not necessary to reschedule hemodialysis periods or attempt to normalize the bleeding time. However, it is a good idea to avoid aspirin for several days before and after a biopsy. Coumadin therapy must be interrupted. Coagulation studies should be monitored in patients with known bleeding disorders.

Despite all possible precautions, there are times when a specimen is broken or otherwise damaged. Of course, a qualitative analysis can still be done, but measurements of the cancellous bone area, trabecular spacing, and cortical width may be impossible. In fragmented cores, the bone perimeter may be too disrupted for measurements of the osteoid, osteoblast, osteoclast, and reversal perimeters. However, even in severely damaged cores, the osteoid area/bone area, osteoid width, trabecular width, and the MAR usually remain measurable.

D. Transilial Closed Needle Bone Biopsy

Percutaneous transilial bone biopsy is a simple process that can be learned after observing the procedure and practicing on a cadaver. Orthopedic surgeons may offer to do the biopsy, but are usually unfamiliar with the biopsy trephines used for the investigation of metabolic bone diseases, and are unaware of the necessity to obtain an intact specimen from a standardized location. Experience with at least 25–30 patients is necessary before the operator can reliably obtain bone cores with both cortices and the intervening cancellous bone tissue intact for a quantitative histological analysis. Since approx 0.5 mm of the cylindrical bone biopsy core diameter is damaged by the cutting teeth, the internal diameter of the trephine must be 7.0–8.0 mm to obtain an undamaged core of 6.0–7.0-mm diameter, which is required for measurement of the trabecular microarchitecture. The transilial approach is best, because patient discomfort is minimal and most of the normal tetracycline-labeled reference values have been obtained with this technique.[18] Biopsies obtained through other procedures may yield less ideal specimens. Vertical iliac crest biopsies have only one cortex and a distorted distal end, and are usually only 3–4 mm in diameter. Specimens obtained with an electric drill have as much as 1.0 mm damage at their circumference, and contain smashed bone and bone powder at their proximal and distal margins. If the drill is stuck, the resulting heat may severely damage the core. Wedge sections of the iliac crest are absolutely contraindicated. They are difficult to adequately fix, and cause moderate to severe pain at the biopsy site for more than 1 yr. Rib biopsies are also contraindicated in metabolic diseases of the skeleton because of their paucity of cancellous bone tissue in the specimen and the significant risk of pneumothorax. The author has used the following outpatient transilial closed-needle bone biopsy technique for over 20 years. The procedure is safe, the anterior-superior ilium is easy to anesthetize, and normal data from this site is readily available.[18] Several other techniques have been described,[1,3–5,13–15] but it is apparent that closed-needle biopsy procedures have the lowest rate of complications.[4,13] About 5% of patients may develop a small superficial ecchymosis.

After just a light breakfast, the patient gives a signed informed consent and is premedicated with 50–75 mg of meperidine and 10–15 mg of diazepam (intramuscularly) about 30 min before the procedure. An examination table with foot pedal controls is desirable. The patient must be supine with legs outstretched, elbows touching the table, and hands folded over the chest. The appropriate hip is elevated on several folded sheets placed well under the buttock (Fig. 2). A felt-tip pen is used to mark a point 2.5 cm posterior and inferior to the anterior-superior iliac spine and clearly below the external lip of the iliac crest. A second point is marked 2–3 cm medial to the crest of the ilium in a line with the first point and the opposite elbow. After a povidone-iodine or hexachlorophene scrub,

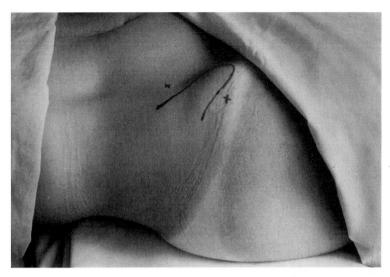

Figure 2. Biopsy site and patient positioning. The patient's hip is elevated on several folded sheets placed under the buttock. The biopsy site (+) is 2.5-cm posterior and inferior to the anterior-superior iliac spine and clearly below the external lip of the iliac crest. A second point (+) is marked 2–3 cm medial to the crest of the ilium in a line with the first point and the opposite elbow to facilitate anesthesia of the medial iliac periosteum.

drapes are applied and a skin wheal is made at both marked points with 0.5% lidocaine without epinephrine and a 0.5-in. 25–gauge needle on a 3-mL syringe. The subcutaneous tissue, fascia, and lateral iliac periosteum are anesthetized with 5–10 mL of 0.5% lido-caine and a 1.5-in. 18-gauge needle on a 10-mL syringe. With a 10-mL three-finger con-trol syringe and a 5-in. 20-gauge anesthesia needle inserted at the second point, the medial iliac periosteum is explored, and if there is no blood return, anesthetized with an additional 5 mL of lidocaine. Next, with a No. 3 knife handle and No. 15 blade, a 1.5–2.0 cm incision is made parallel to the iliac crest at the first point. After incising the superfi-cial fascia, a single stab incision is made and extended down to the lateral periosteum. Enough lidocaine should be used so that the patient is unable to feel pain during this part of the procedure. The outer sleeve of the biopsy needle is placed over the large trocar and delivered to the lateral periosteum with a gentle twisting motion until the teeth of the sleeve rest on the ilium. The trocar is then withdrawn, and the outer sleeve is aimed toward the contralateral elbow and anchored to the lateral ilium by a few taps with the handle of the large trocar.

The patient is told, "You will hear a knock, like a knock at a door, but it will not hurt." With the sleeve held down firmly to act as a guide for the trephine, the cutting trephine is slowly inserted with a gentle to-and-fro rotary motion until it has transfixed the inner cor-tex and the hub of the trephine meets the top of the outer sleeve. Heavy pressure on the trephine must be avoided. If the medial iliac periosteum has not been completely anes-thetized, the patient will feel a momentary pain at the time the inner cortex is penetrated. Excessive penetration is prevented by the hub of the trephine. The trephine is then rotated 360° several times to separate the specimen from the underlying tissue. With the operator's thumb held tightly over the distal opening of the trephine, the instrument is slowly withdrawn, 1–2 mm at a time, with the same rotary motion that was used for insertion.

The long, thin, blunt trocar is then used to gently push the bone core out of the trephine and into the cold fixative. If the specimen does not come out of the trephine easily, a few light taps with the handle of the large trocar will suffice to expel it. If the core does not have both cortices or is otherwise inadequate, a second try should be made through the same incision. A 0.5 × 3 in. piece of absorbable hemostat gauze (oxidized regenerated cellulose, Surgicel®) is placed into the biopsy hole with the small trocar, and then the small trocar, and outer sleeve are withdrawn. The wound is closed with two or three 3-0 nylon sutures, and after application of benzoin, a pressure dressing is made with fluffed gauze and an elastic bandage. The procedure takes about 30–45 min, and blood loss is usually less than 1 mL. The patient is instructed to turn over and lie on the pressure dressing for about 1 h, after which the dressing is removed, a small adhesive gauze pad is applied, and the patient may go home. The wound should stay dry for 48 h, and sutures are removed in 1 wk. Most patients do not require more than 2–3 d of acetaminophen for analgesia, and readily agree to a second biopsy. A repeat biopsy to evaluate the response to therapy or to reveal the natural course of a disorder must be done on the opposite side. The first side should be avoided as a biopsy site for at least 1 yr.

E. Bone Biopsy Specimen Handling Procedures

- 7-mm transiliac bone cores will be fixed in about 50 mL of 4°C Millonig's buffered formalin (please check that the pH=7.4).
- After 20–24 h in cold Millonig's, transfer the core to a clean 20-mL glass vial filled with 70% ethanol and keep at 4°C.
- Put a 1 × 4 cm strip of index card with the subject's name, allocation number, and the date of biopsy written in pencil inside the vial with the specimen, tighten the cap, and seal with several wraps of lab film.
- Wrap the vial with padding, surround it with mailer ice packs and send by Federal Express.
- Include a sheet with the tetracycline regimen dates, subject's name, investigator's name, and FAX number.

The freshly obtained bone core is fixed in approx 50 mL of 4°C Millonig's buffered formalin[**] at pH 7.4 (also available from Fisher Scientific or SurgiPath). An emesis basin filled with ice can be used to keep the fixative cold in the procedure room, after which the container should be placed in a refrigerator. The cortices of a well-obtained specimen display a parallelogram appearance (Fig. 3). After 20–24 h in cold Millonig's, the core is gently transferred with a small pickup or jeweler's forceps to a clean 20-mL glass vial filled with 70% ethanol, and kept at 4°C. To ensure that identification is maintained, a 1 × 4 cm strip of index card with the subject's name, allocation number and the date of biopsy is written in pencil (to avoid dissolution by the fixatives) is placed inside the vial with the specimen. After tightening the cap and sealing the top with several layers of labfilm, the vial is swaddled with bubble wrap and surrounded with mailer ice packs before shipping by express mail. A sheet with the tetracycline regimen dates, subject's name, investigator's name, telephone, and fax number in a waterproof plastic bag is included in the package.

[**] Millonig's Fixative: 100 mL 37% formalin in 900 mL distilled water containing 18.6 g NaH_2PO_4, 4.2 g NaOH and 5 g sucrose. Adjust pH to 7.4 with a few drops of 1 N NaOH.

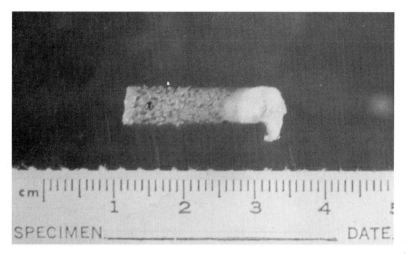

Figure 3. A freshly obtained transilial bone biopsy core showing the typical parallelogram appearance of an adequate specimen.

Acknowledgments: This work was supported by the National Institutes of Health (PO1-AG13918 and RO1-AR46191) and VA Merit Review and Research Enhancement Award Program (REAP) Grants from the Veterans Administration.

REFERENCES

1. Byers PD: The diagnostic value of bone biopsies. In: Avioli LV, Krane SM, eds: *Metabolic Bone Diseases, Vol 1*. Academic Press, New York, NY, 1977;183–236.
2. Frost HM: *Bone Remodeling and Its Relationship to Metabolic Bone Diseases*. Charles C. Thomas, Springfield, IL, 1973.
3. Hodgkinson A, Knowles CF: Laboratory methods. In: Nordin BEC, ed: *Calcium, Phosphate and Magnesium Metabolism: Clinical Physiology and Diagnostic Procedures*. Churchill Livingstone, New York, NY, 1976:516–524.
4. Hodgson SF, Johnson KA, Mults JM, et al: Outpatient percutaneous biopsy of the iliac crest: methods, morbidity and patient acceptance. *Mayo Clin Proc* 61:28–33, 1986.
5. Jowsey J: *The Bone Biopsy*. Plenum Press, New York, NY, 1977:59–89.
6. Kleerekoper M, Villanueva AR, Stanciu J, et al: The role of three-dimensional trabecular microstructure in the pathogenesis of vertebral compression fractures. *Calcif Tissue Int* 37:594–597, 1985.
7. Malluche HH, Faugere MC: Renal osteodystrophy. *N Engl J Med* 321:317–318, 1989.
8. Merz WA, Schenk RK: Quantitative structural analysis of human cancellous bone. *Acta Anat* 75:54–66, 1970.
9. Parfitt AM, Podenphant J, Villanueva AR, Frame B: Metabolic bone disease with and without osteomalacia after intestinal bypass surgery: a bone histomorphometric study. *Bone* 6:211–220, 1985.
10. Parfitt AM, Drezner MK, Glorieux FH, et al: Bone histomorphometry: standardization of nomenclature, symbols, and units. *J Bone Miner Res* 2:595–610, 1987.
11. Parfitt AM, Foldes J: The ambiguity of interstitial bone thickness: a new approach to the mechanism of trabecular thinning. *Bone* 12:119–122, 1991.
12. Podenphant J, Engel U: Regional variations in histomorphometric bone dynamics from the skeleton of an osteoporotic woman. *Calcif Tissue Int* 40:184–188, 1987.

13. Rao DS: Practical approach to bone biopsy. In: Recker RR, ed: *Bone Histomorphometry: Techniques and Interpretation.* CRC Press, Boca Raton, FL, 1983:3–11.

14. Rasmussen H, Bordier P. *The Physiological and Cellular Basis of Metabolic Bone Disease.* Williams & Wilkins, Baltimore, MD, 1974:57–69.

15. Recker RR, ed. *Bone Histomorphometry: Techniques and Interpretation.* CRC Press, Boca Raton, FL, 1983.

16. Reid IR, Nicholson GC, Weinstein RS, et al: Alendronate in Paget's Disease. *Am J Med* 101:341–348, 1996.

17. Weinstein RS, Hutson MS: Decreased trabecular width and increased trabecular spacing contribute to bone loss with aging. *Bone* 8:137–142, 1987.

18. Weinstein RS, Bell NH: Diminished rates of bone formation in normal black adults. *N Engl J Med* 319:1698–1701, 1988.

7

Biopsy Issues for Bone and Cartilage Tumors

John L. Eady

Department of Orthopaedic Surgery, University of South Carolina
School of Medicine, Columbia, SC, USA

I. INTRODUCTION

Biopsy of soft tissue and osseous musculoskeletal lesions is the final step in the staging workup of an unknown tumor, and the first step in therapeutic management.[4,10,19,21] Because of this overlapping role, biopsy is arguably the most critical process in the management of musculoskeletal tumors.[4,10,14,15] Inappropriate biopsies result in the need for more extensive surgical procedures than initially required, and can be the direct cause of death in patients with musculoskeletal tumors.[9,13,14,15] Two well-documented reports in the literature spaced 14 years apart[13,14] show that biopsies for musculoskeletal tumors continue to be inappropriately planned, placed, and utilized. When this occurs, patients with malignant musculoskeletal tumors need limb amputations instead of salvage procedures for appropriate tumor control, and 4.5% of the time, the ill-planned and executed biopsy is the direct cause of amputation of the patient's limb and can contribute to the patient's death.[4,11,13,14,18] For these reasons, it is important to revisit the issue of the biopsy, focusing on the types of biopsy, appropriate evaluations prior to the biopsy, technical aspects of this procedure, and consequences of the ill-planned or executed biopsy. At the end of this chapter, an outline for appropriate uses of this important tool is provided.

II. CONSEQUENCES OF AN INAPPROPRIATE BIOPSY

The consequences of inappropriate biopsy are numerous. Local consequences have been mentioned in Section I, and include complication rates as high as 19.3% and unnecessary amputations as high as 4.5%. Mankin et al. reported these findings in 1982 and in 1996.[13,14] Simon,[21] in a second study of patients who underwent biopsy for bone or soft-tissue sarcomas, showed that the differences in patient function and survival outcome between referring and oncology centers were unchanged. Therefore, if one wishes to prevent major errors in the diagnosis of 13–18% and complication rates of 15–17%, as well as unnecessary amputations of 3–5%, one should avoid the inappropriate biopsy at all costs. The following errors represent the spectrum of biopsy errors, but are not all-inclusive.

From: *Handbook of Histology Methods for Bone and Cartilage*
Edited by: Y. H. An and K. L. Martin © Humana Press Inc., Totowa, NJ

A. *Local and Systemic*

1. Excessive bleeding—most high-grade sarcomas bleed profusely when cut into, so be prepared to control bleeding with measures including a watertight layered closure at the completion of the procedure. For bone biopsies, be prepared to plug the hole with methyl methacrylate (MMA) to help control the bleeding.

2. Multiple-compartment contamination[4] may be caused by crossing more than one compartment while performing the biopsy. Usually this is a result of the operating surgeon's adherence to routine surgical principles of dissecting between intermuscular planes to avoid blood loss. This habit should be avoided without exception. It is rarely necessary to violate more than one compartment to obtain a proper specimen.

3. Inadequate sampling resulting from inappropriate sampling.[19] This is often caused by sampling of the necrotic portion of a highly malignant sarcoma in which over 90% of the tumor has infarcted and the only viable portion of the lesion is a thin rim (<1 cm) of peripheral tissue. Another example is sampling the reactive but normal periosteum (Codman's Triangle) over an intraosseus malignancy, either primary or metastatic. This type of material can be inappropriately misinterpreted by the most experienced pathologist, with over- and under-diagnoses.

4. Propagation of metastatic foci, usually resulting from repeated manipulations of neoplastic processes. This can occur with benign as well as malignant lesions. For example, it is adequately documented that repeated manipulations of a giant-cell tumor raise the risk of chest metastases.

5. Inappropriate placement/orientation of biopsy sites, causing greater loss of function of the extremity or even death of the patient.[4,13,14,15] Transverse incisions on an extremity, incisions parallel to major neurovascular bundles (exceptions—neural tumors or hemangiomatous lesions) and in major joint creases (popliteal fossa, antecubital fossa, axillary and antecubital fossa) create, at the very least, the necessity for large soft-tissue resections to eliminate the contaminated biopsy site, thereby eliminating function, which could be salvaged safely with the definitive procedure. This type of biopsy management can even result in amputation of the limb to eliminate the contaminated biopsy tract with the actual tumor. Death of the patient can also be the result of an inappropriate biopsy.

III. USES OF THE BIOPSY

The casual observer or infrequent performer of the biopsy can be misled into believing that the biopsy is useful only for diagnostic purposes. Although a biopsy is diagnostic in most cases, its value in present-day management of musculoskeletal lesions is much more critical and detailed.[3,6,8]

Biopsy uses include: diagnostic, assay, confirmatory, and therapeutic applications. Obtaining tissue for diagnostic purposes is the most frequent use of the biopsy, but the assay, confirmatory, and therapeutic biopsies are equally important, although less often employed. For instance, the nonossifying fibroma (also known as fibrous cortical defect), enchondroma, osteochondroma, bone infarct, hemangioma, fibrous dysplasia, multiloculated cyst, and osteomyelitis can often be reasonably and safely diagnosed, with a careful history, physical exam, and knowledgeable interpretation of appropriate laboratory and radiographic material.[4] Even some of the soft-tissue lesions such as hemangioma, myositis ossificans, traumatic muscle rupture, neurilemmoma, lipoma, and neurofibroma can be sorted out without employing the biopsy.[16,17]

However, each of the conditions noted here may require a biopsy to firmly diagnose because it does not "fit" the established (historical), expected, predictable behavior patterns or have acceptable radiographic and/or laboratory findings for its presentation in a specific patient.[16,17]

It is important to note that all of these lesions were routinely biopsied during some period in the past until enough information was collected from these biopsies and the radiographic material to safely and reasonably confirm that routine biopsy was not required, as long as the presentation "fit" expected clinical behavior as well as appropriate laboratory and radiographic findings. Even today, a definitive diagnosis of musculoskeletal lesions can only be confirmed by biopsy—or as one of my more irreverent residents was fond of quoting, "if tumor is the rumor, tissue is the issue." Therefore, the diagnostic biopsy is used to make a definitive diagnosis of the musculoskeletal lesion that cannot be reasonably and safely identified by the clinical behavior and the laboratory and radiographic information collected on it.[16,17]

Although diagnostic biopsy is not required or even necessary in many bony musculoskeletal lesions today, it is more often necessary in soft-tissue musculoskeletal lesions, as both benign and malignant soft-tissue defects can display similar findings on clinical exam and the laboratory/radiographic studies presently available to investigate them.[1,2,7,9,15]

Needless to say, if the history, physical, and laboratory data, including the radiographic and laboratory investigations, remain nebulous in the workup of a musculoskeletal tumor, the diagnostic biopsy becomes necessary. Keep in mind that even when the diagnostic biopsy becomes necessary, it cannot be done without the required pre-operative investigations,[16,17] as the biopsy done without this information can result in the necessity for a more extensive than necessary limb-salvage surgical procedure, amputation, or even the death of the patient during the definitive treatment phase.[4,13,14,15]

There are also several lesions for which biopsy must be avoided. For example, the benign enchondroma of the proximal femur found serendipitously during a routine radiographic evaluation of the area for other reasons (i.e., work-up for pelvic disease) needs no biopsy if the radiographic evaluation shows no evidence of activity of the entity.[16,17] If a biopsy is done without careful consideration of the prebiopsy workup, the histological evaluation of such cartilaginous material will frequently be interpreted by the pathologist as a "disturbing" lesion in which chondrosarcoma cannot be ruled out. This is because even benign cartilage of an enchondroma in the older individual usually has a histological appearance with a number of the characteristics of malignant cartilage ("binucleate cells"), when in fact the changes are caused by "old" cartilage. It is more appropriate to follow the patient with a serendipitous finding of the musculoskeletal tissues with serial radiographs, comparing them at routine intervals for changes in the appearance of the lesion and the bone around it before performing a biopsy.[16,17] If such a biopsy is done, regardless of these precautions, and the histological material is reported as "showing changes in which malignancy can not be ruled out" the patient is at risk of being subjected to a much larger procedure than required, even limb-salvage surgery, which in retrospect was probably unnecessary. Older patients cannot recover their preoperative function when this happens.

The second type of biopsy is the assay procedure. The assay biopsy was often used until recently in postmenopausal women to evaluate their bone for osteoporosis. The data obtained from these studies could then be used to plan appropriate therapy. Recent advances in radiographic evaluation of osteoporotic patients, such as the dual energy X-ray absorptiometry (DEXA) scan, have almost completely eliminated the need of a biopsy for these technically and expensive specialized histological evaluations. Other instances in which assay biopsy has been used include bone biopsy of renal dialysis patients in

Stage I of the disease. Information about aluminum salt deposition in the bone of these patients, from the filters utilized for their dialysis, was needed to determine its effect on bone. This type of assay has also almost been eliminated with recent advances in filter materials and drug management. Other assay biopsies include those needed to determine deposition of heavy metals (i.e., lead and arsenic), radioisotope materials (i.e., strontium-90), or industrial poisons. Forensic pathologists use this information in criminal cases or industrial poisoning incidents. Before an assay biopsy is attempted, pertinent information must be gathered from the investigating agency and receiving laboratory about the amount of material required, selection of site, and any special handling requirements needed for the specimen obtained. For instance, if the investigating agency wishes at least 3 g of bone from the iliac crest transported in glutaraldehyde, it does little good to submit 5 g from the distal femur immersed in phenol.

The confirmatory biopsy is most frequently used to confirm information already obtained by other means. For instance, the patient with carcinoma of breast, lung, kidney, prostate, or gut who has a typical metastatic lesion to the bone requires a confirmatory biopsy of the bony lesion to help guide the medical oncology and radiotherapy treatment plan.[3,5,10,12,21] Metastatic carcinomas to bone are sometimes found primarily by biopsy, but an appropriate investigation of patients older than 50 yr of age with a recently appearing bone defect (which has the typical permeative appearance of metastatic disease) will locate the primary disease more than 80% of the time prior to a biopsy. With one or two exceptions, such as the solitary metastatic renal-cell carcinoma to bone or the isolated initial appearance of myeloma in bone, surgical treatment of metastatic lesions beyond the biopsy is required only for stabilization of impending or actual pathologic fractures. Most of these lesions are treated palliatively with radiation or oncologic therapy.

"Therapeutic" biopsy is probably an overstatement, but excisional biopsy of an osteochondroma is an example of a therapeutic as well as diagnostic procedure. Biopsy of the typical Langerhans histiocytosis lesion (eosinophilic granuloma) is usually therapeutic as well as diagnostic, when biopsy of eosinophilic granuloma is required. Most of the time biopsy in this instance is unnecessary. For instance, once the CBC and/or peripheral smear obtained in a young patient (less than 8 yr old) with vertebra plana confirms that lymphoma or leukemia is not the cause of the vertebra plana (spinal defect), a presumptive diagnosis of eosinophilic granuloma of bone can be made with a high degree of confidence, and no other primary surgical treatment is required at that point. Follow-up is required, with radiographs at regular intervals. In a child less than 8 yr of age, the affected vertebrae will usually reconstitute completely because of continued enchondral ossification of the endplates of the involved vertebrae, and the eosinophilic granuloma will spontaneously heal. The astute reader will rapidly conclude that therapeutic biopsy is most appropriate for benign self-healing lesions, and is indicated primarily for these lesions.

IV. TYPES OF BIOPSY

A. Technical

1. Small Needle Biopsy

The small needle (18-, 23-, or 25-gauge) aspirate is gaining popularity in major centers today, primarily because it can be done in the outpatient setting, is cost- and time-efficient, and provides rapid diagnosis of musculoskeletal lesions.[2,3,5,7,12,22–24] This particular type of biopsy lends itself well to soft-tissue lesions, but can also be utilized for bony ones.[24] Most centers across the country that use this technique find the fine-needle aspirate to be highly dependent upon the confidence and experience of the pathologist interpreting the limited amount of material obtained by the process.[2,3,12,22–24] Even those who use it would agree that the small-needle aspirate is a useful tool to determine benign from malignant and metastatic vs primary lesions. Further characterization of the material obtained is necessarily limited by the amount of material obtained. This can lead to errors in diagnosis when the material is insufficient for diagnosis, and complications do occur with this method.[11,18]

2. Core Needle Biopsy

The core needle biopsy, done with the Craig Core Needle, Biomet hand-driven core needle, or Zimmer counter-rotating instruments, provides more tissue for diagnosis and is minimally more invasive than the fine needle.[3,12] The Craig needle is the author's personal preference for this task, but the Biomet and Zimmer counter rotating needle are also very helpful in obtaining appropriate tissue for this type of biopsy. The Biomet hand-driven core needle biopsy instrument is especially useful in the author's hands. Any of these instruments will usually (95% diagnostic accuracy)[19] obtain enough material from any bony or soft-tissue location for an appropriate diagnosis. If three cores are taken using any of these instruments, adequate material can also be obtained for additional histological studies most of the time.[19] Depending on the skill of the person doing the biopsy, the location of the cores taken, and the viability of the tissue in the area where the material is obtained, the yield of such biopsies can be inaccurate as much as 40% of the time, according to some published reports.[19] In experienced hands, the expected accuracy of this procedure can be in the 64–96% range.

3. Open Biopsy

Open biopsy is the most appropriate technique if 98% diagnostic accuracy is the goal and material for additional studies such as histochemical stains, electron microscopy, or cell cultures is needed. However, open biopsy has shortcomings. It creates a larger incision than the other methods, results in more blood loss, exposes the patient to major nerve or blood vessel injury, can create iatrogenic assisted pathologic fracture (if the lesion is in bone), and result in contamination of tissue planes not otherwise at risk with poorly planned procedures. Despite these limitations, the open biopsy still remains the gold standard against which all other techniques are measured, because of its high degree of diagnostic accuracy and the amount of material that can be obtained for other studies. If open biopsy is chosen, the person doing the biopsy must carefully pre-plan the location of the biopsy, limit contamination of tissue compartments by following proper incisional techniques, and maximize the information gained while minimizing exposure to further risks for the patient.[4,20,21]

B. Medical

1. Incisional Biopsy

An incisional biopsy is a procedure that removes a portion of the tumor for study, but leaves gross tumor behind. Depending on the diagnosis of the lesion, that portion which remain in the patient may require further surgical management. An incisional biopsy is

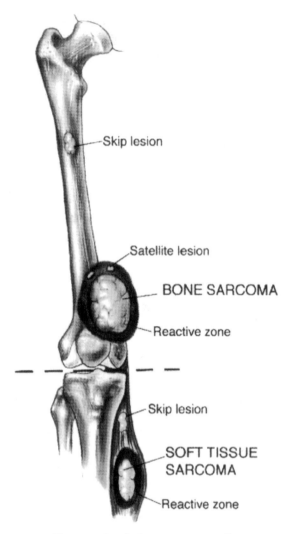

Skip lesion

Satellite lesion

BONE SARCOMA

Reactive zone

Skip lesion

SOFT TISSUE
SARCOMA

Reactive zone

Figure 1. Growth pattern of bone and soft-tissue sarcomas. Sarcomas grow in a centripetal fashion, with the most immature part of the lesion at the growth edge. A reactive zone is formed between the tumor and the compressed surrounding normal tissues, and may be invaded by tumor nodules that represent microextensions of tumor (satellites) and are not a metastatic phenomenon. High-grade sarcomas may present with tumor nodules that grow outside the reactive zone (skip lesions), but within the same anatomic compartment in which the lesion is located. Used with permission.[4]

appropriate for the patient with *any* soft-tissue lesion greater than 5 cm in diameter and a bony one that is potentially malignant. In general, the cells at the margin of a malignant musculoskeletal tumor are the most highly (high-grade) malignant portion of the lesion (Fig. 1). For the infrequent user of biopsies, it is recommended that the incisional biopsy always be planned as the procedure of choice for musculoskeletal lesions that are potentially malignant, since excisional biopsies of actual or potentially malignant musculoskeletal tumors are not the standard of care.[4,10,13,14,20,21] It is more appropriate to require that a second operative procedure be performed on an undiagnosed mass that proves to be benign at biopsy but which showed signs of potential malignancy on the prebiopsy studies, instead of inappropriately managing the malignant or potentially malignant one. "Shelling out" a malignant tumor opens up vascular channels and interfascial planes to the most aggressive cells of the mass, making the definitive surgical procedure planning and execution much more difficult and sometimes impossible.

The incisional biopsy should be appropriately placed through one compartment, and the biopsy site should be closed watertight in layers to help control the inevitable hemorrhage that occurs from surgical manipulation of high-grade musculoskeletal lesions.[10,20,21]

2. Excisional (Marginal) Biopsy

Excisional biopsy (marginal excision) is resection of a musculoskeletal lesion around its margin or pseudo-margin that *always* leaves microscopic portions of the tumor behind. It is not the appropriate surgical procedure for malignant or potentially malignant lesions of the musculoskeletal system.

The musculoskeletal soft-tissue lesion that is 5 cm or less in size (benign or malignant), and is located in its host tissue so that it can be successfully removed with a circumferential/hemispherical 2–3 cm cuff of normal tissue around it, can be safely removed with a wide excision as the primary procedure in experienced hands. Note that this is not an excisional biopsy (marginal excision), but a formal wide excision. Malignant musculoskeletal lesions are rarely found when they are less than 5 cm in diameter or confined to an easily expendable muscle such as the sartorius, gastrocnemius, or biceps. As such a wide excision is rarely done for these tumors as the initial definitive procedure, even by the most experienced surgeon.

Excisional biopsy should be reserved for benign or self-healing lesions of the musculoskeletal system. Such examples include the osteochondroma, osteoid osteoma, lipoma, eosinophilic granuloma, nonossifying fibroma, and the myxoma of muscle, to name a few. Needless to say, one must have clear evidence that the diagnosis of the benign lesion is precisely what one thinks it is prior to performing an excisional biopsy, and the tumor is clearly a benign or self-healing—for example, one such as the ganglion cyst, lipoma, osteochondroma, nonossifying fibroma, or chondroblastoma.

V. APPROPRIATE EVALUATION PRIOR TO BIOPSY

As noted in the introduction, biopsy is the last step in the pre-operative staging of a patient with a musculoskeletal tumor, and the first step in the therapeutic management regardless of what that management requires.[4,10,13,14,20,21] Therefore, the biopsy should be carefully planned, placed, and executed by an experienced member of the musculoskeletal team. It should not be left to the least knowledgeable or skilled member of the team to perform as an afterthought. The history and physical exam may not provide diagnostic information, but can provide major clues for appropriate diagnosis of such lesions as myositis ossificans, a stress fracture, and a fracture of insufficiency in the osteoporotic patient. For instance, in the patient with chronic alcoholism who is found to have a bone-forming density in the medial femoral neck that radiographically would represent a number of different diagnoses, the history of the patient's alcoholism and evolution of the patient's symptoms can be extremely helpful in making a diagnosis of an insufficiency (Milkman's) fracture. It is also important to discuss the critical value of radiographic investigations. The plain film is the indicated diagnostic tool[16,17] for appropriate diagnosis of bony lesions. Although the bone scan, computerized tomography (CT) scan, and magnetic resonance imaging (MRI) may give helpful confirmatory information about many lesions, it is critical that plain films be made of any bony defect in humans, as it is the tool on which all diagnostic information hangs. The bone scan is helpful in providing an approximation of the local extent of the bony defect, but is most useful in determining the presence of distant disease or multiple bone involvement. The CT scan is most helpful in evaluation of the cortical extent of bone tumors. Even in the age of the MRI, the CT scan remains the most appropriate diagnostic adjunct determining cortical involvement of a lesion. For instance, the osteoid osteoma located in cortical bone is best identified and characterized using the CT scan in conjunction with the plain film and not the MRI. The MRI is appropriate for evaluation of primary soft-tissue lesions as well as the marrow and/or soft-tissue extent of a lesion with its epicenter in bone. It is inadequate to use for diagnosis of all but the most obvious of musculoskeletal lesions, such as the lipoma, hemangioma, and endochondroma on the MRI. Finally, appropriate laboratory data must be performed when infection, myeloma, parathyroid (primary or secondary) or Cushing's disease are part of the differential diagnosis.

Once appropriate evaluations have been accomplished, the technical aspects of the last step in evaluation and first step in therapy must be organized in an effort to gain optimum information from the biopsy.

VI. TECHNICAL ASPECTS

A. Location of the Biopsy

The location of the biopsy is critical to the ultimate success of future surgical therapy. In the appendicular skeleton, the location of the biopsy site must be contained within one compartment, with care taken to avoid crossing multiple compartments to get to the lesion. The incisional site on the appendicular skeleton must always be parallel to the axis of the involved part so that the biopsy track can be excised with the definitive procedure. Any transverse incision across the upper arm, forearm, thigh, knee, ankle, or foot is always inappropriate biopsy placement[4] (Fig. 2), because definitive management of this inappropriate site placement will require extensive resection of tissue, loss of function, and transposition of bone and soft tissues not otherwise required. On the central axis of the skeleton, biopsy sites must follow the same principles: always going through a single compartment to reach the tumor, not located along "fault lines" of the body, to allow complete resection of the biopsy tract during the definitive procedure. For instance, a transverse or even vertical incision directly over the gluteus maximus of the hindquarter for a lesion deep within the buttock would require almost certain resection of the entire gluteus and a quadriceps rotational flap to close the huge defect required for resection of the tumor and its biopsy tract. The same considerations must be made for incisions around the shoulder (Fig. 3). An incision following but inferior to that of a formal hemi-pelvectomy resection outline would be a more appropriate choice for biopsy of a pelvic lesion, although the distance to the lesion may be further away than the easier, direct approach. In these areas, a needle biopsy proves to be the most helpful in minimizing the complications of the biopsy site. Remember, the open biopsy site always requires resection to eliminate residual tumor along its tract,[11,13,14,18] and the inappropriately placed site can result in the loss of the ability to completely eradicate the tumor. Finally, it is important to reemphasize that

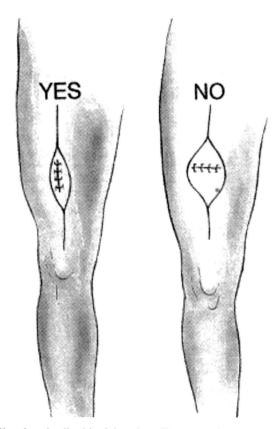

Figure 2. The smallest longitudinal incision that allows an adequate specimen to be obtained should be used. A transverse biopsy incision requires a wider resection of soft tissues at the time of the definitive surgery. Used with permission.[4]

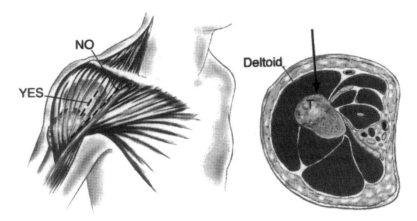

Figure 3. Biopsy tract, proximal humerus: The deltoid must be resected with most primary bone sarcomas of the proximal humerus. A transdeltoid approach through the anterior third of the muscle is used. The traditional deltopectoral approach requires wider resection of the pectoralis major muscle, compromises its use for soft-tissue reconstruction, and may contaminate the main neurovascular bundle of the upper extremity. Used with permission.[4]

appropriate biopsy is accomplished only with careful planning and awareness of the definitive surgical procedure that will be required, once the diagnosis is confirmed.

B. Proper vs Improper Incisional Techniques

Skin incisions for the open biopsy should always be parallel to the axis of the limb part in the appendicular skeleton.[4] The intervening muscle must be incised directly, and no attempt must be made to dissect between interfascial planes of muscles, as this will open up long expanses of tissue to the potential hematoma that forms from the open biopsy. When this hematoma develops, it can potentially spread malignant cells along the course of the interfascial planes of the entire limb compartment. Bone should be incised directly if it is soft enough to cut (which is usually the case with high-grade musculoskeletal lesions). When the bone is "hard", an oval window is made in the bone to extract material from its interior (Figs. 4, 5).[4] Once the material in question is obtained from the bone, the window must be plugged with cement to help prevent further bleeding and/or spread of hematoma into the soft tissues from intramedullary cavity bleeding. Muscles should be closed with a watertight process in layers, and the skin should be closed with a subcuticular suture or a suture very close to the margins of the skin.[10] The need for excision of large amount of tissue with the biopsy tract is thereby kept to a minimum, when definitive surgical treatment is required for a malignant tumor.

C. Amount of Material Required

Present-day staining techniques require enough material to do histochemical staining, electron microscopy (if a small-cell tumor), and cell cultures for certain research protocols. If the material obtained is taken from the necrotic center of a malignant fibrous histiocytoma, for example, the only information the pathologist can provide is nondiagnostic. Conversely, cutting out the plump center of a maturing area of myositis ossificans creates a risk of the histological interpretation of the material is an osteosarcoma by the uninformed or unaware pathologist. Therefore, enough tissue must be obtained to satisfy these needs, no matter which method is used. This involves consultation with the pathologist prior to, or during, the biopsy.

VII. OUTLINE FOR APPROPRIATE BIOPSY

Biopsy must be planned based on the potential diagnoses of the specific lesion being investigated. In many musculoskeletal tumors, especially the intraosseous cartilage lesions, myositis ossificans, osteoid osteoma, histiocytosis X, myeloma, lymphoma, and metastatic diseases, to name only a few, the histological diagnosis is directed by the pre-biopsy clinical, laboratory, and radiographic material.[10,20,21] Beyond that, some additional rules are advisable to follow:

1. Never biopsy musculoskeletal tumors if you are not prepared to perform definitive surgery for the unexpected as well as the anticipated result.
2. Never make transverse biopsy incisions on any extremity. Always make incisions parallel to the limb, and always remain in one soft-tissue compartment when biopsying a lesion.
3. Never dissect between intermuscular planes to reach a tumor, soft tissue, or bony lesion. Go directly through the muscle of one compartment to reach a soft tissue or bony lesion.
4. Always work to get a watertight closure of the biopsy site. Use methyl methacrylate (MMA) to plug a bony window biopsy.

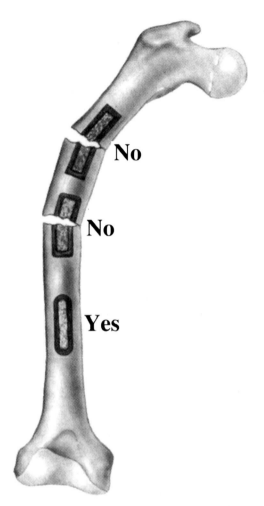

No

No

Yes

Figure 4. An oblong cortical window with rounded ends affords the greatest residual strength and is recommended for biopsy of purely intraosseous lesions. Used with permission.[4]

5. Perform a needle biopsy in difficult sites. This technique depends on the expertise of the entire team that uses it. The author's preference of devices is the Craig Core Needle. However, the Biomet hand-held needle and Zimmer counter-rotating needle are useful when hard bone must be sampled, as the Craig needle is not sturdy enough to perform this function. The Craig needle can be used to sample vertebral body lesions from T8 to the sacrum, the ilium, the proximal humerus and femur, the proximal and distal tibia, the proximal ulna, and distal radius and the os calcis.

6. When doing an open biopsy, avoid taking material exclusively from obviously necrotic areas in soft-tissue tumors and obviously reactive areas in bone, as shown by pre-operative staging studies.

7. Take enough tissue with the needle or open biopsy, usually $2 \times 2 \times 2$ cm, with biopsy, so the pathologist can perform adequate sampling and special studies on the material. Sometimes this is not possible, especially when the tumor is necrotic (Ewings, MFH), but it should be done where possible. Also remember that the zonal pattern of myositis ossificans can be confidently diagnosed by the pathologist using a wedge of tissue from the periphery to its core.

MEDIAL LESIONS   LATERAL LESIONS

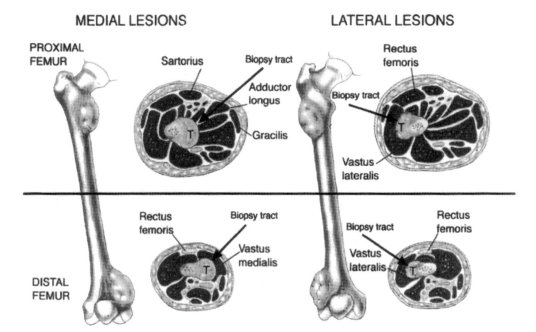

Figure 5. Biopsy tract, proximal and distal femur: A distinction is made between lateral and medial lesions. Because most primary bone sarcomas have an extraosseous extension, the muscle underlying the tumor has to be resected with the specimen. This principle applies to all anatomic locations. Used with permission.[4]

8. *Never* send a biopsy specimen to any pathologist without discussing the pre-operative staging with that expert. As noted in the text, the diagnosis of a number of musculoskeletal tumors is aided by this pre-operative staging information.[16,17]

9. Avoid excisional biopsy of soft-tissue musculoskeletal tumors greater than 5 cm in diameter (based on clinical and MRI findings), unless there is clear evidence from appropriate staging studies, that the tumor is benign (lipoma, mature myositis ossificans).

10. While performing an excisional biopsy for what one believes is a benign soft tissue or bony musculoskeletal tumor and the lesion encountered is an unexpected one, immediately discard all plans for the excisional biopsy and perform an incisional one, closing the wound to be as watertight as possible. Take a sample of the material to the pathologist with the information available at that point, and wait on the histologic results. Promptly inform the patient of the problems and explain the need to await definitive pathologic information before proceeding further. Do any necessary additional laboratory studies, but avoid initiating the MRI, bone scan, or CT scan in the immediate postoperative period, as the inflammatory reaction from the biopsy surgical procedure will obscure the results.

11. For the assay biopsy, obtain guidance from the pathologist for proper handling of the tissue—for example, muscle biopsy handling requires special techniques to preserve the length and morphology of the tissue.

12. The confirmatory biopsy is usually done to confirm metastatic disease, so a needle biopsy will usually obtain adequate tissue for this purpose. However, as with all needle biopsies, take at least three cores when possible[19] (one exception is spine biopsies), so that adequate tissue is available to the pathologist.

13. Therapeutic biopsies are most often excisional, and are done for benign lesions. The most important principle to remember when doing this is that complete excision of the tumor is

required to be therapeutic. Leaving bits and pieces of a cartilaginous tumor in the soft tissues (if an osteochondroma) or the bone (if an enchondroma) gives rise to misinterpretation of these remnants when viewed radiographically or even histologically at a later date.

14. Finally, if the pathologist's interpretation does not "fit" with the prebiopsy workup, especially the radiographic data, do not proceed with definitive treatment. Redo the biopsy, if necessary, to get a clear histological diagnosis that "fits" all the data. For instance, if the material obtained from the fine or core needle biopsy is so limited that the pathologist can report only individual cell types and not the pattern/behavior of the biopsy, the operating surgeon must obtain more tissue, even if this requires a formal open biopsy. Some examples of histological diagnoses that will not justify proceeding with the definitive procedure are:

   a. "Multiple giant cells, inflammatory cells, and necrotic debris most likely representing a Giant Cell Tumor" from the fine-needle aspirate of a destructive lesion causing a pathologic fracture of the femur of a 50-yr-old patient who had removal of a kidney 10 yr ago for renal cell carcinoma. The prebiopsy workup, including the patient's age, clearly suggests a metastatic cause for this problem, not a Giant Cell Tumor.

   b. Another example would be a histological report of "histiocytes, blood, a thin lining of endothelial-like cells containing scattered inflammatory cells, and fibroblasts representing a simple cyst," in an adolescent patient with an eccentrically (not concentrically) located metaphyseal Enneking Grade 3 (not III) lesion on radiographs that is a dead ringer for a Giant Cell Tumor of bone.

In both of these examples, no prebiopsy coordination was done with the pathologist, leading to the report rendered.

   c. One final example is that in which a well-planned and executed fine or core needle biopsy produces a histological diagnosis of "large amount of necrosis and scattering of viable cells consistent with a sarcoma," where the prebiopsy staging shows simultaneously bone formation and destructive lesion that is most likely an osteogenic sarcoma, but could be a Ewings tumor. It goes without saying that more material, even if it requires an open biopsy, is required to clearly identify the cell type and pattern of this tumor before any other actions are taken.

In conclusion, it is appropriate to re-emphasize that biopsy is the last step in the staging workup, and the first in definitive treatment of musculoskeletal lesions not confidently diagnosable by other means. Careful attention to the principles in this chapter will prevent unnecessary errors in the management of patients with these conditions.

REFERENCES

1. Akerman M: The cytology of soft tissue tumors. *Acta Orthop Scand* 273(Suppl):54–59, 1997.
2. Akerman M, Rydholm A, Persson BM: Aspiration cytology of soft tissue tumors. The 10-year experience at an orthopedic oncology center. *Acta Orthop Scand* 56:407–412, 1985.
3. Ayala AG, Ro JY, Fanning CV, et al: Core needle biopsy and fine needle aspiration in the diagnosis of bone and soft-tissue lesions. *Hematol Oncol Clin North Am* 9:633–651, 1995.
4. Bickels J, Jelinek JS, Shmookler BM, et al: Biopsy of musculoskeletal tumors. *Clin Orthop* 368:212–219, 1999.
5. Bommer KK, Ramzy I, Mody D: Fine needle aspiration biopsy in the diagnosis and management of bone lesions: A study of 450 cases. *Cancer* 81:148–156, 1997.
6. Chang AE, Sondak VK: Clinical evaluation and treatment of soft tissue tumors. In: Enzinger FM, Weis SW, eds: *Soft Tissue Tumors.* CV Mosby, St Louis, MO, 1995:17–38.
7. Costa MJ, Campman SC, Davis RL, et al: Fine-needle aspiration cytology of sarcoma: retrospective review of diagnostic utility and specificity. *Diagn Cytopathol* 15:23–32, 1996.

8. Eady JL: Pre-operative evaluation of bone tumors. Orthopaedic Audio—Synopsis Continuing Medical Education. Vol.18, Lecture 8, April 1986–May 1987.

9. Eady JL: Pitfalls in musculoskeletal tumor management. Scientific Exhibit, AAOS 50th Annual Meeting, Anaheim, CA, February, 1991.

10. Enneking WF: General principles of musculoskeletal tumor surgery. In: Enneking WF, ed: *Musculoskeletal Tumor Surgery, Vol 2.* Churchill-Livingstone, New York, NY, 1983:3–27.

11. Ferrucci Jr JT: Malignant seeding of needle tract after thin needle aspiration biopsy: a previously unrecorded complication. *Radiology* 130:345–346, 1979.

12. Heslin MJ, Lewis JJ, Woodruff JM, et al: Core needle biopsy for diagnosis of extremity soft tissue sarcoma. *Ann Surg Oncol* 4:425–431, 1997.

13. Mankin HJ, Lange TA, Spanier SS: The hazards of biopsy in patients with malignant primary bone and soft tissue tumors. *J Bone Joint Surg [Am]* 64:1121–1127, 1982.

14. Mankin HJ, Mankin CJ, Simon MA: The hazards of biopsy, revisited. *J Bone Joint Surg [Am]* 78:656–663, 1996.

15. Noria S, Davis A, Knadel R, et al: Residual disease following unplanned excision of soft-tissue sarcoma of an extremity. *J Bone Joint Surg [Am]* 78:650–655, 1996.

16. Resnick D: Tumors and tumor-like lesions of bone: radiographic principles. In: Resnick D, ed: *Diagnosis of Bone and Joint Disorders, 3rd ed.* W.B. Saunders Company, Philadelphia, PA, 1996:3613–3627.

17. Resnick D, Kyriakos M, Greenway GD: Tumors and tumor-like lesions of bone: imaging and pathology of specific lesions. In: Resnick D, ed: *Diagnosis of Bone and Joint Disorders, 3rd ed.* W.B. Saunders Company, Philadelphia, PA, 1996:3628–3638.

18. Schwartz HS, Spengler DM: Needle tract recurrences after closed biopsy for sarcomas: three cases and review of the literature. *Ann Surg Oncol* 4:228–236, 1997.

19. Skrzynski MC, Biermann JS, Montag A, et al: Diagnostic accuracy and charge-savings of outpatient core needle biopsy compared with open biopsy of musculoskeletal tumors. *J Bone Joint Surg [Am]* 78:644–649, 1996.

20. Simon MA: Biopsy. In: Simon MA, Springfield D, eds: *Surgery for Bone and Soft-Tissue Tumors.* Lippincott-Raven, Philadelphia, PA, 1998:55–65.

21. Simon MA:Biopsy of musculoskeletal tumors. *J Bone Joint Surg [Am]* 64:1253–1257, 1982.

22. White VA, Fanning CV, Ayala AG, et al: Osteosarcoma and the role of fine-needle biopsy: a study of 51 cases. *Cancer* 62:1238–1246, 1988.

23. Will'en H: Fine needle aspiration in the diagnosis of bone tumors. *Acta Orthop Scand* 273(Suppl):47–53, 1997.

24. Will'en H, Akerman M, Carl'en B: Fine needle aspiration (FNA) in the diagnosis of soft-tissue tumours: a review of 22 years experience. *Cytopathology* 6:236–247, 1995.

8

Tissue Harvesting and Fixation

Linda L. Jenkins and Karen J. L. Burg

Department of Bioengineering, Clemson University, Clemson, SC, USA

I. INTRODUCTION

Fixation is the chemical or physical process that allows tissue sections to be viewed in a close approximation to the living tissue.[1] Histological fixation practices have been derived from many other fields, such as the leather tanning industry. Fixation is the single most important factor in achieving a well-prepared section for microscopic analysis. Fixation processes should be standardized so that subtle changes in microanatomy may be detected by comparing similarly fixed sections. When tissue is removed from the host, a good fixative will stop autolysis (the dissolution of cells by intracellular enzymatic digestion) and putrefaction (the breakdown of tissue by bacterial action) by inactivating the enzymes, bacteria, and molds that begin to form immediately after death. It will also protect the tissue from excessive shrinkage and swelling, and it will not dissolve or distort the tissue. Dehydrating agents and clearing agents can cause distortion of tissue, so the chosen fixing agent will also protect the cellular constituents so that they will not be altered by these chemicals.[2] The fixative must also protect the tissue during the embedding process, which involves polymer impregnation at a high temperature. Finally, it must protect the tissue during sectioning, where the potential for mechanical damage is high.

Before any tissue is harvested, many factors must be considered. First of all, a basic understanding of human anatomy or the research model is essential; therefore, an extensive list of anatomical terms including diagrams has been included in this chapter. A sample dissection and processing documentation form is also included. Fixative, fixation methods, processing chemicals, embedding medias, and sectioning techniques must be selected well in advance of harvesting. Fixative selection is discussed in detail in this chapter, and special emphasis is placed on perfusion fixation as the method of choice. A table detailing stain-fixative interactions is given (*see* Table 4), and common fixative formulations are presented in the Appendix (*see* Appendix C).

II. DISSECTION TECHNIQUES

It is strongly recommended that the researcher meet with the histology lab personnel to develop a specific harvesting and processing protocol. Once the fixative has been selected, the fixation technique should be planned. It is also recommended that perfusion fixation

From: *Handbook of Histology Methods for Bone and Cartilage*
Edited by: Y. H. An and K. L. Martin © Humana Press Inc., Totowa, NJ

be considered, as it will greatly enhance tissue processing and improve the quality of the final tissue section.[3] All implants and surrounding tissue should be well-documented; a sample "Dissection and Processing Protocol Form" is included in Appendix A. With the advent of digital cameras, it is very easy, and highly recommended, to take a picture of the implant site as well as the implant. Photographs should be taken of the implant immediately after dissection and again just prior to histological processing. Additionally, the orientation of the specimen should be noted with respect to the surrounding tissues and organs. It is useful, particularly with multiple implants, to include a schematic denoting implant locations. Documentation of all dissections should include at least the following items: date and investigation title, investigator name, type of implant material and material sensitivities, animal model and I.D. number, date of initial surgery, date of sacrifice, location of the implant, and any gross observations that indicate a pathological condition such as effusion, hematoma, or scar.[4]

A. Anatomical Terminology

In order to properly document location, it is necessary to understand the anatomical terminology. Four imaginary anatomical planes pass through the human body. These are the median, sagittal, coronal, and horizontal planes. The planar locations are depicted according to an upright body position, with legs together, arms at body sides. Anatomical planes in a four-legged animal are similarly located, based on the animal in an upright position, standing on its hind legs. The median plane is an imaginary vertical plane that passes longitudinally through the middle of the body from front to back, dividing it into left and right halves. A sagittal plane is a vertical plane that runs parallel to the median plane, but does not necessarily pass through the body's midline. Thus, the median plane is a specific type of sagittal plane. The coronal plane is a vertical plane that is perpendicular to the median and sagittal planes, passing from side to side through the body. It is sometimes referred to as the frontal plane. The horizontal plane, or transverse plane, is a plane that splits the body or body part in question into upper and lower parts. Fig. 1 shows each of these planes in the goat model, as this animal is often used for orthopedic studies. Directional terms are also used to describe tissue location. Table 1 describes various directional terms.

III. FIXATION

In clinical pathology as well as many research programs, fixation with neutral buffered formalin (NBF) is the method of choice. The term "formalin" is often incorrectly interchanged with "formaldehyde." Formalin (formol) is a trade name for the liquid resulting from the combination of formaldehyde gas and water.[5] The solubility limit of formaldehyde gas in water is 40%. Ten percent NBF is comprised of 10 mL of formalin and 90 mL of water. Thus, a 10% NBF solution contains approx 4% formaldehyde. Ten percent NBF is suitable for standard paraffin processing with a hematoxylin and eosin (H&E) end point. When processing undecalcified bone, it is important to select a fixative that will not decalcify the specimen or remove bone labels. However, fixative selection is complicated by the development of novel procedures, such as *in situ* hybridization, that rely on the recovery of intact messenger ribonucleic acids (mRNA) and/or deoxyribonucleic acids (DNA). NBF can crosslink DNA and RNA to nearby proteins, causing difficulties in extraction of mRNA and DNA.[6] Recommended fixatives include 4% paraformaldehyde,

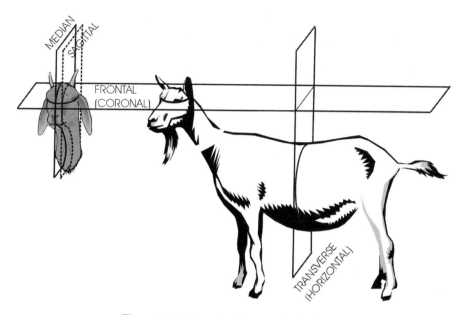

Figure 1. Schematic of anatomical planes.

Table 1. Common Directional Terms

Directional term	Description
Superior	Toward the head or upper part of body
Inferior	Away from the head or toward the lower part of the body
Anterior (ventral)	Toward or at the front of the body
Posterior (dorsal)	Toward or at the back of the body; behind
Medial	Toward or at the midline of the body
Lateral	Away from the midline of the body
Ipsilateral	On the same side of the body
Contralateral	On the opposite side of the body
Proximal	Closer to the point of attachment of an extremity to the body trunk; closer to the origin of the body part (e.g., the knee is proximal to the foot)
Distal	Further from the point of attachment of an extremity to the body trunk; further from the origin of the body part (e.g., the hand is distal to the elbow)
Superficial	Toward or at the body surface
Deep	Away from the body surface; more internal

2% glutaraldehyde, or ethanol/acetic acid (95:5).[7] Since there is a huge amount of data in archived NBF fixed tissues, it is critical to develop better analysis techniques that will accommodate them for future processing and analysis.

A. Fixatives

Improvements and new demands in tissue processing have mandated the evolution of fixatives. One of the earliest attempts at fixation was the use of chromic acid as a "hardening agent" in 1833.[8] Shortly thereafter, combinations of blood, serum, water, and amniotic fluid were used. Yet these "fixatives" did not prevent autolysis of the tissue. To address tissue autolysis, a series of chemicals was developed and, in 1896, formaldehyde was tested as a fixative.[8,9] Later, the efficacy of different staining techniques following formaldehyde fixation was demonstrated.

Many tissue components are water-soluble, so it is critical that they should not be lost from the tissue section, in order to maintain the highest staining quality. A fixative stabilizes the protein so that it can withstand autolysis or treatment by processing reagents. A good fixative will preserve cellular structure without damaging cellular chemistry. Fixatives may be physical or chemical, or a combination of the two.[1] Physical fixation includes heating, microwaving, desiccation, and freeze-drying. Chemical fixation is far more reliable, and generally involves treatment of the tissue in an aqueous or alcoholic base. Most medical techniques rely on chemical fixation as the main mode, with physical fixation incorporated to enhance the rate of fixation. There are many chemical fixatives, and each has attributes as well as drawbacks (Table 2). Crosslinking chemical fixatives (such as formaldehyde and glutaraldehyde) form covalent crosslinks between proteins and between proteins and nucleic acids. Dehydration chemical fixatives, such as ethanol, methanol, and acetone, remove free water from tissues and thus precipitate and coagulate proteins.[10] Other chemical fixatives, such as acetic acid and zinc acetate, cause shifts in pH or salt concentration and therefore denature proteins and nucleic acids.[11] Some fixatives, such as alcoholic formalin, fix by crosslinking and dehydration methods.

Many textbooks mention 70% ethanol as the ideal "fixative" for long-term storage of bone. This does not mean that the original specimen is initially fixed in this solution. Alcohol is rarely used as an initial fixative and only for select histological applications; e.g., 70% alcohol is excellent for fixation of cytology smears, touch preparations, and fine-needle aspirate. Bone should be adequately fixed in NBF or an alternate fixative and then stored in 70% ethanol. Ethanol storage is used to eliminate the effects of decalcification, which are sometimes found with long-term storage in formalin-based fixatives.

Chemical fixation may be enhanced by the use of physical fixation, such as heat and vacuum. Heat fixation is used to precipitate proteins, rendering them less soluble in water. Heat is generally used to accelerate fixation and not as a stand-alone method. The diffusion of molecules increases with increasing temperature, so penetration of a tissue by a fixative is increased with temperature. Heat causes protein coagulation, and thus it also causes undesirable distortions. Microwave fixation is also used to enhance chemical fixation, reducing fixation time. Freeze-drying is used to fix highly soluble materials.

Fixatives have varying ingredients or components, including those shown in Table 3. It is reported that select additives (sucrose, dextran, detergent, calcium chloride, potassium thiocyanate, ammonium sulfate) may also improve fixation in specific cases.[13] These additives inhibit denaturation through reaction with proteins, fixative, or cellular components.

Concentrations of fixatives are also very important.[15] This will be determined by the cost, the solubility, and the necessity. For example, a formalin concentration over 10% causes unnecessary hardening, while an ethanol concentration below 70% does not satisfactorily dehydrate. Osmolality or ionic concentration will also influence fixation. Hypertonic solutions will lead to shrinkage, while hypotonic solutions will lead to swelling. Recommended solutions are mildly hypertonic.[1] Essentially, the ionic concentration

Table 2. Common Fixatives: Advantages and Disadvantages[1,2,12]

Fixative	Advantages	Disadvantages
10% neutral buffered formalin (NBF)	Best all-around fixative. Preserves mucopolysaccharides.	If no buffer is used will form a "formalin pigment" artifact. Not suitable for certain special stains.
Formalin ammonium bromide (FAB)	Good for central nervous system tissue when stained with gold or silver.	
10% alcoholic formalin	Cuts fixation time in half. Preserves glycogen.	Dissolves fat and lipids. Does not preserve iron-bearing pigments. Tissue must be placed in 70% ethanol for long-term storage.
Zenker's fluid	Tissues stain brilliantly and is compatible with most staining techniques. Often used as mordant.	Contains mercury. Prolonged treatment makes sections brittle. Rinsing in alcoholic iodine is necessary before staining in order to remove mercuric chloride crystals.
Helly's fluid (Zenker-Formol)	Basically the same as Zenker's fluid with the addition of improved penetration and fixation.	Contains mercury. Prolonged treatment makes sections brittle. Rinsing in alcoholic iodine is necessary before staining in order to remove mercuric chloride crystals.
Bouin's fluid	Used for glycogen fixation. Intensifies staining.	Lipids are altered and decreased. Solution must be removed by thorough rinsing.
Gendre's fixative	Used for glycogen fixation.	
Carnoy's fluid	Quick-acting and penetrating. Preserves glycogen and chromosomes.	Contains chloroform. Suitable only for small pieces of tissue.
Acetone	Acetone (~4°C) is used for fluorescent antibody techniques and for preservation of some enzymes, especially phosphatases and lipases.	Some shrinkage and distortion may occur.

Table 3. Common Fixative Components and Their Function[2,14]

Fixative component	Function
Cupric salts	Combine with hematoxylin to form an insoluble compound.
Zinc salts	May be added to 10% formalin to enhance nuclear detail; especially recommended for immunohistochemistry.
Mercuric chloride	Coagulant used in conjunction with other chemicals. Renders tissues receptive to dyes, producing a pigment that must be extracted prior to staining.
Picric acid	Coagulant used to preserve glycogen. Leaves yellow color that must be extracted prior to staining.
Glutaraldehyde	Crosslinks proteins. Preserves ultrastructure very well.
Paraformaldehyde	Powdered form of formaldehyde.

should be as close to physiologic values as possible. Several common fixative formulations are given in Appendix C.

B. Fixation Time

Most of the fixation times in the currently available reference books are for routine soft tissue. A standard processor schedule, for example, is designed for formalin fixation and for samples of 4 mm or less.[17] The most common fixative is 10% NBF, sometimes with zinc or mercury additives. It is important to remember that undecalcified bone is much denser than soft tissue, and fixation times should be adjusted accordingly. Bone is a composite material; a given sample may contain cortical bone, trabecular bone, and marrow. In fact, it has been shown that the time required to fix bone marrow roughly approximates that for normal soft tissue.[18] For samples containing trabecular bone and marrow, a rule of thumb is penetration of 10 mm per 24 h at ambient pressure and room temperature.[19] A sample with cortical bone will have a much slower fixation rate, estimated at approx 2 mm per 24 h.[20] Explants may contain soft tissue (skin, muscle) as well as bone and bone marrow.

Some basic guidelines for the use of any fixative are as follows:[2]

- Use at least 15–20 volumes of fixative for every volume of tissue.
- No fixative will penetrate more than 2–3 mm of solid tissue or 0.5 cm of porous tissue in a 24-h period. Allow at least 1 wk for a 3–4 mm cube of compact bone to adequately fix.
- Thickness will depend on the type of tissue, but no specimen should be thicker than 4 mm for good fixation; 3 mm is preferable.
- Fix at room temperature unless otherwise specified. Heat will increase the rate of fixation, but it also increases the rate of autolysis. Raising the temperature from 25°C to 37°C can double the fixation rate.
- Vacuum can increase fixation rate at room temperature by about 2.5×.

C. Overfixation and Underfixation of Samples

Overfixation is a term that is widely debated. Many feel that this term is often confused with over-dehydration. Regardless of the terminology, the results are the same—overfixation can result in specimens that are difficult to cut (for example, shattering may occur) and sections that are not receptive to immunohistochemical or histological staining. There are chemical means to salvage overfixed tissue specimens, including the use of antigen retrieval kits, which will break protein bonds and thus facilitate immunohistochemical staining. Depending on the amount of overfixation, the fixation may only be partially reversible.

Underfixed tissue may also be problematic. Underfixation of bone may be characterized by bloodiness or gumminess, and a lack of rigidity and difficulty in sectioning. After harvesting, the tissue should be trimmed and exposed to the fixative as quickly as possible. Holes may be drilled into samples in order to facilitate fixation, a particularly useful technique for those samples that have not been perfusion-fixed. Following the requisite fixation time, the tissue will be trimmed to the embedding size. If the tissue is soft or gummy at this point, it should be fixed further. If an underfixed specimen is inadvertently embedded, it may be possible to remove the resin and further fix the tissue. Glycol methacrylates and polymethylmethacrylates (PMMA) may be removed by placing the embedded tissue in the respective monomer. Following initial removal of the embedding resin, the tissue must be washed in the appropriate solvents to remove the residual liquid monomer. The tissue then may be further fixed. The success of this will be variable, and it is certainly preferable to adequately fix the tissue prior to the initial embedding stage.

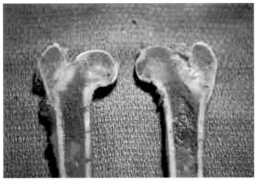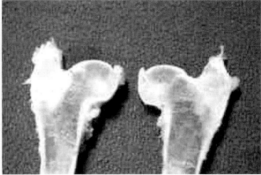

Figure 2. Immersion fixed goat femur on left and perfusion fixed goat femur on right. Note darker color of immersion fixed tissue indicating unfixed tissue.

When handling bone, it is very important to not rush the fixation process. Epoxy resins may not be readily removed.

One technique that can speed up the fixation rate is perfusion fixation. Perfusion-fixed tissue will not require the extended fixation times post harvesting that non-perfused tissue will require. If tissue must be shipped from the harvesting site to the histological processing site, it may be most safely shipped in 70% ethanol following fixation in formalin. It is important to note that ethanol treatment is for shipping purposes only, and is not a replacement method for fixation.

D. Perfusion Fixation

Traditional methods for specimen retrieval call for the placement of the excised tissue and implant into a container of fixative (immersion fixation). Fixation of tissue is then accomplished via diffusion of the fixative into the tissue. This technique is adequate for small to medium-size soft-tissue specimens; however, the rate of diffusion is relatively slow for undecalcified tissue and large soft-tissue specimens. An explanted biomaterial may be surrounded by soft and hard tissue, and some large or dense specimens may need weeks to adequately fix. The combination of slow fixation and continued enzymatic activity may result in cellular necrosis and/or degradation. Thus, the slides produced from the specimen may produce misleading data or obscure the host reaction.

By using the circulatory system to aid in the fixation process, the amount of post-mortem necrosis and degradation can be greatly reduced. Specifically, while the animal is under general anesthesia, catheters are threaded into an artery and its adjacent vein. The blood is then replaced with heparinized saline, followed by formalin. Appendix B details a procedure for perfusion fixation of the lower extremities of goats which has shown excellent fixation.[3] Fig. 2 shows fresh goat femur and a perfused goat femur, demonstrating that perfusion fixation is a superior method for bone preservation, guaranteeing almost instant fixation.

E. Fixatives and Stains

Many stains are fixative-dependent.[1,2] Stains and fixatives should be carefully considered prior to harvesting and processing. Table 4 lists various stains, the recommended fixatives for each, and fixatives to avoid, if applicable.

Table 4. Selected Stains and Fixative Constraints[1,2,16]

Stain	Recommended fixative	Fixatives to avoid
for Calcium		
Von Kossa	Alcohol or 10% NBF	
Alizarin Red S	10% NBF	
for Carbohydrates—Polysaccharides		
Periodic acid-Schiff	10% NBF, Zenker's, Bouin's	
Periodic acid-silver methenamine	10% NBF, Carnoy's	
for Carbohydrates—Glycogen		
Bauer-Feulgen	Carnoy's, Gendre's	Aqueous fixatives
Periodic acid-Schiff	Absolute ethanol, Carnoy's	Aqueous fixatives
Best's carmine	Absolute ethanol, Carnoy's	Aqueous fixatives
for Carbohydrates—Mucoproteins and Mucopolysaccharides		
Mayer's mucicarmine	Any	
Alcian blue	10% NBF, Bouin's	
Masson's trichrome	Bouin's	10% NBF without mordanting
for Carbohydrates—Acid Mucopolysaccharides		
Thionin	Any	
Periodic acid-Schiff	Any except glutaraldehyde	Glutaraldehyde
Müller-Mowry colloidal iron	Alcoholic formalin, Carnoy's	Chromates
Mowry's alcian blue	10% NBF, Bouin's	
Alcian blue – Periodic acid-Schiff	10% NBF, Bouin's	
Alcian blue – Feulgen	10% NBF, Bouin's	
for Connective Tissue		
Wilder's reticulum	10% NBF, Zenker's, Helly's	Picric acid
Foot's modification	Any	
Gridley's modification	10% NBF	
Laidlaw's method	Bouin's, 10% NBF	
Snook's reticulum	10% NBF	
Van Gieson's picric acid-acid fuchsin	Any	
Masson's trichrome	Bouin's	10% NBF without mordant
Mallory's aniline blue	Zenker's	All except Zenker's
Gomori's trichrome	Any	
for Elastic Fibers		
Gomori's aldehyde fuchsin	10% NBF	Orth's or Möller's (note that mercury fixatives result in lavender background)
Orcinol new fuchsin	Any	
Verhoeff-Van Gieson	10% NBF, Zenker's	
Weigert's resorcin fuchsin	10% NBF	
for Fats and Lipids		
Oil red O (frozen section)	10% NBF	Zenker's, Helly's
Sudan black B (frozen section)	10% NBF	Zenker's, Helly's
Nile blue sulfate (frozen section)	Formol calcium	All except formal calcium
Osmic acid (frozen section)	10% NBF	All except 10% NBF
Luxol fast blue	10% NBF	
Smith-Dietrich (frozen section)	Formol calcium	All except formol calcium
Baker's acid hematin (frozen section)	Formol calcium	All except formol calcium
Fischler's (frozen section)	10% NBF	All except 10% NBF

(Continues)

Table 4. *(Continued)*

Stain	Recommended fixative	Fixatives to avoid
for Fibrin		
Mallory's phosphotungstic acid hematoxylin	Zenker's	Bouin's
Weigert's	Absolute ethanol, Carnoy's, alcoholic formalin	Bouin's
for Fungi		
Brown-Brenn modified	10% NBF, Bouin's, Zenker's, Helly's	
Gridley's	Any	
Grocott's	10% NBF, Bouin's	
Periodic acid-Schiff	10% NBF, Bouin's, Zenker's	
Hotchkiss-McManus Periodic acid-Schiff	10% NBF, Bouin's, Zenker's	
for Copper		
Mallory-Parker	95% or absolute ethanol	
Mallory's	Ethanol-based	10% NBF
Rhodanine	10% NBF	
Rubeanic acid	10% NBF	
for Gold		
Hydrogen peroxide	10% NBF	
for Iron		
Mallory's	Ethanol-based	10% NBF
Prussian blue	10% NBF	
Turnbull's blue	10% NBF	
for Lead		
Mallory-Parker	95% or absolute alcohol	
for Hematins		
Acid hematin	10% NBF	
Malarial pigment	10% NBF	

F. Fixation and Explanted Biomaterials

Many factors should be considered before selecting the appropriate fixative and processing chemicals, especially when working with biomaterial implants. Not only is fixation of the cells important, but it is also crucial to retain the original shape of the implant and the delicate tissue-biomaterial interface. An orthopedic explant, for example, will usually include the biomaterial, bone, and soft tissue. When working with absorbable polymers, it is necessary to perform a pilot study in which the implant material is submerged in all of the proposed chemicals (i.e., formalin, alcohol, and xylene) for the allocated processing times and temperatures. The absorbable material will then be evaluated for degradation and/or distortion, and the processing method may be modified.

G. Fixative Safety Issues

Fixation requires handling of biohazards and chemical hazards. Safe handling of these materials is beyond the scope of this chapter, but is overviewed elsewhere.[21] However, it is important to remember that formalin is a carcinogen.

REFERENCES

1. Eltoum I, Fredenburgh J, Myers RB, et al: Introduction to the theory and practice of fixation of tissues. *J Histotechnol* 24:173–190, 2001.
2. Sheehan D: *Theory and Practice of Histotechnology, 2nd ed.* Battelle Press, Columbus, OH, 1980:44–58.
3. Jenkins L, Claassen E: Perfusion fixation. *National Society for Histotechnology Hard Times Communiqué.* April, 1992.
4. von Recum AF: *Handbook of Biomaterials Evaluation. Scientific, Technical & Clinical Testing of Implant Materials, 2nd ed.* Hemisphere Publishing Corporation, Philadelphia, PA, 1998.
5. Preece A: *A Manual for Histologic Technicians.* Churchill, London, Great Britain, 1972:31–55.
6. Frost AR, Sparks D, Grizzle WE: Methods of antigen recovery vary in their usefulness in unmasking specific antigens in immunohistochemistry. *Appl Immunohistochem Mol Morph* 8:236–243, 2000.
7. Grizzle WE, Manne U, Jhala NC, et al: The molecular characterization of colorectal neoplasia in translational research. *Arch Path Lab Med* 125:91–98, 2001.
8. Bricegridle B: *History of Microtechnique, 2nd ed.* Science Heritage Limited, Chicago, IL, 1987.
9. Fox CH, Benton C: Formaldehyde: the fixative. *J Histotechnol* 10:199–201, 1987.
10. Grizzle WE, Myers RB, Manne U, et al: Immunohistochemical evaluation of biomarkers in prostatic and colorectal neoplasia. In: Hanausek M, Walaszek Z, eds: *Methods in Molecular Medicine Series—Tumor Marker Protocols.* Volume 14. Humana Press, Totowa, NJ, 1998.
11. Arnold MM, Srivastava S, Fredenburgh J, et al: Effects of fixation and tissue processing on immunohistochemical demonstration of specific antigens. *Biotech Histochem* 71:224–230, 1996.
12. Gray P: *The Microanatomist's Formulary and Guide, 3rd ed.* McGraw-Hill, New York, NY, 1954.
13. Hayat MA: *Principles and Techniques of Electron Microscopy Biological Applications, 2nd ed.* Vol. 1. University Park Press, Baltimore, MD, 1981.
14. Jones ML: To fix, to harden, to preserve—Fixation: a brief history. *J Histotechnol* 24:155–162, 2001.
15. Fox CH, Johnson FB, Whiting J, et al: Formaldehyde fixation. *J Histochem Cytochem* 33:845–853, 1985.
16. Kiernan JA: *Histological and Histochemical Methods: Theory and Practice, 3rd ed.* Butterworth-Heinemann, Oxford, UK, 1999.
17. Skinner RA, Hickmon SG, Lumpkin CK, et al: Decalcified bone: twenty years of successful specimen management. *J Histotechnol* 20:267–277.
18. Robb-Smith AH, Taylor CK: *Lymph Node Biopsy.* Oxford University Press, London, UK, 1981.
19. Luna LG: *Histopathological Methods and Color Atlas of Special Stains and Tissue Artifacts.* American Histolabs, Gaithersburg, MD, 1992:1–27.
20. Lillie RD: *Histopathologic Technique and Practical Histochemistry, 3rd ed.* McGraw-Hill, New York, NY, 1965.
21. Titford M: Safety considerations in the use of fixatives. *J Histotechnol* 24:165–171, 2001.
22. Carson F: *Histotechnology, A Self-Instructional Text.* ASCP Press, Chicago, IL, 1990:1–22.
23. Luna L: *Manual of Histologic Staining Methods of the Armed Forces Institute of Pathology, 3rd ed.* McGraw-Hill, New York, NY, 1960:1–6.

APPENDIX A
DISSECTION AND PROCESSING FORM

Investigator: _____

Project: _____

Animal Number: _____

Date of Surgery/Date of Sacrifice _____

Bone Labels: _____

Perfusion fixed/Immersion Fixed/Fresh (circle one)

Gross Observations: _____

Tissue(s) Submitted/Location of Tissue: _____

Implant Material: _____

Material Sensitivities (i.e., chemical, temperature, etc.) _____

_____

Histological Objectives: _____

HISTOLOGICAL METHODS

	Paraffin	Frozen Section	Plastic
Fixative			
Dehydrant			
Clearing			
Embedding Media			
Sectioning			
Staining			

ESTIMATED NUMBER OF SPECIMENS: _____

ESTIMATED NUMBER OF BLOCKS: _____

TIME FRAME: (INDICATE DATE)

Specimens harvested by: _____

Specimens fixed by: _____

Specimens embedded by: _____

Specimens sectioned by: _____

Specimens stained by: _____

Specimens mounted by: _____

MICROSCOPY NEEDS: _____

Transmitted _____

Reflected _____

UV _____

Image Analysis _____

Photomicrographs _____

OTHER NEEDS: (Radiographs, decal, etc.) _____

COST ESTIMATE: _____

APPENDIX B
PERFUSION FIXATION FOR LOWER EXTREMITIES[3]

Materials:

5 L 10% neutral buffered formalin (NBF)

5 L saline

Heparin

Lidocaine

Roller pump

Five feet Tygon® tubing (1/4″ O.D., 1/8″ I.D.)

10 feet Tygon® tubing (1/4″ O.D., 1/8″ I.D.)

Pre-Surgical Preparation

Heparinized saline is prepared by combining 2000 units of heparin per L of saline (lactated Ringer's solution can be substituted). 10% NBF is also prepared. Approximately 3–5 L of each solution is necessary for a 60-lb animal. A roller pump is used to force the solutions through at a constant speed (Fig. 2). The 5-foot piece of tubing is used for venous output and the 10-foot length of tubing is used for the arterial feed. Each of the catheters should be beveled on one end, and small holes should be cut in the back of the arterial catheter (Fig. 3) to allow even perfusion of both legs. The arterial catheter is then threaded through the pump, as seen in Fig. 2. The unbeveled end of the arterial catheter will be placed first in the saline and then in the formalin and may need a small weight attached to prevent it from floating (a pair of scissors works well).

Surgery

The animal, under general anesthesia, is placed in dorsal recumbency on the table. Heparin (350 μ/kg) and lidocaine (2 mg/kg) are given intravenously (iv) to prevent blood clotting and promote vasodilatation, respectively. An abdominal approach is used to gain access to the aorta and vena cava just above the point where they bifurcate into the legs. A detailed outline of the surgical procedure can be found in *Handbook of Biomaterials Evaluation.*[4] Once good exposure has been obtained, the vein is catheterized using the 5-ft segment of Tygon® tubing. The unbeveled end of the venous catheter is directed into an appropriate waste container. The arterial catheterization is performed next, with its free end already routed through the roller pump and into the heparinized saline. The pump is turned on and approximately 3–5 L of saline are pumped in as the blood is allowed to flow out of the venous catheter into the waste container. Manual pumping of the legs in a bicycling motion has been found to increase the depth of penetration of the saline. When the fluid in the venous catheter becomes clear, place the free end of the arterial catheter into the 10% NBF and repeat the procedure. The venous catheter is rerouted into a suitable

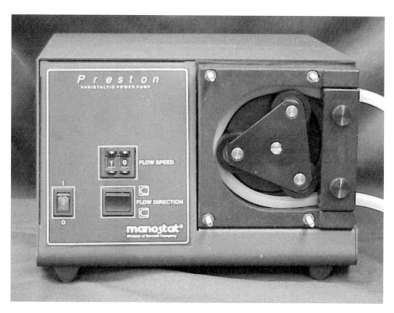

Figure 3. Perfusion pump with silicone tubing.

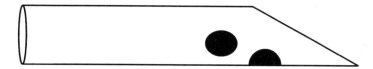

Figure 4. Catheter with bevel.

disposal container for formalin. As the legs are bicycled and the formalin enters the tissue via the blood vessels, an increased rigidity and a decrease in temperature of the thigh muscles is felt. Approximately 5 L of 10% NBF is necessary, although complete fixation of the adipose portions of adult bone marrow requires 1–2 L more. When the muscle feels hard, stop the pump and remove the desired specimens, leaving catheters in place (removal of the catheters results in a large geyser of blood and fluid). When all specimens have been taken, remove catheters and dispose of carcass appropriately. Specimens should be placed in containers of 10% NBF for storage.

APPENDIX C
COMMON FORMULATIONS FOR FIXATIVES[5,22,23]

10% Neutral Buffered Formalin

Formaldehyde solution, 37–40%	100.0 mL
Distilled water	900.0 mL
Sodium phosphate monobasic	4.0 g
Sodium phosphate dibasic (anhydrous)	6.5 g

Bouin's Solution

Picric acid, saturated aqueous solution	750.0 mL
Formaldehyde solution, 37–40%	250.0 mL
Acetic acid, glacial	50.0 mL

Fix tissues from 4–12 h depending on size. Rinse in 50% alcohol until solution stays clear. If any residual picric acid is left in the tissue, deleterious effects can occur many months later if recuts are required. Store in 70% ethanol.

Calcium Formalin

Formaldehyde, 37–40%	100.0 mL
Calcium chloride	10.0 g
Distilled water	900.0 mL

Carnoy's Fluid

Absolute ethyl alcohol	60.0 mL
Chloroform	30.0 mL
Acetic acid, glacial	10.0 mL

Fixation should occur within 3–4 h. Tissue is then transferred to absolute alcohol.

Formalin Alcohol

Formaldehyde solution, 37–40%	100.0 mL
Ethanol, absolute	650.0 mL
Distilled water	250.0 mL

Formalin Ammonium Bromide

Formaldehyde solution, 37–40%	150.0 mL
Ammonium bromide	20.0 g
Distilled water	850.0 ml

Gendre's Fixative

95% ethanol saturated with picric acid	80.0 mL
Formaldehyde solution, 37–40%	15.0 mL
Acetic acid, glacial	5.0 mL

Fix for 1–4 h. Rinse thoroughly in 95% ethanol to remove excess picric acid.

Modified Millonig's Formalin

Formaldehyde solution, 37–40%	100.0 mL
Distilled water	900.0 mL
Sodium phosphate, monobasic	18.6 g
Sodium hydroxide	4.2 g

Zenker's and Helly's Stock Solution

Distilled water	1000.0 mL
Mercuric chloride	50.0 g
Potassium dichromate	25.0 g
Sodium sulfate	10.0 g

Zenker's Working Solution

Stock solution	95.0 mL
Acetic acid, glacial	5.0 mL

Helly's Working Solution

Stock solution	95.0 mL
Formaldehyde solution, 37–40%	5.0 mL

This is not a stable solution. Prepare immediately before use.

Note: Tissues should not be fixed for longer than 24 h in either Zenker's or Helly's solutions. After fixation the tissues should be washed in running water and stored in 70–80% ethanol. Mercury pigment must be removed before staining.

9

Common Fixatives In Hard-Tissue Histology

Antonio Scarano, Giovanna Iezzi, and Adriano Piattelli

Dental School, University of Chieti, Chieti, Italy

I. INTRODUCTION

Fixation is the most important step in obtaining a good histological specimen. Its goal is to block all lytic enzyme activity as well as the activity of bacteria and other infectious agents in order to preserve the constituents of a tissue as they were in the living state. In implant histology, fixation is carried out with chemical compounds without using physical processing such as heating or freezing of the specimen, because these treatments cause contraction and/or expansion of tissues and biomaterials and may give rise to artifacts at the interface. The artifacts are produced by the difference in the coefficients of thermal expansion between hard/soft tissues and biomaterials.[8,11] If mistakes occur during fixation, there can be problems with the subsequent infiltration of the resin. The portions of the specimens that are not well-infiltrated tend to detach from the histological slide and prevent optimal focusing and evaluation of the specimen.[1–6]

The most common solutions employed for fixation include 10–30% formalin, glutaraldehyde, paraformaldehyde, and alcohol-based solutions. Tissue is fixed by crosslinkages formed in the proteins, particularly between lysine residues. This crosslinkage does not harm the structure of proteins greatly, so that antigenicity is not lost. Formalin penetrates tissues well, but its action is relatively slow. The standard solution used is 10% neutral buffered formalin (NBF). A buffered solution prevents acidity, which would promote autolysis, causing precipitation of formol-heme pigment in the tissues.

The alcohol-based solutions have the advantage of preserving numerous enzymes, allowing the performance of many histochemical studies. All these fixatives are known as primary, and other fixatives are known as secondary. The latter are obtained by mixing together several primary fixatives (e.g., Bouin's fixative containing picric acid, formalin, and glacial acetic acid), in order to use the different advantages presented by each component.

The hard tissues have a compact (mineralized) structure that renders the penetration of the fixative difficult. When fixation of large anatomical specimens is attempted, usually only the most peripheral portion undergoes adequate preservation, whereas there are lytic changes of the areas closer to the center of the section that prevent a good infiltration by resin. Thus, if we need to process specimens of large dimensions, it is advisable to either perform a prefixation in 30% formalin for 1 h, or to carry out the fixation by intravascular

From: *Handbook of Histology Methods for Bone and Cartilage*
Edited by: Y. H. An and K. L. Martin © Humana Press Inc., Totowa, NJ

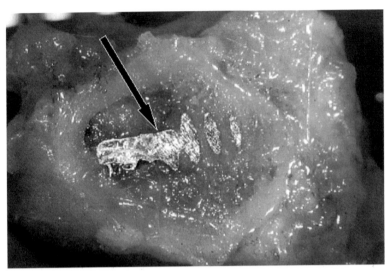

Figure 1. Bone tissue has been reduced in order to allow fixative penetration. The titanium implant is visible.

perfusion. It is also important to reduce the size of the specimens (Fig. 1) to allow better fixation: the best size of the specimens appears to be 4–5 mm.

Although formaldehyde is the best fixative, it is not perfect. Therefore, a variety of fixatives are available for use, depending on the type of tissue we want to study and on the features we want to analyze.[9,10,12,13] For specimens with a diameter larger than 4–6 mm, glutaraldehyde and formalin are suggested, while for specimens smaller than 1–3 mm, alcoholic fixatives may be used.

There are five major groups of fixatives, classified according to the mechanism of action:

- Aldehydes—formaldehyde (formalin) and glutaraldehyde;
- Mercurials—B-5 and Zenker's;
- Alcohols—alcohol (methanol) and ethyl alcohol (ethanol);
- Oxidizing agents—potassium permanganate, dichromate fixatives (potassium dichromate), and osmium tetroxide;
- Picrates—picric acid.

Primary fixatives may be classified as precipitant or non-precipitant, according to their effects on tissue protein (Table 1).

A number of factors affect the fixation process:

- Buffering—to avoid the formation of pigments, the fixative must have pH of 6–8, which is obtained using buffers such as phosphate, bicarbonate, cacodylate, and barbital.
- Penetration—the tissue penetration of a fixative depends on its intrinsic capability to diffuse. Formalin and alcohol have the best penetration, and glutaraldehyde has the worst. Mercurials and other fixatives are somewhere in between.
- Volume—the ideal ratio of fixative to tissue should be 10:1.
- Temperature—increasing the temperature increases the speed of fixation, taking care not to exceed 37°C. In this regard, a recently published study increased the speed of fixation by using microwave irradiation.[7]

Table 1. Primary Fixatives Classified as Precipitant (P) or Non-Precipitant (NP)

Precipitant fixatives (P)	Non-precipitant fixatives (NP)
Chromium trioxide	Acetic acid
Ethanol	Formalin
Mercuric chloride	Osmium tetroxide
Methanol	Potassium dichromate
Picric acid	

- Concentration—increased concentration (within limits) will reduce the length of time needed for fixation.
- Time interval—the length of time in which the tissues remain in the fixative is important. Usually 12–24 h are necessary for the fixative to penetrate completely, depending on the size of the specimens. For large samples, 2–3 d of fixation can be required, changing the solution every 24 h.

Fixatives will: i) confer chemical stability to the tissues; ii) harden the tissues, helping with further handling; iii) block enzyme autolysis; iv) block bacterial putrefaction; and v) enhance later staining techniques.

II. FORMALIN

Formalin is the most commonly used fixative. It acts by binding to the aminic groups of the protein lateral chains, forming a proteic network and modifying in a substantial way the tertiary structure of the protein component of tissues. Formalin-fixed specimens have a higher affinity for basic dyes than for acid dyes, and for this reason, no histochemical studies can be carried out. However, the formalin-fixed specimens may be treated by heating or enzymatic digestion in order to break down the proteic network (aminic binding) and make the proteins available for histochemical reactions.

Fixation is optimally carried out at close to neutral pH, in the range of 6–8. Hypoxia of tissues lowers the pH, and thus, the fixative must have a buffering capacity to avoid the excess of acids. Acidity increases the formation of formalin-heme pigments, which appear as black deposits in the tissues. These deposits can be observed under polarized light, and prevent a good evaluation of the specimen. Common buffers include phosphate, bicarbonate, cacodylate, and barbital.

When exposed to sunlight, fixatives undergo modifications. For example, formalin tends to form higher dimension polymers that have a low penetration capability. Thus, it must be kept in the dark at 4°C. Potassium dichromate and acetic acid bind to lipids, and they cause cells to swell slightly so they can be added to other fixatives to counteract their shrinking effects.

To reduce costs, formalin should be used at the lowest possible concentration. It is usually used in a 10% aqueous solution. It is always buffered with sodium phosphate dibasic and sodium phosphate monobasic in the following proportion:

- Formalin   100 mL
- Distilled water   900 mL
- Sodium phosphate dibasic   4 g
- Sodium phosphate monobasic   6.5 g

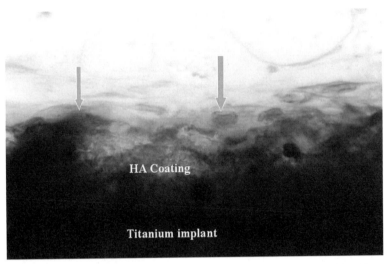

Figure 2. A well-performed fixation gives a good detail of the cells positive for acid phosphatase (arrows) at the bone-implant interface. Magnification ×1200. (*See* color plate 9 appearing in the insert following p. 270.)

This solution diffuses into the tissue at 1–4 mm every h. Non-buffered formalin reacts with oxygen, forming formic acid, which has a low pH (about 4).

Specimens must be placed in buffered formalin for 12–24 h. There should be a 10:1 ratio of fixative to tissue. Agitation of the specimen in the fixative will also enhance fixation. Formalin-fixed specimens stain very well with toluidine blue and acid fuchsin. For histochemistry, it is important to conserve cell structures as well as the proteic structures (Fig. 2).

Formalin is carcinogenic, irritant, corrosive, and toxic. It must be used in well-ventilated areas, and goggles and gloves must always be worn. Formaldehyde is toxic, and the exposure limit is 2 ppm for 10 min every 8 h. Containers of formaldehyde solutions should only be opened in a designated ventilated area. Goggles, gloves, and an apron should be worn over the laboratory coat. Gloves, goggles and apron must also be worn over the laboratory coat when making up formol saline or changing the formalin on specimens. This procedure should be performed in a designated ventilated area.

Formaldehyde is corrosive, and is a severe eye and skin irritant. It is also a sensitizer by skin and respiratory contact, and is toxic when ingested or inhalated. Its target organ is the respiratory system.

III. ALCOHOLS

Some fixatives, like ethanol, act by coagulation and precipitation of the proteins and dissolution of lipids, and have a small penetration capability because of the coagulation of the superficial protein layer. Alcohols such as methanol and ethanol are protein denaturants, and are not used routinely for tissues because they cause excessive brittleness and hardness. However, they are very good for small specimens. Ethanol is preferred for low cost and low toxicity.

With alcohols, the external tissue layers will be fixed in a short time (generally only a few minutes), whereas a longer time period will be needed for the central layers because of the diminution of the fixative penetration. These fixatives may be used when studying enzymatic activity, such as acid and alkaline phosphatases, and when specimens of small dimension are to be investigated. However, if used in elevated concentrations, they tend to shrink the cells. Thus, 70% alcohol is used with some drops of glacial acetic acid or potassium dichromate to prevent cells from shrinking.

There should be a 10:1 ratio of fixative to tissue. Agitation of the specimen in the fixative will also enhance fixation. The specimen must be immersed in alcohol for 1–2 h; a longer time period could cause cell shrinkage. Alcohol-fixed specimens are more easily infiltrated by resins.

Methanol is flammable and is toxic when ingested.

IV. GLUTARALDEHYDE

Glutaraldehyde binds with phospholipids and with DNA, and is mainly used for transmission electron microscopy (TEM). Glutaraldehyde causes deformation of the alpha-helix structure in proteins, and thus is not a good choice for immunoperoxidase staining. It penetrates very poorly, yet fixes very quickly, providing the best overall cytoplasmic and nuclear detail.

The concentration of glutaraldehyde should be adjusted down to the lowest level possible to reduce costs. The routinely used concentration is 1% for small specimens, and 2.5% for large specimens. If it comes in a concentration of 50%, the 2.5% final solution must be prepared in the following way:

- 50% glutaraldehyde   5 mL
- Phosphate-buffered saline (PBS)   95 mL

Glutaraldehyde must be stored at 4°C. There should be a 10:1 ratio of fixative to tissue. Agitation of the specimen in the fixative will also enhance fixation.

Glutaraldehyde is toxic by ingestion and inhalation, and is a sensitizer by skin and respiratory contact. Its target organ is the respiratory system.

V. BOUIN'S SOLUTION

Bouin's solution has a high penetrating capability, and can be used also for larger specimens that must be immersed in the solution for 12–24 h. It is a popular fixative for embryonic tissues and skin, because of its excellent preservation of nuclei and chromosomes. Bouin's is very compatible with the trichrome stain. Its mechanism of action is unknown. It does almost as well as mercurials with nuclear detail, but does not cause as much hardness. Picric acid, in dry form, may pose an explosive hazard. As a solution, it stains everything it touches yellow, including skin.

Bouin's solution is used for the fixation of small, calcified specimens. However, poor results are obtained with large specimens. The solution is composed of:

- Aqueous saturated solution of picric acid   15 mL
- Formalin   5 mL
- Glacial acetic acid   1 mL

Picric acid gives a yellow background stain to specimens. This yellow color can create problems for the staining of slides and for their further evaluation. To avoid the yellow background stain, the specimens must be repeatedly washed for 1–2 d with a solution of alcohol and lithium carbonate. However, for specimens measuring more than 10×10 mm, the complete removal of the picric acid can be impossible.

If the use of Bouin's solution is not frequent, the purchase of small quantities of this prepared fixative is recommended. This reduces hazardous waste, removes the picric acid hazard and ensures the presence of a fresh fixative. There should be a 10:1 ratio of fixative to tissue. Agitation of the specimen in the fixative will also enhance fixation.

Formalin is carcinogenic, corrosive, toxic, and a severe eye and skin irritant. Work must be done in a well-ventilated area, wearing goggles and gloves. It is a sensitizer by skin and respiratory contact and toxic by ingestion and inhalation. The target organ is the respiratory system. Picric acid crystals can become explosive if allowed to dry out, so purchasing saturated picric acid solution is recommended. Picric acid is toxic through skin exposure. Acetic acid is corrosive, and the target organ is the respiratory system.

VI. POST-FIXATION TREATMENT AND SPECIMEN STORAGE

The fixed specimen must be washed in phosphate buffered saline (PBS) or running water to completely remove all the fixative solution, which could affect the staining procedure. Washing in PBS is performed by immersing the specimen for 1 d in PBS, and changing the solution several times.

Fixed specimens can be stored in alcohol or fixative for several weeks, but longer periods in alcohol tends to shrink the cells, altering the morphology. For large specimens, water tends to separate from alcohol and the latter also evaporates, leaving a large portion of the tissue under water and without alcohol. Formalin, after long time periods, tends to lose its fixing capability. If specimens must be preserved for more than several weeks, the best way is to infiltrate and embed them in resin. In this case, there is no time limit.

REFERENCES

1. Bergroth V, Reitamo S, Konttinen YT, et al: Fixation-dependent cytoplasmic false-positive staining with an immunoperoxidase method. *Histochemistry* 73:509–513, 1982.
2. Eggert FM, Linder JE, Jubb RW: Staining of demineralized cartilage. I. Alcoholic versus aqueous demineralization at neutral and acidic pH. *Histochemistry* 73:385–390, 1981.
3. Holund B, Clausen PP, Clemmensen I: The influence of fixation and tissue preparation on the immunohistochemical demonstration of fibronectin in human tissue. *Histochemistry* 72:291–299, 1981.
4. Lee TH, Kato H, Pan LH, et al: Localization of nerve growth factor, trkA and P75 immunoreactivity in the hippocampal formation and basal forebrain of adult rats. *Neuroscience* 83:335–349, 1998.
5. Liem RS, Jansen HW: The use of chromic potassium sulphate in bone electron microscopy. *Acta Morphol Neerl Scand* 22:233–243, 1984.
6. Koen Bos P, van Osch GJ, van der Kwast T, et al: Fixation-dependent immunolocalization shift and immunoreactivity of intracellular growth factors in cartilage. *Histochem J* 32:391–396, 2000.
7. Massa LF, Arana-Chavez VE: Ultrastructural preservation of rat embryonic dental tissue by rapid fixation and dehydration under microwave irradiation. *Eur J Oral Sci* 108:74–77, 2000.
8. Margo CE, Lee A: Fixation of whole eyes: the role of fixative osmolarity in the production of tissue artifact. *Graefes Arch Clin Exp Ophthalmol* 233:366–370, 1995.
9. Mepham BL: Influence of fixatives on the immunoreactivity of paraffin sections. *Histochem J* 14:731–737, 1982.

10. Mrini A, Moukhles H, Jacomy H, et al: Efficient immunodetection of various protein antigens in glutaraldehyde-fixed brain tissue. *J Histochem Cytochem* 43:1285–1291, 1995.

11. Naganuma H, Murayama H, Ohtani N, et al: Optically clear nuclei in papillary carcinoma of the thyroid: demonstration of one of the fixation artifacts and its practical usefulness. *Pathol Int* 50:113–118, 2000.

12. Ramos-Vara JA, Beissenherz ME: Optimization of immunohistochemical methods using two different antigen retrieval methods on formalin-fixed paraffin-embedded tissues: experience with 63 markers. *J Vet Diagn Invest* 12:307–311, 2000.

13. Tahan SR, Wei Y, Ling P, et al: Influence of formalin fixation time and tissue processing method on immunoreactivity of monoclonal antibody PC10 for proliferating cell nuclear antigen. *Mod Pathol* 8:177–182, 1995.

10

Decalcification of Bone Tissue

Robert A. Skinner

Center for Orthopaedic Research, University of Arkansas for Medical Sciences, Little Rock, AR, USA

1. INTRODUCTION

Bone is among the hardest, most dense tissue encountered at the bench by histotechnologists. In order to achieve acceptable 3–6-μm sections of bone, the technologist surrounds and infiltrates the material with a media of relatively similar density to form a more homogenous construct. For studies involving mineralization, the technologist may choose one of several polymer resins, which produce a block close to the hardness of the bone itself. For studies of intracellular detail in which extremely thin sections of marrow are preferred, the technologist may choose a "softer" polymer that can readily produce sections of bone marrow at 1.5–2 μm. Frozen sections of some samples can also be achieved using very cold temperatures and harder tungsten carbide blades. These are usually specialized procedures, which are not available to most histopathology laboratories. Because paraffin processing of tissue is the most widely used methodology in histologic slide preparation, procedures have been developed to allow specimens to conform to this routine histologic preparation. In order to accomplish this, bone specimens must be made compatible with the embedding media and sectioning apparatus associated with this process. Because the paraffin used in this process is significantly softer than most bone, the bone sample must be treated to take on this softer characteristic in order to be sectioned. This treatment known as decalcification.

II. DECALCIFICATION

The composition of bone can be represented by the equation:

$$\text{Crystals of Inorganic Salts (Calcium)} + \text{Organic Matrix} = \text{BONE} \tag{1}$$

A simplified definition derived from classic and current texts describes decalcification as the removal of the inorganic components from the hard tissue. In more technical terms, it is the dissolution of the hydroxyapatite complex, $Ca_{10}(PO_4)_6(OH)_2$, and can be represented by the following equation:

$$Ca_{10}(PO_4)_6(OH)_2 + 8H^+ \Leftrightarrow 10Ca^{+2} + 6HPO_4^{-2} + 2H_2O \tag{2}$$

Once the removal of these salts has been accomplished, the process of decalcification reaches its "end point." The end point of decalcification is the moment when all inorganic

From: *Handbook of Histology Methods for Bone and Cartilage*
Edited by: Y. H. An and K. L. Martin © Humana Press Inc., Totowa, NJ

material is removed from the tissue, leaving the remainder of the organic matrix intact. Precise determination of this end point is critical to optimal staining, and in some cases higher-level analyses. Post-end-point decalcified tissue, consisting of the cellular components and organic matrix, should theoretically be soft enough for paraffin processing by routine means and sectioning with standard equipment. Additional exposure to a solution that is more acidic than the remaining organic matrix will at some point begin to extract organic components from the tissue, especially from cells. This is the primary connection between poor staining and overdecalcification. Because stronger acids decalcify in less time, there may be a greater risk of overdecalcification because the window of opportunity to arrest the process at the optimal time of the precise end point is shorter.

Choices of decalcifying fluids are numerous, as are the factors that influence their selection. Making the sample soft enough for sectioning is not the only consideration. The concept that more decalcification is better does not make for the best preparation. Post-decalcification staining quality for routine as well as specialized protocols is becoming an increasingly significant factor in decalcifant choices for both research and clinical studies. The additional turnaround time added by the decalcification step is often the most significant contributor to poorly decalcified tissue. Speed vs the textbook-perfect preparation plays a major role in compromise and corner cutting. Literature and textbook reviews present numerous approaches and protocols for decalcification, with equally as many levels of complexity and accuracy. Principles and practices that will produce the best results tailored to the mission of the laboratory are most often distilled from hands-on experience. Attention to detail and the practical application of prior success can be most valuable in setting up a decalcification regimen.

III. DECALCIFIER COMPONENTS/ACTION

The usual mechanism for decalcification is immersion in an acid solution, a chelating solution, or a solution consisting of an acid-chelator complex. This immersion may be augmented by heat, ultrasonic stimulation, vacuum, or agitation to decrease the time for complete calcium removal. Chelators used in decalcification are usually specific for removal of calcium ions from the surface of the sample. Whatever the acid solution involved, it will initially have a pH lower than that of the immersed bone. It is this lower pH solution that will cause the hydroxyapatite to dissolve and move the calcium from the mineral/organic matrix composite to the surrounding liquid. The exact pH of the decalcifant and the difference in pH between the solution that is in contact with the sample and the sample itself are controlled by several factors. These factors include constituent components of the solution, solution strength, and the availability of fresh, active liquid.

A. Acid Decalcifiers

Acids are nominally categorized as either strong or weak. Strong acids commonly used for decalcifiers are hydrochloric acid and nitric acid, usually employed in aqueous solutions of concentrations ranging from 5–10%. Decalcifying acids classified as weak acids are formic acid, picric acid, and acetic acid. Of these weaker acids, formic acid is the one used principally as a stand-alone reagent or in consort with a buffer (usually sodium citrate) in aqueous solutions from 5–15%. Acetic acid in aqueous solutions of 5–10% was once a popular choice, but in recent times has gone the way of picric acid as a fixation additive to provide mild decalcification properties.

B. Chelators

A chelator is an organic chemical that bonds with and removes free metal ions from solutions. Chelating agents (sometimes referred to in the older literature as "complexing agents") react with one of the ionic species, derived from the substance to be dissolved, and form a stable complex with the substance, reducing the concentration of the free ions in the solution to the point where the target substance dissolves. Ethylenediamine tetraacetic acid (EDTA) is a chelating agent that reacts with calcium. It is the most widely used chelator for decalcification in concentrations of up to 14%.

There are over 50 formulae of decalcifiers or decalcifier/fixative solutions based in some manner on these components. Stronger acids or stronger concentrations of a given weaker acid will promote faster decalcification because the resultant pH is relatively lower. With strong, rapid-acting solutions, there is the danger of having the tissue immersed in the solution past the precise end point of decalcification. This overdecalcification robs protein from the remaining cells and organic matrix, making for a smoothly cut yet poorly stained section. The concept of decalcification up to its end point and no further is universally important to the best possible slide preparation. There are four generalized methods for establishing a decalcification end point worthy of examination. They are radiography, timed immersion, probing or bending, and chemical testing.

IV. END POINT DETERMINATION

A. Radiography

Radiography can determine whether the calcium has been removed from a specimen. It is described by Carson[5] as "the most accurate method of determining the completeness of decalcification." But in order to ensure this, a pre-decalcification exposure to establish baseline readings and relative settings is suggested to maximize this accuracy (Fig. 1). This additional step and the process of developing the film makes it time-consuming. In addition to the costs of the generating unit and developer plus chemicals, the price of the film puts the cost of mere end point determination beyond the reach of most laboratories unless it is incorporated into a study data collection or an overall documentation regime.

B. Manipulation (Probing and Bending)

Probing or bending is generally the most commonly described method for end point determination. This may be a misnomer, as it is actually a method to determine whether the section is soft enough to section. This method is adequate for determining when a sample is ready to be sectioned, but by the time the sample is deemed pliable enough for sectioning, it can be well past the optimal end point for staining. At the opposite end of the spectrum, samples containing large percentages of dense cortical bone may be flexible, but still harbor centralized areas of undecalcified material (Fig. 2). Probing with a sharp object, such as a needle or a scalpel blade, can leave undesirable artifacts.

C. Timed Immersion

Timed immersion can be relatively successful with like-kind samples. For example, a manufacturer may state that the average bone *marrow* biopsy will be completely decalcified after x amount of time in 20 calcified tissue volumes of their product. Or your laboratory may establish its own protocol, as ours did: "a 5 mm slab of femoral head will be

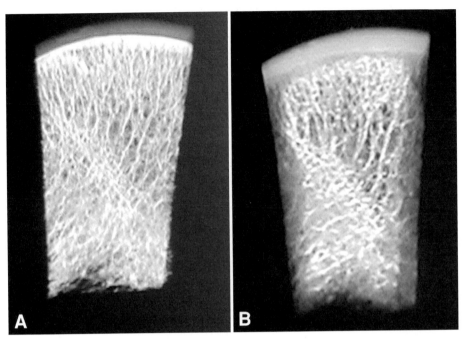

Figure 1. (A) Radiograph of a selected sample of 5-mm-thick slab of femoral head prior to decalcification. (B) Radiograph of same sample after suggested 5 h of decalcification illustrating central portion of sample still not fully decalcified.

adequately decalcified to do full face sectioning after 24 hrs in 250 mL of a 1.35N hydrochloric acid/chelator solution." Again, this will ensure adequate sectioning, but may provide less than optimal staining, depending on the density and the exact calcium content of the sample.

D. Chemical Testing

Chemical testing for the presence of calcium in the solution used is the most accurate method. Daily testing is preferred, with a weak acid such as formic acid. Bancroft[3] suggests weekly testing for EDTA. Not all acids and acid-chelator combinations are conducive to convenient chemical testing; thus, the choice of decalcifant can be a limiting factor in using this method. Specific methods in chemical end point determination will be dealt with in depth in the subsection *"Chemical End Point Determination."*

V. SPECIMEN PREPARATION/MANAGEMENT

In order to optimize the information obtained from decalcified specimens, attention must be given to a wide range of issues which begin with specimen management at the grossing table. Specimens requiring decalcification cannot be simply resected and placed directly into the decalcifant. All specimens destined for paraffin processing require some type of fixation. One of the most overlooked factors contributing to less than optimal results from decalcified tissue begins with poor fixation. Although detailed fixation practices are discussed at length in Chapter 8 of this book, overlapping princi-

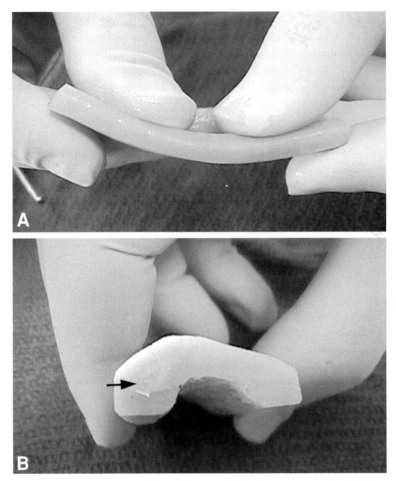

Figure 2. (A) Portion of human tibia during decalcification, apparently pliable enough for sectioning. (B) Cutting 5 mm into the end of the sample reveals a centralized, sequestered area of calcification (arrow).

ples for both processes, which are not stand-alone concepts, must be considered. Thicker, denser specimens take longer to fix throughout, regardless of the fixative employed. These specimens experience relatively the same types of penetration impediments to the decalcifying fluids as are presented to the fixation fluids. Therefore, although the overall size of the sample is important, the most important parameter to be considered is sample thickness, although there is evidence to support the concept that the penetration characteristics of decalcifying fluids are not the same as those of fixatives. Although Lillie[14] states that formalin penetrates in a uniform fashion, Brain[4] suggests that there are rate differences as well as qualitative differences, which take place at "minimum diffusion distance" thresholds of 1.5 mm and 3.0 mm. These measurements coincide with specimen thickness of 3.0–6.0 mm. Specimens up to 3.0 mm in thickness decalcify evenly and rapidly. Specimens from 3.0 to 6.0 mm thick exhibited even decalcification, although the rate was slower than anticipated. Specimens thicker than

6.0 mm—especially those with very dense centralized areas—seemed to actually resist the action of the decalcifying reagent.

Taking these concepts to the grossing table will help to promote optimal decalcification. Bone marrow core biopsies for hematopoetic analysis, decompression bone cores for osteonecrosis studies, and much debridement material are generally submitted in a ready fashion for fixation and decalcification. Femoral heads, osteoarticular constructs, and bone/tumor composites generally must be downsized prior to processing. Options for downsizing large samples include the fine-toothed hand saw, Stryker type oscillating saw, and various types of band saws. Multiple parallel slabs of equal thickness can be made so that a representative slab can be submitted. Care must be taken when using aggressive toothed blades, no matter what type of saw is employed, so that potential architectural damage is minimized. Some pathologists insist on allowing specimens to fix before sawing to help minimize this damage. In cases of large tumor/bone composites, where a confident diagnosis has been made through small-piece sampling and the balance of the composite is submitted for teaching or research purposes, the specimen may be frozen prior to slabbing and the resulting slabs warmed in 37°C formalin to minimize the freeze artifact.[11] It is during this stage of downsizing the specimen into a manageable sample size that the first of many potential compromises is encountered.

Because of the systematized automation of today's routine pathology labs, sample size is generally dictated by the size of the standard cassette, which is 4 mm deep. This nominal thickness has become the relative standard for average non-mineralized tissue in an overnight processing scheme. Since thinner samples will fix and decalcify more rapidly, the inclination is to saw the sample down to the thinnest possible size—i.e., 4 mm or less. Although this will promote more rapid fixation and decalcification, it may not be the best practice for ensuring optimal quality sections. Dense samples with a large surface-area cutting face are prone to being lifted out of the paraffin block by the physical forces generated by the ensuing microtomy. Thus, although a 2-mm-thick sample of a femoral head or a cortical bone/tumor composite may be desirable for rapid turnaround, the potential risk of a poorly sectioning block may make a 4–5-mm-thick sample more appropriate if there is available time. Because our lab does specimen radiography on most bone samples, we slab our samples to a consistent 5-mm thickness, which meets all our needs. In a case such as this, the compromise is between least turnaround time and the concepts of adequate vs optimal.

VI. CHOOSING A DECALCIFIER

For some specimens, for which the most critical issue is the turnaround time, or when the specimen is thin and not very dense—as in the case of a bone-marrow core biopsy—several combination "fixative-decalcifiers" are commercially available. They are usually a combination of formic acid plus formalin in proprietary percentages, depending on the manufacturer. Manufacturers tout products of this nature as being able to fix and decalcify standard bone-marrow needle biopsies in as little as 20 min to 4 h, and to fix and decalcify "larger specimens" overnight. End point determinants range from "decalcification is complete when the specimen floats" to specific chemical tests,[7,17] encompassing a wide range of completion possibilities. These products generally produce serviceable sectioning once experience with the product and familiarity with the impact of the density of varying samples has been attained. Staining can be of variable quality if samples are not sufficiently monitored. If the conventional "fix first, then decalcify" mode is employed, once the sample thickness is established and the specimen is fixed, choosing a decalcifying agent is the next critical step.

The primary consideration in choosing a decalcifant should be which types of analyses will be performed on the resulting slides. If the primary consideration is merely to make the sample soft enough to acquire a face-cut section followed by a machine-stained H&E, then any decalcifier will fill the need if properly used. However, if the sample in question requires extremely fine intracellular detail, multiple special stains, or immunohistochemical or molecular biology procedures, then it is more important to determine the type of decalcifant chosen as well as how decalcifant of choice is monitored.

A. Strong Acid Decalcifiers—Hydrochloric and Nitric Acid

When speed is the primary consideration, the first choices of decalcifier are usually solutions, with the active decalcifying agent being either nitric acid or hydrochloric acid. Both are considered to yield adequate results when the size of the tissue allows for decalcification to end point in less than 48 h, even in solutions of 5% concentration. Nitric acid in a 5% aqueous solution is often touted in the older literature for its speed and its ability to avoid tissue swelling. Luna[16] states that by making the 5% solution in 80% ethanol, the decalcification process can be accelerated because the ethanol simultaneously removes fat, which may impede the dissolution of the hydroxyapatite. Hydrochloric acid in concentrations from 8–15% is arguably the most widely used of the mineral acids for rapid decalcification. Much of this usage can be attributed to the recent market expansion of commercially produced, prepackaged decalcifiers. Hydrochloric acid with or without a chelator is the component of choice in commercially available "rapid" decalcifiers. Urban,[23] Brain,[4] and Sheehan and Hrapchak[18] all caution the user about the hydrolysis of the bone matrix and tissue swelling associated with overexposure as the primary drawbacks of using hydrochloric acid. However, Sheehan and Hrapchak describe the addition of salt (15% solution of NaCl) to a hydrochloric acid decalcifier (3% HCl) to reduce this deleterious swelling. The commercially available HCl/chelator solutions provide this rapid demineralization and reduced swelling effect with prepackaged proprietary chemistry, which in some cases can decalcify a 2-mm bone marrow core in a little as 15 min. Whether using a hydrochloric acid solution by itself or in combination with a chelator, it should be noted that combining hydrochloric acid vapors and formaldehyde vapors reportedly form a potent carcinogen, bischloromethyl ether. It has been strongly recommended that samples fixed in formalin should be washed in water prior to hydrochloric acid decalcification to avoid this problem[2,5] By fine-tuning the package directives, applying them to the routine specimens received, and close monitoring of the process to end point, quality serviceable results with routine stains can be consistently obtained in the shortest time. It must be remembered that the primary drawback with the mineral acid decalcifiers is the very small time window when decalcification reaches the precise end point. With some of these solutions, 60 min too early can leave the tissue difficult to section; 60 min too late can have significant negative effects on even the simplest of routine stains. When the need for optimal staining in the absence of intensive monitoring outweighs the need for rapid turnaround, the acid decalcifant of choice is generally formic acid.

B. Weak Acid Decalcifiers—Formic Acid

Aqueous formic acid in concentrations from 5–10% is generally considered to be the best overall choice for decalcification, considering the balance between reproducible optimal quality of the stained section and turnaround time from specimen to slide. It is touted as delivering excellent morphological detail, with little or no tissue distortion.[23] Increasing the concentration to from 15% to as much as 25% may subject the material to staining pitfalls similar to those associated with the stronger acids.[6] A solution of 5% formic acid is mild enough to allow for a longer cushion between the time of precise decalcification and the point when proteins are detrimentally removed from the matrix. This helps to reduce the severity of accidental overdecalcification. Decalcification with 5% formic acid is slower than similar-strength nitric or hydrochloric acid solutions, and slower than most commercial decalcifiers. Experience with well-fixed bone/tumor and bone/biomaterial composites has shown serviceable staining with sections from samples that have been immersed in 5% formic acid for more than 30 d.[20] Established literature, much of it based on the work of Lillie,[15] states that 5% formic acid can be used to yield overall excellent staining results with the exceptions of Fuelgen nuclear staining, which is rendered "unsatisfactory" and the impairment of Van Gieson's and Masson's staining.[18] A significant portion of this Masson staining impairment can be consistently corrected by careful monitoring of post-decalcification washing and careful monitoring of the Bouin's step in the Masson's trichrome procedure. These variations have yielded preferred results for numerous specimens.[1,9,10,22] Reports in the new literature have stated that certain immunohistochemical procedures can be done on tissues subjected to decalcification in 5% formic acid for up to 25 d.[24] Additionally, mounting evidence suggests that exposing tissues to formic acid in concentrations from 1–5% can serve as an epitope enhancement procedure.[14,19] However, even with this new information, when specimens are taken with a strong possibility of requiring immunohistochemical or enzyme histochemical analysis, the leading decalcifant of choice is the chelator EDTA.

C. Chelators—EDTA

EDTA is a chelating agent that reacts with calcium by binding the ionized calcium on the outer layer of the apatite crystal, thus reducing the size of the crystal as the process continues. Because of the specificity of the chelating reaction, the EDTA has virtually no effect on surrounding tissues or tissues depleted of calcium, as do acid decalcifiers. Therefore, many enzymes that are altered by acid decalcification remain intact. Decalcification in EDTA can be a very slow process in comparison to acid decalcification, and has been described by Brain[4] as taking up to eight times longer than with 4N formic acid. There are several protocols for concentration and pH of EDTA solutions, ranging from mainstream to obscure. The two most popular formulae seem to be a 5% solution, pH 7.0, and a 10% solution, pH 7.0–7.4.

VII. CONCEPTS COMMON TO ALL DECALCIFIERS

A. Decalcifant Fluid Volume and Change Intervals

All the techniques described in Section VI share common concepts. The most rapid turnaround time, regardless of the modality, will be accomplished by immersion in the "freshest," "most active" solution, regardless of the initial strength. The generally accepted volume of decalcifant is 10–20× the volume of the tissue, with the 10× volume applying to the strong acid decalcifiers and the 20× volume applying to weak acids, especially 5% formic acid. In order to ensure "freshness" or availability of specific ions, or lower pH fluid, the solution should be changed on a regular basis. This allows the calcium ions to more freely migrate out of the material and into the surrounding decalcifying fluid. Brain[4] suggests that the decalcifying acid diffuses into the tissue, and the soluble products of decalcification diffuse toward the area of lower pH. This would suggest that as the pH of the solution rises, the transport of calcium into the solution is decreased, thus the need for fresh solution surrounding the specimen. Recommendations for changing the decalcifant vary with the decalcifant selected. Tissues should not remain in nitric or hydrochloric acid for more than 48 h, so it stands to reason that unless directed otherwise by the manufacturer of a rapid decalcifier, the solution should be changed at lest twice daily for the short duration. The recommendation for formic acid in 5–10% concentrations is to change the fluid daily until the end point is achieved.[20] The recommendations for EDTA vary from daily to weekly.[3,18]

B. Suspension, Heat, Agitation and Vacuum

To ensure complete surrounding with the freshest possible fluid, suspending the sample is optimal. Although this is optimal, it is not necessary, and in many instances the practicality of not suspending the sample outweighs the gain in using this process. I have successfully decalcified femoral head slabs sitting on the bottom of the container for 20 years, and cannot recall a complaint associated with this practice. I make up for the omission of the suspension of large slabs by turning them over when changing the fluid. In addition to surrounding the specimen with fresh active fluid, the action of the chosen decalcifier can be expedited by heat, agitation, or a combination of both. Intermittent and constant vacuum has been evaluated with mixed results, but from a practical standpoint, it is not reasonable.[4] Although it is universally accepted that heat will accelerate the process, there is a significant risk involved in employing acid decalcifiers at temperatures above 37°C. The risk of tissue swelling and danger of tissue digestion demand close monitoring if the use of heat is implemented. Several studies indicate that EDTA decalcification at temperatures up to 60°C could cut the time to end point by 50%, and show little or no negative impact on staining.[4] Agitation of any decalcifant will prevent the stagnation of ion transport into the surrounding solution. However, what is interesting about the concept of agitation as a decalcification enhancement is that studies reported by Brain[4] and Bancroft[3] indicate that agitation does not significantly increase the diffusion of the calcium ions through the bone to the outside fluid. So, with large samples, as the surface and "outer core" of calcium is eliminated, the rate of decalcification of the "inner core" is then governed by the diffusion rate. Thus, with large samples, the ultimate gain in turnaround time is not significant. With this in mind, the minimum daily agitation is recommended to be "manually, two to three times a day." We have found it to be more convenient to place out samples on an orbital type shaker and turn it on after the fluids have been changed, and then turn it off with the lights at the end of the day.

C. Chemical End Point Determination

The most critical common concept, regardless of the decalcifant employed, is that the best sectioning and staining will be obtained from tissue that has been decalcified to its precise end point. Considering that chemical end point testing is the most practicably accurate end point determination method, it is important to remember that different modalities require particular tests. Although the testing procedures may vary, the bottom line is that if the tested solution yields a precipitate (usually calcium oxalate), the solution contains calcium, and therefore the end point has not been definitively established.

1. Strong Acid Decalcifiers—Hydrochloric and Nitric Acid

For decalcifiers that contain strong acids such as nitric or hydrochloric acid, there is a chemical test cited by Bancroft and Stevens,[3] Carson,[5] Kiernan,[12] and Sheehan and Hrapchek[18] among others, which calls for the neutralization of the decalcification fluid with ammonium hydroxide until it tests neutral with litmus paper, then proceeds with the addition of 5 mL of saturated ammonium oxalate to 5 mL of the neutralized solution, which is then allowed to sit for 30 min. A simplified version of this test, touted by Luna,[15] calls for 5 mL of the decalcifying solution, adding 5 mL of 5% ammonium hydroxide and 5 mL of 5% ammonium oxalate and letting stand for 15 min. In both cases, if the solution is clear, theoretically all the calcium has been removed from the specimen and the end point has been achieved. If a precipitate forms, the solution should be changed and the test should be repeated after the tissue is further exposed to the decalcifier fluid. This type of test accurately detects the presence of calcium oxalate in the solution. However, there are no clear-cut directives for when the test should be administered. Testing the solution used to decalcify a bone sample of undetermined density after 1 h will yield a precipitate. But if the calcium was removed at the 40-min mark, and your test registers the product of hydroxyapatite dissolution from time 0–40 min, you may already be in danger of significantly detrimental overdecalcification. If you change this solution at the 60-min mark and then retest after an arbitrarily selected time of an additional 20 min, the test will confirm that the end point has been reached. The sample will most likely cut satisfactorily, but what negative effects on the staining of the section will be realized as a result of this overdecalcification? Chemical end point testing of individual variable samples in high-volume environments may not be practical as the best defense against overdecalcification because of the factors of short-increment multiple testing. In these scenarios it, may be best to develop a customized time format for end point estimation. Reference points for time estimation are generally provided by the manufacturers of proprietary decalcifiers.[2,7,8,17] Chemical testing of decalcification solutions with concentrations of mineral acids higher than 10% is not as accurate, and is therefore not recommended as a sole determinant of end point.[3]

2. Weak Acid Decalcifiers—Formic Acid

The chemical test for formic acid decalcifiers is 1 part 5% aqueous ammonium oxalate poured into 5 parts "spent" formic acid. This test works best for 5% solutions. Positive precipitate may form quickly or instantaneously. If the sample is close to the end point, the precipitate may form slowly (15 min), and may only be detectable by the precipitate that adheres to the sides of the test tube. If no precipitate forms after 15 min, the sample is deemed clear and the end point has been reached. As stated earlier, formic acid is slow-acting in comparison to the hydrochloric acid solutions. As such, the recommended time increment for changing the solution is daily. With some exceptionally thick samples, we may start off by changing twice daily at the beginning. Chemical end point testing should be done at the time of change, but common sense based on experience dictates that a 5-

mm-thick slab of femoral head will not be completely decalcified in 1 wk using 5% formic acid. For samples which we are confident will take at least "x" number of days to achieve end point, we adjust our testing regimen accordingly. Thus, for the sake of convenience, we may do a "change only" and omit the test for those "x" number of days. We have also observed that with certain types of standard samples, once established, we can reduce the total decalcification time in 5% formic acid by approx 30% by changing the solution twice daily during the early stages of the process.

With exceptionally thick or dense samples, our group will also reduce the volume of fluid from the suggested 20× volume of 5% formic acid to the minimum amount of fluid required to submerse the specimen as the sample gets closer to the end point. This will concentrate any potential precipitate to reduce the possibility of false-negative results because of what Brain[4] describes as "calcified residue" in the central areas caused by ineffective ion transport out of the sample. It is suggested that in the absence of a radiographic backup for the confirmation of suspected "false-negatives" in specimens thicker than 6.0 mm, a secondary gross cut be performed after the end point is suspected. Because 5% formic acid is relatively mild, there is a relatively large "margin for error" leading to the detrimental effects of overdecalcification. This is especially true for excessively thick or dense samples. If there is any doubt as to the result of the test, there is virtually no harm in leaving the tissue in the same formic acid for an additional 24 h.

3. Chelators

The most reliable chemical end point test for EDTA decalcified material is the same neutralization of the decalcification fluid with ammonium hydroxide until it tests neutral with litmus paper, then adding 5 mL of saturated ammonium oxalate to 5 mL of the neutralized solution and allowing to sit for 30 min as previously described. Recommendations for testing range from every day to every 5 d. Because of the chelating action of EDTA, the sample can be left for several days after end point with no harmful effects.

Another common concept involves the "optimal end point determination window" and the margin for error associated with this concept, as applied to extra-thick and composite specimens. For the purpose of illustration, we will define a composite specimen as one that must be decalcified because of its bone content, but also contains a substantial amount of surrounding soft tissue. Examples of this are tumors attached to or incorporated into bone, muscle, connective tissue associated with whole mounts of animal knees in arthritis studies, or what I consider to be the ultimate challenge—whole rodent heads. Whole rodent heads contain what are considered by many to be the two extremes of difficulty in tissue processing—bone and brain. While the decalcifant is removing and transporting the calcium ions out of the central areas of the skull, the delicate tissues of the brain are exposed to the same fluids for what in some cases are very extended periods of time. Even in the case of a 5-mm-thick slab of femoral head, although the surface 500 μm will decalcify rapidly, by the time the interior calcium has been removed, the surface face is well past end point, yet face-cut sections will still yield superior staining.[1,10,12,22] It is this consideration which has made 5% formic acid the most widely touted general decalcifier of choice for decades.

Using the extremes of tissue examples cited here, from the 2-mm bone marrow biopsy core to the whole gerbil head, general practical suggestions for decalcified specimen management follow in Section VIII.

VIII. WORKING EXAMPLES

A. Bone Marrow Biopsy

Gross—The sample is already small enough for processing.

Decalcifant—This specimen offers many choices for decalcification. A proprietary fixative/decalcifant may be appropriate for the fastest turnaround time, especially if the study does not extend beyond routine staining. This solution should be used as per the instructions or modified, as per experience. If the specimen is fixed as an initial independent step, a proprietary rapid decalcifier (most likely with hydrochloric acid as the primary active ingredient) may be appropriate, again for the fastest turnaround time, especially if the study does not proceed beyond routine staining. This will most likely be used as per the instructions or experience for end point determination, but can be used with the chemical end point test. If more intricate special stains and immunostaining procedures are anticipated, it may be in the best interest of optimization to fix the sample as appropriate, then use 5% formic acid. This solution will generally decalcify a 2-mm bone marrow core to yield satisfactory sections overnight to 18 h. If a more precise end point is required, the ammonium oxalate test is employed. This strategy requires more time, but will potentially yield more diverse information with consistent textbook-quality sections throughout the sample. Some facilities will gross off a representative sample from the received biopsy for the slower treatment, while putting through the majority of the specimen for rapid routine processing. Depending on the type of studies and procedures required, this representative sample may be decalcified in either 5% formic acid or EDTA.

B. Femoral Head

Resected femoral heads are difficult specimens to deal with. Within the confines of today's laboratory business structure, they are sometimes difficult to justify as more than the "gross only" specimen, and are routinely treated as such by many institutions. For this example we will consider the scenario of a freshly received femoral head with an atypical form of osteonecrosis slated for both routine and special paraffin-embedded studies in an institutional setting equipped to perform staining procedures from routine H& E to complex immunohistochemistry.

Gross—The grossing regimen for optimal sectioning would be to serially gross cut the specimen into 5-mm-thick slabs ideally using a band saw (Fig. 3). Visually or radiographically select the slab that is best suited for whole mount section and place it into fixative. Select the slab from either side of the chosen one, which contains an area of interest which will fit into a cassette. (It is recommended to have a supply of "double thick" 10-mm-deep cassettes to accommodate the thicker samples.) "Chisel out" the appropriate area by means of a hammer and disposable high-profile microtome blade (Fig. 4). Place the cassette in fixative. After adequate fixation appropriate for each ensuing processing procedure (*see* Chapter 8), the appropriate decalcifier can be selected.

Decalcifant—Because of the thickness and density of this type of specimen, a combination fixative/decalcifier is not recommended unless only a surface section is desired. A well-fixed cassette-sized sample placed in a proprietary hydrochloric acid decalcifier for the recommended 5 h was satisfactorily decalcified to be "face sectioned" approx 1/3 into the block (Fig. 1). My personal preference for processing this type of specimen is to use a nominal 10% hydrochloric acid/chelator proprietary decalcifier overnight, wash the spec-

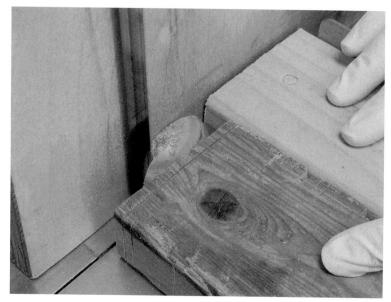

Figure 3. Gross slabbing of femoral head using a band saw. Note the utilization of wood blocks to hold the sample in place.

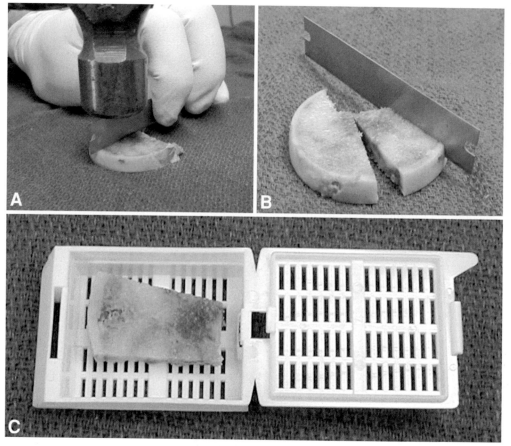

Figure 4. (A,B) Driving disposable microtome blade with hammer through undecalcified 5-mm slab of femoral head. (C) Resulting cassette-sized sample ready for radiography and decalcification (*see* Fig. 1).

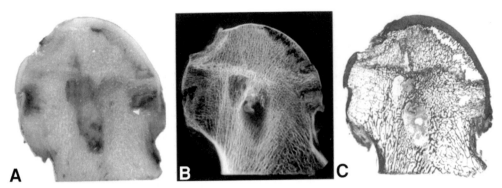

Figure 5. (A) 5-mm gross slab of femoral head. (B) Radiograph of slab that assisted in selection of specific slab for processing. (C) Resulting 5-μm micron Masson's trichrome-stained section. This specimen had been previously cored for osteonecrosis treatment, and ultimately resected because of collapsing of the cartilage cap.

imen through most of the following work day, and then run it through the processor the following evening. For the whole-mount slab section, the option that will provide optimal sections and a broad range of available tests in a reasonable amount of time is 5% formic acid (Fig. 5). EDTA is an option, but the time expenditure for a specimen of this size is severe. Unless there is a specific reason for decalcification in EDTA, the 5% formic acid would be my choice.[21]

C. Composite Bone/Soft Tissue

Gross—The complex structure of a composite specimen dictates that in order to preserve architecture and orientation, the best approach would be to throughly fix the sample as received prior to downsizing, especially if a band saw will be utilized. Depending on the percentage of soft tissue per bone, as in with whole rodent heads, it may be better to fix and decalcify as received in order to preserve architecture and orientation. After decalcification, the sample can be gross cut to the appropriate plane or size, using a high-profile disposable microtome blade (Fig. 6).

Decalcifant—As previously examined, composite tissues are not suitable for strong mineral acid decalcification, and would best be decalcified in 5% formic acid unless specific reasons for EDTA exist (Fig. 7).

IX. POST-DECALCIFICATION

Once a specimen has been satisfactorily decalcified, regardless of the decalcifier employed, it is imperative that the samples be thoroughly washed after the end point is achieved. This not only arrests the decalcification process, but also eliminates any residual decalcifier solution that could interfere with subsequent processing and staining. Recommendations for washing range from "brief washing in water" for bone marrow biopsies to overnight for large slab specimens. Naturally, the thickness and density of the specimen will dictate the amount of washing needed. There is evidence to support that adequate elimination of the decalcifier takes place during the dehydration/clearing steps with automated vacuum processors. Much of this is anecdotal and relates to the concept that specimens are removed from decalcifier and combined with the rest of the daily specimens to

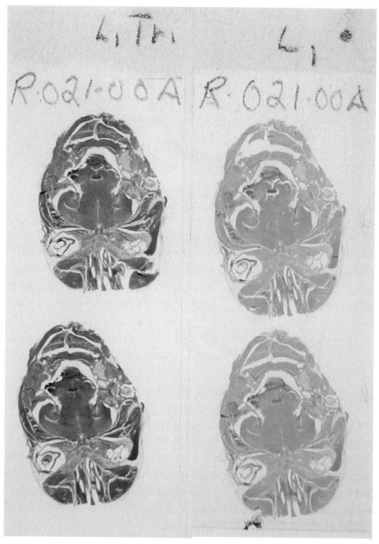

Figure 6. Resulting slides of 5-μm sections from formalin-fixed rodent heads decalcified 20 d in 5% formic acid prior to grossing. Left: Masson's trichrome stain; Right: Gill's II H&E stain.

be processed with no complaints. If the "holding vessel" or initial station on the automated processor is 50–70% ethanol, this could serve as an acceptable decalcifant removal option for routine or rapidly processed samples. As previously stated, hydrochloric acid vapors combined with formalin vapors reportedly produce bischloromethyl ether, which is a carcinogen. To avoid any possibility of mixing these vapors, the standard recommendation is that samples decalcified with hydrochloric acid should not be placed directly into formalin for holding prior automated processing without washing in water first to remove any residual HCl. However, a closer examination of this postulate suggests that this vapor production occurs when high concentrations of the chemicals are involved.

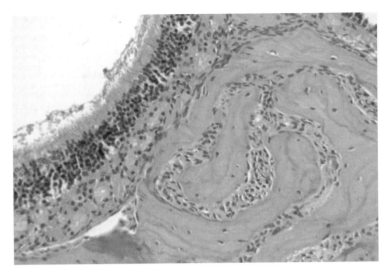

Figure 7. Bone/mastoid cavity junction from gerbil head decalcified in 5% formic acid for 20 d prior to grossing. This field exhibits quality staining of cells and osteoid seams in the bone as well as the non-calcified soft tissues of the epithelial lining of the cavity. Gill's II H&E. Original magnification ×100.

Therefore, the "usual" concentrations of hydrogen chloride (approx 10%) and formaldehyde (10%) used in everyday decalcification and fixation are not strong enough to produce the reported carcinogenic substance when used in a prudent manner.[13]

At this point, properly decalcified tissue is ready to process, section, and in many instances, stain to yield results consistent with soft tissues.[3] Options for dehydration fluids and schedules, clearing agents, embedding media, microtome design, blade engineering, and section thickness can all have a qualitative influence on the final product. But unless the specimen is optimally decalcified, the possibility for optimal sections is significantly reduced.

This chapter has focused on practical concepts and methodologies that allow for applicable flexibility, which can be incorporated into the routines of a wide variety of laboratory settings for the production of optimally as well as adequately decalcified tissues. There are specific application procedures such as ion-exchange procedures and electrical augmentation, which are also available. At the time of this writing, decalcification via microwave or microwave augmentation is in the developmental stages and is mentioned as such because of the vast array of procedures and results currently being considered. Expediting the decalcification process via sonication is also being scrutinized with more interest.

Although the basic chemistry behind the decalcification process has not changed significantly since the 1930s, the commercial manufacturers of decalcifants are constantly fine-tuning their proprietary chemistry to meet the demands of the market, which at this time appears to be focused on volume and speed. In this arena, the conceptual differences between simultaneous fixation/decalcification vs the fix before decalcification preference is evident by the fact that some manufacturers offer both, and some offer only one. These concepts should drive a wider variety of product introductions, including the development of fixatives specifically tailored for tissue to be decalcified, perhaps via a decalcifant specifically developed to work in consort with that fixative. The further demands for sophisticated immunohistochemical and *in situ* reverse-transcriptase polymerase chain reaction (RT-PCR) procedures to be performed on decalcified bone will either drive the decalcifant preference back to the basics of EDTA or lead to the development of decalcifiers not yet available. It is certainly incumbent upon the histologist to be aware of these overlapping concepts and determine how their foundations will impact upon their resulting product.

Acknowledgments: The author wishes to thank Dr. Leon Sokoloff for his ongoing constant guidance in large sample decalcification and processing; Dr. Carl L. Nelson, Dr. Aubrey J. Hough, Dr. Richard W. Nicholas, Dr. Michelle L. LaCroix, and Dr. Edward K. Gardner for specimen and interpretive support; Donna C. Montague, Sandra G. McLaren, and Vincent J. Della Speranza for reference resource support; and William R. Hogue for his photographic and computer-related contributions.

REFERENCES

1. Ackerman LV: Personal communications during the production of conference and teaching slides.
2. Apex Engineering Products Corporation, RDO Rapid Decalcifier Supplemental Instruction Sheet/Technical Memo. Deerfield IL, 2000.
3. Bancroft JD, Stevens A: *Theory and Practice of Histological Techniques, 4th ed.* Churchill Livingstone, New York, NY, 1996:314–320.
4. Brain EB: *The Preparation of Decalcified Sections.* Charles C. Thomas, Springfield, IL, 1966:69–143.
5. Carson FL. *Histotechnology A Self Instructional Text.* ASCP Press, Chicago, IL, 1997:38–40.
6. Culling CF. *Handbook of Histopathological and Histochemical Techniques, 3rd ed.* Butterworths, Boston, MA, 1975:63–72.
7. Decal Chemical Corporation. Supplemental Data Sheets, Congers, NY, 2000.
8. Delta Medical, Inc. Supplemental Data Sheets. Aurora, IL, 2000.
9. Hough AJ: The pathology of osteoarthritis. In: Moskowitz RW, Howell DS, Altman RD, et al: *Osteoarthritis—Diagnosis and Medical/Surgical Management, 3rd ed.* WB Saunders, New York, NY, 2001:69–100.
10. Hough AJ. Pathology of osteoarthritis. In: Koopman WJ, ed: *Arthritis and Allied Conditions: A Textbook of Rheumatology, 14th ed.* Lippincott, Williams & Wilkins, Philadelphia, PA, 2001:2167–2194.
11. Hough AJ: Personal communications during the production of conference and teaching slides.
12. Kiernan JA: *Histological and Histochemical Methods Theory and Practice, 3rd ed.* Butterworth Heinemann, Oxford, UK, 1999:33–36.
13. Kiernan JA: Re: Bleach + formalin + tissue. *Histonet.* July 9, 2000. Personal communication. October 10, 2000.
14. Kitamoto T, Ogomori K, Tateishi J, Prusiner SB: Formic acid pretreatment enhances immunostaining of cerebral and systemic amyloids. *Lab Invest* 57:230–236, 1987.
15. Lillie RD: *Histopathologic Technique and Practical Histochemistry, 2nd ed.* McGraw-Hill, New York, NY, 1954:423–428.
16. Luna LG: *Histopathological Methods and Color Atlas of Special Stains and Tissue Artifacts.* American Histolabs, Inc., Gaithersburg, MD, 1992:103–121.
17. Poly Scientific R&D Corporation. Supplemental Data Sheet. Bay Shore, NY, 2000.
18. Sheehan DC, Hrapchak BB: *Theory and Practice of Histotechnology, 2nd ed.* CV Mosby, St. Louis, MO, 1980:71.

19. Shibata Y, Fujita S, Takahashi H, et al: Assessment of decalcifying protocols for detection of specific RNA by non-radioactive in situ hybridization in calcified tissues. *Histochem Cell Biol* 11:153–159, 2000.
20. Skinner RA, Nicholas RW, Stewart CL, et al: Processing of resected allograft bone containing an expanded polytetrafluoroethylene implanted prosthetic ligament: comparison of paraffin, glycol methacrylate and Exakt grinding system. *J Histotech* 16:129–137, 1993.
21. Skinner RA, Hickmon SG, Lumpkin Jr., CK, et al: Decalcified bone: twenty years of successful specimen management. *J Histotech* 20:267–277, 1997.
22. Sokoloff L, Fincham J, Du Toit G: Pathologic feature of the femoral head in Mseleni disease. *Human Pathol* 16:117–120, 1985.
23. Urban K: Routine decalcification of bone. *Laboratory Medicine, American Society of Clinical Pathologists.* 12:4 207–212, 1981.
24. Weinstein RS, Nicholas RW, Manolagas SC: Apoptosis of osteocytes in glucocorticoid-induced osteonecrosis of the hip. *J Clin Endocrinol Metab* 85:2907–2912, 2000.

11

Principles of Embedding and Common Protocols

Yuehuei H. An,[1] Patricia L. Moreira,[1] Qian K. Kang,[1] and Helen E. Gruber[2]

[1]*Orthopaedic Research Laboratory, Medical University of South Carolina, Charleston, SC, USA*
[2]*Orthopaedic Research Biology, Carolinas Medical Center, Charlotte, NC, USA*

I. INTRODUCTION

Embedding techniques were first developed in the mid 1800s in response to the significant improvements in light microscopy. As the resolution of microscopy increased, so did the need for improved quality of the tissue specimens to be analyzed. The specimens needed to be cut in much thinner slices, which could only be done if embedded in a suitable medium supporting the material and providing the hardness required for thinner sectioning. Edwin Klebs introduced the paraffin-embedding methodology in 1869.[18] However, at that time, the material was not completely infiltrated with paraffin and the sections were cut freehand with a razor.

Since then, embedding techniques using waxes and resins have been developed and perfected for different specific aims and different types of specimens. Paraffin is most suitable for embedding soft tissues and decalcified hard tissues for thin sections of 3–6 μm, and is the most widely used embedding method. Celloidin is a better option when working with large, harder, and more fragile tissues. Depending on the size of the specimen, sections of 3–12 μm can be cut. Hard embedding materials such as glycol methacrylate, methyl methacrylate (MMA), or Spurr's resin are chosen for undecalcified hard tissue embedding suitable for heavy-duty sectioning or ground sectioning. Sections from the latter method are relatively thick, ranging from 50–200 μm.

Before embedding, the specimens require a lengthy time for fixation, decalcification (although not for ground sectioning), dehydration, clearing, and impregnation or infiltration. Each step is interdependent, and failure in one of these will directly affect both the ease of sectioning and the quality of the sections. Thus, it is important that all the steps of processing be carried out by a patient, careful, and responsible technician. More recent findings show that use of a microwave may significantly reduce the time for fixation, dehydration, clearing, infiltration, and even staining, with no obvious adverse effects on the tissue structure.[2,7,16]

Bone tissue can be decalcified before embedding in paraffin, celloidin, and some other resins. The details of this process are discussed in Chapters 10 and 13. When embedding in methacrylates, Spurr's media, or other resins or plastics for ground sectioning, it is not necessary to decalcify the tissue.[17]

From: *Handbook of Histology Methods for Bone and Cartilage*
Edited by: Y. H. An and K. L. Martin © Humana Press Inc., Totowa, NJ

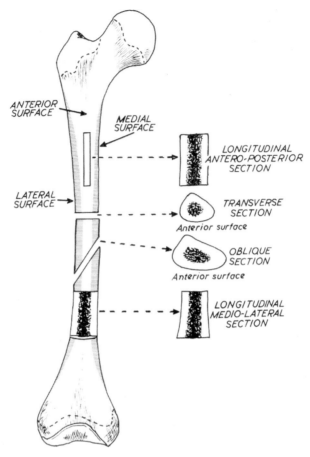

Figure 1. Illustration of sectioning planes in a cylindrical specimen.

The principles of embedding and routine procedures, including paraffin, cellodin, and plastic embedding, are described in this chapter. For serious readers, there are many references in the literature about hard-tissue processing.[3,4,6,8,14,19] Readers may refer to Chapter 12 for more embedding protocols used in undecalcified tissues.

II. SPECIMEN ORIENTATION, TRIMMING, FIXATION, AND DECALCIFICATION

In bone histology, the planes of sectioning are referred to as longitudinal, cross-sectional or oblique as shown in Fig. 1.[3] Often the desired sectioning plane of a bone specimen is very difficult to obtain unless the precise plane was carefully preserved and indicated before and during tissue harvesting and processing. Once the plane is chosen, the specimen should be trimmed to provide a flat surface (for sectioning). This can be done before or after decalcification, or before dehydration for undecalcified bone tissues. There are no ideal material dimensions, since these are completely dependent on the specimen to be analyzed. However, smaller samples are processed more quickly and easily than larger ones. Bone samples can be cut into slices on a band saw with a fine

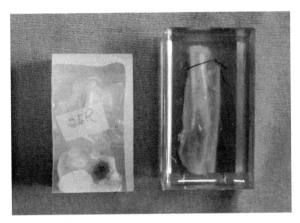

Figure 2. (Left) A pencil-written label was embedded in the block. (Right) A black silk suture was tied on the proximal side of a segment of the forelimb bones of a rabbit.

metal-cutting saw blade. Also, specimens can be trimmed or reduced using a wheel grinder. Smaller pieces may be reduced by carefully grinding away superfluous tissues with a turning hand piece mounted with a carborundum wheel or a burr. After trimming, the precise sectioning plane (not necessary for plastic embedding) of the specimen should be noted, properly labeled, and recorded. A pencil-written label on solute-resistant paper with the specimen number or identifier can be placed in the embedding medium so it stays permanently in the tissue block. Sometimes, a silk suture tag on the specimen helps to identify the sectioning surface and the prior position or orientation of the specimen in the living body (Fig. 2). Colored dyes may also be used to mark specific areas of a specimen.

Proper fixation is the first key step in bone histological processing (*see* Chapter 8). If at all possible, reduce the specimen size before fixation, as this dramatically improves fixation. Make sure the volume ratio between the fixative and specimen is large enough (>10:1). Drilling holes in the cortex of large specimens helps with fixation and later infiltration. For large specimens, perfusion fixation is recommended.

Very often, bone tissues are decalcified, embedded in paraffin or celloidin, and cut using a rotary microtome or a sliding microtome. For principles and detailed techniques of decalcification, one may refer to the literature[3,4,8,19,21] or Chapters 10 and 13 in this book.

III. DEHYDRATION

After trimming, fixation, and decalcification, the specimens should be completely dehydrated for further processing, including clearing, infiltration, and embedding in paraffin, celloidin, plastics, or resins. Because many of the embedding media are not miscible with water, removal of the fixatives should be thorough.

The most common reagent used for dehydration is alcohol (ethanol). Through a graduated series of increasing alcohol concentrations, usually ranging from 70% through 95% to absolute, all the water in the specimen can be removed. The specimens should remain in each concentration until complete saturation, as sudden excessive immersion in higher con-

Table 1. Dehydration of 3-mm-thick Soft and Hard Tissues

Dehydration agent	Soft tissue	Hard tissue
Alcohol 70%	1–3 h	up to 1 d
Alcohol 70%	1–3 h	up to 1 d
Alcohol 95%	1–3 h	up to 1 d
Alcohol 95%	1–3 h	up to 1 d
Alcohol 100%	1–3 h	up to 1 d
Alcohol 100%	1–3 h	up to 1 d

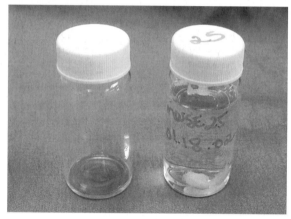

Figure 3. Small glass bottles can be used for tissue dehydration, clearing, and infiltration until embedding in a mold, or the tissue can stay in the bottle for embedding.

centrations of alcohol can result in too much shrinkage and hardening of the tissue. A dehydration protocol is listed in Table 1 for cancellous bone samples approx 3 mm in thickness.

Other dehydration agents such as acetone and dioxane (diethylene dioxide) can also be used. Although the latter is miscible with both water and paraffin and does not require the use of a clearing agent, its fumes are extremely toxic, and it does not permit good trimming of the sections. Alcohol and other reagents should be used at a ratio at least of 10:1 volume ratio of alcohol:tissue. Agitation is recommended for thorough dehydration.

Small glass bottles can be used for dehydration until the embedding step, or in some cases (such as plastic embedding) the specimen can stay in the bottle for embedding (Fig. 3). If a large number of specimens are processed at one time, plastic cassettes may be used for individual specimens, and all cassettes can be placed in one beaker for solution changes until embedding (Fig. 4). Modern automated tissue processors allow multiple programs of varying infiltration schedules.

IV. CLEARING, INFILTRATION, AND EMBEDDING IN PARAFFIN

A. General Aspects

Clearing is the process in which the dehydration fluid in the specimen is replaced with a substance that is miscible with alcohol and the embedding medium. There are

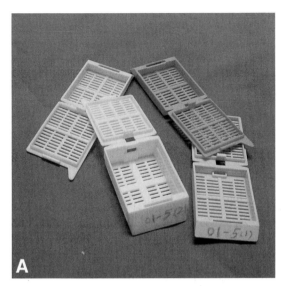
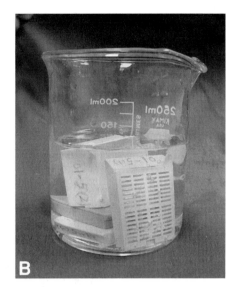

Figure 4. Tissue cassettes of different sizes are available (A), and multiple plastic cassettes containing tissues can be put in one container for processing (B).

many clearing reagents available, but most routine laboratories rely on only a few, such as xylene, toluene, or benzene. Every clearing reagent has its advantages and disadvantages. Toluene and benzene cause less hardening of tissue than xylene. Xylene is the most commonly used reagent in most laboratories, but one should bear in mind that xylene tends to make most tissue brittle, a fact that is compounded when used with already harder decalcified bone. Brain[3] and Skinner[20,21] suggest the use of cedar wood oil and methyl salicylate, which does not cause brittleness even after prolonged clearing time. A 50:50 dehydrating and clearing agent step is recommended prior to immersion in a pure clearing agent.[3]

Paraffin is available in a wide range of melting points, ranging from 45–60°C, and in recent years some additives have been used in order to improve the cutting qualities of the wax, thus providing a greater adhesive property. Paraplast® (Fisher Scientific) is a widely used mixture of paraffin and several plastic polymers that are responsible for its elasticity improvement. The same methodology employed for paraffin infiltration and embedding should be used for Paraplast®. Infiltration of the samples with paraffin before embedding includes several changes (normally 2 h infiltration with one change of fresh paraffin at 1 h) of fresh wax in a 60°C oven until the clearing agent is completely removed. The use of vacuum during infiltration will eliminate the potential for bubble entrapment and speed the infiltration of the wax into the tissue.

Following infiltration, the sample is embedded by immersing in fresh molten paraffin (5–10°C above its melting point) in embedding molds and then cooled quickly at approx −5°C on the cold surface of an embedding center. Care should be taken to ensure the correct orientation of the cutting surface in the block. There are many different kinds of molds available. Some common ones for paraffin are made of stainless steel, which is fitted with a plastic top known as an embedding ring (Fig. 5). The more common ones, of various sizes, are completely plastic. Once wax is poured in, the specimen is immersed in

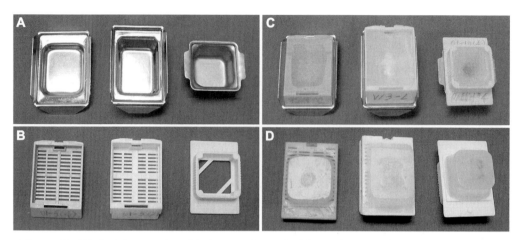

Figure 5. (A) Stainless steel molds for paraffin embedding. (B) An embedding ring with two tissue cassette bottom portions for adding to the block for fixation onto the microtome. (C) Completed embedding with all parts still in place. (D) Completed tissue blocks.

Table 2. Protocol for Paraffin Embedding of 3-mm-thick Decalcified or Soft Tissues (Omit the Decalcification Step for Soft-Tissue Processing)

Steps	Procedure	Time
1	Fix tissue in 10% NBF	At least 1 d
2	Immerse in decalcification solution	Overnight to several days (frequent radiography is needed)
3	70% ethanol	1 h
4	95% ethanol	1 h
5	Fresh 95% ethanol	1 h
6	100% ethanol	1 h
7	Fresh 100% ethanol	1 h (if tissue is >5 mm thick, use a third 100% ethanol rinse for 1 h)
8	Xylene	1 h
9	Fresh xylene	1 h
10	Paraffin (in 60°C oven with vacuum)	1 h
11	Fresh paraffin	1 h
12	Embed in paraffin	

the melted wax and the blocks are allowed to harden and then the mold is removed. This type of tissue block has the advantage of not requiring any kind of mounting prior to sectioning. Automatic embedding centers are available which can provide reproducible quick specimen embedding.

B. Routine Protocol

A routine protocol for processing decalcified specimens used in the authors' laboratory is given in Table 2.

Table 3. A Protocol for Processing 5-mm-thick Decalcified Bone Specimens

Steps	Procedure	Time
1	Dehydration in a series of ethanol: 70%, two changes of 95%, two changes of 100%.	Hours to overnight for each concentration
2	Infiltration in increasing concentrations of celloidin solutions 2%, 4%, 6%, 8%, 10%, 12%.	3–7 d for each concentration
3	Embedding: Place specimen in a glass dish filled with 15–20% celloidin solution. Place gently in the solution to avoid air bubbles. The surface to be sectioned should be face down. Cover the dish, but do not seal it so that the solution will slowly evaporate. When the periphery of the block becomes solid and as hard as rubber, separate the edge from the dish with a knife, and fill the dish with 80% ethanol for 3–5 d to make the block homogenously hard as rubber.	3 d to 1 wk
4	Trim the block leaving a celloidin margin about 2–3 mm thick around the specimen. Store the block in 80% ethanol until sectioning.	Stored in 80% ethanol

V. INFILTRATION AND EMBEDDING IN CELLOIDIN

A. General Aspects

Celloidin is a purified form of nitrocellulose (gun cotton), and is very useful when embedding hard or delicate samples.[3] It provides greater support for tissues than paraffin, so much larger specimens can be embedded in it. When embedding bone, it causes little shrinkage and hardening of the tissue, as no heat is involved at the process. However, the infiltration is measured in days and weeks rather than in hours, and sections are normally more than 10 μm in thickness. Moreover, the blocks should be kept in 70% alcohol, even during sectioning.

Following dehydration, the tissue should be placed into equal parts of ether and alcohol for 12–24 h for clearing. Then the samples should be placed in a series of celloidin solutions (2, 4, and 8% in equal parts of ether and alcohol) for 5–7 d at each concentration.

Embedding is performed with 8% celloidin and the blocks are left to harden, which can take several days. Paper boats should be used as a mold. When the embedding process is complete, the blocks should be stored in 70% alcohol. Before cutting, the tissue blocks should be mounted on a vulcanite or wooden support block using 2% celloidin. The two blocks should be clamped together for at least 1 h and then immersed in a 70% alcohol solution for 30 min until the seal hardens.

For cutting celloidin-embedded specimens, commonly used microtomes include sledge, sliding, and heavy-duty rotary microtomes. If the specimen is small, a basic rotary microtome can also be used.

B. Routine Protocol

A protocol for celloidin infiltration and embedding of 5-mm-thick decalcified specimens is listed in Table 3 (also *see* Chapter 38).[3] The steps are carried out at room temperature. Celloidin solutions are prepared by adding celloidin to absolute alcohol and then adding ether to the mixture. The alcohol:ether ratio is always 50:50 by volume. For example, 100 mL 10%

celloidin is a mixture of 10 g celloidin, 45 mL alcohol, and 45 mL ether. Both ether and dry celloidin (low-viscosity nitrocellulose) are explosive and flammable, so care should be taken during handling. The dry celloidin can be kept moist with butyl alcohol.

VI. INFILTRATION AND EMBEDDING IN PLASTICS

A. General Aspects

Some of the plastics or resins used today include methyl methacrylate, glycol methacrylate, Araldite, Bio-Plastic, Technovit, L-R White, Osteo-bed, Epon, and Spurr's medium. The most commonly used plastic-embedding media include methyl and glycol methacrylate, and Spurr's medium. Glycol methacrylate embedding provides good infiltration and embedding of cartilage and good preservation of certain enzymes such as alkaline phosphatase (ALP). Methyl methacrylate (MMA) embedding provides better preservation of alkaline phosphatase in osteoblasts and cartilage matrix and of acid phosphatase in osteoblasts.[12] MMA-embedding results in a harder block, which provides better support for cortical and trabecular bone.[14] Spurr's medium, an epoxy resin, has been reported to prevent artifacts because of the separation of different tissue layers through its low viscosity which allows good tissue penetration and minimal shrinkage during polymerization.[22,24] Spurr's is a hard embedding medium that is suitable for cortical bone and bone containing metal implants.[10,11]

Embedding in plastic provides many advantages in hard-tissue histology. Using a sliding or heavy-duty rotary microtome, thin sections (several microns in thickness) can be made because of the better support given by the media to cellular components. When choosing a plastic-embedding medium, the goal is to match the hardness of the embedding medium to the hardness of the bone or cartilage in order to produce successful sections. Theoretically, during sectioning, separations between hard and soft components in the tissue and fractures of hard structures will occur if there is a mismatch between the hardness of the tissue and the embedding media. For example, glycol methacrylate has a low viscosity that allows fast and complete infiltration and forms a relatively soft block, so it is suitable for embedding soft tissues, cartilage, and cancellous bone. In contrast, MMA has an initial low viscosity that also provides a rapid infiltration, but has high hardness after polymerization. Thus, it is suitable for studying hard tissues such as cortical bone and bone containing hard implants; and it is also excellent for trabecular bone.

Dehydration using serial alcohols is routine practice in most laboratories. The time needed for dehydration will vary depending on whether the tissue has been previously decalcified and also on the size of the specimen. Undecalcified samples should be placed in increasing concentrations of the dehydration agent for several hours to 24 h at each concentration. Agitation is always helpful for solution exchange. Sometimes, clearing is used before infiltration using clearing agents such as xylene[9] or ClearRite 3 (Richard-Allan, Kalamazoo, MI).[17]

For the best penetration and to prevent bubble formation, dehydration and infiltration are better carried out in a vacuum dessicator or in a vacuum oven set at room temperature. An improved routine method for embedding tissue, especially hard tissue, in polymethyl methacrylate (PMMA) was reported by Buijs and Dogterom.[5] The improvements include: i) the final dehydration step before MMA infiltration was performed with methanol; ii) the stabilizer hydroquinone was not extracted from the monomer (MMA); and iii) the ini-

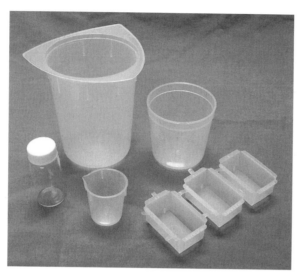

Figure 6. Containers which can be used for plastic embedding, including polyethylene cups, glass bottles, and Peel-A-Way molds.

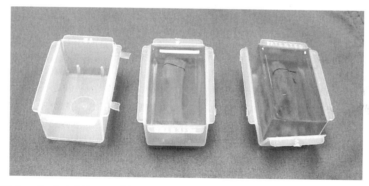

Figure 7. Using Peel-A-Way molds, a segment of rabbit radius and ulna was embedded in Spurr's medium.

tiator, benzoyl peroxide, was replaced by Perkadox 16, *bis* (4-tert-butylcyclohexyl)peroxydicarbonate. The modified method created almost no bubbles.[5] The use of Perkadox 16 is less hazardous and is time-saving, although it is difficult to obtain (only from Akzo Nobel Chemicals, Dobbs Ferry, NY).[17]

When using methacrylates as embedding media for large specimens or composite tissues (containing soft tissue, bone, and implants), such as a canine vertebral body or distal femur, the time intervals for fixation, dehydration, and infiltration should be increased, and a heat sink or infiltration and polymerization in hotter or cooler temperatures may be used.[9,13,23]

The most popular plastic- or resin-embedding mold is the polyethylene Peel-A-Way (Polysciences, Inc., Warrington, PA), which is available in several sizes. Small plastic containers or even glass bottles can also be used as molds for plastic embedding (Fig. 6). Once the embedding media hardens, the mold can be peeled off or removed to release the tissue-media block (Fig. 7, 8).

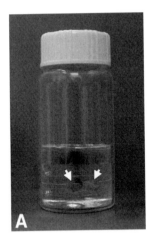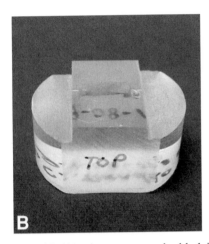

Figure 8. Using a small glass bottle as the mold (A), tissue was embedded in a glycol methacrylate block (B).

Table 4. Glycol Methacrylate Infiltration Schedule for Small Bone and Cartilage Specimens*

Step	Solution	Time/Condition
1	70:30 Solution A:dH$_2$O	Overnight/shaker in cold room
2	85:15 Solution A:dH$_2$O	2–3 h/shaker in cold room
3	95:5 Solution A:dH$_2$O	2–3 h/shaker in cold room
4	10 mL Solution A+ 0.09 g catalyst	2–3 d infiltration on shaker in cold room
5	Embedding medium (5 mL Solution A + 0.045 g catalyst + 0.1 mL Solution B)	Embed (4–5 h at room temperature)

* This table is adapted from Gruber HE, Stasky AA: Histological study in orthopaedic animal research. In: An YH, Friedman RJ, eds. *Animal Models in Orthopaedic Research.* CRC Press, Boca Raton, FL, 1999: 115–138.

B. Protocols

Many protocols for hard-tissue processing have been developed. Two protocols used in the authors' laboratory are given in Section VI, B1, for glycol methacrylate and Spurr's medium. The reader may refer to Chapter 12 for more details on plastic-embedding techniques.

1. Glycol Methacrylate for Smaller Bones and Cartilage

This method utilizes the "JB-4" kit (a glycol methacrylate-based polymer) available from Polysciences, Inc. (Warrington, PA). The infiltration solution (monomer) is a water-soluble medium, which does not require dehydration to absolute alcohol except for large, dense, or fatty-tissue specimens. After fixation and dehydration, the infiltration and embedding schedule are carried out as in Table 4. Be sure that specimen containers are well-capped during processing.

To make the embedding media, mix the JB-4 catalyst (benzoyl peroxide, plasticized) into JB-4 embedding solution A (monomer) until completely dissolved. Add JB-4

Table 5. Preparation of Spurr's Media

Solution	Quantity				
	100 mL	150 mL	200 mL	250 mL	300 mL
ERL 4206/VCD (4-vinylcyclohexene dioxide)	25 g	35 g	47 g	59 g	71 g
DER 736 (epoxy resin)	15 g	21 g	28.2 g	35.4 g	42.6 g
NSA (nonenyl succinic anhydride)	65 g	91 g	122.2 g	153.4 g	184.6 g
DMAE (2-dimethylaminoethanol)	1 g	1.4 g	1.88 g	2.36 g	2.84 g

Note: The reagents are measured in gram, not mL. Mix in the order listed.

Table 6. Embedding Protocol for Spurr's Medium

Step	Solution	Time for rabbit distal femur	Time for soft tissue containing metal
1.	70% ethanol	1 d	1 or more hours
2.	70% ethanol	1 d	1 or more hours
3.	95% ethanol	1 d	1 or more hours
4.	95% ethanol	1 d	1 or more hours
5.	100% ethanol	1 d	1 or more hours
6.	100% ethanol	1 d	1 or more hours
7.	100% acetone	1 d	1 or more hours
8.	100% acetone	1 d	1 or more hours
9.	50% Spurr's + 50% acetone	1 d	1 or more hours
10.	75% Spurr's + 25% acetone	1 d	1 or more hours
11.	100% Spurr's—Vacuum	1 d	1 or more hours
12.	100% Spurr's—Vacuum	1 d	1 or more hours
13.	Embed: 100% Spurr's—40°C—Vacuum	2–3 d	2–3 d

embedding solution B (accelerator), mix for 1 min and start the embedding procedure by pouring the embedding medium into a mold containing a well-oriented specimen. Polymerization will be complete at room temperature in 4–5 h (let sit overnight for best results). Successful embedding produces blocks with no bubbles formed during polymerization. All methacrylates should be handled under a fume hood.

2. Spurr's Resin for Embedding Small to Medium-Sized Specimens

Spurr's resin has been used successfully in hard tissue processing for many years.[22] The kit can be purchased from Electron Microscopy Sciences (Fort Washington, PA). The typical uses of Spurr's medium are small-tissue embedding for ultrathin sectioning and evaluation with electron microscopy, and medium-size bone-tissue embedding for preparing ground sections.[1,11,15,25] For undecalcified bone embedding, Spurr's resin can be prepared as shown in Table 5.

Bone specimens measuring up to 10 mm thick and 30 mm long (such as whole rat femur, rabbit distal femur, segmental rabbit radius or ulna, or even canine femoral slices) can be successfully embedded using Spurr's resin. A routine protocol used in the authors' laboratory for processing rabbit distal femur (18 mm long, 18 mm wide, and 14 mm thick) and soft tissue containing metal implants (5 mm thick) is given in Table 6.

Routinely, the Spurr's-embedded blocks will be cut into slices (300–500 μm in thickness) using a diamond wheel saw or a diamond wire saw. The bone slices are hand-ground on a wheel grinder to make 75–150-μm-thick sections. They are commonly stained with Cole's hematoxylin & eosin (H&E), Cole's hematoxylin, or toluidine blue.

Acknowledgments: Patricia L. Moreira is a visiting PhD candidate from Biologic Sciences of Biology Institute at the State University of Campinas (UNICAMP), Campinas SP, Brazil. Her fellowship was jointly supported by the Brazilian Government (Fundação Coordenação de Aperfeiçoamento de Pessoal de Nível Superior (CAPES PDDE Proc. number BEX 0121/01-0)) and the Orthopaedic Research Laboratory at the Medical University of South Carolina.

REFERENCES

1. Blomlof L, Lindskog S, Appelgren R, et al: New attachment in monkeys with experimental periodontitis with and without removal of the cementum. *J Clin Periodontol* 14:136–143, 1987.
2. Boon ME, Kok LP, Ouwerkerk-Noordam E: Microwave-stimulated diffusion for fast processing of tissue: reduced dehydrating, clearing, and impregnating times. *Histopathology* 10:303–309, 1986.
3. Brain EB: *The Preparation of Decalcified Sections.* Charles C. Thomas, Springfield, IL, 1966.
4. Brown GG: *An Introduction to Histotechnology.* Appleton-Century-Crofts, New York, NY, 1978.
5. Buijs R, Dogterom AA: An improved method for embedding hard tissue in polymethyl methacrylate. *Stain Technol* 58:135–141, 1983.
6. Clayden EC: *Practical Section Cutting and Staining.* Churchill Livingstone, Edinburgh and London, 1971.
7. Cunningham 3rd, CD, Schulte BA, Bianchi LM, et al: Microwave decalcification of human temporal bones. *Laryngoscope* 111:278–282, 2001.
8. Drury RAB, Wallington EA: *Carleton's Histological Techniques.* Oxford University Press, Oxford, UK, 1980:199–220.
9. Emmanual J, Hornbeck C, Bloebaum RD: A polymethyl methacrylate method for large specimens of mineralized bone with implants. *Stain Technol* 62:401–410, 1987.
10. Friedman RJ, An YH, Jiang M, et al: Influence of biomaterial surface texture on bone ingrowth in the rabbit femur. *J Orthop Res* 14:455–464, 1996.
11. Friedman RJ, Bauer TW, Garg K, et al: Histological and mechanical comparison of hydroxyapatite-coated cobalt-chrome and titanium implants in the rabbit femur. *J Appl Biomater* 6:231–235, 1995.
12. Gruber HE, Marshall GJ, Nolasco LM, et al: Alkaline and acid phosphatase demonstration in human bone and cartilage: effects of fixation interval and methacrylate embedments. *Stain Technol* 63:299–306, 1988.
13. Gruber HE, Stasky AA: Large specimen bone embedment and cement line staining. *Biotech Histochem* 72:198–201, 1997.
14. Gruber HE, Stasky AA: Histological study in orthopaedic animal research. In: An YH, Friedman RJ, eds: *Animal Models in Orthopaedic Research.* CRC Press, Boca Raton, FL, 1999:115–138.
15. Horton WA, Dwyer C, Goering R, et al: Immunohistochemistry of types I and II collagen in undecalcified skeletal tissues. *J Histochem Cytochem* 31:417–425, 1983.
16. Kahveci Z, Minbay FZ, Cavusoglu L: Safranin O staining using a microwave oven. *Biotech Histochem* 75:264–268, 2000.
17. Sanderson C: Entering the realm of mineralized bone processing: a review of the literature and techniques. *J Histotechnol* 20:259–266, 1997.

18. Sanderson C, Emmanuel J, Bnanual J, et al: A historical review of paraffin and its development as an embedding medium. *J Histotechnol* 11:61–63, 1988.
19. Sheehan DC, Hrapchak BB, eds: *Theory and Practice of Histotechnology.* Battelle Press, Columbus, OH and Richland, WA, 1980:89–117.
20. Skinner RA: The value of methyl salicylate as a clearing agent. *J Histotechnol* 9:27–28, 1986.
21. Skinner RA, Hickmon SG, Lumpkin CK, et al: Decalcified bone: twenty years of successful specimen management. *J Histotechnol* 20:267–277, 1997.
22. Spurr AR: A low-viscosity epoxy resin embedding medium for electron microscopy. *J Ultrastruct Res* 26:31–43, 1969.
23. Steflik DE, McKinney RV, Jr., Mobley GL, et al: Simultaneous histological preparation of bone, soft tissue and implanted biomaterials for light microscopic observations. *Stain Technol* 57:91–98, 1982.
24. Watts RH, Green D, Howells GR: Improvements in histological techniques for epoxy-resin embedded bone specimens. *Stain Technol* 56:155–161, 1981.
25. Weaker FJ, Richardson L: A modified processing and sectioning technique for hard tissues. *Am J Med Technol* 44:1030–1032, 1978.

12

Infiltration Techniques and Results in Different Types of Resin

Antonio Scarano, Giovanna Orsini, and Adriano Piattelli

Dental School, University of Chieti, Chieti, Italy

1. INTRODUCTION

Plastic-embedding technique generally does not require the removal of the resin before staining, a process that could introduce artifacts at the tissue-implant interface. The presence of the resin in the sections makes the staining procedures different from routine paraffin-embedded tissues, and achieving satisfactory staining is more difficult. An exception is methyl methacrylate (MMA) which is removed from the sections after cutting to permit staining. Embedding in MMA requires the removal of the resin with solvents. Glycol methacrylate cannot be removed because of the high number of crosslinking binding sites present in the chains of the glycol methacrylate polymer.[7,8]

Sectioning of blocks containing hard endosseous biomaterials can be made easier by the use of a system consisting of a special glycol methacrylate resin (Technovit 7200 VLC, Kulzer, Wehrheim, Germany), which provides good infiltration, polymerization, and subsequent easy sectioning by cutting and grinding the specimens. Although this system allows the precise observation of an intact interface between bone and endosseous biomaterials, the hardness of glycol methacrylate and its permanence in the tissues make any routine staining procedure very difficult.[10,15]

During the last three decades, the increase in the use of medical and dental implants and techniques of bone regeneration has underlined the importance of the histological evaluation of the tissue-implant interface. Conventional methods of microscopic examination have been shown to be inappropriate for studying undecalcified bone, implants, and biomaterials. Thus, various plastic-embedding methods have been used to produce sections in which both the implant material and the adjacent tissues are intact. Many biomaterials cannot be infiltrated with conventional embedding media, and they can be more resistant to grinding than the embedding media and/or the surrounding hard tissues, producing sections of uneven thickness. Plastic embedding allows a distinction between mineralized bone and unmineralized osteoid, with an excellent preservation of the cellular structures. Because of the importance of the processes of bone apposition and bone resorption in the growth of osseous tissue around dental implants, we have tried to develop a reproducible technique for the simultaneous localization of these mechanisms

From: *Handbook of Histology Methods for Bone and Cartilage*
Edited by: Y. H. An and K. L. Martin © Humana Press Inc., Totowa, NJ

at the bone-implant interface of undecalcified specimens using the embedding medium Technovit 7200 VLC.

It must be kept in mind that histological detail is critical for the morphometrical evaluation, diagnosis, and study of the bone pathology.[5] For optimal and reproducible processing of the specimens, the following steps are necessary:

- Optimal procurement of the specimen
- Proper fixation
- Proper embedding
- Proper sectioning
- Proper staining

Methacrylate-embedding media are the methods of choice for the study of bone.[1] Glycol methacrylate-embedding provides good infiltration of cartilage and good preservation of osteoblast-associated alkaline phosphatase (ALP). Methyl methacrylate (MMA) produces a harder plastic that provides a superior support for cortical and trabecular bone and allows a better preservation than glycol methacrylate of ALP in cartilage matrix and of acid phosphatase (ACP) in osteoclasts.[2] The use of MMA as an embedding medium has made possible the study of semi-thin sections of mineralized bone.

II. PRINCIPAL STAGES OF HISTOLOGICAL SPECIMEN PREPARATION

A. Dehydration

Dehydration follows fixation, and it has the goal of removing all the water contained within the specimen to allow uniform penetration of the resin. It also allows the penetration of resin into any biomaterial present. The dehydration process is essential because the resins employed are not water-soluble. The water is removed by immersing the specimen in alcohol solutions of increasing concentration. The time for each step will vary (from 15 min to 24 h), depending on the size of the specimen. The alcohol concentrations used are as follows:

- 30% alcohol
- 50% alcohol
- 70% alcohol
- 90% alcohol
- 100% alcohol
- 100% alcohol

The time required for dehydration may be reduced when vacuum is applied. The dehydration process hardens the tissues, making resin penetration more difficult. To avoid this problem, a few drops of glacial acetic acid may be added to the 70% alcohol solution. For some resins, acetone dehydration can be performed.

B. Infiltration

Resins commonly used for infiltrating and embedding are:

- Technovit 7200 Kulzer
- Technovit 8100 Kulzer
- Technovit 9100 Kulzer
- Epon
- L-R White
- Other MMA resins
- Spurr's resin

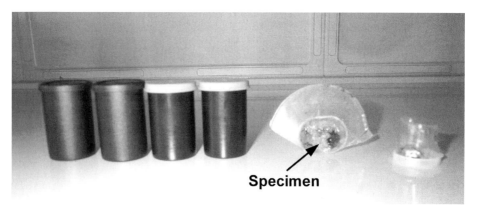

Figure 1. Resin is put in appropriate embedding containers (arrow) that do not react with the resin.

All these resins are initially fluids, and solidify during polymerization. Resin embedding produces hard blocks containing the tissues to be trimmed and cut for examination. The resins must be put in appropriate embedding molds that do not react with the resin (Fig. 1).

III. METHODS FOR COMMONLY USED PLASTIC RESINS

A. *Technovit 7200 Kulzer*

Technovit 7200 Kulzer is a methacrylate-based resin which polymerizes with exposure to light, so infiltration must be performed in a dark environment. Technovit 7200 Kulzer penetrates hard and soft tissues completely. Following dehydration, infiltration of specimens is carried out in mixtures of alcohol and resin, beginning with 30% resin and 70% alcohol and ending with 100% resin. The infiltration process requires 3–4 d. However, as with the dehydration process, this time may be reduced if performed under vacuum (Fig. 2). Sometimes, the resin cannot penetrate into the internal portion of large specimens, and this is particularly true in the case of bone with large marrow spaces (Fig. 3).

1. Dehydration

Dehydration is carried out with a graded alcohol series. Acetone must not be used, as it may alter the resin's properties, modifying the polymerization and the staining procedures.

2. Infiltration

The infiltration protocol is relatively short. The samples with resin must be in dark bottles, as light may start the polymerization process. Heating facilitates the polymerization process. The protocol is as follows:

- Day 1: 50% resin/50% alcohol
- Day 2: 70% resin/30% alcohol
- Day 3: 90% resin/10% alcohol
- Day 4: 100% resin
- Day 5: 100% resin

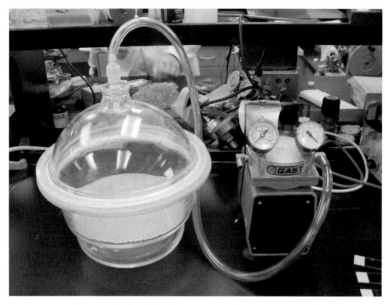

Figure 2. Vacuum can be applied to facilitate better infiltration of the resin and prevent air-bubble formation.

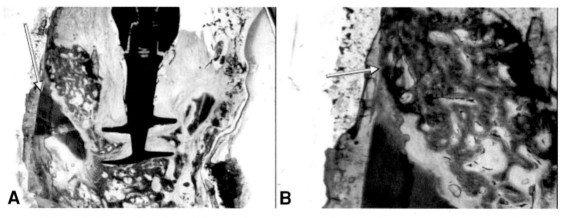

Figure 3. Poor infiltration of the specimen can cause its detachment from the glass slide (arrows). (A) low magnification; (B) high magnification.

The bottles must be put under vacuum to remove the air bubbles contained in the specimen. If allowed to remain, these air bubbles will damage the specimen.

3. Embedding and Polymerization

After embedding, polymerization is performed for about 6–8 h at a temperature not exceeding 40°C. The polymerized resin is very hard, and it is possible to cut and grind the specimen in a very uniform way with no alteration of the histological features, especially at the tissue-implant interface.

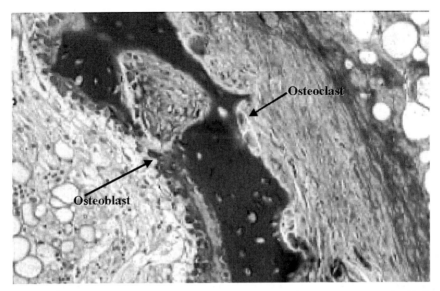

Figure 4. A specimen of mineralized tissue which has been properly embedded. Acid fuchsin-toluidine blue. Magnification ×200.

Polymerization may be accomplished either by using light polymerization or autopolymerization, depending on the type of resin used.

Once the block is obtained, for light microscopy observation, it can be glued to either a base of Plexiglas or a clean glass slide. Several types of glue are suitable (e.g., Technovit 4000, Attack, Vitroresin). The surface to be examined must be positioned uppermost. Excess resin is removed in order to obtain a free surface of the specimen parallel to the holding slide. At this stage another slide is glued to the free surface.

However, the most superficial portion of the resin usually remains fluid as the presence of oxygen in the air inhibits the polymerization process. This excess resin is removed with a knife or by grinding and the clean glass slide can be attached with glue.

4. Staining

Toluidine blue, acid fuchsin, silver nitrate, acid and alkaline phosphatase are routinely used staining agents with this resin (Fig. 4). Acid solutions may alter the resin properties, and can produce a background staining that does not allow an accurate morphologic evaluation.

B. Technovit 8100 Kulzer

This is a very fluid glycol methacrylate resin, exhibiting a low viscosity that allows fast and complete infiltration of the specimens. This resin has been proposed for the study of soft tissues, but it can be used successfully also for the processing of mineralized tissues. Compatibility with histo-and cytochemical techniques is well-documented.

1. Dehydration and Infiltration

Specimens are dehydrated through a graded alcohol series at room temperature.

The infiltration starts in a resin and alcohol solution and progresses to 100% pure resin concentration. Each step must last at least 1 d.

2. Embedding and Staining

After embedding, the 8100 resin is hardened by polymerization at 4°C. Sectioning is performed using a cutting system. Semi-thin sections are cut, stained for light microscopy, and observed.

C. Technovit 9100 Kulzer

This is a MMA-based resin, which is obtained by mixing the monomer, a catalyst, and an initiator. The MMA monomer should be stored in a cool place because of its high flammability. Mixing the MMA monomer with the catalyst activates the resin. The quantity of the catalyst controls the final hardness. The blocks obtained are transparent and allow an accurate morphological analysis. Mineralized specimens can also be embedded with this resin. Technovit 9100 Kulzer has been successfully used for light and electron microscopy, as its initial low viscosity provides a rapid infiltration and high hardness after polymerization.

1. Dehydration and Infiltration

Dehydration is carried out through graded alcohol or acetone series at room temperature. The time required will vary depending on the size of the specimen, taking from 1 h to 3–4 d. Infiltration is performed using graded resin/alcohol or resin/acetone series.

2. Embedding

During the embedding procedure, special care must be taken so as not to inhibit the polymerization process. It is important to avoid all potentially interfering substances that could eventually change the color of the hardened resin. Indeed, before use the resin must be tested. Once the resin has been activated, ultraviolet light and room temperature should be avoided.

3. Staining

Semi-thin sections are cut. All the routine staining methods for light microscopy can be utilized. These sections show a more detailed morphology than those obtained by embedding with 7200 Kulzer resin.

D. Epon

Epon is an epoxydic resin containing a mixture of glycosidic ethers and polyossihydrilic phenols, which derives from a reaction of polycondensation between phenols, polyvalent alcohols and other substances having an ossiethilenic group (epichlorine). The major components are dodecenyl succinic anhydride (DDSA) and nadic methyl anhydride (NMA). The activators of the reaction are 2,4,6-tri-(dimethylaminomethyl) phenol (DMP-30) and benzyldimethylamine (BDMA), used in a concentration of 1–2%. Epon can be prepared as follows:

- Epon 812 (from kit)   23.5 mL
- Dodecenyl succinic anhydride (DDSA)   12.0 mL
- Nadic methyl anhydride (NMA)   14.0 mL
- 2,4,6-tri-(dimethylaminomethyl) phenol (DMP-30)   0.75 mL

The resin is made by gently mixing Epon 812 with DDSA, NMA and DMP-30. The resulting mixture has an orange-brown color and must be put under vacuum before using to remove air bubbles.

1. Dehydration and Infiltration

Dehydration is carried out through graded alcohol or acetone series at room temperature. Epon resin has the highest viscosity of all the resins described in this chapter and must not be used to infiltrate specimens of a size bigger than 4–5 mm^3.

2. Embedding and Staining

Extreme care must be taken during the embedding procedure to avoid the formation of air bubbles. This resin is difficult to manipulate because it is sticky and viscous. However, during the polymerization, which is carried out at 60°C for 12–24 h, there is no deformation or shrinking.

Toluidine blue and acid fuchsin are routinely used, as other staining agents do not yield good results. For this reason, Epon is not usually used to embed undecalcified tissues. Epon resin offers a very high quality morphological detail, but can interfere with some histo- and cytochemical techniques.

E. LR White Resin

LR White Resin is available in soft, medium, and hard forms (London Resin, Berkshire, UK). For osseous tissue infiltration, hard or medium consistency is advisable. It is an easy resin to manipulate, and has the advantage of being compatible with histo- and cytochemical techniques. The hardened blocks can be trimmed and cut without any difficulties.

1. Dehydration and Infiltration

Dehydration is carried out through graded alcohols at room temperature (alcohol 30%, 50%, 70%, 90%, one change each; 100%, 2 changes). The infiltration times are relatively long, and are influenced by the dimension and the consistency of the specimen. Usually, the steps are the following: 1:1 resin/alcohol; 2:1 resin/alcohol; 100% resin, repeated twice. Each step can last from 1 h to 1–2 d. It is advisable to perform infiltration at 4°C.

2. Embedding and Staining

Once infiltration has been completed, the specimens are correctly oriented and embedded in plastic capsules. Polymerization is carried out between 60°C and 68°C for 48–72 h. It is important that the resin containers have a lid to prevent oxygen from inhibiting the polymerization process on the superficial layer. The resin-embedding capsules used must be previously tested, to ensure that there is no reaction between the resin and its material. Gelatin capsules have been documented to work well for embedding small specimens with LR White.

A polymerization accelerator can also be used (use one drop for every 10 mL of resin). If too much accelerator is used, the reaction takes place too rapidly and the inner part of the block remains soft, making trimming and sectioning difficult. Moreover, a section derived from a specimen that is not well-polymerized cannot be properly stained and is difficult to examine microscopically. For staining, all the agents previously described can be used (Fig. 4).

F. Spurr's Resin

Although Araldite and Epon are the most popular epoxy resins, Spurr's resin is very useful for penetrating dense specimens, like mineralized tissues, because it is a low-viscosity-embedding medium. Its major component is the epoxy resin ERL 4206 (vinyl-4-cyclohexene dioxide, VCHD), but the presence of the flexibilizer DER 736 (epichlorohydrin-polyglycol epoxy resin) may be responsible for its low viscosity. It also contains the hardener NSA (nonenyl succinic anhydride) and the accelerator DMAE (2-dimethylaminoethanol), which both have a low viscosity. Moreover, aside from the good and rapid infiltration in the tissues, Spurr's resin shows a high resistance to the electron beam, the ultrathin sections are very stable, and for this reason they can be collected on uncoated grids. However, Spurr's resin is more carcinogenic and toxic than the other epoxy resins, and it should be handled with extreme caution—using gloves and mask, always under a fume hood.

REFERENCES

1. Bennett HS, Wyrick AD, Lee SW, et al: Science and art in preparing tissues embedded in plastic for light microcopy, with special reference to glycol methacrylate, glass knives and simple stains. *Stain Technol* 51:71–97, 1976.
2. Berger-Gorbet M, Broxup B, Rivard C, et al: Biocompatibility testing of Ni-Ti screws using immunohistochemistry on sections containing metallic implants. *J Biomed Mater Res* 32:243–248, 1996.
3. Botti F, Ragazzoni E, Pilloni A, et al: Assessment of the acrylic resin Technovit 7200 VLC for studying the gingival mucosa by light and electron microscopy. *Biotech Histochem* 72:178–184, 1997.
4. Caropreso S, Bondioli L, Capannolo D, et al: Thin sections for hard tissue histology: a new procedure. *J Microsc* 199:244–247, 2000.
5. Clark, G: *Staining Procedures Used by the Biological Stain Commission, 3rd ed.* Williams and Wilkins, Baltimore, MD, 1973:15–25.
6. Fricain JC, Rouais F, Dupuy B: A two-step embedding process for better preservation of soft tissue surrounding coral implants. *J Biomed Mater Res* 33:23–27, 1996.
7. Frosch D, Westphal C: Choosing the appropriate section thickness in the melamine embedding technique. *J Microsc* 137:177–183, 1985.
8. Luna LG: *Manual of Histologic Staining Methods of the Armed Forces Institute of Pathology, 3rd ed.* McGraw-Hill, New York, NY, 1968:37–42.
9. Noorlander C: Deplasticizing of thick Epon sections involving a new adhesive technique and staining of nervous tissue. *Acta Morphol Neerl Scand* 24:133–138, 1986.
10. Odgaard A, Andersen K, Melsen F, et al: A direct method for fast three-dimensional serial reconstruction. *J Microsc* 159:335–342, 1990.
11. Preece A: *A Manual for Histologic Technicians, 3rd ed.* Little, Brown, Boston, MA, 1972.
12. Rappay G, Van Duijn P: Chlorous acid as an agent for blocking tissue aldehydes. *Stain Technol* 40:275–277, 1965.
13. Tenorio D, Germain JP, Hughes FJ: Histochemical studies of acid and alkaline phosphatases in rat tooth germs with undecalcified resin-embedded specimens. *J Histochem Cytochem* 40:1229–1233, 1992.
14. Watts RH, Green D, Howells GR: Improvements in histological techniques for epoxy-resin embedded bone specimens. *Stain Technol* 56:155–161, 1981.
15. Westphal C, Frosch D: Fracturing of melamine-embedded cells and tissues: a new technique for studying cell membranes. *J Microsc* 137:17–23, 1985.
16. Spurr AR: A low viscosity resin embedding medium for electron microscopy. *J Ultrastruct Res* 26:31–43, 1969.

IV Sectioning Techniques

13

Histological Techniques for Decalcified Bone and Cartilage

Qian K. Kang,[1] Jackie C. LaBreck,[1] Helen E. Gruber,[2] and Yuehuei H. An[1]

[1]*Orthopaedic Research Laboratory, Medical University of South Carolina, Charleston, SC, USA*
[2]*Orthopaedic Research Biology, Carolinas Medical Center, Charlotte, NC, USA*

I. INTRODUCTION

Bone tissues are often processed to produce undecalcified sections, or ground sections. These sections range from 50–150 μm in thickness and are used for common histomorphometric studies, yielding poor cellular detail. To better observe the details of cellular components, thinner sections of single-cell thickness (ideally 4–6 μm) are preferred. Several methods are available for making such sections, including plastic-embedded sectioning with a sliding microtome (*see* Chapter 14) and decalcified paraffin- or celloidin-embedded sectioning with routine rotary microtome or a sliding microtome. Decalcified paraffin-embedded sectioning has been widely used because of its simplicity. It can be performed in most routine histological laboratories without the need for special equipment such as a diamond-coated saw or a grinder.

More detailed information on bone decalcification and verification can be found in Chapter 10 in this book. The basic principles and routine methods used in the authors' laboratory are provided here with attention paid to general information about the whole process of tissue preparation, including rough cut, fixation, decalcification, dehydration, infiltration and embedding (using paraffin), sectioning, and staining. There are some good resources in the literature for serious readers, such as the book by Brain,[3] several book chapters,[4,5,8,15] and journal articles.[17]

II. ROUGH CUT AND FIXATION

Rough cut and fixation is first step in the preparation of decalcified sections. Fixation is the process of rapid preservation of the tissue, thus maintaining its existing form and structure and all of its constituent elements. In order to obtain the best result, it is essential to place the tissue into a large volume of fixing fluid at the earliest possible moment after it has been removed from the body.

According to the requirement of the specific project, rough cut the specimen into the smallest possible size to facilitate the best fixation and decalcification. It is customary in histology to refer to the planes of sectioning as "longitudinal, oblique, and transverse."

From: *Handbook of Histology Methods for Bone and Cartilage*
Edited by: Y. H. An and K. L. Martin © Humana Press Inc., Totowa, NJ

Once the plane of sectioning and the area of interest have been chosen, the specimen should be trimmed to the smallest size possible, according to the purpose of the study and to provide a flat surface in the sectioning plane. This procedure should preferably be done before decalcification, although it can be done afterward. One advantage of trimming the specimen after decalcification is the ease of cutting, as completely decalcified tissue can be easily cut with a scalpel or razor blade.

The most popular agent for fixing gross specimens before decalcification is 10% neutral buffered formalin (NBF), but the quality of the decalcification depends on the decalcifying agent, the size of the specimen, the specimen:fixative volume ratio, the ambient temperature, and the length of fixation.[17] The smallest possible specimen size is preferred for fixation. Fixation for light microscopy is usually carried out at room temperature. The volume ratio between the specimen and the fixative must be at least 1:10 to 1:20. The most common reason for inadequate fixation may be an insufficient volume of fixative. Penetration can be hastened by pulling a vacuum on the specimen in the fixative solution. The length of time that tissue should left in the fixative depends on the rapidity of penetration of the fixative and on the thickness of the tissue. For most small bone specimens (less than 5 mm in thickness) 24–48 h fixation is enough. For larger specimens or small dense bones at least 48–72 h fixation is needed. However, long fixation times may compromise the ability to localize enzymes (such as alkaline phosphatase or tartrate-resistant acid phosphatase) and immunolocalization. For extremely large specimens such as canine or goat femoral heads or femoral condyles, perfusion fixation is necessary before specimens are harvested.

III. DECALCIFICATION

Decalcification is the process of complete removal of calcium salt and mineral from the bone tissue following proper fixation (*see* Chapter 10). Without decalcification, sectioning is nearly impossible unless the specimen is embedded in a plastic medium and cut with a heavy-duty rotary microtome. Decalcification using acid-decalcifying solutions and/or chelating agents is the most commonly used method. Other methods, such as ion-exchange resins and electrolytic methods, are rarely used.[8,15]

The most widely used decalcification procedures use either acids, which react with the calcium in bone to form soluble calcium salts, or chelating agents, which complex the calcium ions. Acid-decalcifying agents are known to have the drawback of altering the staining properties of bone.[3,4] Some decalcifying solutions also contain formalin, and thus increase the possibility of aldehyde groups in the tissue and blocking reactions. Commonly used decalcification solutions include formic acid (5–10% in saline),[3,4,9,11,178] ethylenediamine tetraacetate acid (EDTA),[3,4,8,11] and several commercially available decalcifying solutions. A 5-mm slice of bone can be decalcified with 10% formic acid in 3–7 d and by EDTA in 7–21 d.[4,5] A commercially available decalcification solution used in the authors' lab is Cal-Ex® (Fisher Scientific), which is an aqueous solution of 1.35 N hydrochloric acid and 0.003 M sodium EDTA, a chelating agent. This product can decalcify a 5-mm-thick bone within 24–48 h. It appears that the use of a combination of acid and chelating agent contributes the features of faster decalcification and limited tissue damage. However, the concentration of the hydrochloric acid in this product is relatively high, which may make it unsuitable for some applications. Other acid decalcification solutions include nitric acid, sulfurous acid, chromic acid, trichloroacetic acid, and trifluoroacetic acid.[4,5,15]

Whether one should use solutions prepared in the laboratory or a commercial product is a matter of personal choice. Different formulations of decalcifying fluids have varying lengths of decalcification time, and there are many commercially available decalcification solutions offering a wide range of decalcification times. It is important to remember that many commercial products have been developed for rapid decalcification of large specimens in the clinical pathology lab; these products should not automatically be assumed to be suitable for specialized orthopedic research applications. Therefore, a careful test run should be always done before using a new commercial decalcifying solution. The Cal-Ex® we routinely use in our laboratory is a fast decalcifier and causes no obvious harmful effect to the animal bones we study. Even for induced bone nodules harvested from nude mice, the cellular details are not altered using stains such as H&E (hematoxylin and eosin), safranin O, and fast green. Frequent monitoring using X-rays helps to prevent over-decalcification.

If the experiment involves specialized histology, such as localization of tartrate-resistant acid phosphatase or alkaline phosphatase, or *in situ* hybridization studies, it is important that the decalcification method employed is compatible with the special techniques. Although rapid decalcification solutions are quick, there is a danger that they may destroy the ability to localize key enzymes or to perform other special procedures on the decalcified tissue. An alternative to paraffin-embedding of decalcified tissue is embedment in glycol methacrylate, which always provides crisper resolution of cellular detail and is an often overlooked method. It is again advisable that a pilot study be used to ensure compatibility of the chosen decalcification and embedment method with the desired histological outcome.[9]

For best results, gauze-wrapped bone tissue can be suspended in the center of the decalcifying fluid.[15] Placing the specimen in the decalcifying solution on a slow-moving shaker or periodic manual agitation will help the speed of the decalcification.[8,12] Frequent changes of the solution are also important.

Although raising the temperature can hasten decalcification, it also may further deteriorate cell and tissue details. At 55–60°C the loss of calcium occurs rapidly, followed by swelling and hydrolysis of collagen, resulting in complete digestion of the tissue.[4,5,15] The swelling changes the original structure of the specimen and may also impair staining by H&E as well as some other stains.[4,5,15] However, more recent findings show that microwaving significantly reduces decalcification time, with no obvious adverse effects on the structure and antigenicity.[2,7,10] Microwaving also reduces the time taken for fixation, dehydration, infiltration, clearing, and staining.

IV. TESTING FOR COMPLETION OF CALCIFICATION

Blocks should be removed from decalcifying solution immediately on the completion of process. Treatment beyond this point will not improve cutting qualities, and will adversely affect staining; too short an exposure will result in residual calcium. A satisfactory decalcifying procedure should ensure: i) complete removal of calcium salts: ii) lack of distortion of cells and connective tissue; and iii) absence of harmful effects on staining reactions.[8]

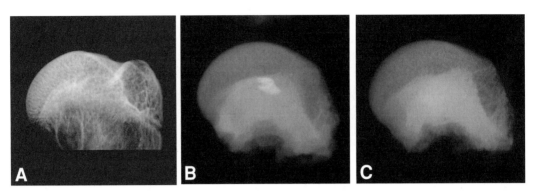

Figure 1. Radiographs taken before decalcification (A), after incomplete decalcification (B), and after decalcification is completed (C).

Several methods are useful to determine whether a specimen has been completely decalcified and is ready for embedding, including: cutting the specimen with a scalpel, radiography, and chemical methods.[3,4,11,15]

For bones of small mammals or relatively loose bone or immature bone—such as a bone nodule formed in subcutaneous tissue induced by a osteogenic implant—testing can be done by cutting the specimen with a scalpel or sticking a needle into the tissue. If the tissue is easily cut or pierced, decalcification can be assumed to be complete. Experience is needed for this kind of test. Another physical test, which also relies on the experienced technician's sense of touch in determining when tissue is decalcified, is performed by bending the tissue. However, using this method may leave residual calcium in the tissue, and the resulting artifacts will destroy important detail necessary for diagnosis.

For larger or dense bone specimens, an X-ray should be taken before and after decalcification. In an appropriately decalcified specimen, the bone should have radiological contrast similar to that of the surrounding muscle. It is important to obtain specimen radiographs before demineralization, particularly when the whole specimen is to be processed as it provides some idea of the type of tissue present. This information may help determine the orientation of pieces for embedding and also help to evaluate the approximate period required for decalcification. The use of X-ray as a routine measure to establish the presence of calcified remnants in biopsy material is valuable; it forms a permanent record that is ideal for ready reference. X-ray examination is the most reliable method for determining the completion or progress of decalcification, as even the smallest pocket of calcium (Fig. 1) can be detected with a modern high resolution X-ray machine such as a Faxitron.

Chemical testing relies on the detection of calcium in the used decalcifying solution; a negative result during calcification indicates completion of decalcification.[5,15] The general method is to add concentrated ammonia, drop by drop, to 5 mL of decalcifying solution, until the fluid is neutralized (i.e., pH = 7). If the solution becomes cloudy (because of the formation of calcium hydroxide), decalcification is not complete. If the solution remains clear, add 0.5 mL saturated ammonium oxalate. If the solution becomes cloudy (because of the formation of calcium oxalate), the decalcification is incomplete. If the solution remains clear for 30 min, it can be determined that the decalcification is complete.

In general, the specimen should be placed in a fresh solution of decalcifying fluid and testing repeated after a suitable interval (24–48 h) before the fluid is to be discarded.

V. FURTHER PROCESSING OF TISSUE

The steps for further processing the decalcified tissue include dehydration, clearing, infiltration, and embedding until a solid block of paraffin containing the decalcified tissue is obtained. The decalcified tissue can be transferred into 70% ethanol for dehydration toward the eventual infiltration and embedding in paraffin or celloidin.[8] Tissues can also be placed in 70% ethanol for long-term storage.

For dehydration, the three most common reagents are alcohol, acetone, and dioxane. Of these, the most commonly used dehydrating agent is ethanol (alcohol). There are no significant differences between the dehydration of decalcified tissues and other soft tissues. Dehydration is carried out in stages using increasing strengths of alcohol—e.g., 70% alcohol, 95% alcohol, and absolute (100%) alcohol, generally two changes for each concentration.

Clearing is the replacement of dehydration fluid in the specimen with a substance that is miscible with the embedding medium to be employed. There are many clearing reagents available, but most laboratories rely on only a few, such as xylene, toluene, and benzene. Every clearing reagent has its own advantages and disadvantages. In the case of decalcified tissues, xylene is still the most common one. One should bear in mind that xylene tends to make most tissue brittle, which is compounded when used for the already harder decalcified bone. Brain[3] and Skinner[16,17] suggested the use of cedar wood oil and methyl salicylate which do not make tissue brittle, even after prolonged clearing time. A 50:50 mixture of dehydrating and clearing agent is recommended prior to immersion in pure clearing agent.[3]

Infiltration displaces the clearing agent from the tissues and allows the tissue to be completely permeated by the paraffin, which is subsequently allowed to harden (embedding), thereby producing a block from which sections may be cut. It may be necessary to use vacuum infiltration, to remove potentially trapped air bubbles in the specimens.

Following infiltration of specimens with paraffin, the specimen is transferred into a mold and fresh wax added, then the molten wax containing the specimen is allowed to harden. These steps are known as embedding. When embedding, it is very important to ensure that the specimen is in the desired orientation, with the chosen cutting plane parallel to the face of the block.

A. A Sample Protocol for Processing Small Decalcified Bone Specimens

A practical protocol employed in the our laboratory for processing small decalcified bone specimens (2–3-mm-thick slabs of rabbit distal femoral bone) is as follows:

- Fix specimens (preferably for at least 24 h) in 10% NBF.
- Rinse the specimens in distilled water and then place them in decalcification solution (Cal-Ex®, Fisher Scientific) overnight (18–24 h). Remember that this is a fast decalcifier, and frequent monitoring should be performed using either X-rays or a chemical method.
- Rinse the specimen with distilled water and place it in 70% ethanol. X-ray the specimens to determine whether there are any calcium deposits (this is very important!). If you see any residual calcium, place the specimens back in decalcifying solution and repeat until there is no calcium in the specimen. Rinse with distilled water and continue to the next step.
- More trimming as needed.

- Immerse the specimen in 70% ethanol for 1 h with agitation.
- 95% ethanol for 1 h with agitation.
- Fresh 95% ethanol for 1 h with agitation.
- 100% ethanol for 1 h with agitation.
- Fresh 100% ethanol for 1 h with agitation.
- If tissue is large (more than 4 mm thick), use an additional 100% ethanol step for 1 h with agitation.
- Xylene for 1 h.
- Fresh xylene for 1 h.
- Paraffin (in 65°C oven) for 1 h under vacuum.
- Fresh paraffin (in 65°C oven) for 1 h under vacuum.
- Embed in paraffin.

VI. SECTION CUTTING AND PRECAUTIONS

There are several differences between cutting paraffin-embedded soft tissue and decalcified hard tissues. Only routine equipment for sectioning soft-tissue blocks is needed. For decalcified specimens, rotary microtomes are adequate to cut 6–10-μm-thick sections. However, for preparing blemish-free sections from decalcified bone tissues, the following are the fundamental requirements:

1. Proper fixation.
2. Complete decalcification.
3. Sufficient dehydration.
4. Good infiltration and embedding.
5. A suitable microtome in well-maintained condition.
6. Cold working temperature (let the paraffin block sit face down on ice prior to sectioning).
7. Sharp knives or blades.
8. Experienced and patient hands.

Surface decalcification and water softening can be very useful to solve the most common problem in decalcified tissue sectioning: a hard cutting surface resulting from incomplete decalcification and/or incomplete dehydration or clearing of the specimens. When cutting a tissue block, the feeling of scraping and tears seen in the section may mean incomplete decalcification. This also damages the knife's cutting edge. A hard cutting surface makes satisfactory sectioning impossible. Surface decalcification may be used to deal with this problem. One method is the use of a pad of cotton or sponge soaked with decalcifying solution (Cal-Ex®, 1% hydrochloric acid solution in 70% ethanol,[4] or 10% formic acid[8]) placed over the surface of the block face for 10 min. Another method of surface decalcification is to simply immerse the block in one of the decalcifying solutions for 30–60 min.[8] These steps may result in progressive decalcification and tissue softening (Fig. 2), with little or no adverse effect on subsequent staining. Often, even a well-decalcified bone may still need some "surface decalcification" before each round of a serial cut. Water also has a softening effect. An exposure of 15–30 min to water (attaching a wet sponge or placing in water) allows water to enter the exposed tissue, often softening it for a depth of up to 500 μm.[11]

Cartilage is composed largely of macromolecular sugars, but often also contains insoluble calcium salts. Cartilage can be softened to some extent by decalcification in acids or chelating agents.[11]

Low working temperature makes the paraffin harder, and the water shed by melting ice softens the tissue surface, making a more homogenous composite surface, which reduces

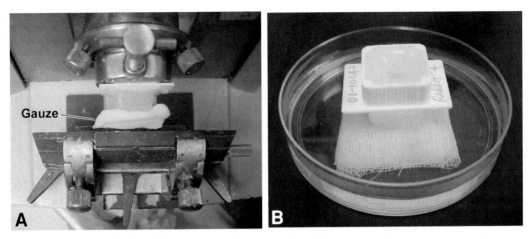

Figure 2. Surface decalcification by covering the face of the block with a gauze soaked with decalcifying solution (A) or by immersing the block face in decalcifying solution (B).

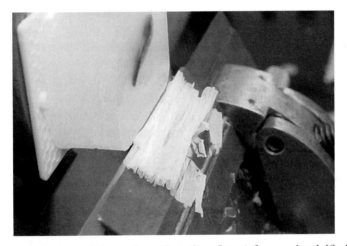

Figure 3. Photograph shows thin sections (less than 5 μm) from a decalcified tissue block are sometimes difficult to obtain because of significant compression.

chattering.[3,17] The ambient temperature should be adjusted to be as cool as possible. More importantly, cutting should be carried out on a cold tissue block. It is a good idea to store tissue blocks in a refrigerator before a cutting session. Immediately before sectioning, the temperature of the block and the knife can be lowered by using Freeze' it spray (Fisher Scientific), which can quickly freeze the local area to –60°C.

Thickness of the section is an essential issue to be addressed for each project. For studies that require more cellular detail, such as cell identification, cellular activities at tissue-implant interface, or tumor diagnosis, 3–6 μm is preferred. However, in practice sections this thin from a decalcified tissue block may be difficult to obtain because of significant compression (Fig. 3).[3] Often, a limited number of satisfactory sections can only be achieved with numerous cuts and by a patient technician. For low-magnification histomorphometric

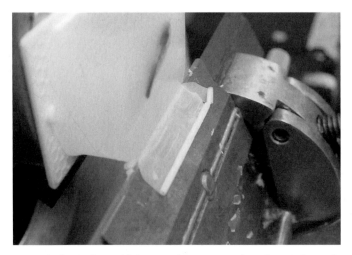

Figure 4. Photograph shows how thicker sections (more than 8 μm) from decalcified tissue tend to curl up.

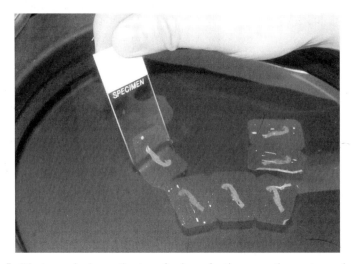

Figure 5. Photograph shows the transferring of a tissue section onto a microslide.

analysis, thicker sections of more than 10 μm may be sufficient. Such sectioning is relatively easy to accomplish. One potential problem is the curling phenomenon (Fig. 4).[3] With examination under a stereomicroscope, it can be seen that the surface next to the blade is smooth and glossy, although the upper surface appears dull and granular.

Section flattening and mounting is the last step before deparaffinizing and staining.[3] After satisfactory sections are cut, they are transferred into a flotation bath using a jewelry forceps or a fine brush for flattening and for mounting onto microslides (Fig. 5). The bath is usually set at 45–50°C, which is good for flattening sections with a thickness less than 6 μm. For thicker sections, a warmer temperature of 50–60°C may be used.

VII. STAINS AND RESULTS

Many of the routine trichrome stains, H&E, toluidine blue, safranin O, and fast green, and other stains have been adapted for studying decalcified bone and cartilàge in paraffin sections.[1,17] The most commonly used staining techniques include H&E, safranin O/fast green,[18] and Goldner's trichrome.

Methylene blue/basic fuchsin and other metachromic stains are useful if one wishes to view entire long bones with epiphysis, physis, and metaphysis present in one specimen. If the cartilage matrix components are of interest, the metachromic stains, including azure A and the critical electrolyte staining series with alcian blue, are very valuable.[13] Periodic acid–Schiff can be applied both to decalcified and plastic-embedded specimens to investigate the mucopolysaccharide content of cartilage.[14]

The potentially harmful effect of fast-acting decalcifying solutions on the staining of cellular details, especially nuclear staining, is again worth emphasizing.[4] If the purpose of the study is low-magnification histomorphometric or structural evaluation, rapid decalcification may be used and the sections stained with a monocolor stain, such as toluidine blue, hematoxylin, or methylene blue/basic fuchsin. If the purpose of the study is to observe cellular details, however, a slow-acting weak acid (formic acid) or EDTA should be used. Simply choosing a slow decalcifier, such as 5% formic acid or EDTA, is a relatively safe choice, and can be a standard for many research purposes. However, a careful and well-tested decalcification protocol should be established for each type of specimen, and the time frame for a specific decalcification process should be strictly observed.

Another potential problem is that when specimens have been decalcified in a harsh manner or over-decalcified, enzyme or other biochemical localizations may not be possible. There are set methods for processing tissues for demonstrating different enzymes or biochemicals, such as those for acid phosphatase, alkaline phosphatase, and glycogen.[15] For example, to demonstrate acid phosphatase, tissue should be fixed for no more than 24 h in 10% neutral formalin and a decalcifying solution of sodium citrate-formic acid (20% sodium citrate 50 mL, formic acid 2.5 mL, dH_2O 47.5 mL, pH 4.2) should be used. After decalcification, frozen sections are prepared.[15]

Below is a practical staining protocol of safranin O/fast green stain[6,18] used for decalcified rabbit femoral condyle in the our laboratory:

A. Safranin O/Fast Green Stain

1. Reagents

- 1.5% aqueous safranin O: 1.5 g safranin O (C.I. 50240) in 100 mL distilled water.
- 0.02% alcoholic fast green: 0.02 g fast green (C.I. 42053) in 100 mL 95% ethanol.
- 1% acetic acid (always use fresh): 5 mL glacial acetic acid in 495 mL distilled water.

2. Procedure

- Deparaffinize sections in 3 changes of xylene, 5 min each.
- Rinse in 2 changes of 100% ethanol, 1 min each to remove the xylene.
- Hydrate in 2 changes of 95% ethanol, 1 min each.
- Finish hydration with 3 changes of distilled water, 1 min each.
- Put slides in 1.5% safranin O for 40 min.
- Rinse in 3 changes of distilled water, 6 dips each. Make sure to immerse entire slide. Do not leave slides in water for excessive amounts of time, which will wash out the safranin O.

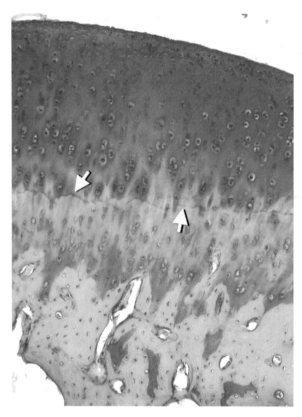

Figure 6. Safranin O and fast green staining of rabbit femoral condyles. Articular cartilage is stained red because of its content of proteoglycan, subchondral bone is stained green, and calcified cartilage between them is stained light pink. The latter is actually a mixture of red and green. The arrow indicates the tidemark separating the calcified and non-calcified portions of the cartilage. (*See* color plate 10 appearing in the insert following p. 270.)

- Dip slides in 0.02% alcoholic fast green for 30 s.
- Dip slides in fresh 1% acetic acid solution, 8 dips.
- Rinse quickly in distilled water, 6 dips.
- Quickly dip slides in 95% ethanol, 6 dips.
- Dehydrate in 2 changes of 100% ethanol, 8 dips each.
- Rinse one slide in xylene for 1 min and check the staining under the microscope. If the stain is good, proceed with the next step; if it is not good, rinse the checked slide in 100% ethanol to remove xylene and go back to either water or the stain. Water will take out stain that is too dark or re-stain if the result was too light. Clear in three changes of xylene, 1 min each.
- Cover slip.
- Result: Articular cartilage is stained red because of its proteoglycan content, subchondral bone stained green, and calcified cartilage in between stained light pink (Fig. 6).

One may also want to test the 30-s claimed time for staining cartilage sections using safranin O and fast green with the aid of a microwave.[10]

REFERENCES

1. Bancroft JD, Stevens A: *Theory and Practice of Histological Techniques.* Churchill Livingstone, New York, NY, 1982:313.
2. Boon ME, Kok LP, Ouwerkerk-Noordam E: Microwave-stimulated diffusion for fast processing of tissue: reduced dehydrating, clearing, and impregnating times. *Histopathology* 10:303–309, 1986.
3. Brain EB: *The Preparation of Decalcified Sections.* Charles C. Thomas, Springfield, IL, 1966.
4. Brown GG: *Primer of Histopathologic Techniques.* Appleton-Century-Crofts, New York, NY, 1969:38–51.
5. Brown GG: *An Introduction to Histotechnology.* Appleton-Century-Crofts, New York, NY, 1978:39–51.
6. Bulstra SK, Drukker J, Kuijer R, et al: Thionin staining of paraffin and plastic embedded sections of cartilage. *Biotech Histochem* 68:20–28, 1993.
7. Cunningham CD, III, Schulte BA, Bianchi LM, et al: Microwave decalcification of human temporal bones. *Laryngoscope* 111:278–282, 2001.
8. Drury RAB, Wallington EA: *Carleton's Histological Techniques.* Oxford University Press, Oxford, UK, 1980:199–220.
9. Gruber HE, Stasky AA: Histological study in orthopaedic animal research. In: An YH, Friedman RJ, eds. *Animal Models in Orthopaedic Research.* CRC Press, Boca Raton, FL, 1999:115–138.
10. Kahveci Z, Minbay FZ, Cavusoglu L: Safranin O staining using a microwave oven. *Biotech Histochem* 75:264–268, 2000.
11. Kiernan HA: *Histological and Histochemical Methods: Theory and Practice.* Pergamon Press, Oxford, UK, 1990:32–35.
12. Lillie RD: *Histopathologic Technic.* McGraw-Hill, Philadelphia, PA, 1948.
13. Scott JE, Dorling J: Differential staining of acid glycosaminoglycans (mucopolysaccharides) by alcian blue in salt solutions. *Histochemie* 5:221–233, 1965.
14. Scott JE, Dorling J: Periodate oxidation of acid polysaccharides. III. A PAS method for chondroitin sulphates and other glycosamino-glycuronans. *Histochemie* 19:295–301, 1969.
15. Sheehan DC, Hrapchak BB, eds: *Theory and Practice of Histotechnology.* Battelle Press, Columbus, OH and Richland, WA, 1980:89–117.
16. Skinner RA: The value of methyl salicylate as a clearing agent. *J Histotech* 9:27–28, 1986.
17. Skinner RA, Hickmon SG, Lumpkin CK, et al: Decalcified bone: twenty years of successful specimen management. *J Histotech* 20:267–277, 1997.
18. Thompson Jr., RC, Oegema Jr., TR, Lewis JL, et al: Osteoarthrotic changes after acute transarticular load. An animal model. *J Bone Joint Surg [Am]* 73:990–1001, 1991.

14

Techniques for Sectioning Undecalcified Bone Tissue Using Microtomes

William L. Ries

Departments of Stomatology and Pediatrics,
Medical University of South Carolina, Charleston, SC, USA

I. INTRODUCTION

The first "cutting machine" for preparing sections of soft tissues was introduced by Cummings in 1770. The prototype, a metal cylinder that contained the specimen, usually a plant, was screwed by hand into the path of a knife to make a tissue slice. In 1835, Pritchard clamped a similar instrument to a table for greater stability. A section was then prepared with a two-handled knife by cutting across the specimen. Eventually, Chevalier introduced the name "microtome" for these devices in 1839. The development of a sliding mechanism for cutting machines began as early as 1798 as a method to section large tissue specimens. With hand-held knives barely adequate for cutting small specimens, rotary microtomes were introduced by scientific investigators in 1883 and 1886 for greater precision and uniform section thickness. In this case, the specimen passed through into a stable stationary knife. The Spencer Lens Company, between 1901 and 1910, manufactured the first clinical microtome and a larger, precision laboratory microtome.[8] However, these early devices were inadequate for sectioning mineralized tissues unless the mineral could be removed by a decalcification process. At the time, mineralized bone had to be cut with a saw into relatively thick sections, and ground to a desired thickness.

Significant advances in the histological study of bone tissue were not made until the early 1960s. To make thin sections prior to that period, the next step after fixation of osseous tissue was usually the removal of the most important component—the mineral—with acids or chelators of calcium ions. The decalcified bone structures were then subject to deformation during embedment. In addition to the difficulty in accurately assessing the microanatomy, the study of the dynamics of bone could not be totally appreciated or measured when mineral was removed. The advent of acrylic and epoxy resin-embedding materials, and the introduction of heavy-duty microtomes equipped with knives having edges of tungsten carbide, eventually made it possible to examine mineralized bone tissue in semi-thin sections.[11]

Numerous techniques have been reported that describe the preparation of nondemineralized bone specimens for study at both the light and electron microscopic levels. It is not

From: *Handbook of Histology Methods for Bone and Cartilage*
Edited by: Y. H. An and K. L. Martin © Humana Press Inc., Totowa, NJ

the purpose of this chapter to contrast and compare all of these techniques. Most of the techniques in specimen preparation prior to sectioning have been covered thoroughly in the earlier chapters. A claim will not be made here to describe the "best" techniques. Each individual investigator and laboratory specialist should develop their own individual approaches to deal with the problems involved in sectioning undecalcified bone specimens. The major focus of this chapter is to provide a guide to the potential pitfalls common to this challenging investigative endeavor.

It is important to emphasize that caution should be used with the chemicals, devices, and equipment mentioned in the chapter because of the potential hazards they present if misused. For this reason, it is highly recommended that you read and observe all warnings and cautions provided by the manufacturers for each product mentioned before initiating a procedure.

II. BONE PREPARATION TO ENHANCE SECTIONING

A. *Fixation and Dehydration*

1. *Fixation*

Fixation to preserve microscopic structural details is the first step in the adequate preparation of nondemineralized bone specimens for sectioning. The most commonly used fixatives for bone in light microscopic studies—10% neutral buffered formalin (NBF) and 40–70% ethanol—must be treated differently at the completion of fixation. The difference becomes clear prior to initiating tissue dehydration, which is usually done with graded ethanols. When ethanol is the fixative, dehydration in ethanol may begin immediately. On the other hand, an overnight or longer (depending on the specimen size) washing step in water is required after formalin fixation. Besides the additional time needed, the washing step may introduce tissue swelling, followed by contraction during dehydration. These processes may cause excessive tissue separation at the bone marrow-to-bone interface.[1] Another potential problem with formalin is its ability at low pH to remove mineral, which can extract tetracycline labels. To overcome this problem, phosphate-buffered formalin at pH 7.1 is recommended.[5] Although relatively slow and weak compared to formalin, ethanol fixation does not remove calcium.[9] Ethanol will penetrate quickly into small pieces of bone. However, infiltration with 40% ethanol is faster then 70%, and large bone specimens take 12 h and 1 wk, respectively (Technovit 9100, Heraeus Kulzer GmbH, D-61273 Wehrheim/Ts., instructional insert). Some large specimens may need to be halved to allow thorough penetration. Bone specimens may be stored for long periods of time in a sufficient volume (10–20 times the volume of the bone sample) of NBF or 70% ethanol. However, the maximum storage period in 40% ethanol is 2d.[1] Storage in ethanol should be at 4°C, and room temperature is adequate for NBF[1]

Other fixatives for bone include 4% paraformaldehyde used for enzyme and immunohistochemistry (Technovit 9100), 50% acetone in water[12] and slowly penetrating 2.5% glutaraldehyde in 0.05 M phosphate-buffered saline (PBS) plus 0.1% sucrose (Technovit 9100) for electron microscopic study. Fixative infiltration through dense or sclerotic bone may be hastened by reducing the specimen size and/or by agitation with a mechanical stirrer or rotator. For fragile specimens, agitation should be done with caution to avoid bone fragmentation.

2. Dehydration

Acrylic[1,9] and epoxy[12] resins used for embedment are immiscible in water. Therefore, all water must be extracted for thorough infiltration of undecalcified bone by these resins. Improperly dehydrated specimens cannot be cut into intact thin sections because of voids in the resin. The most common method of dehydration uses graded concentrations of ethanol. However, dehydration in acetone has been recommended prior to infiltration with epoxy resins.[12] In general, each concentration of the dehydration agent should be changed at least twice over the course of the procedure. The time of dehydration depends on the size of the specimen and bone density. For example, thin (100-μm width) trabeculae infiltrate faster than dense cortices. For small specimens (with the exception of dense or sclerotic bone), 2 h for each concentration with three solution changes in between should be adequate. The temperature at which the dehydration is done varies according to the procedure. The majority of dehydration protocols proceed at room temperature. However, a temperature of 4°C has been recommended for dehydration in ethanol.[1] Specimens in absolute ethanol at 4°C should be brought to room temperature before any solution change, particularly in humid climates, to avoid water droplet condensation on the inside of the container or cap. In addition to agitation and a low temperature for the solutions, another recommendation to improve infiltration has been to remove air bubbles trapped in the specimens by application of a vacuum. Air bubbles block liquid infiltration to portions of the specimen. No more than 1 h in a vacuum should be a sufficient time to allow any trapped air to escape.

Acrylic resin monomer infiltration may proceed directly from absolute alcohol at the end of dehydration. However, a "clearing" step with several changes of xylene or acetone at room temperature to remove fat tissue may be included following alcohol dehydration. A brief period in a vacuum after each liquid change also is recommended during this step.

B. Resin Infiltration

For safety reasons all handling of liquid plastic monomers is done under a fume hood. The first infiltration of a resin plus a plasticizer (softener) at 4°C actually completes the dehydration process.[3] Several changes of the resin mixture take place over the course of the infiltration along with up to 1 h exposure to a vacuum at each change. To prevent any moisture contamination caused by condensation on the container surfaces, the specimen container should be brought to room temperature before opening. Addition of a catalyst/activator to the final change of fresh monomer and plasticizer at the embedment step initiates the polymerization of the resin. Once polymerized, the resin should exhibit a degree of hardness similar to that of bone. This similarity in hardness will prevent specimen tears during sectioning with the microtome knife. The hardness of the resin should be adjustable by varying the amount of plasticizer. Another requirement is that the polymerized resin be dissolvable in available solvents prior to staining of the sections.

Methyl methacrylate (MMA) and glycol methacrylate—both acrylic resins—and Spurr's, an epoxy resin, have the necessary characteristics for infiltration and embedment of bone for light microscopic study. Spurr's medium has been reported to prevent artifacts because of the separation of different tissue layers through its low viscosity for good tissue penetration and minimal shrinkage during polymerization.[12] Both resin and activator should be stored at 4°C. Before use, they should be brought to room temperature prior to mixing to avoid water contamination from condensation on glass container surfaces.[3]

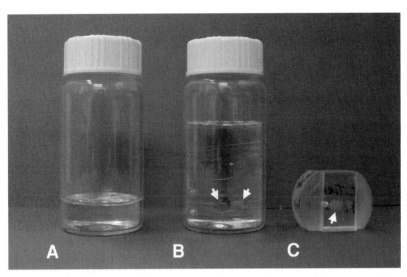

Figure 1. Glass scintillation vial (25 mL) mold with a 5-mm-thick polymerized methyl methacrylate (MMA) acrylic base (A). Embedded bone specimen with excess acrylic for block fabrication (B). Trimmed acrylic block with 3-mm-diameter bone core (C). Arrows indicate bone specimens.

C. Embedding

Commercially available molds to contain the bone specimen and the plastic embedment during the polymerization process are currently limited for light microscopic studies. One popular mold is the 25-mL glass scintillation vial. Other types of useful molds are often made of polystyrene (Peel-A-Way). The walls of molds should be thin enough to allow the heat generated by the exothermic polymerization reaction to be dispersed quickly. Deep embedding molds (approx 50-mm deep) allow for an extra layer of plastic that can be trimmed and clamped directly into the microtome chuck (Fig. 1). Before embedding the specimen in a glass or polystyrene vial, a layer of resin or acrylic approx 5 mm thick is polymerized at the bottom to form a base (Fig. 1). The base layer allows an embedded bone specimen to be oriented in a desired plane before beginning to trim the block to fit the microtome chuck. Capping the vial tightly helps the polymerization of the surface layer of plastic by excluding some air. The presence of air will inhibit the completion of the polymerization process at the surface. Alternatively, flushing the vial with a gentle stream of nitrogen gas for 10–20 s before immediately applying the cap removes most of the air, resulting in a fully polymerized base layer.

To embed the specimen, a mold with a polymerized base is first filled nearly full with freshly mixed plastic monomer, plasticizer, and catalyst. Nearly filling the mold will displace most of the air. Most infiltrated bone specimens can be carried into the filled mold with a metal forceps. However, for fragile bone cores that may be crushed with a forceps, a laboratory micro-spoon, bent at a right angle to the handle, or similar instrument can be used to cradle the specimen into the mold. The mold is placed in a vacuum for a half hour to remove any air trapped in the specimen during transfer. Once removed from the vacuum, center the specimen in the mold using a glass rod and cap tightly.

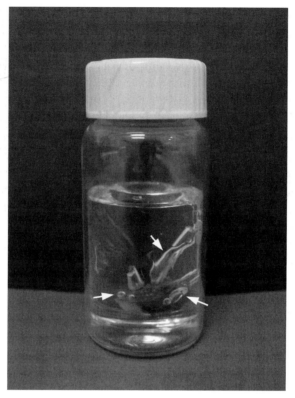

Figure 2. Gas bubbles in a polymerized MMA embed (arrows).

The polymerization reaction is hastened by heating the monomer in a water bath to temperatures as high as 48°C.[7] The water bath actually tempers the heat generated by the exothermic polymerization reaction. The high temperature reached during polymerization (up to 92°C) is the major reason for the generation of gas bubbles in the resin (Fig. 2). If multiple molds go into a water bath, adequate space is needed between them to account for an additional increase in bath temperature immediately around the molds. As the high temperature speeds the hardening process, gas bubbles become trapped in the block. The trapped gas introduces holes in the sections as they come off the microtome, and could interfere with their adhesion to glass slides prior to staining. Depending on the plastic-embedding technique used, the completion of polymerization may take 1–4 d. As mentioned previously, the final degree of hardness of the embedding plastic should approach the hardness of bone.

D. Block Trimming

Once polymerized, the blocks must be removed from their molds. Glass vials should be broken with caution. To avoid injury from flying pieces of glass, vials should be covered with cloth or paper towels before striking with a mallet or similar instrument. Also, the glass pieces should be discarded in an appropriate container for broken glass. Before trimming the plastic block, you should determine the orientation of the specimen in the block to the microtome blade. For example, a transiliac bone biopsy core should have both cortices oriented perpendicular to the knife edge to spread the stress to the blade over a wider sector and reduce the chances of edge damage.[1] First, a cylindrical block containing a bone core is flattened on a plane parallel to the length of the core. Flattening can be done on a grinder/polisher machine (Buehler Ltd, Lake Bluff, IL) with coarse silicon carbide paper. The grinding paper should be flushed with a stream of water to prevent plastic particles from clogging the paper. A drill press vice (Palmgren Steel Products, Inc., Chicago, IL) can be used to hold the plastic cylinder in the correct orientation during grinding. The vice also provides a flat surface to grind against. Second, with the previously flattened surface of the block on the cutting platform of a band saw (10-inch model with regular saw teeth, 15 teeth per inch for plastic) two cuts are made, one on each side of the bone core. Leave at least 1 mm of plastic between each cut and the bone specimen. To remove the excess plastic on the sides of the specimen, two more cuts are made, each perpendicular to the end of the first two cuts. Next, with the aid of the drill press vice, grind a plane parallel to the first flattened side of the block. Finally, cut away the base layer on which the bone core rested initially. This layer can be removed with a precision slow-speed saw (Buehler Ltd.) equipped with a diamond wafering blade oriented parallel to the length of the bone core. Removal of the base layer with the saw reduces the amount of trimming with the microtome knife, increasing the longevity of the knife-edge sharpness. An example of a trimmed block is shown in Fig. 1.

E. Microtome Sectioning

1. Microtome Types for Sectioning Bone

Microtomes generally produce two movements: the cutting movement of the knife along the desired plane, and the feeding movement of the specimen block perpendicular to the cutting plane. Microtomes of good quality have precise adjustable movements. Most microtomes from well-known manufacturers meet these demands. Large, non-demineralized bone specimens should be sectioned with a sliding (known as the Schantz microtome after the original German model[6]) or base sledge[2] microtome, where in either case the specimen block remains stationary while the knife is passed through it. The knife is fastened in a holder, which slides back and forth on rails with the cutting edge of the blade in the lead. The specimen is advanced in small increments at a right angle into the path of the oncoming knife-edge. As the knife sweeps past the specimen, a thin slice or section is made. The uniform thickness and flatness of the section is determined by the sharpness of the blade, the stoutness of the cutting-edge, the steadiness of the knife motion, and the ability of the apparatus to absorb vibration. For this purpose, these microtomes are stable and robust, and are motorized to provide a slow and steady cutting motion.

A rotary microtome (Spencer[6] or Minot[2] microtomes named after the originators) is only robust enough to cut small bone specimens (Fig. 3). By the rotation of a handwheel, the block, clamped in a chuck, moves vertically downward nearly 7.5 cm in the cutting-stroke through a stationary knife and upward on the return stroke retracted away from the blade. At each rotation of the handwheel, the block also moves forward in micrometer increments through the action of a micrometer screw, which gives the tissue sections the desired thickness. A motorized version of the rotary microtome is essential for a controlled, slow cutting speed.

Microtomes should rest on a stable laboratory table. Any large appliances, such as refrigerators or freezers, should not be in proximity to a microtome because of the vibrations they

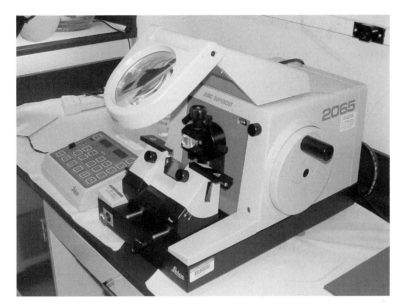

Figure 3. Motorized rotary microtome with microprocessor controls.

introduce to nearby objects. A microtome that vibrates produces wrinkled sections as a result of knife chatter. Wrinkled sections flatten with difficulty, and tend to lift from slides in staining solutions.

2. Microtome Knives

Microtomes require tungsten carbide-tipped knives to section undecalcified bone embedded in plastic. In addition, the blade must be stout to withstand damage at the cutting edge by mineralized tissues. A C profile knife, used for cutting sections of soft tissues and decalcified bone embedded in paraffin blocks, has a relatively small wedge angle of approx 17° and a 29° facet angle (Fig. 4A). The C profile knife-edge would be rapidly dulled by mineralized bone. A D profile knife has a tooled edge[2] that provides a stout wedge angle of approx 36° and a facet angle of 45° honed at the edge (Fig. 4B). As a general rule, the harder the tissue specimen to be cut, the greater the knife angle should be. However, the wider the angle, the more change in direction the section must take to pass over the knife. This greater direction change can cause tearing of the section[1] by vibration of the knife-edge or chattering.

The microtome should have a knife holder that tightly pins the knife into a stable position. A coin is often inserted between the tip of the screw pin and the blade to broaden the pinning force for increased blade stability (Fig. 5). Instability can induce chatter, and can also damage the fine knife-edge in a number of ways.

Sharpness of the knife is critical to successful sectioning of undecalcified bone. Blunt knives slide over the block face, compressing the block. The next cutting stroke following compression produces a thick section. Knives are dulled by frequent cutting of hard tissues, blade corrosion, accumulation of resin on the edge of the blade, and incidental contact of the knife-edge with instruments while retrieving sections. The importance of proper care of the knife cannot be overemphasized.[8] Block-face lubricants/moisteners,

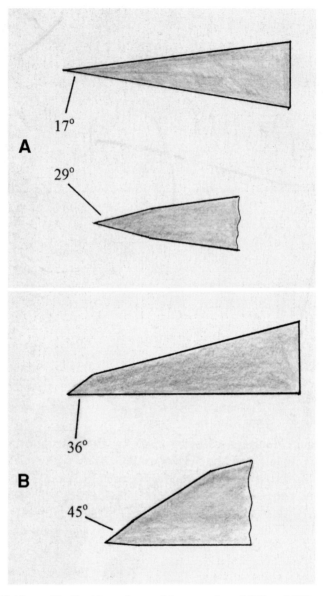

Figure 4. (A) Knife-profile *C* with wedge and facet angles of 17° and 29°, respectively. (B) Knife-profile *D* with tool edge and facet angles of 36° and 45°, respectively.

such as water and diluted ethanol that collect on the knife-edge, should be wiped away to avoid knife-edge corrosion. These substances are removed carefully with cotton-tipped applicators and tissue wipes by wiping the knife in a direction away from the edge. This direction lessens the chance of injury to fingers and the possibility of denting the knife-edge. Resin accumulation can also be removed by a wiping action with a cotton-tipped applicator moistened in xylene. To protect the knife against dents or nicks from metal instruments, remove tissue sections with a fine paintbrush instead of a forceps. Nicks in a knife-edge manifest themselves as striations in the sections and on the surface of the

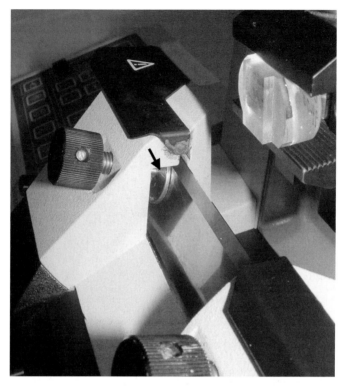

Figure 5. Profile D knife pinned securely to the holder back of a rotary microtome with a coin (arrow).

block face. These linear scratches damage the microstructure of the tissues in a section. Even the keen edges of tungsten carbide are dulled rapidly when cutting mineralized bone, and frequent sharpening is necessary. Sharpening may be done in your own laboratory or commercially (e.g., Delaware Diamond Knives, Inc., 3825 Lancaster Pike, Wilmington, DE). Either way, a sharpening technique that will not damage the knife-edge further requires the skills of an expert.

When not in use, the knife should be stored in its case, and not be left on the microtome where the knife-edge could corrode with exposure to humidity. The knife should be cleaned with xylene on a tissue wipe and then wiped dry.[8] After smearing a light coating of anti-corrosive oil over the knife, it should be stored in its case.[2] Any oil should be carefully removed before the knife is used again.

3. Section Preparation

The trimmed specimen block (*see* Section IID *"Block Trimming"*) must be held tightly in position by the microtome chuck. Most rotary microtome models have a chuck attached to an adjustable holding adapter that orients the block face both horizontally and vertically to the knife-edge.

After aligning the block with the knife-edge, the next adjustment sets the "knife angle" to the block face. Knife holders should allow for the adjustment of the angle the knife-edge makes with the block face known as the "clearance angle" (Fig. 6). Adjustment of

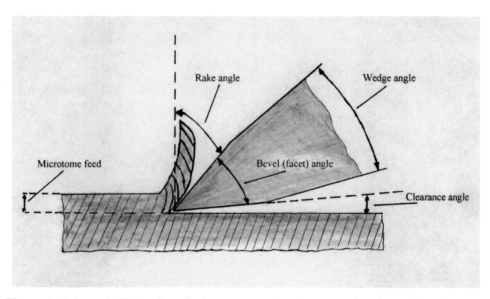

Figure 6. Schematic illustration of microtome cutting, demonstrating the angles relevant to the process.

the clearance angle can prevent excessive compression of the block face, which may introduce tears in the sections. Compression of the block produces alternate thick and thin sections, none of which are at the thickness desired. The only method to judge whether or not the proper clearance angle has been selected is to examine the sections as they come off the knife. A clearance angle that is too large scrapes the section off the block face instead of cutting it. This scraping action curls the sections into a scroll and gives them a wrinkled appearance when attempting to flatten them. If the clearance angle is too small, the blade compresses the block face. The next cutting stroke will produce an overly thin section followed by a thick one. To select a clearance angle, it is advisable to start at 0° and increase the angle in approx 2° increments until flat sections come off the knife.

Hard-tissue specimens, such as bone, are cut best at a slow speed.[9,10] High-speed sectioning induces knife chatter that wrinkles and tears the section. Knife-chatter noise resembles the sound made by a damp finger rubbed on a pane of glass. When the correct speed is reached, sectioning should become inaudible. As sections come off the knife, they should be kept moist with either water or ethanol (40–70%). The liquid is applied to the block face with a soft paintbrush. Ethanol moistens the sections, and temporarily lubricates and softens the block face to reduce curling. Another technique to decrease section curling—particularly when using a base sledge microtome for large specimens—is to cool the block face with a brief aerosol spray of the cryogen—ethyl chloride—just before cutting (F.A. Young, personal communication, Medical University of South Carolina, Charleston, SC).

As the sections come off the knife, care must be taken not to damage the knife-edge with any instruments used to lift the sections onto glass slides. Metal instruments such as a forceps may knick or dent the edge. The bristles of a fine paintbrush are safest for lifting sections. Even with the best sectioning technique, thin plastic sections require further flattening to enhance adherence to glass slides. To facilitate flattening, the sections are kept moist in 50–95% ethanol. Another liquid to use for flattening is a mixture of three parts butylglycol:two parts 70% ethanol.[7] Unfolding is done with a fine paintbrush and the tip of a dissecting needle or microfiber applicator. Avoid contact with the thin, fragile bone section by stretching the plastic at the borders around the specimen.

Plastic sections may be lost during staining because of poor adherence to glass slides. To reduce loss, slides may be coated with gelatin[9] or albumin[3] alone and air-dried. Additives to the gelatin solution have been suggested such as glycerin, approx 15%, with 1.0% gelatin and 2% phenol crystal preservative (Haupt's solution).[4] Another slide treatment for section adhesion uses 4% w/v chromium-alum solution with 0.5% gelatin (w/v).[1] Glass slides are dipped in these solutions, and are air-dried before proceeding with the attachment of plastic sections. Uncurl and stretch out the section, as described previously, on an adhesive-coated slide. Next, cover the slide with a sheet of polyethylene film (Saran wrap) or a clear, thin plastic strip the size and shape of a slide.[1] A piece of coarse filter paper may be placed over the film wrap or strip. Using a wallpaper seam roller or a rubber photoroller[1,3] compress the slide on an absorbent benchtop paper to remove excess ethanol. This procedure flattens the plastic section further. To assure that the sections remain flattened against the glass as they dry, the plastic wrap-covered slides are stacked together and held in place with gentle pressure by two C-clamps[1,3] or a similar slide press. Additionally, two blocks of wood approx 1 cm thick, cut to the dimensions of the slides, may be inserted under the clamps to distribute the pressure evenly and lessen the chance of breaking the slides.[1] As the sections dry overnight stacked in a slide press, either at room temperature or in an oven at 40–56°C, eventually they should adhere tenaciously to the glass. This strong attachment should prevent the sections from detaching in storage or floating away in agents for dissolving the plastic prior to staining. Regardless of the precautions taken, sections may detach from the slides while the plastic is being removed.[10] An alternative approach includes floating sections during certain staining procedures. Masson's and Goldner's trichrome,[10] von Kossa,[10] and hematoxylin (Cole's) and aqueous eosin[2] staining methods work well with the floating technique. Part V (Staining Techniques) of this book includes a thorough review of stains used for histological study of bone and the methods of preparation.

REFERENCES

1. Baron R, Vignery A, Neff L, et al: Processing of undecalcified bone specimens for bone histomorphometry. In: Recker RR, ed: *Bone Histomorphometry: Techniques and Interpretation.* CRC Press, Boca Raton, FL, 1983:13–35.
2. Drury RAB, Wallington EA: *Carleton's Histological Technique, 5th ed.* Oxford University Press, Oxford, UK, 1980:77, 78, 83, 84.
3. Emmanual J, Hornbeck C, Bloebaum RD: A polymethylate method for large specimens of mineralized bone with implants. *Stain Technol* 62:401–410, 1987.
4. Galigher AE, Kozloff E: *Essentials of Practical Microtechnique, 2nd ed.* Lea & Febiger, Philadelphia, PA, 1971:241.
5. Glorieux FH, Travers R, Taylor A, et al: Normative data for iliac bone histomorphometry in growing children. *Bone* 26:103–109, 2000.
6. Gray P: *Handbook of Basic Microtechnique, 3rd ed.* McGraw-Hill, New York, NY, 1964:145–190.
7. Hahn M, Vogel M, Delling G: Undecalcified preparation of bone tissue: report of technical experience and development of new methods. *Virchows Archiv A Pathol Anat* 418:1–7, 1991.

8. Humason GL: *Animal Tissue Techniques, 2nd ed.* WH Freeman and Company, San Francisco, CA, 1967:47–54.

9. Malluche HH, Faugere M-C: *Atlas of Mineralized Bone Histology.* Kargar, Basel, Switzerland, 1986.

10. Page KM, Stevens A, Lowe J, et al: Bone. In: Bancroft JD, Stevens A, eds: *Theory and Practice of Histological Techniques, 3rd ed.* Churchill Livingstone, New York, NY, 1990: 309–341.

11. Recker RR: Introduction. In: Recker RR, ed: *Bone Histomorphometry: Techniques and Interpretation.* CRC Press, Boca Raton, FL, 1983:1–2.

12. Watts RH, Green D, Howells GR: Improvements in histological techniques for epoxy-resin embedded bone specimens. *Stain Technol* 56:155–161, 1981.

15

Cutting and Grinding Methods for Hard-Tissue Histology

Thomas W. Bauer and Diane Mahovlic

Orthopaedic Pathology and Biomaterials Laboratory, Departments of Pathology and Orthopaedic Surgery, The Cleveland Clinic Foundation, Cleveland, OH, USA

I. INTRODUCTION

A necessary step in the development of a new biomaterial, and an important step in evaluating the efficacy of an existing biomaterial, is to histologically evaluate the interface between the material and host tissue. Although many sophisticated and expensive techniques have emerged in recent years, conventional light microscopy has proven to be an extremely valuable and cost-effective tool that provides important information about biocompatibility and host response. However, the histologic evaluation of ossified specimens, especially those containing synthetic biomaterials, is a difficult technical challenge. Whether the sample is from a prospective experimental study involving laboratory animals or a human device retrieved at autopsy or after clinical failure, the specimens are often relatively large, and usually contain materials of different hardness, making the preparation of adequate microscope slides difficult. Many methods have been developed to meet this challenge, and some of these are described elsewhere in this volume. The purpose of this chapter is to describe how our laboratory prepares microscope slides of biomaterials, mostly those intended for use in orthopedic applications.

II. SPECIMEN ACCESSIONING

The first step in evaluating a tissue specimen is to "accession" it into the laboratory. Although not often discussed, it is of critical importance to be able to track a specimen from the moment it leaves an operating room until it is filed as one or more microscope slides. A competent laboratory should be able to document at each stage of sample processing, and several organizations have published guidelines for specimen documentation.[1] Our laboratory receives samples either from operating rooms (human or animal) at the Cleveland Clinic Foundation, or by mail. In either case, the first step is to record basic information about the specimen in a log book and in a centralized computer system. The information recorded for each sample includes patient name or animal designation, source of specimen, date received, gross description of the specimen, and any other information available. Each specimen is given a unique accession number that is retained

From: *Handbook of Histology Methods for Bone and Cartilage*
Edited by: Y. H. An and K. L. Martin © Humana Press Inc., Totowa, NJ

throughout sample processing, so that the identity of any sample can be precisely determined at any time.

III. SPECIMEN DISSECTION

Once accessioned, the specimen is usually photographed, radiographed, and dissected. Our laboratory now exclusively uses digital gross photography. Gross images are captured with a Sony DFW-V300 Digital Interface camera, and stored on a microcomputer using dedicated software (ImageQUEST, Visual MED, Inc., Fort Mill, SC). Images are also often obtained with the use of a stereomicroscope (Wild M3Z) and the same camera. A local area network (LAN) is used to transport images between different workstations. Images are archived on a LAN that is backed up nightly; selected images are also stored on compact discs. The numbering system for the images corresponds to the specimen reference numbers to allow easy image retrieval. Radiographs are also commonly obtained using a tabletop radiography system (Model Micro 50: MicroFocus Imaging, Hagerstown, IN). Some specimens are dissected free of soft tissue, or may be cut with a band saw into smaller segments to facilitate fixation and subsequent processing. Specimen radiographs or prints of digital photos are often used to "map" the orientation of histologic sections. India ink of varying colors is also used to help with specimen orientation (Triangle Biomedical Sciences, Durham, NC), and is available through the major clinical laboratory supply companies. For example, the superior surface of a complex specimen may be marked with ink of one color, and the anterior surface may be marked with ink of another color. The ink will be retained through tissue processing, and can be seen on the surface of the final microscope slides, thereby confirming that the sample has retained orientation throughout processing.

IV. FIXATION

Regardless of subsequent processing, adequate initial tissue fixation is critical to preserving good morphology. The choice of fixative is determined by the nature of the material and the overall plan for future analysis. Ten percent neutral buffered formalin (NBF) is the most versatile fixative, with adequate penetration for most samples. It is important that the formalin is buffered to neutral, because many calcium phosphates (such as hydroxyapatite, tricalcium phosphate, or calcium sulfate) are soluble in acid, and would dissolve in unbuffered formalin. Furthermore, it should be recognized that buffered formalin contains salts that can precipitate on a tissue if it is allowed to dry. Although this should not be a problem for the usual histology specimen, if one performs chemical or scanning electron microscopic (SEM) analysis of such a sample crystals from the buffer may be present on the device surface.[11] These should be recognized as an artifact and not attributed to crystal growth in vivo. As an alternative to formalin, tissues can be fixed in 70% ethanol. We recommend ethanol fixation if the specimen has received intravital fluorochrome labeling or if it contains calcium phosphate biomaterials; otherwise, we usually use formalin. Other fixatives, for example, glutaraldehyde or paraformaldehyde, can be useful for electron microscopy or for histochemistry, but these fixatives do not penetrate tissue as well as formalin and are not as useful for most routine histology. It should also be recognized that good fixation by immersion requires an adequate volume of fixative. For example, formalin should be used in a ratio of 10–20 volumes fixative to one volume

Table 1. Dehydration and PMMA Embedding

 1. Specimen is received in 70% ethyl alcohol and placed into fresh 70% ethyl alcohol overnight.
 2. 50% Acetone—8 h.
 3. 50% Acetone—overnight.
 4. 75% Acetone—8 h.
 5. 75% Acetone—overnight.
 6. 100% Acetone—8 h.
 7. 100% Acetone—overnight.
 8. Acetone/Monomer (50:50)—24 h.
 9. Monomer—24 h.
10. Embed in polymer:
    a. Fill a glass vial with polymer and label with accession number.
    b. Insert the bone specimen with the side to be sectioned facing DOWN.
    c. Cover with foil and place in explosion-proof refrigerator for 48 h.
    d. Remove from refrigerator and check orientation.
    e. Allow vial to remain at room temperature until polymerization occurs (usually 3–7 d). Once polymerization occurs to a level slightly above the specimen (check hardness with a teasing needle), place the vial into a 37°C incubator overnight to complete polymerization of the polymer.
11. Place specimen in a plastic bag and hit carefully with a mallet to crack and shatter glass vial. Carefully remove block and rinse in running water. Affix a new accession label to the block. Cover label with tape. Trim excess plastic from block with the Isomet saw.

of tissue. Even formalin has a limited ability to penetrate large specimens, so it is often desirable to use a band saw to trim the specimen before fixation. The duration of fixation varies, largely based on specimen size, and may range from overnight to more than 1 wk. When permitted by experimental procedures, fixation by perfusion is often desirable. Methods for fixation by perfusion have been described in detail by Plenk.[14]

V. DEHYDRATION AND EMBEDDING

After fixation, it is important to rinse the specimen to remove residual fixative. Many questions in orthopedic biomaterials can be addressed with the use of decalcified, paraffin-embedded processing, but the implant must be removed before sectioning decalcified tissues. Many different plastics are being used for undecalcified tissue processing, and some are summarized elsewhere in this volume. Our laboratory uses polymethylmethacrylate (PMMA) for relatively small samples that will be cut with the use of a motorized microtome, and Spurr's plastic for specimens that will be rough cut with a special saw and hand-ground for sections. Each of these methods is summarized in Sections V, A and B.

A. Polymethylmethacrylate (PMMA)

The use of PMMA for embedding undecalcified specimens has been described in detail by Plenk.[14] We use PMMA primarily for biopsies related to metabolic bone disease,[17] and relatively small orthopedic specimens, usually those without metal or ceramic. Specimens are dehydrated in a graded series of acetone and infiltrated with PMMA as shown in Table 1. Once the plastic has polymerized, the block can be trimmed with an Isomet Low Speed saw (Buehler Ltd., Lake Bluff, IL). Blocks can be either sectioned with the use of a heavy-duty, motorized microtome (Jung, Model K) yielding sections approx 5 µm in

Table 2. Dehydration and Spurr's Embedding

The use of a mechanical shaker to enhance solution penetration is recommended.

1. Two changes of 95% ethyl alcohol—8–24 h each.
2. Two changes of 100% ethyl alcohol—8–24 h each.
3. Two changes of acetone—8–24 h each.
4. Two changes of acetone/Spurr's resin (50:50)—24 h.
5. Place specimen in fresh 100% Spurr's resin—24 h each (use intermittent vacuum as needed).
6. Embed in prepared aluminum foil baking pans with fresh Spurr's resin.[a] Place in vacuum oven (25 PSI) for 24–48 h at room temperature. Turn oven on (37–40°C) for 48–72 h to facilitate polymerization.
7. After polymerization is complete, the aluminum pan is carefully peeled away from the specimen block. The excess plastic is trimmed from the block using a band saw.

[a] Specimens are embedded in disposable, aluminum foil baking pans into which a layer of Spurr's resin has been pre-polymerized. Paper labels with the accession number are embedded along with the implant to ensure correct identification.

thickness, or hand-ground to approx 35 μm in thickness. The resulting sections can be stained with any one of a variety of stains. These undecalcified sections are excellent for evaluating cellular morphology as well as for the process of bone mineralization.[8]

B. Spurr's Plastic

Originally developed for use in transmission electron microscopy (TEM),[16] we have found Spurr's plastic to be highly satisfactory for large specimens containing combinations of bone, soft tissue, and orthopedic biomaterials.[2–7,9,12,15] Our dehydration and embedding protocol is shown in Table 2. Embedded samples are then rough cut with the use of a Buehler Isomet 2000 Precision saw (Figure 1), yielding specimens 1–2 mm in thickness. These samples are then mounted to Plexiglas slides (manufactured for us in-house, but available from a variety of suppliers), and ground using a series of graded abrasive sand papers. We do most grinding by hand using a Buehler Polimet I grinding table. It is difficult to hand-grind sections evenly, especially when the tissue contains materials of different levels of hardness (e.g., a metal implant surrounded by cancellous bone and bone marrow). To help overcome this difficulty, some investigators prefer to use automated grinding instruments (Exakt Apparatebau GMBH, Norderstedt, Germany) equipped with silica carbide blocks that help limit the extent of grinding and help ensure planar grinding. Sections are then polished using a Buehler Ecomet IV Polisher. During the grinding and polishing process, section thickness should be monitored regularly with the use of calipers (Mitutoyo Digital, Kanagawa, Japan). Sections can be stained with a variety of stains, but our standard stains are either hematoxylin and eosin (H&E) or, at the recommendation of Professor Hans Plenk Jr., Giemsa (Tables 3 and 4). Although some investigators use surface stains and transmitted or reflected light without cover slips,[10] we prefer the use of transmitted light and cover slips for most specimens.

VI. INTERPRETATION

Many questions related to biomaterials can be answered by qualitative review of sections processed using the methods described above (*see* also Figs. 2–6). When comparing different experimental groups, however, it is often desirable to use histomorphometry to

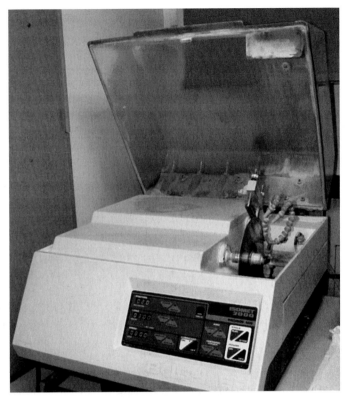

Figure 1. Buehler Isomet 2000 Precision saw used to trim embedded tissue blocks.

Table 3. Spurr's Resin

Spurr's Low Viscosity Embedding Kit (catalog #14300) is purchased commercially from Electron Microscopy Sciences, P.O. Box 251, Fort Washington, PA 19034.

The kit contains the following and is mixed in the following proportions:

TO PREPARE	320 mL	200 mL	160 mL
ERL 4206 (vinylcyclohexane dioxide)	80 mL	50 mL	40 mL
DER 736 (diglycidyl ether polypropylene)	40 mL	25 mL	20 mL
NSA (nonenyl succinic anhydride)	200 mL	125 mL	100 mL
DMAE (dimethylaminoethanol)	1.6 mL	1.0 mL	0.8 mL

Add each component in turn to a disposable beaker. Measure accurately (this is especially important with the DMAE). Gently mix. Add catalyst (DMAE) last and mix vigorously. Refrigerate any unused solution and use ASAP.

Table 4. Giemsa Stain

Prior to staining, the slides are cleaned in a 30% alcohol solution in an ultrasonic cleaner for approx 5 min. The plastic is allowed to "soften" in the alcohol for an additional 5–10 min. The slides are rinsed in running water.

To facilitate staining, the plastic is etched with a 0.5% formic acid solution for 10 min, and rinsed well in distilled water. We routinely stain sections with a Giemsa stain. We purchase commercially prepared Giemsa stock staining solution (Romanowski modification) from Newcomer Supply, Middleton, WI (catalog #1121). The working solution is made by adding 5 mL of the stock solution to 245 mL of distilled water.

The slides remain in the staining solution for 18–36 h and are then decolorized in two changes of 95% alcohol followed by two changes of 100% alcohol. The excess alcohol is blotted with absorbent towels, and the sections are allowed to air dry for several hours before dipping in xylene and cover slipping with Permount.

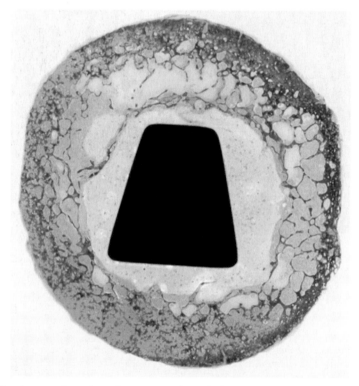

Figure 2. Hand-ground section of a cemented total hip prosthesis retrieved at autopsy after 20 yr of satisfactory clinical use. The PMMA bone cement has dissolved from the section, but the space occupied by the cement and adjacent tissue is well-visualized (Spurr's plastic embedding, H&E stain).

quantify various observations. Although morphometry by point-counting and ocular grid methods are valid,[13] they are time-consuming and difficult. The use of a microcomputer with dedicated image-analysis software has facilitated histomorphometry for many laboratories. Our laboratory uses a conventional light microscope equipped with a camera (Sony CCD-IRIS Video) interfaced with a microcomputer with a digital capture board and appropriate image-analysis software (BioQuant, R&M Biometrics, Nashville, TN) to cap-

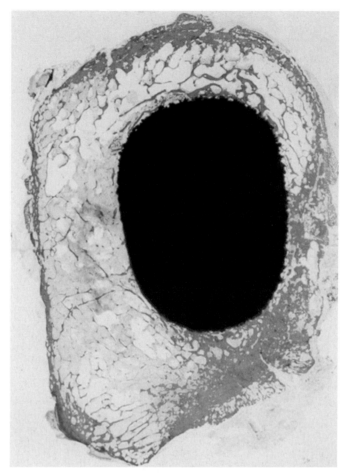

Figure 3. Hand-ground section of an uncemented, extensively porous coated femoral component of a hip prosthesis (Spurr's plastic embedding, H&E stain).

ture and quantify images. The details of histomorphometry are beyond the scope of this chapter, but this software allows either interactive or automated quantification. Although the quality of our microscope slides is good, an important feature of morphometry software is the ability to omit selected areas of the image that contain artifacts of histologic processing. The results of morphometry are filed using a numbering system that matches our specimen accession log, and can be exported to other programs for statistical analysis. This integrated system allows construction of a final report that includes specimen identification information, gross description, a description of methods, digital gross and light microscopic images, histomorphometry results, and qualitative interpretation, all of which can be recorded onto a compact disk.

VII. SUMMARY

The nature of the specimen and the specific goals of the study should determine the most appropriate methods of fixation, embedding, sectioning, and staining. Many of the

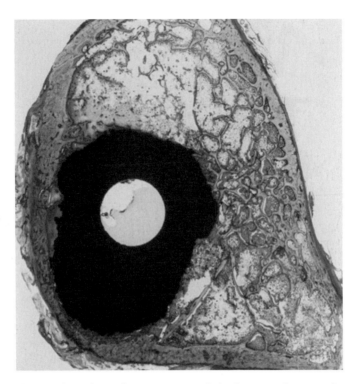

Figure 4. Hand-ground section of an uncemented, hydroxyapatite-coated canine femoral component of a hip prosthesis (Spurr's plastic embedding, Giemsa stain).

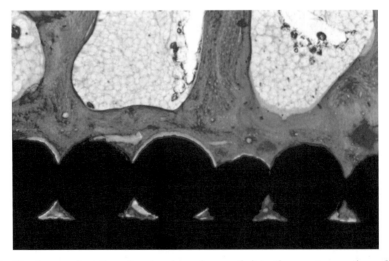

Figure 5. Hand-ground section showing bone ingrowth into the porous coating of an uncemented, metal-backed patellar component of a human total knee prosthesis (Spurr's plastic embedding, H&E stain).

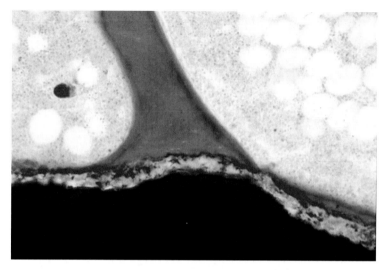

Figure 6. Hand-ground section showing extensive bone apposition to a hydroxyapatite-coated canine total hip prosthesis after 26 wk in vivo.

questions posed by contemporary orthopedic biomaterials studies can be addressed by using a combination of decalcified and undecalcified sections along with appropriate photography and histomorphometry. Although a number of different methods are being used for preparing sections of undecalcified tissues and implants, we have found ethanol or formalin fixation, plastic embedding, and hand grinding to be cost-effective methods for many types of specimens.

REFERENCES

1. *Practice for Retrieval and Analysis of Implanted Medical Devices and Associated Tissues.* American Society for Testing and Materials (ASTM), West Conshohocken, PA, 1998:1–14.
2. Bauer TW, Geesink RC, Zimmerman R, et al: Hydroxyapatite-coated femoral stems. Histological analysis of components retrieved at autopsy. *J Bone Joint Surg [Am]* 73:1439–1452, 1991.
3. Bauer TW, Muschler GF: Bone graft materials. An overview of the basic science. *Clin Orthop* 371:10–27, 2000.
4. Bauer TW, Schils J: The pathology of total joint arthroplasty. I. Mechanisms of implant fixation. *Skeletal Radiol* 28:423–432, 1999.
5. Bauer TW, Schils J: The pathology of total joint arthroplasty. II. Mechanisms of implant failure. *Skeletal Radiol* 28:483–497, 1999.
6. Bauer TW, Stulberg BN, Ming J, et al: Uncemented acetabular components. Histologic analysis of retrieved hydroxyapatite-coated and porous implants. *J Arthroplasty* 8:167–177, 1993.
7. Collier JP, Bauer TW, Bloebaum RD, et al: Results of implant retrieval from postmortem specimens in patients with well-functioning, long-term total hip replacement. *Clin Orthop* 274:97–112, 1992.
8. Frankenburg EP, Goldstein SA, Bauer TW, et al: Biomechanical and histological evaluation of a calcium phosphate cement. *J Bone Joint Surg [Am]* 80:1112–1124, 1998.
9. Friedman RJ, An YH, Ming J, et al: Influence of biomaterial surface texture on bone ingrowth in the rabbit femur. *J Orthop Res* 14:455–464, 1996.
10. Gross UM, Strunz V: Surface staining of sawed sections of undecalcified bone containing alloplastic implants. *Stain Technol* 52:217–219, 1977.

11. Kieswetter K, Bauer TW, Brown SA, et al: Alteration of hydroxylapatite coatings exposed to chemicals used in histological fixation. *J Biomed Mater Res* 28:281–287, 1994.
12. Larsson S, Mattsson P, Bauer TW: Resorbable bone cement for augmentation of internally fixed hip fractures. *Ann Chir Gynaecol* 88:205–213, 1999.
13. Merz WA, Schenk RK: A quantitative histological study on bone formation in human cancellous bone. *Acta Anat* 76:1–15, 1970.
14. Plenk Jr., H: The microscopic evaluation of hard tissue implants. In: Williams DF, ed: *Techniques of Biocompatibility Testing.* CRC Press, Boca Raton, FL, 1986:35–81.
15. Schildhauer TA, Bauer TW, Josten C, et al: Open reduction and augmentation of internal fixation with an injectable skeletal cement for the treatment of complex calcaneal fractures. *J Orthop Trauma* 14:309–317, 2000.
16. Spurr AR: A low-viscosity epoxy resin embedding medium for electron microscopy. *J Ultrastruct Res* 26:31, 1969.
17. Vigorita VJ: The bone biopsy protocol for evaluating osteoporosis and osteomalacia. *Am J Surg Pathol* 8:925–930, 1984.

Bone Sectioning Using the Exakt System

Karl Donath[1] and Michael Rohrer[2]

[1]*Department of Oral Pathology, University of Hamburg, Hamburg, Germany*
[2]*Division of Oral and Maxillofacial Pathology, University of Minnesota School of Dentistry,*
Minneapolis, MN, USA

1. INTRODUCTION

A description of a method for successful preparation of histological slides from previously nonsectionable ceramic or metallic material in bone and soft tissue was published by Donath and Breuner in 1982.[2] Further development of instruments that were specifically designed for this method by Biermann (Exakt, Hamburg-Norderstedt, Germany) beginning in 1983 has made it possible for many laboratories throughout the world to easily perform hard-tissue histotechnology.[6,8,9]

In some centers of dental research sections of mineralized bones or teeth had already been used for histologic studies.[1,10] However, this routine method of sectioning non-demineralized enamel-free teeth or bones was not free of artifacts and could not be used for teeth with enamel, teeth with metallic fillings, crowns or bridges, or bones with ceramic or metallic implants. In 1977, Gross and Strunz, using an annular saw, made hard-tissue sections of mineralized tissue that were 50–200 µm in thickness with inclusion of metallic or ceramic implants.[7] The Säge-Schliff (sawing and grinding) technique was developed by the Donath group to permit the histological study of mineralized jawbones with teeth or implants of metallic or ceramic materials.[2–5] The goal was to retain dental restorations, crowns, bridges, enamel with calculus, and plaque *in situ,* and also to preserve the tissue adjacent to the implant and to the teeth. It was also important that the equipment should be as economical as possible, and the technique itself should be simple so that reasonable numbers of specimens could be processed and examined.

II. STEPS BEFORE ACTUAL BONE SECTIONING WITH THE EXAKT SYSTEM

The quality of the final histological slide depends on the correct performance of many procedures. These are primarily the selection of the tissue, dehydration, and resin infiltration. When selecting tissue from a surgical specimen or autopsy specimen, proper size is important for good fixation and infiltration. Fresh or recently fixed tissues are initially sectioned to a thickness of 2–4 mm by means of the Exakt band-cutting system (Exakt

From: *Handbook of Histology Methods for Bone and Cartilage*
Edited by: Y. H. An and K. L. Martin © Humana Press Inc., Totowa, NJ

300 or 310). The dehydration and resin infiltration is performed in the completely closed "Exakt 510 Dehydration and Infiltration System" with constant agitation and the possibility of connection to a vacuum pump. The embedded specimen is polymerized by photopolymerization in the "Exakt 520 Light Polymerisation Unit" with blue light of 450-nm wavelength. The temperature of the specimen never rises above 40°C.

III. STEPS OF BONE SECTIONING

Bone sectioning from the tissue block to the final histological slide consists of eight steps:

1. Producing completely smooth and parallel (plane parallel) upper and lower surfaces of the tissue block with the Exakt cutting-band system using the precision parallel control (CL—contact line or CP—contact point).
2. Parallel mounting of the block on a Plexiglas slide using Exakt vacuum system 401.
3. Preparation of the surface of interest by grinding with the Exakt 400CS or 420CL grinding system to the desired level of tissue and biomaterial.
4. First measurement of the thickness "A" (block + Plexiglas slide + glue) and the thickness "B" of the plane parallel Plexiglas slide.
5. Affixing a plane parallel Plexiglas slide onto the ground-tissue surface to be studied using the "Exakt Precision Adhesive Press 402."
6. Second measurement of the total thickness "C" (thickness A + glue + plane parallel Plexiglas slide).
7. Sectioning of the embedded tissue to a thickness of 100–200 μm using the Exakt cutting-band systems Exakt 300 CL or CP or 310 CL or CP.
8. Grinding of the final thin section by the "Exakt 400 CS or 420 CL grinding systems."

IV. MAJOR EQUIPMENT

A. Exakt Band Cutting System

The Exakt band-cutting system resembles a band saw with a diamond- or carborundum-coated cutting band. The cutting-grinding apparatus is available in two sizes. The smaller Exakt 300 (with 300 CP or 300 CL) has its application in dental research. The larger Exakt 310 (with 310 CP or 310 CL) evolved from the need within orthopedic research to cut the same type of samples on a larger scale.

Both cutting systems have a precision paralleling guide, an advancing screw system, and a cooling/flushing system. Stainless-steel cutting bands of 0.1–0.3 mm may be used. The precision parallel guide moves along linear bearings that are free of side-to-side play, permitting operation with very low friction. This low friction allows a very small constant feed force to be maintained using a gravity-feed weight system (Fig. 1). This constant force, produced by weights rather than by a mechanical drive, allows the diamond- or carborundum-coated band to move slowly through hard tissue such as cortical bone and metallic material, and faster through soft tissues and medullary bones, preventing directional deviation of the band and burning of the specimen. Feed force is the major factor in surface quality, interface preservation, and material stress. By adding an arcing motion to the precision parallel guide CL (CL—contact line), Exakt has been able to further reduce the required feed force and improve many aspects of the sectioning process. Oscillating the sample reduces the actual contact between the sample and the band. The light-polymerizing plastic-embedding medium, with its glasslike hardness, prevents clogging of the diamond particles of the band with precision parallel guide CL (contact line). The devel-

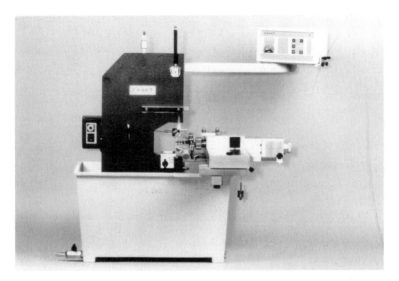

Figure 1. Exakt 300 CP band system with precision parallel unit.

opment of the precision parallel guide CP (contact point) has also made it possible to use methacrylate as an embedding medium. This plastic-embedding medium is also used in the "hard-cutting technique." It can be deplasticized when mounted on glass slides, and such sections make immunohistochemical investigations possible.

An advancing screw system is used, with a universal clamp or vacuum plate to move the specimen toward the cutting band. The clamp grasps unembedded fresh or fixed tissue, allows the tissue to be sectioned in a vertical plane, and results in parallel slices of predetermined thickness. The vacuum plate for slides of either 25×100 mm or 50×100 mm is used to separate a parallel section of predetermined thickness from the mounted tissue block.

B. Exakt 400 CS and 420 CL Grinding Systems

The Exakt 400 CS microgrinding system (Fig. 2) consists of a circular grinding plate and a vacuum attachment that holds the specimen. This attachment travels reciprocally in a horizontal plane over the rotating grinding plate, and uses water to cool and clean the grinding apparatus and specimen. Adjustable weights control the grinding pressure and allow great variability for different specimen types. The actual grinding of a sample can be automatically controlled with the optional AW 110 Electronic Measuring and Control System. Because sample sizes always vary, the AW 110 is equipped with an algorithm for setting a reference point before grinding each sample. Cued by the electronic display, the technician is guided through a series of steps that determine this reference point. Once electronically entered, the AW 110 can be set so that Exakt 400 CS removes a precisely determined amount of sample. When this is accomplished, the AW 110 will automatically shut off the grinding and oscillating functions. The grinding platform is diamond-coated, and may be covered by a variety of grinding papers and films. Ranging in grit from 320 to 4000, papers and films provide a stepped progression of grinding that ends with a polished surface that is suitable for staining. The grinding papers and films are held on the disk by surface tension.

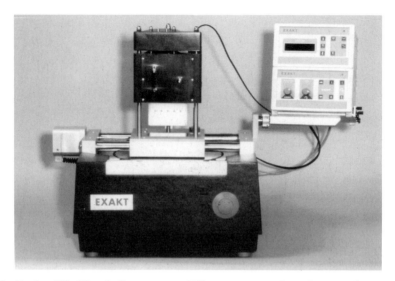

Figure 2. Exakt 400 CS grinding system (CS—contact surface, i.e., continuous grinding over the complete sample surface).

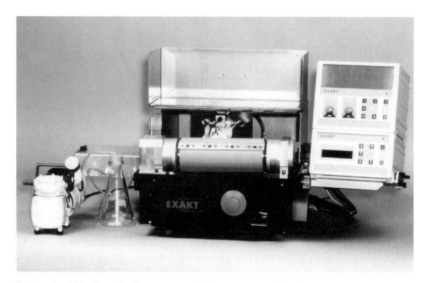

Figure 3. Exakt 420 CL grinding system (CL—contact line, i.e., continuous grinding over only a line section of the sample surface).

The Exakt 420 CL precision grinding system (CL—contact line; Fig. 3) offers a solution for grinding samples with large metal components by reducing the grinding forces. These decreases in the forces acting on the sample surface further reduce the risk of losing parts of the sample during the grinding process. Unlike the Exakt 400 CS, the grinding platform of the 420 CL is a roller and not a disk. The small contact area and the abbreviated contact time further reduce any thermal impact on the sample components

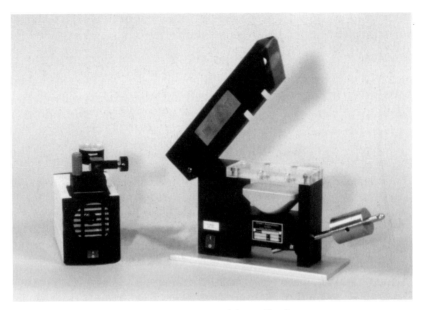

Figure 4. Exakt 402 precision adhesive press.

and the amount of grinding debris that is generated. This technology enables one to use methacrylate as the embedding medium, resulting in a high-quality surface after grinding.

C. Vacuum-Adhesive System (Exakt 401)

The vacuum-adhesive system is made up of an upper and a lower plate, and is used to mount a slide onto the polymerized tissue block. The slide must be mounted opposite to the surface of interest. It provides the means of mounting in order to produce the thin, perfectly parallel final specimen section which will be achieved by the band system and grinding system. The vacuum keeps the slide on the upper plate, and is only necessary for the primary contact of autopolymerizing mounting resin and tissue block.

1. Possible Problems

The Plexiglas may bend after mounting when the proportion of monomer is too high.

The bent slide cannot be kept on the vacuum plate; careful grinding of the bent slide might help.

D. Precision Adhesive Press (Exakt 402)

The precision adhesive press affixes a plane parallel Plexiglas slide with a photo-polymerizing glue onto the ground-tissue surface to be studied (Fig. 4).

The Plexiglas slide is held by vacuum on the thick, translucent upper plate. The tissue block with the cleaned surface of interest is placed on the weight-loaded moveable section. The photo-polymerizing glue is applied to the cleaned surface, and is slowly moved to the Plexiglas slide under the translucent upper plate. Upward pressure is applied by the weight-loaded part. As soon as the tissue block and Plexiglas slide contact each other, the vacuum pump can be switched off. After 5–10 min, when the glue has distributed itself into a thin film (10–20 µm) between the tissue block and the Plexiglas slide and no air bubbles are visible, the blue light starts the photo-polymerization. If air bubbles are present, the Plexiglas slide must be removed and the gluing procedure must be repeated.

1. Possible Problems

The tissue block with the Plexiglas slide cannot be removed—too much glue was used, and it seeped between the translucent upper plate and the Plexiglas slide.

The Plexiglas slide cannot be held by vacuum—polymerized glue on the translucent upper plate prevents a vacuum seal.

E. Digital Readout Micrometer

A digital micrometer is essential for accurate measurements of slide, and tissue block.

V. DISPOSABLE MATERIALS

A. Embedding Media

Many kinds of resin on the market can be used as embedding medium for the hardcutting technique. For the cutting-grinding technique, we use a light-polymerizing resin of glasslike hardness, Technovit 7200 VLC, (Kulzer & Co GmbH, Friedrichsdorf, Germany.) For special investigations such as enzyme- and immunohistochemistry, the sectionable new Technovit 9100 is used.

Technovit 4000 (Kulzer & Co GmbH, Germany)—for mounting of the tissue block on the Plexiglas slide.
Technovit 7230 VLC (Kulzer & Co GmbH, Germany)—photo-polymerizing precision glue.
Light-transparent mold (Exakt).
Plexiglas slides (plane parallel) Exakt.
Sandpaper (Exakt)—diamond-coated grinding plate.

VI. PROCEDURE

A. Producing a Plane Parallel Block

The shape of the polymerized tissue block is dependent on the embedding mold used. The tissue side of interest has only a small film of resin on top. The opposite side of the tissue contains a thick layer of resin. To smooth the surfaces and make the two sides of the block parallel, several procedures may be used. One method is to use the Exakt band-cutting system. The tissue block is held by the advancing screw system and supported by the moving table. The first cut is done on the side of interest; the second parallel cut is made on the opposite side after moving the advancing screw system with the tissue block toward the band the distance necessary for the desired thickness of the block. After mounting the resin surface of the tissue block on a Plexiglas slide, less grinding and polishing of the surface of interest are required before gluing on the final Plexiglas slide.

Another method for making the surfaces of the tissue block plane parallel is to remove the thin film of resin on the tissue side by grinding while keeping the block in the hand (this presents danger for the fingers and often results in non-parallel facets on the grinding side). It is more effective to mount the tissue block with the resin side on a Plexiglas slide, grind the tissue side plane parallel, and polish the final Plexiglas slide with the Exakt 400 CS Micro Grinding System or Exakt 420 CL Precision Grinding System.

B. Mounting of the Block With Plane Parallel Surfaces

The plane parallel tissue block made by the Exakt band-cutting system with the precision parallel control, or the tissue block that was prepared by hand, are mounted on the Plexiglas slide using the Exakt Vacuum Adhesive Unit. The Plexiglas slide is held by vacuum to the upper plate and the block lies on the lower plate with mixed Technovit 4000 on top of the block. The upper plate with the attached slide (which is parallel to the surface of interest) is moved down to the block until an adequate contact with Technovit 4000 occurs. The plate is then secured with a screw. The Technovit 4000 must be mixed using the correct proportion of monomer and polymer. Free monomer reacts with the Plexiglas, and the result is a bent slide.

As soon as the polymerization is finished, the block is ready to be ground and polished with the Exakt Grinding System.

C. Preparation of the Surface of Interest By Grinding With the Exakt Grinding System 400CS or 420CL

The block mounted on the Plexiglas slide is placed on the vacuum plate attachment, which travels reciprocally in a horizontal plane over the rotating grinding plate. The grinding table is covered with sandpaper. The quality of the sandpaper is important because single oversize grits may tower above the others and destroy the surface by creating deep grooves. The grinding process is complete when all the tissue and biomaterial segments to be studied are exposed to the surface. Simultaneously, the surface of the block must be parallel with the Plexiglas slide. Unevenness within the surface of the block can be seen with a straight edge. Differences of 3–5 μm are tolerable when large specimens of approx 90—100-mm length are used. After the definitive surface of the block is reached it is finished with 4000-grit sandpaper to make the surface as smooth as possible.

D. First Measurement of the Thickness "A"

For the determination of the thickness of the light-polymerizing precision glue, it is necessary to measure the tissue block with the Plexiglas slide "A" as well as the plane parallel slide "B" for the final slide.

E. Affixing a Plane Parallel Plexiglas Slide on the Block Surface to be Studied

The parallelism of the final slide and the block with mounted slide must be verified. If discrepancies are present, both the plane parallel final slide and the block must be adjusted with the Exakt 400 CS microgrinding system. When parallelism is obtained, 4000-grit sandpaper is used to smooth the surface of the slide. The final thickness of the slide is recorded. Before the precision affixing, the surfaces of the slide and tissue block are cleaned with petrol-benzene. The cleaned slide is placed onto the upper vacuum plate of the precision press with the side to be glued facing down. The precision adhesive (Technovit 7230 VLC; Kulzer & Co GmbH) is delivered (thin) onto the prepared block surface. The prepared tissue block with the primary slide is put on the lower movable plate. The lower plate is pressed by an adjustable counterbalanced weight toward the upper plate after loosening the safety device and pressure is maintained. If bubbles appear in the glue, the slide and block are separated. The gluing sides of the block and the slide are cleaned using petrol-benzene. The same procedure can be repeated. When perfect mounting occurs, a uniform distribution of the precision adhesive in the space between the Plexiglas slide and the tissue block will occur within 2–5 min. After that time, photo-polymerization is initiated by activating the curing light. The polymerization is completed within 15–20 min. The excess glue, which flows out from the glue space, remains soft because of the influence of the air (oxygen) and therefore, can be removed easily from the slide.

F. Second Measurement of the Total Thickness "C"

Before sectioning is started, the glue thickness must be calculated by measurement of the whole tissue block with two slides "C" minus the final Plexiglas slide "B" and minus tissue block with the first slide ("A").

$$\text{Precision glue thickness } (X) = C - (A+B)$$

G. Sectioning of the Definitive Tissue Portion Using the Exakt Band System

All Band Systems (Exakt 300CL, 300CP, 310CL, 310CP) have a vacuum apparatus on the precision-parallel unit. It is possible to place either the first or final slide onto the vacuum apparatus attached to the cutting band. Because the photo-polymerized adhesive area remains visible, it is advisable to select the final parallel slide. It is helpful to use a paper sticker (100 μm) on the edge of the slide to adjust the chosen thickness. Using the parallel slide at the vacuum plate allows one to cut further specimens with a parallel slide of the same thickness without changing the distance between the vacuum appratus and the cutting band.

How to find the distance of the cutting band to the final slide for sectioning 100-μm-thick sections:

While the sawband is slowly moving, the vacuum plate with the specimen is moved horizontally toward the band by using the screw with a micrometer scale until the paper sticker barely touches the band without being damaged. The anticipated thickness is about 100 μm, including the thickness of the glue. Weights of 50–100 g are sufficient during the cutting process for moving the precise-parallel unit. Less weight is needed when the precision-parallel-unit CP is used. It is important to know that every interruption of the cutting process will cause unevenness on both surfaces that are produced.

1. Possible Problems

The new surfaces are steplike—a clogged band of the precise-parallel unit (CL type) causes this.

Only half of the specimen contains tissue—the cause could be that either the ground surface of interest was not completely in the tissue or the precise adhesive was not equally distributed when the polymerizing procedure was started.

H. Microgrinding and Polishing of the Final Thin Section

The Exakt 400 CS microgrinding system works with great success when the resin has a glass-like hardness (Fig. 5).

The thickness of the section is calculated by subtracting the thickness of the parallel slide, including of the thickness of the glue, from the thickness of the total specimen. The calculated thickness is considered as the reference point for the digital micrometer of the Exakt 400CS microgrinding system. Before starting the grinding procedure, the zero point is determined. In order to do this, the slide with the specimen is placed on the vacuum

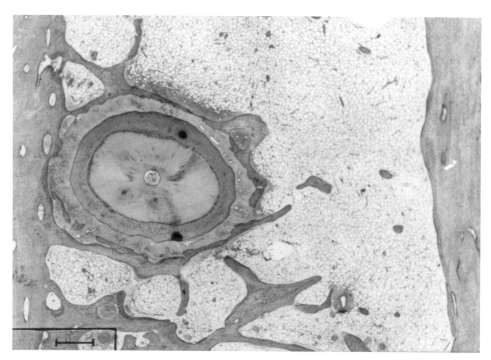

Figure 5. Final result of microgrinding: a root with the periodontal ligament, alveolar bone, and fatty bone marrow of the mandible.

block. The grinding table is covered with sandpaper. The vacuum block with the slide is carefully lowered until the electric current for grinding and parallel movement is interrupted. The digital micrometer is corrected to zero. A control light will indicate that the zero point is established. This procedure is performed while the motors are running, and the actual amount to be ground away is programmed into the digital micrometer. The apparatus will be stopped automatically after the programmed thickness is removed.

Sandpaper cannot be used in every case. Specimens with hard metal surrounded by bone and soft tissue show in the light microscope sharpness of either the metal rim or the adjacent bone or soft tissue. This different level of focus arises during grinding with wet sandpaper. The hard metal is pressed into the sandpaper, and grinding continues more aggressively in the border region. Also, metal may be reduced at the interface. The solution in such cases is the coated grinding table. The final treatment of the surface is with 4000-grit sandpaper.

If the tissue is embedded in a sectionable resin such as Technovit 9100 NEW (Kulzer & Co GmbH) which is used for enzyme- and immunohistochemistry, the Exakt 420 CL microgrinding system should be used for a good grinding result.

REFERENCES

1. Delling G, Schulz A, Seifert G: Fortschritte in der Morphologie und Diagnostik von Osteopathien und Knochentumoren. *Radiologie* 16:45–53, 1976.
2. Donath K, Breuner G: A method for the study of undecalcified bones and teeth with attached soft tissues. *J Oral Pathol* 11:318–326, 1982.

3. Donath K. The diagnostic value of the new method for the study of undecalcified bones and teeth with attached soft tissue. *Pathol Res Pract* 179: 631–633, 1985.

4. Donath K: Die Trenn-Dünnschliff-Technik zur Herstellung histologischer Präparate von nicht schneidbaren Geweben und Materialien. *Der Präparator* 34:197–206, 1988.

5. Donath K: Preparation of histologic sections by the cutting grinding technique for hard tissue and other material not suitable to be sectioned by routine methods. EXAKT-KULZER-PUBLICATION, Norderstedt, 1–15, 1988.

6. Gotfredsen K, Budtz-Jörgensen E, Jensen LN: Method for Preparation and staining of histological sections containing titanium-implants for light microscopy. *Stain Technol* 64:121–128, 1989.

7. Gross UM, Strunz U: Surface staining of sawed sections of undecalcified bone containing alloplastic implants. *Stain Technol* 52:217–219, 1977.

8. Johansson CB, Hansson HA, Albrektsson T: Qualitative interfacial study between bone and tantalium, niobium or commercially pure titanium. *Biomaterials* 11:277–280, 1990.

9. Rohrer MD, Schubert CC: The cutting-grinding technique for histologic preparation of undecalcified bone and bone-anchored implants. Improvements in instrumentation and procedures. *Oral Surg Oral Med Oral Pathol* 74:73–78, 1992.

10. Schoenfeld C, Boesmann K: Eine Methacrylateinbettung zur histologischen Untersuchung entkalkter wie such unentkalkter Präparate von Zähnen mit umgebenden Parodont. *Dtsch Zahnaerztl Z* 35:789–794, 1980.

17

Bone Sectioning Using a Modified Inner Diamond Saw

Joop G. C. Wolke,[1] Jan-Paul C. M. van der Waerden,[1] Christel P. A. T. Klein,[2] and John A. Jansen[1]

[1]Department of Biomaterials, University Medical Center Nijmegen, Nijmegen, The Netherlands
[2]Central Animal Facility, University Groningen, Groningen, The Netherlands

I. INTRODUCTION

The availability and application of medical implants has increased dramatically during the last two decades, and the broad variety of implants ranges from knee prostheses to heart valves, and from pacemakers to breast prostheses. With increased life expectancy, it is further believed that the application of implants will progressively increase. Implants are partially or totally placed into the body for prosthetic, therapeutic, diagnostic, cosmetic, or experimental purposes. Biomaterials play an important role in many of these implants. The required properties of a material used for an implant can be classified roughly under the categories of biocompatibility, implant construction, and biomechanics.[11] Biocompatibility refers to the interfacial reactions between biomaterials and tissue. Implant construction involves the engineering of the implant as well as its mechanical properties, such as hardness and strength. Biomechanics is concerned with the mechanical-dynamic properties of an implant and surrounding tissues. This chapter focuses on the sectioning of biomaterials used for hard-tissue implantation.

Bone and dentine are difficult tissues to study histologically using conventional methods because of the calcified ground substance, which obscures cells and vessels. Histological evaluation of bone generally involves prior decalcification, which significantly alters the structural integrity of the bone. Decalcification using acid solutions such as formic acid causes the loss or denaturation of many organic components and damages the ultrastructure of the tissue.[6,10,12,13] The resulting sections are usually thicker than those from soft tissues that have not been subjected to acid decalcification. If undecalcified bone specimens are investigated, sectioning artifacts must be considered. Because bone and other calcified structures are hard and angular, their presence in specimens results in ragged sections and damaged microtome knives. This may especially hamper compatibility studies of biomaterials implanted in bone that require thin, undecalcified sections of high quality without damage to the interface between bone and implanted material.

Several methods have been developed to prepare thin sections of hard tissue. Early studies used unembedded specimens, which were reduced in thickness by hand-grinding.[1]

From: *Handbook of Histology Methods for Bone and Cartilage*
Edited by: Y. H. An and K. L. Martin © Humana Press Inc., Totowa, NJ

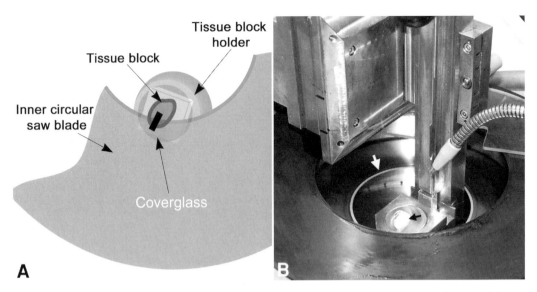

Figure 1. (A) Schematic view of the inner circular diamond saw. (B) A close-up image of the central part of the sawing system. The white arrow indicates the circular saw blade and the black arrow indicates the specimen.

However, these sections were not thin enough for histological analysis, and the grinding process affected them adversely. Embedding hard tissue within a matrix of wax and polymer improves the quality of the sections, and sections of approx 100—200 μm can be achieved using a diamond-blade saw. These sections are reduced in thickness by grinding and polishing to approx 30-μm thickness. However, scratches on the surface of the sections, extrusion of the implanted material, and uneven section thickness result in poor cellular detail. Grinding and polishing machines such as the Exakt system are routinely used in histological evaluation of biomaterials.[3] The time needed for preparation as well as the quality of a section are strongly influenced by the skill of the operator. Therefore our laboratories designed and developed a new saw system that produces one-step thin-sections (<10 μm) of fresh bone/dentine and plastic-embedded bone tissue with or without metallic biomaterials.[9]

II. MATERIALS AND METHODS

A horizontal rotation-sawing machine was developed with a 101-mm-long diamond cutting edge on the inside diameter (Fig. 1, modified from a model manufactured by Fijnmetaal Techniek, Amsterdam, The Netherlands). The inside diameter diamond saw blade consists of a thin circular steel core, which is tensioned at its outer edge in two clamping rings. A rigid and vibration-free assembly is required to obtain exact thickness of the sections. A powerful and silent motor drives the saw. Samples of bone containing implanted biomaterials are embedded in methyl methacrylate, as described by Buijs and Dogterom.[2] After polymerization, the blocks are trimmed and firmly fixed to a flattened ball. The ball is tightly clamped into an arm-type holder that moves toward the diamond saw with a force of 0.2–2 Nm, using a 1:1 (v/v) glycerin/water mixture as a cooling lubricant. The block is fixed in the holder at a defined angle (free motions of 360° horizontally and 60° vertically). Thick sections are cut until the desired area of the specimen is reached, then the surface is etched for 30 s with 1% ethanol-HCl solution and rinsed with water. The surface of the sample is stained with methylene blue (1 min) and basic fuchsin blue (30 s). After staining the surface is rinsed with water and is carefully dried, then a glass cover slip is glued to the stained surface with a thin layer of UV adhesive (Permacol type 370, Permacol®, Ede, The Netherlands); this coverslip stabilizes the thin section during the sectioning process. The block is raised using a high-quality micromanipulator (Mikrocontrol UT 100, Elmekanic®, Markelo, The Netherlands) with a reliable read-off system for a precise sample lift of 1 μm, enabling production of sections of exact thickness. After sawing, the previously stained section with cover slip attached is glued to a glass slide with Permacol and is ready for histological evaluation.[7,8,14]

III. RESULTS

A. *Experiment 1*

The purpose of this experiment was to evaluate the bone behavior of TiO_2 grit-blasted implants coated with a thin calcium phosphate (Ca-P) radiofrequency (RF) magnetron sputter coating.[16] Forty-eight commercially pure titanium (cp-Ti) screw-type implants (Astratech, Sweden) were placed in the medial condyle of the left and right hind limbs of 12 goats. Each condyle received two implants, following a balanced split-plot randomization scheme. The implants were grit-blasted with TiO_2 particles. The implants were left uncoated (Ti) or provided with a 4.0 μm Ca-P coating (Ca-P4).

The coating procedure was performed using a commercially available RF magnetron sputter unit (Edwards ESM 100®, A. de Jong T.H. B. V., Rotterdam, The Netherlands). After coating, the implants were subjected to an additional infrared treatment for 30 s at 425–475°C in air. X-ray diffraction patterns demonstrated that the Ca-P4 coatings had an amorphous/crystalline structure. Evaluation of the bone-implant interface was made at implantation periods of 6–12 wk.

1. *Ca-P4 Implants*

By histological evaluation at 6 wk, intimate bone contact with cortical and trabecular bone could be observed. In the area directly adjacent to the implant, new bone formation had occurred on the implant surface without any intervening soft-tissue layer. Also in this area, remodeling lacunae with osteoblasts were visible. No accumulations of inflammatory cells were seen next to the implant. Very rarely, osteoblasts were visible at the bone-implant interface. At the cortical side, the screw threads were almost completely filled with dense bone (Fig. 2). In the femoral trabecular compartment, the bone present at the implant surface had a tentacle-like appearance. The bone attached to one point, mostly at the top of the screw thread, and was growing as a thin layer over the implant surface into the screw thread. At 12 wk, remodeling and compaction of the lamellar bone-implant interface had proceeded. The newly formed bone either could not or could hardly be distinguished from the surrounding "old" bone. The quality of the apposed cortical bone was very similar to the original cortical bone (Fig. 3). Furthermore, bone ingrowth into the screw threads, which were in contact with trabecular bone, had increased. Apparently, the Ca-P surface had acted as a bone-conductive scaffold, as the screws were completely

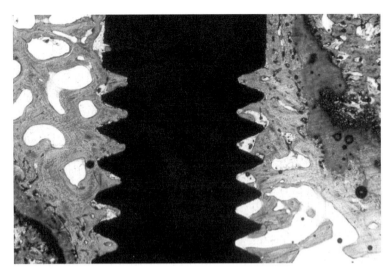

Figure 2. Light micrograph of a Ca-P4 implant after 6 wk. The screw threads were almost completely filled with dense bone. Original magnifaction ×17.5.

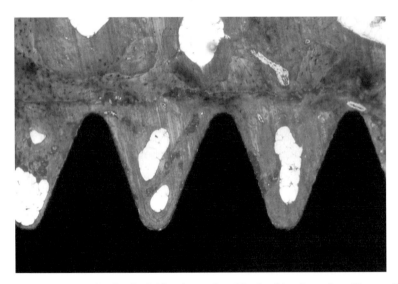

Figure 3. Light micrograph of a Ca-P4 implant, after 12 wk of implantation. The quality of the apposed cortical bone was very similar to the original cortical bone. Original magnification ×70.

covered with bone. This bone was in close contact with the implant surface, with no sign of fibrous tissue formation or inflammatory reaction.

2. Non-Coated Ti Implants

None of the Ti implants showed an adverse bone reaction. The healing process of both cortical and trabecular bone for both implantation periods was almost identical to the Ca-P4 implants. Again trabecular bone ingrowth into the screw threads was very limited.

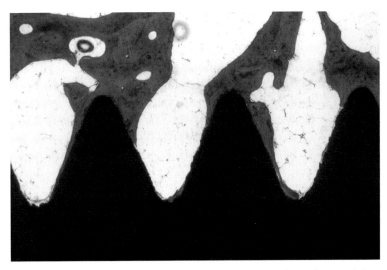

Figure 4. Histological appearance of a Ti implant. Trabecular bone ingrowth into the screw threads was very limited. Original magnification ×70.

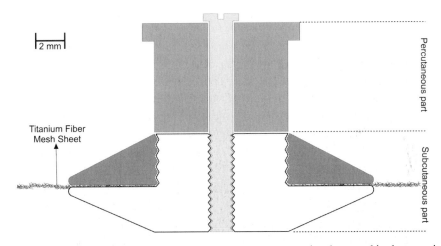

Figure 5. Schematic cross-section of the two-stage percutaneous implant used in the experiment.

If bone apposition still occurred, the newly formed bone was frequently separated from the implant surface by an intervening fibrous tissue layer (Fig. 4).

B. Experiment 2

This experiment focused on the influence of impaired wound healing on the tissue reaction to implantable glucose sensors.[4] Fig. 5 shows a graphical cross-section of the percutaneous implant as used in the experiment. The device consisted of two elements: a flange-shaped subcutaneous component, and a percutaneous component that penetrated the skin. The subcutaneous (sc) component was made of a mesh sheet of sintered titanium fibers (Bekaert Fibre Technologies, Belgium), measuring approx 4 × 4 cm.

Centrally disposed in the sc part was a KEL-F (polychlorotrifluoroethylene) holding element with a threaded hole with a diameter of 0.2 cm. The percutaneous component was a cylindrical structure made of KEL-F with a diameter of 0.9 cm. It could be anchored with a screw thread in the holding element of the sc part. During the first 4 wk of implantation, when only the sc part was implanted, the threaded hole was kept closed with an auxiliary screw to avoid the ingrowth of tissue. The separately inserted sc implant consisted of a titanium fiber mesh sheet similar to the one used to anchor the percutaneous device but without the holding element, measuring approx 1×2 cm.

Female New Zealand white rabbits ($n = 24$), age 3 mo and weight approximately 2–3 kg, were obtained from the animal facility of the University of Nijmegen. In twelve animals, diabetes mellitus was induced with a single intravenous (iv) injection of 100 mg/kg body wt alloxan monohydrate (Sigma-Aldrich Chemicals, Zwijndrecht, The Netherlands) into a marginal ear vein. After injection, the animals were provided with 5% glucose in their drinking water during the critical first 24 h to prevent severe hypoglycemia. All animals remained diabetic for the duration of the experiment. Twelve normal, non-diabetic animals were used as controls.

After the diagnosis of diabetes had been established, the percutaneous devices were inserted in the backs of all rabbits using a two-stage surgical procedure. Before insertion, the implants were sterilized in an autoclave. In the second surgical procedure, separate titanium fiber mesh sheets were also implanted subcutaneously on the opposite site of the spinal column.

Histological evaluation revealed that all the fiber mesh sheets—both the subcutaneously implanted sheets and those used to anchor the percutaneous devices—were surrounded by a relatively thin, fibrous capsule. The porous openings of the fiber mesh were filled with connective tissue containing fibrocytes, small blood vessels, and some inflammatory cells. Furthermore, an effect of the severity of the induced diabetes was observed on the maturity of the connective tissue inside the pores of the mesh. The severely diabetic animals showed ingrowth of immature connective tissue, with little matrix production (Fig. 6). However, in mildly diabetic animals, the mesh pores were filled with more mature connective tissue, comparable to that in control animals. Light microscopic evaluation of the implanted percutaneous devices and their surrounding tissue showed various degrees of epithelial downgrowth, usually with the formation of a small sinus tract. The sinus was filled with keratin. Epidermal downgrowth never extended further than the width of the holding element, and in all cases, epithelial attachment to the implant surface was observed (Fig. 7). None of the implants revealed the presence of a subepithelial inflammatory reaction.

C. Experiment 3

For this experiment, the bone-bonding behavior and coating integrity of hydroxyapatite (HA) coatings were tested in rabbits.[5] Thirty-six specially designed cylindrical cp-Ti implants were made. All implants measured 8.0 mm in length with a diameter of 2.9 mm. The surface of the implants was grit-blasted with Al_2O_3 particles and plasma sprayed with hydroxylapatite, to a thickness of 40–70 μm. Half of the plasma-sprayed implants (HA-PS) were heat-treated (ht) for 2 h at 600°C. The crystallinity of the sprayed HA coating was 60–65%, as measured by X-ray diffraction.

Nine healthy female New Zealand White rabbits (age 3–4 mo) were obtained from the animal facility of the University of Nijmegen. The implants were inserted in both

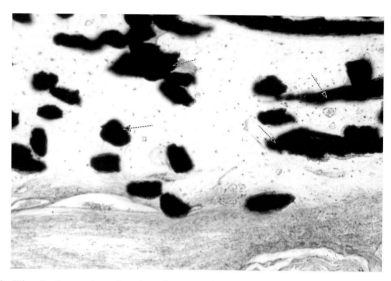

Figure 6. Histologic section showing the porosity of a titanium fiber mesh sheet (arrows) after 4 wk of implantation in a severely diabetic animal. The mesh porosity is filled with immature connective tissue showing little matrix organization, with few small blood vessels. Original magnification ×125.

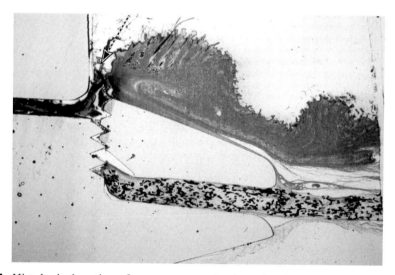

Figure 7. Histological section of a percutaneous implant after 8 wk of implantation showing limited epithelial downgrowth, with the formation of a small sinus tract (arrow). The sinus was filled with keratin. Original magnification ×12.

condyles of each femur. The animals were sacrificed at 3, 6, and 9 wk using an overdose of sodium pentobarbital (Nembutal).

The histological study showed that the coating could easily be detected at all survival times up to 9 wk. Three and 6 wk after insertion a lattice of woven bone was formed around all implants, especially at those sites where the implants were positioned in the

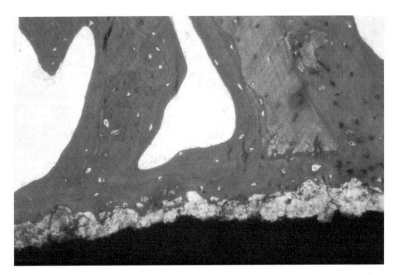

Figure 8. Light micrograph of HA-PS coated implant after 9 wk. Remodeling and compaction of the bone-implant interface. The coating shows no sign of reduction in thickness. Original magnification ×40.

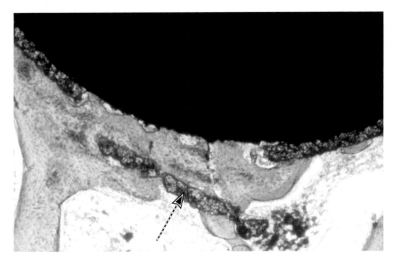

Figure 9. Detail of a HA-PS/ht-coated implant after 9 wk. The arrow indicates a piece of detached coating. Bone formation can be seen in between the detached coating and the implant surface. Original magnification ×40.

trabecular bone or medullar cavity. The coated implants showed no substantial reduction in coating thickness. At 9 wk, remodeling and compaction of the bone-implant interface was occurring (Fig. 8). No difference in bone formation between the various coatings could be seen. Only one of the heat-treated HA-coated implants showed delamination of the coating. Bone tissue was found between the dislodged coating and the implant surface (Fig. 9).

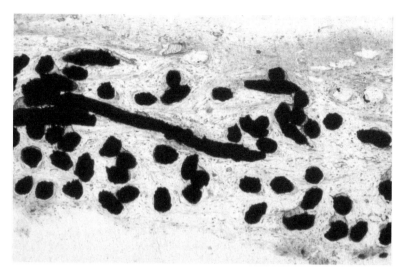

Figure 10. A thin, fibrous tissue capsule surrounds the titanium mesh implant. The dark areas are titanium mesh fibers. No inflammatory cells are visible. Inside the implant, the mesh porosity is filled with fibrous tissue containing capillaries. Original magnification ×10.

Table 1. The Number of Implants in Which Bone Formation Could Be Observed At Different Explantation Periods

Implant	2 wk	4 wk	8 wk
Titanium Mesh	0 (n = 10)	0 (n = 10)	0 (n = 10)
Titanium Mesh + RBM	2 (n = 10)	3 (n = 10)	0 (n = 10)
Titanium Mesh + CaP	0 (n = 10)	0 (n = 10)	0 (n = 10)
Titanium Mesh + CaP + RBM	5 (n = 10)	6 (n = 10)	6 (n = 10)

(n = 10 for each implant at time period.)

D. Experiment 4

The osteogenic activity of porous titanium fiber mesh and calcium phosphate (Ca-P)-coated titanium fiber mesh loaded with cultured syngeneic Fisher 344 male rats was investigated, Ca-P-coated and noncoated porous titanium implants were subcutaneously placed either without or loaded with cultured rat bone marrow (RBM) cells, total seeding density was 200,000 RBM cells per mesh.[15] The rats were sacrificed, and the implants were retrieved at 2, 4, and 8 wk postoperatively. Further, 6 of 10 rats received fluorochrome labeling. The fluorochrome labels tetracycline (yellow), alizarin-complexone (red), and calcein (green) were adminstrated at 2, 4 and 6 wk weeks postoperatively, respectively.

Histological analysis demonstrated that none of the Ca-P-coated and noncoated meshes alone supported bone formation at any time period (Fig. 10). In RBM-loaded implants, bone formation started at 2 wk. At 4 wk, this bone formation increased. However, at 8 wk bone formation was absent in the non-coated titanium implants, while it had remained in the Ca-P-coated titanium implants. Also, in Ca-P-coated implants more bone was formed than in noncoated samples (Table 1). In general, osteogenesis was characterized by the

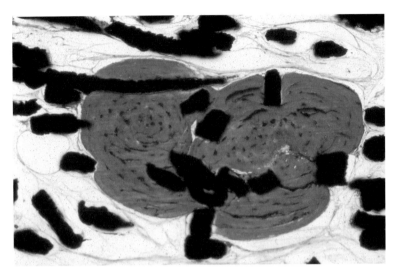

Figure 11. A section of a calcium phosphate-coated mesh loaded with RBM cells (Ti/Ca-P/RBM) 8 wk after implantation. Bone formation is characterized by the presence of randomly distributed multiple spheres in the pores of the Ti mesh. Original magnification ×20.

occurrence of multiple spheres in the porosity of the mesh (Fig. 11). The accumulation sequence of the fluorochrome markers showed that the newly formed bone was deposited in a centrifugal manner, starting at the center of a pore.

IV. DISCUSSION

Several methods have been developed to prepare thin sections of hard tissue. These are mostly based on two steps: relatively thick sections were sawed and reduced in thickness by grinding and polishing. Usually these sections are insufficiently thin for detailed histological analysis and are adversely affected by the grinding process. In addition, this process is laborious, and expert technical skills are required.

The recently developed diamond-blade saw has made it possible to produce thin (ca. 10 μm) slices with good surface qualities. This is because of the minimal tolerances in the rotating machine parts, a flutter-free bearing, and a precise horizontal transposition of the sample holder. The precise tuning of the velocity of rotation and the transverse (perpendicular movement) of the saw block toward the saw blade makes it possible to saw under optimal conditions. The attached cover slip acts as a stabilizing factor, and the precision of the translation stage controlled by an incremental encoder and digital display further enhances sectioning accuracy. The method is based on a one-step procedure in which grinding and polishing are unnecessary. It is easy to perform and takes less time. Presently, the results and the time factor are mainly dependent on the saw-blade type, the block size, and the implant material characteristics.

V. CONCLUSION

The new saw method and apparatus allow the preparation of reproducible 10-μm sections of undecalcified bone tissue containing implant materials such as ceramic, metal, polymer, or composite. The sections have an excellent histological quality. Other interesting applications include advantages for transmission electron microscopy (TEM) preparation techniques and for in vitro bone resorption studies.

REFERENCES

1. Borsboom PC, Wolfs BH, Leydsman H, et al: A machine for sawing 80-micrometer slices of carious enamel. *Stain Technol* 62:119–125, 1987.
2. Buijs R, Dogterom AA: An improved method for embedding hard tissue in polymethyl methacrylate. *Stain Technol* 58:135–141, 1983.
3. Donath K, Breuner GA: Method for the study of undecalcified bones and teeth with attached soft tissues: the Sage-Schliff (sawing and grinding) technique. *J Oral Pathol* 11:318–326, 1982.
4. Gerritsen M, Jansen JA, Lutterman JA: Performance of subcutaneously implanted glucose sensors for continous monitoring. *Neth J Med* 54:167–179, 1999.
5. Hulshoff JEG, van Dijk K, van der Waerden JPCM, et al: Evaluation of plasma-spray and magnetron-sputter Ca-P coated implants: an *in vivo* experiment using rabbits. *J Biomed Mater Res* 31:329–337, 1996.
6. Jande SS, Belanger LF: Electron microscopy of osteocytes and the pericellular matrix in rat trabecular bone. *Calcif Tissue Res* 6:280–289, 1971.
7. Klein CPAT, van der Lubbe HBM, van der Waerden JP: Histological evaluation of "direct" sawed thin sections of undecalcified bony tissue with biomaterials. The 3rd Intl. Symp. on Ceramics in Medicine, Terre Haute, IN, 1990.
8. Klein CPAT, Sauren YMHF, Modderman WE, et al: A new saw technique improves preparation of bone sections for light and electron microscopy. *J Appl Biomater* 5:369–373, 1994.
9. Lubbe van der HBM, Klein CPAT, de Groot K: A simple method for preparing thin (10 μm) histological sections of undecalcified plastic embedded bone with implants. *Stain Technol* 63:171–176, 1988.
10. Luk SC, Nopajaroonsri C, Simon GT: The ultrastructure of cortical bone in young adult rabbits. *J Ultrastruct Res* 46:184–205, 1974.
11. Osborn JS, Newesly H: Dynamic aspects of the implant-bone interface. In: Heimke G, ed: *Dental Implants: Materials and Systems.* Carl Hanser Verlag, Munich, 1980:111–123.
12. Pugliarello MC, Vittur F, de Bernard B: The ultrastructure of cortical bone in young adult rabbits. *J Ultrastruct Res* 12:209–214, 1973.
13. Scott JE, Haigh M: Proteoglycan-type I collagen fibril interaction in bone and non-calcifying connective tissues. *Biosci Rep* 5:71–81, 1985.
14. van der Lubbe HBM, Klein CPAT, van der Waerden JP, et al: A new developed sawing apparatus for direct preparation of thin sections of bone with biomaterials. The 3rd Intl. Symp. on Ceramics in Medicine, Terre Haute, IN, 1990.
15. Vehof JWM, Spauwen PHM, Jansen JA: Bone formation in CaP-coated titanium fiber mesh. *Biomaterials* 21:2003–2009, 2000.
16. Vercaigne S, Wolke JGC, Naert I, et al: A histological evaluation of TiO_2 grit-blasted and Ca-P magnetron sputter coated implants placed in the trabecular bone of the goat. Part 2. *Clin Oral Implants Res* 11:314–324, 2000.

18

Bone Sectioning Using the Precise 1 Automated Cutting System

Antonio Scarano,[1] Manlio Quaranta,[2] and Adriano Piattelli[3]

[1]Dental School, University of Chieti, Chieti, Italy
[2]Dental School, University of Rome, Rome, Italy
[3]Departments of Oral Medicine and Pathology and Dental School,
University of Chieti, Chieti, Italy

I. INTRODUCTION

The possibility of producing thin microscopic slides containing bone, soft tissues, biomaterials and implants in a predictable manner was of great interest to the authors of this chapter. Several techniques that produce very high-quality microscopic specimens and permit evaluation of the bone-biomaterial interfaces have been reported.[1,2,6] In all these techniques, the specimens are cut using a band saw or a metallurgical saw, and are then ground down in different ways to obtain the desired thickness.[3–5,7–9] However, most of these systems had high initial costs and high maintenance costs. In our laboratory, we have developed a low-cost cutting system, using a diamond disc instead of a band diamond saw, capable of giving consistent and predictable results.

II. PRECISE CUTTING SYSTEM

The cutting unit of the Precise system (Assing, Rome, Italy) consists of a mobile diamond cutting disc which produces sections from a block held immobile in a specimen-holding apparatus (Fig. 1). The thickness of the specimen is regulated by the micrometer. Once the cutting thickness has been selected, the slide-holding apparatus and the micrometer are locked in place by two pins to avoid undesirable movements (slipping) that accompany the cutting process. The cutting disc's path is guided by two rails, and thus moves perfectly parallel to the face of the mounted specimen block, with no vibrations that could be detrimental to the cutting precision. The advancing speed of the disc is variable, so it is possible to obtain different cutting forces. The histologic specimen is locked in place by a separate pump-created vacuum. During the cutting procedure, the lower portion of the disc is immersed in water to avoid overheating of the disc and the specimen.

With this system, it is also possible to cut fresh unembedded tissue. Ethanol is used in the bath during cutting so that the histologic specimen remains immersed in the fixative

From: *Handbook of Histology Methods for Bone and Cartilage*
Edited by: Y. H. An and K. L. Martin © Humana Press Inc., Totowa, NJ

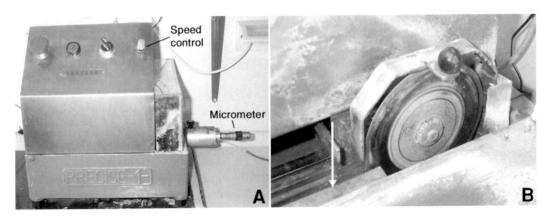

Figure 1. (A) "Precise 1" cutting system. The arrow indicates speed control of the revolution disk. Red arrow: micrometer. (B) Cutting disc and mounted specimen block (arrow).

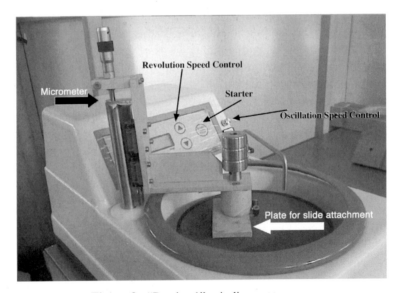

Figure 2. "Precise 1" grinding system.

without the danger of becoming dehydrated, causing subsequent cell lysis. It is not advisable to use other fixatives because of their volatile nature and resulting respiratory hazards.

Daily maintenance of this cutting system simply consists of changing the contents of the water bath. In addition, the disc must be periodically removed and cleaned using alcohol-soaked paper, or alternatively, an ultrasonic apparatus may be used.

III. PRECISE GRINDING SYSTEM

The Precise grinding system consists of a grinding disc, a specimen holder with a micrometer adjustment screw (Fig. 2), and a separate vacuum pump. The disc rotates at a variable speed, up to 400 revolutions per minute. The specimen holder can be adjusted

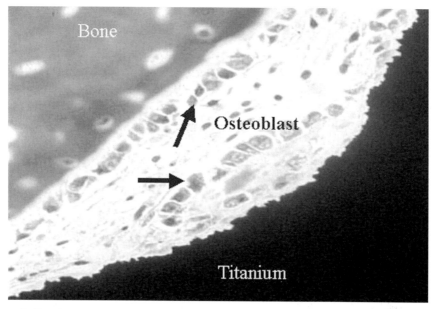

Figure 3. Detailed histological features can be observed in this section containing bone-implant interface.

vertically to place the specimen at the surface of the grinding disc. Weights (up to 70 g) are applied to the specimen holder to calibrate the speed and force of the grinding movement. The amount of weight is related to the shape and the dimension of the specimens. The micrometer screw is used to obtain the desired thickness. The specimen (attached to a slide) is kept in place by a vacuum produced by a pump. Abrasive paper of varying grades is fitted in the disc. These abrasive sheets grind the specimen to an even thickness and reduce the thickness of the histological specimen.

IV. ADVANTAGES OF THE PRECISE SYSTEM

The main difference between this cutting system and previously described systems is that the high-precision diamond disc is mobile, and the material to be cut remains immobile being held in place by a vacuum holder. The cutting pressure is easily regulated by the micromotor. With the Precise 1 Automated System, it has been possible to obtain consistent and reproducible thin (20–30 μm) sections of hard tissues containing biomaterials, which can give good cellular detail (Fig. 3). Many types of materials have been cut using the system, resulting in high-quality microscopic slides. Since the sections produced with the Precise system are reasonably thin, high individual cellular detail is possible, even at higher magnifications (×1200).

The time involved in the specimen cutting is considerably reduced with respect to other systems (Exakt and Buhler); about 15 min are needed to cut a 2 × 1 cm specimen. Moreover, it is possible to obtain about five sections from a specimen block with a minimal tissue loss (150 μm), and these sections can then be stained using different stains.[3]

It is also possible to process soft tissues with the Precise system. In all cases we have been able to obtain a good histological evaluation of the tissue-biomaterial interactions, with fine cellular detail and resolution, and with preservation of specimen and tissue-implant interface integrity.

V. STEPS IN HARD-TISSUE SECTIONING USING THE PRECISE 1 SYSTEM

Bone sectioning from the tissue block to the final histological slide consists of the following steps:

1. Specimens are infiltrated and embedded in resin, producing hard blocks containing the tissues to be examined;
2. Once the block is obtained it is glued to either a base of Plexiglas or a clean glass slide using adherent agents (e.g., Technovit 4000, Attack, or Vitroresin), placing the surface to be examined on the upper side;
3. Excess resin is removed by grinding to make the free surface of the block parallel to the holding slide. At this stage another slide is glued to the free surface;
4. Sectioning of the tissue block at a thickness of 100–200 µm is carried out using the Precise 1 cutting system;
5. Grinding of the final thin section by the Precise grinding systems.

VI. POTENTIAL PROBLEMS AND PRECAUTIONS

Histological preparation of tissues containing metal implants may present some technical difficulties, and problems have been reported with the grinding techniques currently in use.[2,3] Mistakes can occur at every phase of mineralized tissue processing. Here are several potential problems that can be encountered during tissue processing with the Precise 1 system:

1. If there is incomplete polymerization of the resin, cutting and/or grinding of the specimen may be impossible, and there is the possibility of staining artifacts that produce a background stain which obscures the features;
2. If the specimen is overground in an attempt to obtain a thinner section, some of the material may be lost;
3. If an inadequate amount of glue is used, there could be detachment and/or loss of the specimen or empty spaces where parts of the section have detached;
4. During sectioning, a too-thick section (300 µm or more) may result in the loss of an important portion of the specimen, or a too-thin section (10–20 µm) may result in detachment of tissues or biomaterials from the slide;
5. It is very important to control the grinding procedure, because during this phase it is possible to reduce the specimen too much with loss of important parts of the tissue. Also, striations (scratches) may be produced that can mask important features of the specimen;
6. It must also be emphasized that, during grinding, the attrition rates of bone, soft tissues, implant material, and embedding media are different. The implants may remain thicker than the surrounding tissues, with resulting uneven specimen thickness or areas where the material has been lost during grinding;
7. There may be "ledging" at the implant-tissue interface, because of the different rates of grinding attrition for bone and metal. This "ledging" may obscure portions of the implant-tissue interface, and prevent a good interpretation of the structures at the interface.

VII. CONCLUSION

With our system it has been possible to consistently obtain histological slides containing metal implants with a thickness of about approx 20–30 µm, and the grinding process with its inherent problems can be eliminated or considerably reduced. In most of our slides, it has only been necessary to use a precision lapping wheel with very fine sandpaper to polish the specimens. Our system can also be used for processing soft tissues (i.e., in an oral pathology service). In conclusion, this system is easy to use, extremely cost-effective, eliminates the problems connected with grinding, and gives consistent and reproducible results in the observation of biological specimens containing biomaterials.

REFERENCES

1. Donath K, Breuner GA: A method for the study of undecalcified bones and teeth with attached soft tissues. The Sage-Schliff (sawing and grinding) technique. *J Oral Pathol* 1:318–326, 1982.
2. Emmanual J, Hornbeck C, Bloeman RD: A polymethyl methacrylate method for large specimens of mineralized bone with implants. *Stain Technol* 62:401–410, 1987.
3. Gotfredsen K, Budtz-Jorgensen E, Jensen LN: A method for preparing and staining histological sections containing titanium implants for light microscopy. *Stain Technol* 64:121–127, 1989.
4. Gruber HE, Marshall GJ, Nolasco LM, et al: Alkaline and acid phosphatase demonstration in human bone and cartilage: effects of fixation interval and methacrylate embedments. *Stain Technol* 63:299–306, 1988.
5. Hahn M, Vogel M, Delling G: Undecalcified preparation of bone tissue: report of technical experience and development of new methods. *Virchows Arch A Pathol Anat Histopathol* 418:1–7, 1991.
6. Hipp JA, Brunski JB, Lochran GVB: Method for histological preparation of bone sections containing titanium implants. *Stain Technol* 62:247–252, 1987.
7. Murice-Lambert E, Banford AB, Folger RL: Histological preparation of implanted biomaterials for light microscopic evaluation of the implant-tissue interaction. *Stain Technol* 64:19–24, 1989.
8. Steflik DE, McKinney RV, Mobley GL, et al: Simultaneous histological preparation of bone, soft tissue and implanted biomaterials for light microscopic observations. *Stain Technol* 57:91–98, 1982.
9. Van der Lubbe HB, Klein CP, de Groot K: A simple method for preparing thin (10 microM) histological sections of undecalcified plastic embedded bone with implants. *Stain Technol* 63:171–176, 1988.

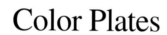

Color Plates

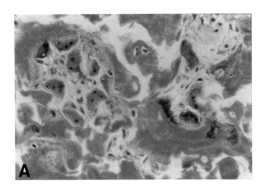
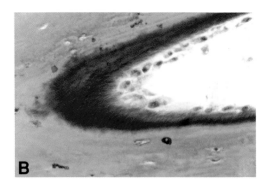

Color Plate 1, Figure 17 (*See* discussion in Chapter 1 and full caption on p. 16). Goldner's trichrome stain of a cutting cone and a filling cone during the process of bone remodeling.

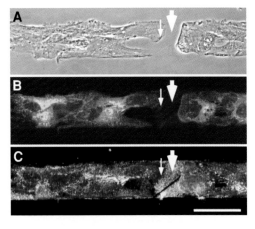

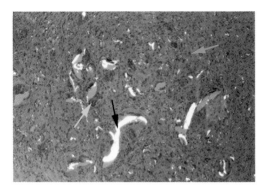

Color Plate 2, Figure 3 (*See* discussion in Chapter 2 and full caption on p. 37). Initial HBD cell attachment and protein profile on EDS/DMS patterned surfaces.

Color Plate 3, Figure 4 (*See* discussion in Chapter 2 and full caption on p. 39). Pseudo-capsule tissue from a revision total shoulder arthroplasty stained with IL-1βcDNA probe.

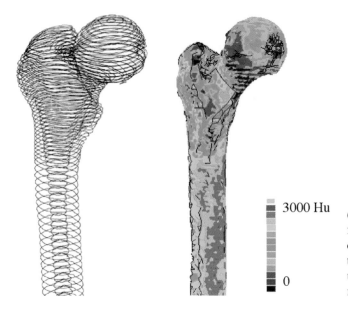

3000 Hu

0

Color Plate 4, Figure 7
(*See* discussion in Chapter 2 and full caption on pg. 41). Extracted computed tomography (CT) contours and the CT data (Houndsfield units, Hu) applied to a finite element (FE) model of the femur.

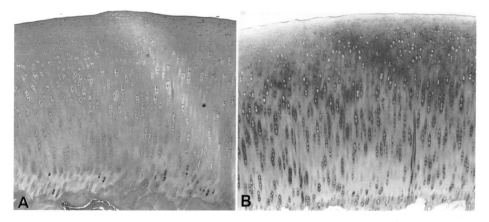

Color Plate 5, Figure 13 (*See* discussion in Chapter 2 and full caption on p. 49). Hematoxylin and esosin (H&E) staining (A) and Safranin O staining (B) of the surface of articular cartilage in an adult sheep distal femur.

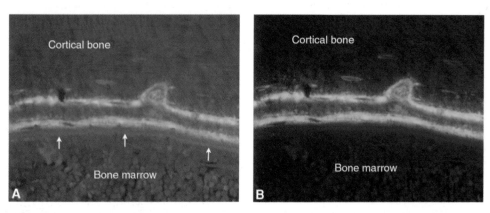

Color Plate 6, Figure 1 (*See* discussion in Chapter 5 and full caption on p. 100). Calcein double-labeling of bone.

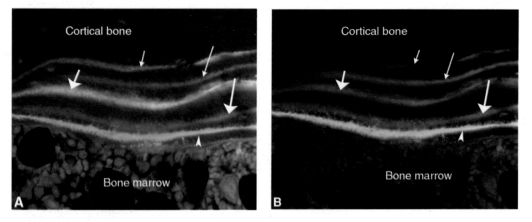

Color Plate 7, Figure 2 (*See* discussion in Chapter 5 and full caption on p. 102). Multiple fluorochrome labeling of bone.

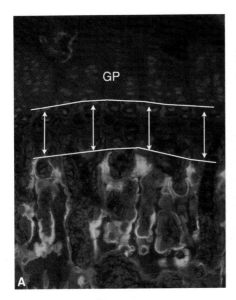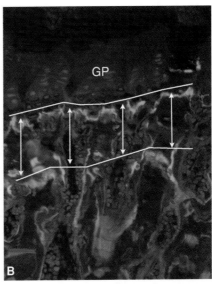

Color Plate 8, Figure 4 (*See* discussion in Chapter 5 and full caption on pp. 112, 113). Measurement of longitudinal bone elongation. These fluorescence photomicrographs show the growth plate (GP) and the metaphysis of proximal tibias from growing rats.

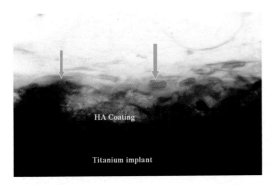

Color Plate 9, Figure 2 (*See* discussion in Chapter 9 and full caption on p. 162). A well-performed fixation gives a good detail of the cells positive for acid phosphatase (arrows) at the bone-implant interface. Magnification ×1200.

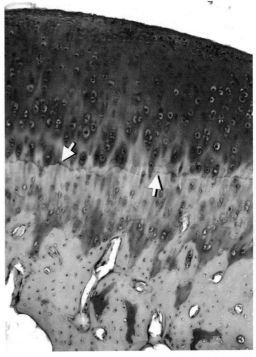

Color Plate 10, Figure 6 (*See* discussion in Chapter 13 and full caption on p. 218). Safranin O and fast green staining of rabbit femoral condyles.

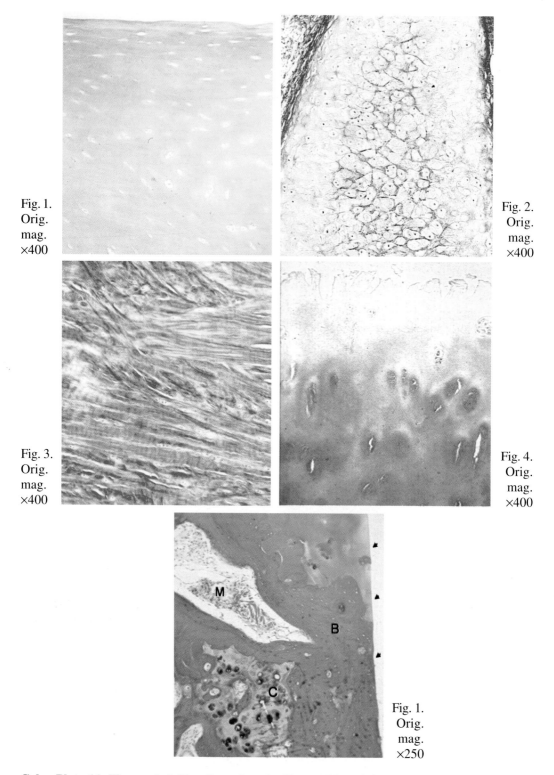

Fig. 1.
Orig.
mag.
×400

Fig. 2.
Orig.
mag.
×400

Fig. 3.
Orig.
mag.
×400

Fig. 4.
Orig.
mag.
×400

M

B

C

Fig. 1.
Orig.
mag.
×250

Color Plate 11, Figures 1–5 (*See* discussions in Chapter 22, and full captions on pp. 302–305). (Figure 1) Normal hyaline cartilage, stained for connective tissue fibers (van Gieson's stain). (Figure 2) Normal elastic cartilage: chondrocytes surrounded by ring-like collagen fibers and tiny elastic fibers. (Figure 3) Fibrocartilage of the meniscus. (Figure 4) Safranin O stain of osteoarthritic hyaline cartilage. (Figure 5) Advanced stages of osteoarthritis.

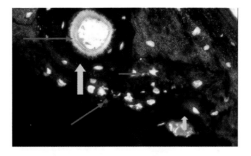

Color Plate 12, Figure 2 (*See* discussion in Chapter 23 and full caption on p. 317). Silver nitrate (von Kossa) and acid fuchsin staining of mineralized bone that appears black.

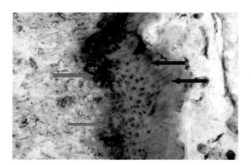

Color Plate 13, Figure 3 (*See* discussion in Chapter 23 and full caption on p. 318). Silver nitrate (von Kossa) and alkaline phosphatase staining.

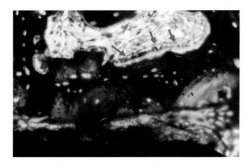

Color Plate 14, Figure 4 (*See* discussion in Chapter 23 and full caption on p. 318). Cartilage of the rabbit femoral metaphysis stained for acid (blue arrows) and alkaline phosphatase (red arrows).

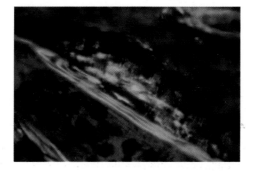

Color Plate 15, Figure 1 (*See* discussion in Chapter 25 and full caption on p. 335). Undecalcified iliac bone double-labeled in vivo with tetracycline and stained in vitro with calcein.

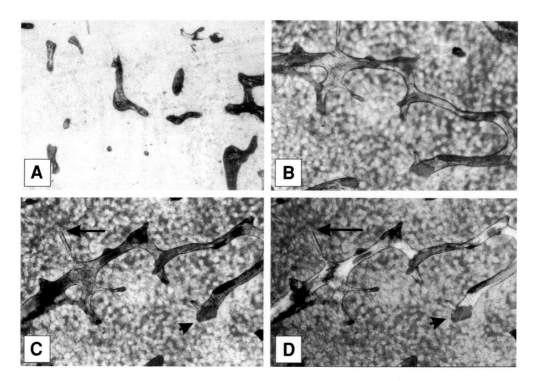

Color Plate 16, Figure 9 (*See* discussion in Chapter 25 and full caption on p. 348). Photomicrographs of cancellous bone in a thin section and a thick slice. (A) A typical 10-μm section stained with toluidine blue contains many apparent termini. In contrast, (B–D) show a 300-μm slice where there are fewer apparent termini; (B) is stained with alizarin red on both surfaces; (C) is stained on one surface with alizarin red and on the other with light green, the color contrast improving separation; (D) is the same as (C) viewed in partially polarized light for clarity. The arrow indicates a real terminus (unstained) within the depth of the slice; these are relatively rare. The arrowhead indicates an apparent terminus (stained). Magnification ×20.

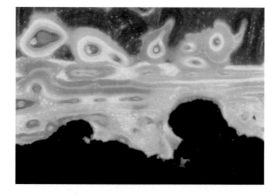

Color Plate 17, Figure 1 (*See* discussion in Chapter 26 and full caption on p. 355). Fluorescence micrograph of bone response to a rough titanium-implant surface. Three labels were administered subcutaneously, i.e., tetracycline (yellow, at 1 wk post-implantation), calcein (green, at 3 wk post-implanation), and alizarin-complexon (red, at 6 wk post-implantation).

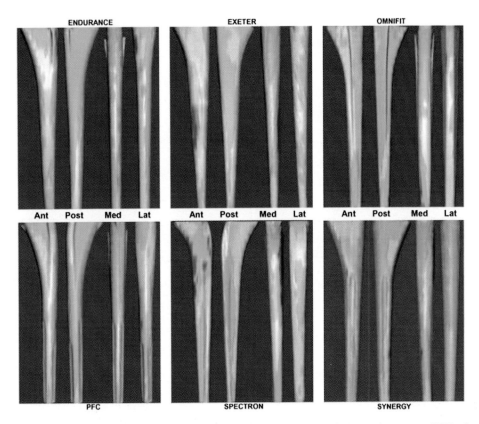

Color Plate 18, Figure 7 (*See* discussion in Chapter 27 and full caption on p. 370). Surface mapping of the cement-mantle thickness. Red <1 mm; yellow 1–2 mm; white 2–4 mm; blue >4 mm.

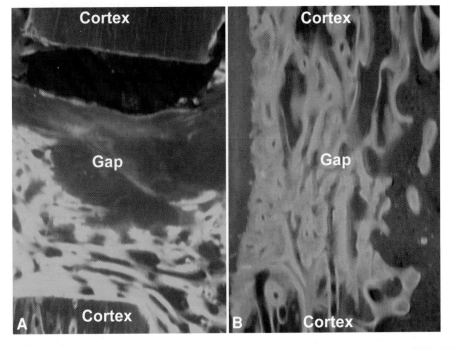

Color Plate 19, Figure 3 (*See* discussion in Chapter 28 and same caption on p. 379). Healing fracture demonstrating continuous bone labeling with oral tetracycline at a dose of 20 mg/kg daily at (A) 4 wk, and (B) 12 wk after osteotomy.

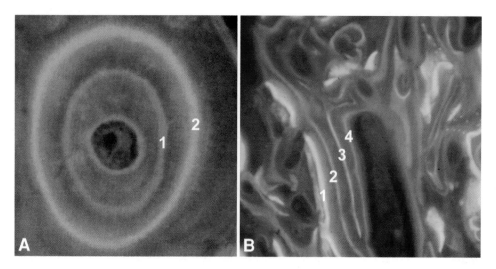

Color Plate 20, Figure 4 (*See* discussion in Chapter 28 and full caption on p. 380). New bone formation demonstrated with (A-1) xylenol orange, and (A-2) tetracycline. (B) section demonstrates quadruple labeling with (1) tetracycline, (2) xylenol orange, (3) calcein red, and (4) calcein blue.

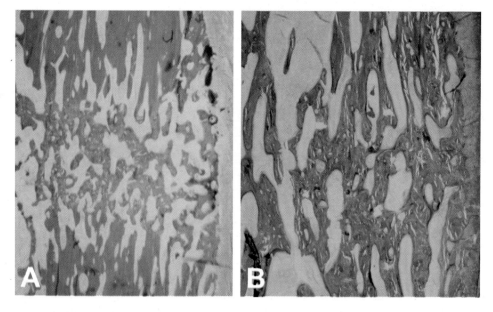

Color Plate 21, Figure 7 (*See* discussion in Chapter 28 and full caption on p. 383). Light microscopy of the osteotomy at (A) 8 wk, and (B) 12 wk following osteotomy. Images demonstrate a decrease in the anisotropy over time as the woven bone within the fracture gap is remodeled. (Goldner's trichrome staining, ×4).

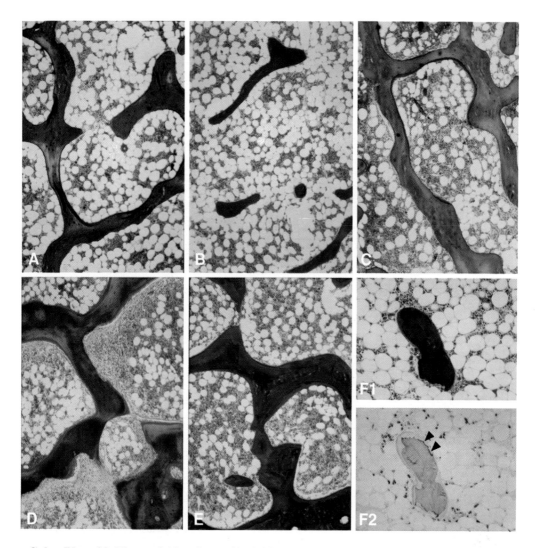

Color Plate 22, Figure 3 (*See* discussion in Chapter 29 and full caption on p. 400). Goldner's trichrome-stained sections from iliac crest biopsies. Goldner's trichrome-stained sections from iliac crest biopsies showing (A) Bone mass, bone turnover, and osteoid thickness from a normal middle-aged person. (B) Osteoporosis with decreased bone mass and disintegrated bone structure. (C) Primary hyper-parathryoidism with increased bone turnover, as judged from the increased erosion and osteoid surfaces. Bone mass and osteoid thickness are within the normal ranges. (D) Secondary hyperparathyroidism with grossly increased bone turnover, foci of increased osteoid thickness, and mineralization defects. The bone marrow shows marked paratrabecular fibrosis. (E) Osteomalacia with very thick osteoid seams covering the entire surface, leaving no bone surfaces for osteoclastic resorption. The interface between mineralized bone and osteoid appears to be irregular. (F1) Aluminum intoxication with normal to low thickness of osteoid seams and an irregular osteiod-bone interface. (F2) Aluminum staining showing deposits of aluminum at the mineralization front (arrow heads).

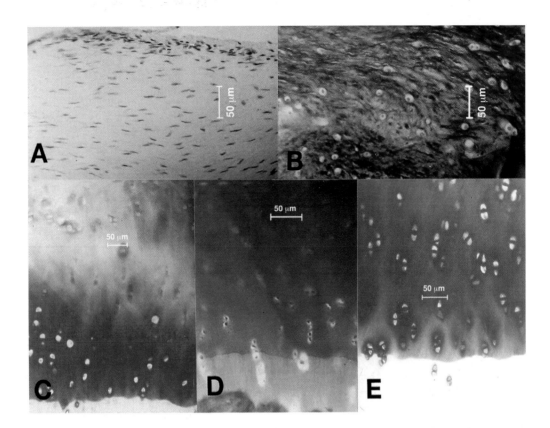

Color Plate 23, Figure 1 (*See* discussion in Chapter 30 and full caption on p. 414). Light micrographs of tissue types found in articular cartilage and healing defects, with the articulating surface at the top and the tidemark at the bottom. Scale bars provided in each panel.

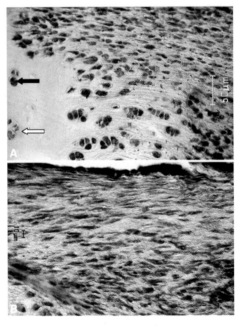

Color Plate 24, Figure 3 (*See* discussion in Chapter 30 and full caption on p. 419). Smooth-muscle actin (SMA) immunohistochemical micrograph of a defect treated with an autologous periosteal cover alone, 6 wk postoperatively. The reddish chromogen labels the SMA.

19

Bone, Cement, and Metal Implant Interface Preparation with a High-Pressure Water Cutter

Jian-Sheng Wang and Lars Lidgren

Department of Orthopaedics, Lund University Hospital, Lund, Sweden

I. INTRODUCTION

Today, many studies in cemented prostheses focus on the interface between bone and cement as well as between cement and stem. Extensive porosity is aggregated at the cement-stem interface in retrieved cement mantle and laboratory-prepared specimens.[2,3,6] Shrinkage of polymethyl methacrylate (PMMA) causes the formation of gaps between the bone and the cement and between the cement and the prosthesis.[9] Hematoma formation during the operation will also cause a gap between bone and cement. Porosity, gap, and bleeding at the interfaces may reduce the initial cemented prosthetic stability and thus the long-term survival rate. Examination of the cement-implant interface from cadaver and experimental samples is essential to understanding and thus improving the interface bonding. Clinical studies cannot provide details about the bone-cement and cement-prosthesis interfaces. To perform such investigations, the most common specimen preparation method is using a cutting technique employing a high-speed, water-cooled, circular saw with a ceramic or diamond blade, which is time-consuming.[10] With continued use, the cutting effectiveness of even a diamond saw gradually declines because the diamond saw wears out.[8] In order to accurately and quickly analyze the interface, we introduced an industrial high-pressure water cutter as a cutting technique for implant and implant-interface investigation. Although the technique has been developed as a cutting tool for soft tissues in visceral surgery[1,4] or bone and cement,[5] it has not been used for bone, cement, and metal together.

II. CUTTING TECHNIQUE OF WATER JET CUTTER

Water Jet cutters (Water Jet Sweden AB, Ronneby, Sweden) are high-technology precision machines which have been used for about 25 years (Fig. 1). A water jet cutting machine is built up around a stiff steel frame. It consists of a cutting table, cutting head for water and abrasive cutting, high-pressure valves, an extraction system, feed turret including pressure vessel, dosing feeder, high-pressure pump, and Computer Numerical Control (CNC) control

From: *Handbook of Histology Methods for Bone and Cartilage*
Edited by: Y. H. An and K. L. Martin © Humana Press Inc., Totowa, NJ

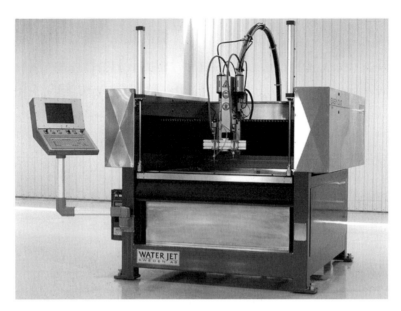

Figure 1. Water Jet Cutter (Water Service AB, Ronneby, Sweden).

(Fig. 2). A CAD/CAM program controls cutting speed and direction. The machine produces water pressure up to 3500 bars through a nozzle. The water cutter can cut through aluminum up to 300 mm, steel up to 150 mm thick, and foam rubber up to 300 mm thick.

The diameters of the nozzles vary from 0.06 mm for water only to 0.68 mm for water with sand. A nozzle can be used for 100 h. To water cut through a metal stem, the water is combined with very fine sand (120 mesh, Oliven, Norway). Water cutting results in a temperature of 30–40 °C at the cutting surface. The position of accuracy is 0.1 mm per M. The speed of the water cutter can be adjusted according to the hardness and thickness of the materials to be cut. The roughness of the cut surface is less than 10 μm (Ra), (Ra = average roughness).

III. CUTTING TECHNIQUE OF CEMENTED METAL IMPLANT

The implanted bone specimen is embedded in gypsum or self-curing acrylic material (Fig. 2). After the material has cured, the embedded specimen is placed on the cutting table and held there tightly by a mechanical clamp to stabilize the specimens. The water cutter is controlled by a computer, which is programmed according to the operator's requirements. For a bone-cement-metal combination, such as cemented hip implant, speeds of around 5 mm to 20 mm per min are suitable. The tip of the water nozzle is placed as close as possible (approx 1–2 mm) above the specimen. Section thicknesses greater than 3 mm are recommended. The cut is about 1 mm thick and, the cut surface is smooth and intact. An even smoother surface may be produced by slowing the forward movement of the water nozzle.

Usually, cemented hip implant with femur is large enough to be cut into 10-mm-thickness sections. If thinner sections (around 3 mm thick) are needed, the specimen should be embedded into harder polymers, and can then be tightly clamped for stability. In cross sec-

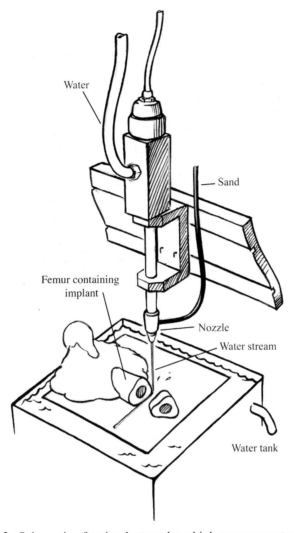

Figure 2. Schematic of an implant cut by a high-pressure water cutter.

tion, the pores and small gaps at the interfaces between the materials can be seen easily (Fig. 3). Gaps between cement and metal that may be caused by cement shrinkage or pores on the interface[7] are not affected by the cutting direction (Fig. 4). The cement penetration into bone trabeculae can be clearly seen under a microscope. The contact between cement and metal prosthesis can be observed with scanning electron microscopy (SEM). (Fig. 5). Quantification of the interface between bone and cement, and between cement and metal, are easily quantified by using a microscope with an image analysis system.

IV. CHARACTERISTICS OF WATER CUTTING

1. High-pressure water cutters significantly reduce cutting time from as much as 1–3 h for common methods to just a few minutes for each section.

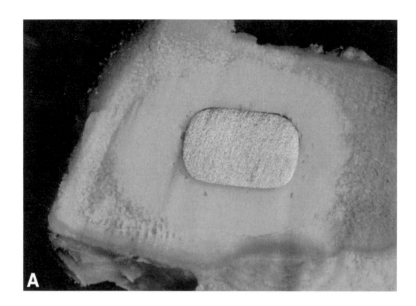

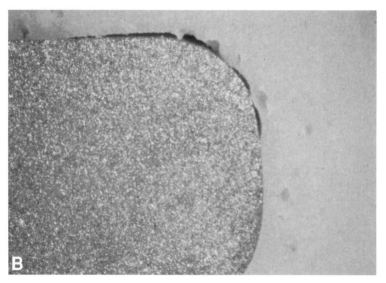

Figure 3. (A). Overview of a cemented stem in the femur cut with a high-pressure water cutter. Magnification ×4. (B) The close-up shows the gap at the cement-stem interface. Magnification ×10.

2. The low temperature reached during the cutting will not change the interface conditions; therefore, this cutting technique is favorable for many biomaterial applications.
3. The cut surface of a cemented prosthesis is comparable to that obtained with a high-speed, water-cooled, circular saw with a diamond blade.
4. If histological examinations must be done for a specific region of the specimen, a slice from the water cutter can be cut by a high-speed, water-cooled, circular saw with a diamond blade to obtain thinner sections.

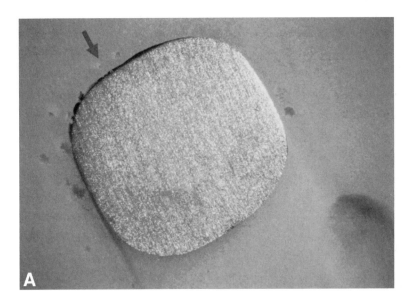

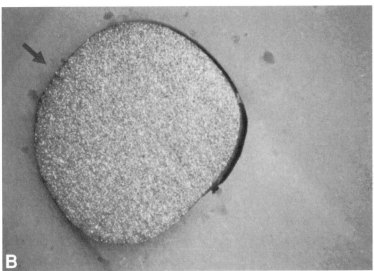

Figure 4. Gaps at the cement-stem interface are not related to the high-pressure water-cutting direction (arrows show the cutting direction. Magnification ×10.

5. The pores, gaps, cement penetration, and contact at the interfaces between bone and cement and between cement and metal can be examined under a microscope with direct light or in a scanning electron microscope.

For investigating a larger series of experiments such as cemented or cementless metal implants in animal bone and clinically retrieval studies (Fig. 6), the water-cutting technique produces minimal artifacts.

Acknowledgment: We thank Water Jet Sweden AB, Ronneby, Sweden, Herman Anderssons Platt AB, Hörby, Sweden, and Jörgen Jönsson, Center for Oral Health Sci-

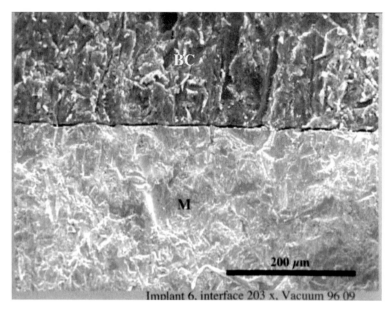

Figure 5. SEM showing gaps between the cement and metal (BC = bone cement, M = metal).

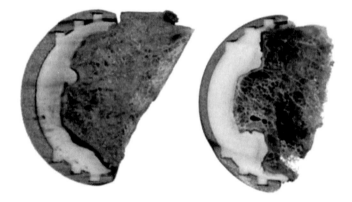

Figure 6. A retrieved shoulder prosthesis cut by a water cutter. At left, there are long gaps at both metal and bone interfaces. The bone was loose from the cement. To the right, there is good contact in most of the area. A large cyst can be seen in the humeral head.

ences, Lund University, Malmö, Sweden, for helping with the cutting of the implants. Financial support was given by the Swedish Medical Research Council (09509).

REFERENCES

1. Basting RF, Corvin S, Antwerpen C, et al: Use of water jet resection in renal surgery: early clinical experiences. *Eur Urol* 38:104–107, 2000.

2. Bishop NE, Ferguson S, Tepic S: Porosity reduction in bone cement at the stem-cement inter-face. *J Bone Joint Surg [Br]* 78:349–356, 1996.

3. Davies JP, Kawate K, Harris WH: Effect of interfacial porosity on the torsional strength of the cement-metal interface. *Transactions 41st Annual Meeting Orthop Res Soc* 1995:713.

4. Hata Y, Sasaki F, Takahashi H, et al: Liver resection in children, using a water-jet. *J Pediatr Surg* 29:648–650, 1994.

5. Honl M, Rentzsch R, Muller G, et al: The use of water-jetting technology in prostheses revi-sion surgery—first results of parameter studies on bone and bone cement. *J Biomed Mater Res* 53:781–790, 2000.

6. James SP, Schmalzried TP, McGarry FJ, Harris WH: Extensive porosity at the cement-femoral prosthesis interface: a preliminary study. *J Biomed Mater Res* 27:71–78, 1993.

7. Jasty M, Maloney W, Bragdon CR, et al: The initiation of failure in cemented femoral compo-nents of hip arthroplasties. *J Bone Joint Surg [Br]* 73:551–558, 1991.

8. Miyawki H, Taira M, Yamaki M: Cutting effectiveness of diamond points on commercial core composite resins and cements. *J Oral Rehabil* 23:409–415, 1996.

9. Wang J-S, Franzen H, Lidgren L: Interface gap after implanation of a cemented femoral stem in pigs. *Acta Orthop Scand* 70:234–239, 1999.

10. Wang J-S, Lidgren L: A new method for cutting metal implants with a high pressure water cut-ter. European Orthopaedic Research Society Meeting, Barcelona, Spain, April 22–23, 1997:249.

V   Staining Techniques

20

Basic Staining and Histochemical Techniques and Immunohistochemical Localizations Using Bone Sections

Helen E. Gruber and Jane A. Ingram

Orthopaedic Research Biology, Department of Orthopaedic Surgery,
Carolinas Medical Center, Charlotte, NC, USA

I. INTRODUCTION

Staining procedures, and more specialized histochemistry and immunohistochemistry, are performed to obtain specific types of information about bone cells, bone, or cartilage extracellular matrix (ECM) and bone formation and mineralization. Unfortunately, all these aspects cannot usually be obtained with one staining procedure or localization method, and thus the specific needs of a project must be clearly defined at the outset of specimen preparation. If bone formation and mineralization are important for the study, then the specimens must be processed in an undecalcified method and sectioned with a special microtome and knives. If more routine histologic stains and localizations are the desired outcome, then routine or specialized decalcification procedures can be performed and the specimen can be embedded in paraffin. We have recently reviewed the technical methods elsewhere.[9] The objective of this chapter is to present technical procedures for the more commonly used bone stains and localizations.

A good experimental plan, which may even include a pilot study, should include a carefully chosen fixative agent. Alcohol retains tetracycline labels, and is still used by some investigators,[13] yet it does not provide good cellular preservation. Ten percent neutral buffered formalin (NBF) is a commonly used fixative, but the length of time that bone is kept in this solution must be carefully controlled because overexposure can block alkaline phosphatase localization in osteoblasts,[7] and may also interfere with specialized immunolocalizations. It is also important to ensure that the fixative penetrates the entire bone specimen. The application of a vacuum can aid in this step. Storage for short periods of time before processing and during transport can usually be carried out in 70% ethanol; higher concentrations tend to make bone more brittle.

II. STAINING TECHNIQUES

Many excellent previous reviews and chapters have presented a variety of staining methods;[1,2,15] however, not all of this important work can be cited here.

From: *Handbook of Histology Methods for Bone and Cartilage*
Edited by: Y. H. An and K. L. Martin © Humana Press Inc., Totowa, NJ

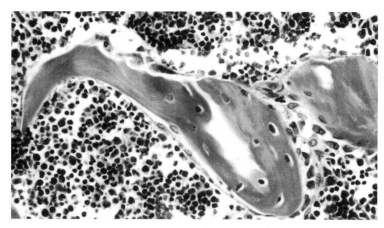

Figure 1. Photomicrograph of Masson's trichrome-stained rat femur. This microscopic field of trabecular bone show the commonly encountered problem of artifactual separation of bone cells away from the bone surface. Magnification ×280.

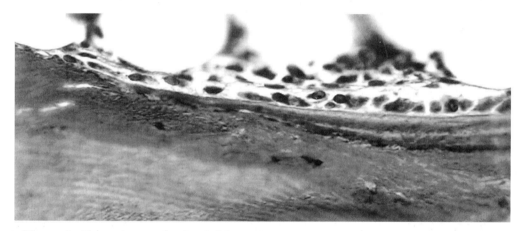

Figure 2. Photomicrograph of a MMA-embedded specimen of human iliac crest bone stained with Goldner's stain. The row of osteoblasts which overlies an osteoid seam shows good morphologic preservation. Magnification ×425.

A. Decalcified Preparations

Most of the routine trichrome, hematoxylin and eosin (H&E), toluidine blue, and other stains have been successfully adapted for study of bone in paraffin sections. Methylene blue/basic fuchsin and other metachromatic stains can be used to view entire long bones with epiphysis, physis, and metaphysis present in one specimen with good distinction of growth plates.

A common problem, even with carefully prepared paraffin bone slides, is the artifactual separation of osteoblasts and osteoclasts away from the bone surface (Fig. 1). This prevents use of such preparations for quantitative histomorphometry. Methyl methacrylate (MMA) (Fig. 2) and glycol methacrylate provide better tissue preservation and detail with osteoblasts and osteoclasts, with better preservation in relation to the bone surface.

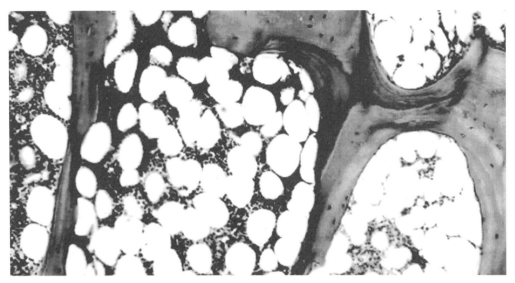

Figure 3. Low-magnification photomicrograph of human iliac crest trabecular bone embedded with MMA and stained with Goldner's stain to differentiate wide osteoid seams (OS). Magnification ×110.

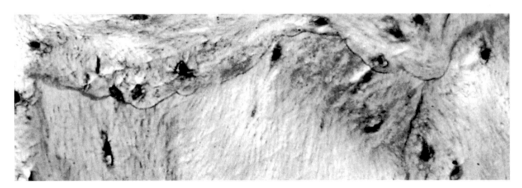

Figure 4. Photomicrograph of human cortical bone embedded in MMA and stained with methylene blue/basic fuchsin for visualization of cement lines (arrow). Magnification ×400.

B. Undecalcified Preparations

In general, staining methods for plastic-embedded tissue require modification because these procedures are usually performed without the removal of the plastic, and thus different timing regimens are utilized. Staining procedures that are commonly used in our laboratory include Goldner's stain[5] and cement line visualization.[4,6,8] Goldner's stain and von Kossa stain both allow differentiation of osteoid from mature mineralized bone matrix (Fig. 3); Goldner's stain (a modified Masson's trichrome) has a hematoxylin component that allows good nuclear cellular staining, as shown in Fig. 2.[5] Cement lines—specialized regions of the bone matrix which mark past sites of bone remodeling—can be stained with a number of procedures, including Stains-All;[4] toluidine blue or methylene blue/basic fuchsin,[6] as shown in Fig. 4; thionine,[3] a combined method using thionine, toluidine blue, methylene blue chloride, or methylene violet;[16] or modifications of Bodian silver stain.[8]

C. Ground Sections

Villanueva et al.[22] developed a method for block staining of the specimen followed by hand-grinding. With other methods, when specimens are not stained *en bloc,* it is usually only the surface of the ground section that absorbs the stain. Large bone blocks embedded in plastic can also be cut, polished, and stained. This may offer an advantage if small rodent long bones are being studied in cross section because the plastic makes the specimen easier to handle, or if very large bones must be visualized intact. Other useful suggestions for the handling and staining of ground sections have been summarized by Schenk et al.[16]

D. Enzyme Histochemistry: Alkaline Phosphatase and Tartrate-Resistant Acid Phosphatase Localization

Enzyme histochemistry has played an important role in the identification and study of osteoblasts and osteoclasts. Two phosphohydrolases have special relevance: alkaline phosphatase, an ectoenzyme present in the osteoblast and in matrix vesicle membranes, and tartrate-resistant acid phosphatase (TRAP), a lysosomal enzyme whose localization provides a sensitive method of osteoclast identification. Three factors influence success in histologically localizing enzymes: optimal procurement of the specimen, proper fixation, and proper embedding. For bone and cartilage, the latter condition can be satisfied by using methacrylate embedding and avoiding decalcification and paraffin processing. Either glycol methacrylate or MMA methods can be used. As with all localization procedures, it is important to include a positive control in all runs with alkaline phosphatase (ALP) and TRAP localizations.

Proper tissue fixation is a very important step in histochemistry. Results from our laboratory have shown that optimal localization of alkaline and acid phosphatase (ACP) in fresh tissue is achieved after fixation not exceeding 15 h in NBF followed by embedment in MMA.[7] As a rule of thumb, 4–6 h provides a safe fixation period. It may sometimes be necessary to retrieve frozen tissue from –70°C collections. When frozen tissue must be used, good localization of both enzymes can be achieved after fixation for 30 min and embedment in MMA or after 5 min fixation followed by embedment in glycol methacrylate.

Cytochemical studies of many enzymes are done on minimally fixed tissue, often sectioned on a cryostat. However, this requires considerable technical skill with fragile growth plates or brittle, large-bone specimens, so it is well worth the effort to define the appropriate fixation period for each enzyme of interest.

E. Immunohistochemistry

Immunocytochemistry and immunohistochemistry are valuable techniques for specialized bone and cartilage matrix and cellular studies. In immunohistochemistry, biologic substances of interest are localized by the precise attachment of a complex or label, which can be subsequently visualized in the cell or tissue of interest. Visualization can be either by bright-field microscopy (viewing of a chromogenic reaction product) or via ultraviolet (UV) microscopy using a fluorescent coupling agent. The visible product binds by the attraction between immunogen (antigen) and immunoglobulin (antibody). Several excellent reviews and instructional texts are available for further study of principles and newer immunologic and non-immunologic visualization methods.[11] For orthopedic research purposes, the specimens are usually either fresh-frozen and cut on a cryostat, or fixed and embedded in paraffin.

Immunohistochemical methods are often technically complex, and most studies on bone have therefore utilized decalcified preparations. However, there are excellent studies using plastic-embedded tissues,[10,12,19] which are best recommended to the more advanced histology laboratory.

As noted here for enzyme histochemical studies of bone, an important initial step in the use of a new antibody localization method is to determine the type of fixation, if any, which is required. Fixatives which maintain excellent morphologic detail in a tissue may not be at all successful in preserving immunoreactivity.[14] For the novice who is investigating an antibody for the first time, testing of fixation agents (1% or 10% NBF, Bouin's fixative, or Zamboni's fixative) is the first step. The reader is referred to detailed texts for further information about fixation types and regimes that may be of interest.[11] Inclusion of a known positive control tissue in each run, and conscientious inclusion of negative controls with each assay run are essential.

Another important step that is critical for successful immunolocalization is proper choice of the method in which the bone specimen was decalcified. The two most commonly used methods are use of ethylendiaminetetraacetic acid (EDTA) and use of formic-citrate.[9] We will initially test an antibody using the formic-citrate decalcification method.

Commonly encountered problems with immunohistochemistry include poor visualization resulting from insufficient specific staining, high levels of nonspecific (background) staining, the inability to achieve localization because of masking by prolonged fixation or embedding methods, and lack of success with initial trials of new antibodies. Thorough rinsing between steps is important to control nonspecific staining. Some investigators have reported success in retrieving antigenicity in specimens fixed for inappropriately long periods (or older archived fixed tissue) with the use of antigen retrieval methodologies as recently reviewed elsewhere.[17,18,20,21,23] These methods include techniques such as enzyme pretreatment of sections and microwave irradiation.

There are other common problems to be resolved when beginning new studies: the first is to identify reliable antibodies for your specific needs, and if the antibody is an anti-human one, to determine whether or not it can be successfully used to localize antigens in non-human tissue if so desired. Secondary antibodies should be chosen from a species that will not cross-react with the tissue of interest. Murine immunocytochemistry has benefited by the recent introduction of commercial kits containing various monoclonal antibodies. It is important to remember that not all commercially available antibodies work equally well, and that there is no certification system for antibodies similar to that which ensures chemical histologic stain quality through the Biological Stain Commission and C.I. (Certification numbers) which are assigned to histologic and cytologic stains.

REFERENCES

1. Anderson C: *Manual for the Examination of Bone.* CRC Press, Boca Raton, FL, 1982.
2. Baron R, Vignery A, Neff L, et al: Processing of undecalcified bone specimens for bone histomorphometry. In: Recker RR, ed: *Bone Histomorphometry: Techniques and Interpretation.* CRC Press, Boca Raton, FL, 1983:13–35.
3. Derkx P, Birkenhäger-Frenkel DH: A thionin stain for visualizing bone cells, mineralizing fronts and cement lines in undecalcified bone sections. *Biotech Histochem* 70:70–74, 1995.

4. Gruber HE and Mekikian P: Application of Stains-All for demarcation of cement lines in methacrylate-embedded bone. *Biotech Histochem* 66:181–184, 1991.

5. Gruber HE: Adaptations of Goldner's Masson trichrome stain for the study of undecalcified plastic embedded bone. *Biotech Histochem* 67:30–34, 1992.

6. Gruber HE, Marshall GJ, Kirchen ME, et al: Improvements in dehydration and cement line staining for methacrylate embedded human bone biopsies. *Stain Technol* 60:337–344, 1985.

7. Gruber HE, Marshall GJ, Nolasco LM, et al: Alkaline and acid phosphatase demonstration in human bone and cartilage: effects of fixation intervals and methacrylate embedments. *Stain Technol* 63:299–306, 1988.

8. Gruber HE, Stasky AA: Large specimen bone embedment and cement line staining. *Biotech Histochem* 72:198–201, 1997.

9. Gruber HE, Stasky AA: Histologic study in orthopaedic animal research. In: An YH, Friedman, RJ, eds: *Animal Models in Orthopaedic Research.* CRC Press, Boca Raton, FL, 1999:115–138.

10. Hermanns W, Colbatzky F, Gunther A, Steiniger B: Ia antigens in plastic-embedded tissues: A post-embedding immunohistochemical study. *J Histochem Cytochem* 34:827–831, 1986.

11. Larsson L-I: *Immunocytochemistry: Theory and Practice.* CRC Press, Boca Raton, FL, 1988.

12. Lucena SB, Duarte MEL, Fonseca EC: Plastic embedded undecalcified bone biopsies: an immunohistochemical method for routine study of bone marrow extracellular matrix. *J Histotech* 20:253–257, 1997.

13. Malluche HH, Faugere M-C: *Atlas of Mineralized Bone Histology.* S. Karger AG, Basel, Switzerland, 1986.

14. Myers JD: Development and application of immunocytochemical staining techniques: A review. *Diagn Cytopathol* 5:318–330, 1989.

15. Page KM: Bone and the preparation of bone sections. In: Bancroft JD, Stevens A, eds: *Theory and Practice of Histological Techniques.* Churchill Livingstone, London, 1982:297–331.

16. Schenk RK, Olah AJ, Herrmann W: Preparation of calcified tissues for light microscopy. In: Dickson GR, ed: *Methods of Calcified Tissue Preparation.* Elsevier, Amsterdam, 1984:1–78.

17. Shi S-R, Cote RJ, Chen T, et al: Antigen retrieval technique: an important approach to standardization of immunohistochemistry. *Cell Vision* 3:235–236, 1996.

18. Shi SR, Cote RJ, Taylor CR: Antigen retrieval immunohistochemistry: past, present, and future. *J Histochem Cytochem* 45:327–343, 1997.

19. Tacha DE, Bowman PD, McKinney L: High resolution light microscopy and immunocytochemistry with glycol methacrylate embedded sections and immunogold-silver staining. *J Histotech* 16:13–18, 1993.

20. Taylor CR, Shi SR, Chen C, et al: Comparative study of antigen retrieval heating methods: microwave, microwave and pressure cooker, autoclave, and steamer. *Biotech Histochem* 71:263–270, 1996.

21. Tsuji Y, Kusuzaki K, Hirasawa Y, et al: Ki-67 antigen retrieval in formalin-or ethanol-fixed, paraffin-embedded tissues: an enhancement method for immunohistochemical staining with autoclave treatment. *Acta Histochem Cytochem* 30:251–255, 1997.

22. Villaneuva AR, Hattner RS, Frost HM: A tetrachrome stain for fresh mineralized bone sections. *Stain Technol* 39:87–94, 1964.

23. Wakamatsu K, Ghazizadeh M, Ishizaki M, et al: Optimizing collagen antigen unmasking in paraffin-embedded tissues. *Histochem J* 29:65–72, 1997.

21

Basic Staining Techniques for Cartilage Sections

Helen E. Gruber and Jane A. Ingram

Orthopaedic Research Biology, Department of Orthopaedic Surgery,
Carolinas Medical Center, Charlotte, NC, USA

I. INTRODUCTION

Historically, growth plate (physeal) and articular cartilage have received greater attention than bone because they can be processed and sectioned more easily following paraffin and glycol methacrylate embedment and because they contain extracellular matrix (ECM) components whose interest and importance is not only confined to the skeleton.[23] Histology has also played a role in defining the cell and matrix degradation that occurs in osteoarthritis and rheumatoid arthritis. Recently, there has been renewed interest in reliable and informative staining methods for articular cartilage, which can be used in the evaluation of tissue-engineered cartilage. The purpose of this chapter is to review the utility of fundamental staining procedures for cartilage specimens.

II. FIXATION, DECALCIFICATION, AND EMBEDDING CHOICES

As summarized in Chapter 20, which focuses on histologic stains for bone, histologic studies of cartilage should be planned to optimize the choice of fixative with a decision as to whether the specimen will be decalcified and embedded in paraffin or whether it will be processed undecalcified and embedded in glycol or methyl methacrylate (MMA).[16] If the evaluation and quantitation of cartilage dynamic mineralization is an important goal, then the specimen must be processed undecalcified. For embryonic or early postnatal animal specimens, with only a small amount of bone present, glycol methacrylate often is a useful embedding medium, and it affords good resolution for cell and matrix morphology (Fig. 1). Older postnatal specimens, specimens from weanling and adult animals, and specimens of healing fracture callus require MMA preparations (Fig. 2) or decalcification (Fig. 3). The choice of fixative is an important consideration which will depend on whether immunolocalization or enzyme histochemistry is required.

Fixative choice is extremely important in studies designed to evaluate ECM components. It has been suggested that conventional histochemical procedures may underestimate some ECM components because elements may not be completely immobilized by protein crosslinking reactions that occur during standard formalin fixation.[14] ECM proteoglycan (PG) macromolecules are easily extracted during conventional histologic aldehyde fixation and during decalcification,[12,30] and 50% ethanol can also contribute to

From: *Handbook of Histology Methods for Bone and Cartilage*
Edited by: Y. H. An and K. L. Martin © Humana Press Inc., Totowa, NJ

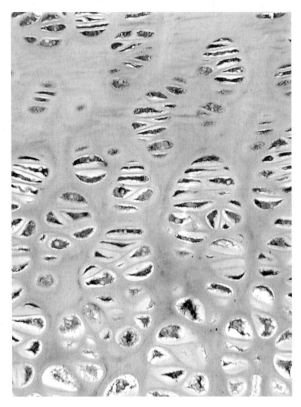

Figure 1. This photomicrograph of a pediatric distal femoral physis illustrates the excellent quality of cellular and matrix preservation afforded by embedding in glycol methacrylate (Toluidine blue). Magnification ×380.

processing changes because it can precipitate glycosaminoglycans (GAGs).[5] Although up to a 40% loss of PG has been seen in arterial smooth-muscle-cell cultures,[3] Kiviranta[12] has found that cubes of articular cartilage have lost little PG when fixed with buffered 4% formaldehyde. Cationic dye supplementation can also improve retention of PG, a process more common to transmission electron microscopy (TEM) than light microscopy. Other methods reported to improve retention include inclusion of 4% buffered formaldehyde or 0.5% safranin O in the decalcification fluid.[11] However, safranin O addition interferes with subsequent immunohistochemistry, so its use should be carefully considered.

Whole specimen *(en bloc)* preparations are sometimes of interest when examining embryos, small vertebrates, and blocks of articular cartilage. This allows visualization of limb and bone patterning throughout the skeleton—a great advantage in assessing changes in transgenic and mutant mouse embryos. Slices of articular cartilage have also been studied using *en bloc* staining with Weigert's iron hematoxylin, Weigert's hematoxylin and eosin (H&E), Harris' hematoxylin, Harris' hematoxylin and eosin, oil red O, and oil red O with Weigert's iron hematoxylin as described by Kincaid and Evander.[10] Specimens were then dehydrated in alcohol and cleared in methyl salicylate, and the suspended specimen was examined with a dissecting microscope. Differential stains for bone

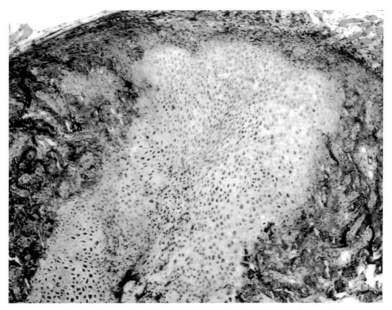

Figure 2. Photomicrograph illustrating a preparation of a rat fibular fracture callus embedded in MMA and stained with Goldner's stain. Magnification ×75.

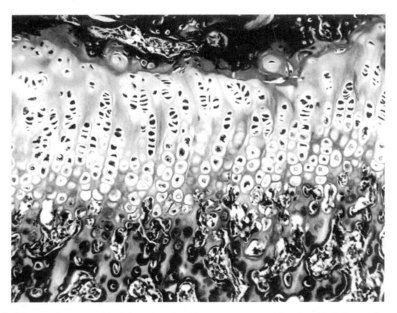

Figure 3. Photomicrograph of the physis of a young rat stained with Masson's trichrome; cartilage appears pale and bone dark blue in the original preparation. (Decalcified paraffin embedment.) Magnification ×190.

and cartilage in whole-mount embryo preparations have also been reported[7,9,19] using alcian blue to stain cartilage and alizarin red S to stain bone.

A final note on specimen preparation concerns the effects of exposure of cartilage to air. Speer et al. have reported that they found depletion of GAGs (as evidenced by loss of surface staining with toluidine blue) in articular cartilage allowed to dry for 1 h during a

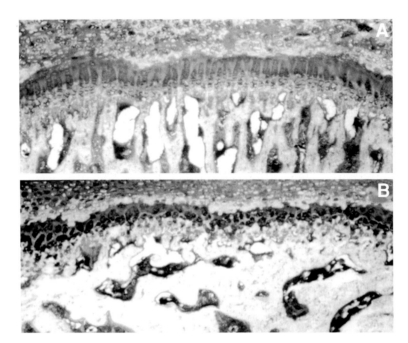

Figure 4. PAS staining in a normal rat physis (A) and a physis from a rat fed a low-magnesium diet (B). Note the abnormal staining pattern, thinner growth plate and irregular column
formation in the experimental specimen from a rat maintained on a low-magnesium diet for 4
wk (MMA embedment). Magnification ×200.

surgical procedure.[29] Based on this finding, it would also be prudent to prevent air-drying
during harvest and trimming of joint specimens prior to fixation.

III. FREQUENTLY USED CARTILAGE STAINS

The major matrix products of cartilage are PGs, collagen, and hyaluronic acid. Scott[23]
has reviewed staining of PGs and related this to the biochemistry of the ECM. Commonly
used procedures for PG staining include the cationic stains toluidine blue and basic
fuchsin. If the cartilage matrix components are of special interest, the metachromatic
stains—including azure A and the critical electrolyte staining series with alcian blue[24]—
are valuable.[18] The alcian blue critical electrolyte concentration method has been applied
to paraffin sections and to Epon-embedded tissue by Mallinger et al.[15] The periodic acid-
Schiff (PAS) method has been used by Kiviranta et al.[13] with quantitative evaluation of
staining with microspectrophotometry. The standard PAS method is believed to stain
oligosaccharides of glycoproteins and other structural cartilage matrix proteins. Since
faint collagen staining is sometimes noted, Scott et al. developed a modified PAS method
for polyuronides.[25–27] This method appears to be specific for chondroitin sulfate, as
shown by histologic studies paired with gas chromatographic analysis.[13] PAS can be
applied to decalcified paraffin-embedded and plastic-embedded specimens to investigate
the mucopolysaccharide content of cartilage.[4] Fig. 4 illustrates the uniform diastase-PAS

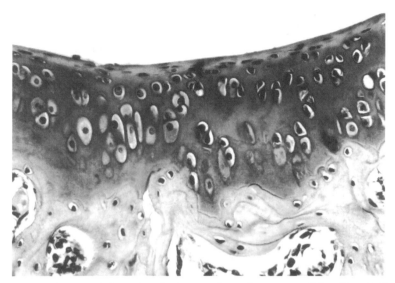

Figure 5. Safranin O staining of articular cartilage from a rat tibia. (Decalcified paraffin embedment.) Magnification ×450.

reactivity seen in normal rat cartilage. In contrast, cartilage from rats on a low-magnesium diet for 4 wk is shown.[4]

Safranin O, a frequently used stain in cartilage studies, is a cationic dye that binds to polyanions but not to collagen (Fig. 5). Chemical studies of this dye show that one molecule of safranin O binds to each negatively charged group of chondroitin 6-sulphate and keratan sulphate.[21] This stain has been used in an automated cartilage histomorphometric analysis method by O'Driscoll et al.[17] However, it is worth noting that there can be problems associated with the interpretation of safranin O staining. It may not be a sensitive indicator of PG content in diseases in which cartilage has a large GAG loss, as noted by Camplejohn and Allard in a comparative study with monoclonal antibodies (MAbs) to specific epitopes of cartilage PG.[1] In our experience, a modification of the safranin O-light green procedure by Jenkins[8] offers more reliable staining of articular cartilage in routine experimental animal specimens.

Masson's trichrome and its variations are also useful for differentiating bone (which stains dark blue) from cartilage (which stains a very pale blue) in decalcified preparations (Fig. 3).

Horton and Rimoin have shown the utility of specialized stains such as von Kossa-trichrome in the identification of inclusion bodies in cartilage from skeletal dysplasia patients.[6]

IV. SEMIQUANTITATIVE GRADING SCALES
FOR CARTILAGE EVALUATION

Experimental histologic studies often need well-designed end points to characterize cartilage healing after surgical creation of defects or following implantation of tissue-engineered implants. Several recent studies have utilized semiquantitative grading scales, which should have value in various types of cartilage studies. Pineda et al. have based their scale on four major outcomes: filling of the defect, reconstitution of the osteochondral junction, matrix staining, and cell morphology.[20] A later modification of the system by Caplan et al. extends the categories with evaluation of surface regularity and bonding of the implant with surrounding cartilage.[2] Other scoring systems have expanded scoring of cellularity, type of cartilage (hyaline or fibrocartilage) and repair features within the implant,[22] and architecture within the entire defect, and replacement of subcondral bone and reformation of the tidemark.[28]

REFERENCES

1. Camplejohn KL, Allard SA: Limitations of safranin O staining in proteoglycan-depleted cartilage demonstrated with monoclonal antibodies. *Histochemistry* 89:185–188, 1988.
2. Caplan AI, Elyaderani M, Mochizuki Y, et al: Principles of cartilage repair and regeneration. *Clin Orthop* 342:254–269, 1997.
3. Chen K, Wright T: Proteoglycans in arterial smooth muscle cell cultures. *J Histochem Cytochem* 32:347–357, 1984.
4. Gruber HE, Massry SG, Brautbar N: Effect of relatively long-term hypomagnesemia on the chondro-osseous features of the rat vertebrae. *Miner Electrolyte Metab* 20:282–286, 1994.
5. Hall D: *The Methodology of Connective Tissue Research.* Joynson-Bruvvers, Oxford, UK, 1976:130.
6. Horton WA, Rimoin DL: Histochemical characterization of the endochondral growth plate: a new approach to the study of the chondrodystrophies. *Birth Defects: Original Article Series* XIV:81–93, 1978.
7. Hu Y, Baud V, Delhase M, et al: Abnormal morphogenesis but intact IKK activation in mice lacking the IKKα subunit of IκB kinase. *Science* 284:316–320, 1999.
8. Jenkins L: Histotechnology of Implant-Tissue Interface: Processing, Resin Selection, Staining, and Immunohistochemistry. http://www.biomaterials.org/online/jhandout.htm. 2000, (UnPub).
9. Kelly WL, Bryden MM: A modified differential stain for cartilage and bone in whole mount preparations of mammalian fetuses and small vertebrates. *Stain Technol* 58:131–134, 1983.
10. Kincaid SA, Evander SA: *En bloc* staining of articular cartilage and bone. *Stain Technol* 60:21–28, 1985.
11. Király K, Lammi M, Arokoski J, et al: Safranin O reduces loss of glycosaminoglycans from bovine articular cartilage during histological specimen preparation. *Histochem J* 28:99–107, 1996.
12. Kiviranta I, Tammi M, Lappalainen M, et al: Fixation, decalcification, and tissue processing effects on articular cartilage proteoglycans. *Histochemistry* 80:569–573, 1984.
13. Kiviranta I, Tammi M, Jurvelin J, et al: Demonstration of chondroitin sulphate and glycoproteins in articular cartilage matrix using periodic acid-Schiff (PAS) method. *Histochemistry* 83:303–306, 1985.
14. Lin WQ, Shuster S, Maibach HI, et al: Patterns of hyaluronan staining are modified by fixation techniques. *J Histochem Cytochem* 45:1157–1163, 1997.
15. Mallinger R, Geleff S, Böck P: Histochemistry of glycosaminoglycans in cartilage ground substance. Alcian-blue staining and lectin-binding affinities in semithin Epon sections. *Histochemistry* 85:121–127, 2000.
16. O'Connor KM: Unweighting accelerates tidemark advancement in articular cartilage at the knee joint of rats. *J Bone Miner Res* 12:580–589, 1997.
17. O'Driscoll SW, Marx RG, Fitzsimmons JS, et al: Method for automated cartilage histomorphometry. *Tissue Eng* 5:13–23, 1999.

18. Page KM: Bone and the preparation of bone sections. In: Bancroft JD, Stevens A, eds: *Theory and Practice of Histological Techniques.* Churchill Livingstone, London, UK, 1982:297–331.
19. Park EH, Kim DS: A procedure for staining cartilage and bone of whole vertebrate larvae while rendering all other tissues transparent. *Stain Technol* 59:269–272, 1984.
20. Pineda S, Pollack A, Stevenson S, et al: A semiquantitative scale for histologic grading of articular cartilage repair. *Acta Anat* 143:335–340, 1992.
21. Rosenberg L: Chemical basis for the histological use of safranin O in the study of articular cartilage. *J Joint Surg [Am]* 55:69–82, 1971.
22. Schreiber RE, Ilten-Kirby BM, Dunkelman NS, et al: Repair of osteochondral defects with allogeneic tissue engineered cartilage implants. *Clin Orthop* 367:S382–S395, 1999.
23. Scott JE: Proteoglycan histochemistry—A valuable tool for connective tissue biochemists. *Coll Relat Res* 5:541–575, 1985.
24. Scott JE, Dorling J: Differential staining of acid glycosaminoglycans (mucopolysaccharides) by alcian blue in salt solutions. *Histochemie* 5:221–233, 1965.
25. Scott JE, Dorling J: Periodate oxidation of acid polysaccharides. III. A PAS method for chondroitin sulphates and other glycosamino-glycuronans. *Histochemie* 19:295–301, 1969.
26. Scott JE, Harbinson RJ: Periodate oxidation of acid polysaccharides. Inhibition by the electrostatic field of the substrate. *Histochemie* 14:215–220, 1968.
27. Scott JE, Harbinson RJ: Periodate oxidation of acid polysaccharides. II. Rates of oxidation of uronic acids in polyruonides and acid mucopolysaccharides. *Histochemie* 19:155–161, 1969.
28. Sellers RS, Zhang RW, Glasson SS, et al: Repair of articular cartilage defects one year after treatment with recombinant human bone morphogenetic protein-2 (rhBMP-2). *J Bone Joint Surg [Am]* 82:151–160, 2000.
29. Speer KP, Callaghan JJ, Seaber AV, et al: The effects of exposure of articular cartilage to air. *J Bone Joint Surg [Am]* 72:1442–1450, 1990.
30. Szirmai J: Quantitative approaches in the histochemistry of mucopolysaccharides. *J Histochem Cytochem* 11:24–34, 1963.

22

Histochemical and Immunohistochemical Staining of Cartilage Sections

Andreas G. Nerlich

Institute of Pathology, Academic Teaching Hospital Munich-Bogenhausen, Munich, Germany

I. INTRODUCTION

The histochemical and immunohistochemical analysis of cartilage tissue provide important information about many physiological and pathological processes in this tissue. This chapter is designed to provide an overview of certain applications and techniques of histochemistry and immunohistochemistry for the study of cartilage. It should be noted that there are several types of cartilage tissue (hyaline, elastic, and fibrocartilage), for which different methods of tissue embedding may be required. There are different staining techniques for the localization of specific structures. This chapter provides a basic overview, and refers those readers who are interested in more specific questions to more specialized literature.

II. TYPES OF CARTILAGE TISSUE

In the human, three basic types of cartilage can be found. Different cartilage types are found at different sites in the body, and show some variation in their molecular composition. The most prevalent type of cartilage tissue—hyaline cartilage—is present in almost all joints, and comprises the cartilage of most laryngeal structures and the trachea, the ribs, and the epiphyses. The only exceptions to this cartilage type in joints are the temporomandibular and sternoclavicular joints, which consist of fibrocartilage. In the larynx, the thyroid, cricoid, triticeal, and arytenoid cartilages are of the hyaline type. Other laryngeal cartilages—such as the epiglottic, corniculate and cuneiform cartilage—are made of elastic cartilage. This cartilage type is also found in auricular and bronchiolar cartilage. Fibrocartilage is found in all discal and meniscal cartilages, the intervertebral discs (except for the end plate, which is made up of hyaline cartilage), the symphyseal and glenoid cartilages, and the joint cartilages of the temporomandibular and sternoclavicular joints.

On the histomorphological level, these three cartilage types differ in the composition and structure of the extracellular matrix (ECM). In hyaline cartilage, the matrix is composed of a collagen network comprised mainly of the cartilage-specific collagen type II along with the minor collagens IX and XI, with collagen VI in the territorial matrix and

From: *Handbook of Histology Methods for Bone and Cartilage*
Edited by: Y. H. An and K. L. Martin © Humana Press Inc., Totowa, NJ

collagen type X in hypertrophic cartilage. Fibrocartilage contains a mixture of the ubiquitous collagen type I with the cartilage collagen type II (along with the other collagen types previously mentioned, plus collagen types III and V). Elastic cartilage also contains elastic fibers.

III. CHOICE OF TISSUE-EMBEDDING PROCEDURE AND SECTION PREPARATION

Before histochemical or immunohistochemical studies can be performed, the type of tissue preparation, and in particular the method of embedding of tissue samples, should be considered. These may be essential for the further design of a study, because some information can only be revealed through the use of special embedding. Generally, three types of embedding procedures must be taken into consideration, and all of these have certain advantages and disadvantages.

A. Frozen Sections

The preparation of frozen sections of cartilage may be particularly useful for the localization of antigens that may be technically difficult to detect—i.e., when the antigen is not retrievable following fixation and paraffin embedding or the available antibody has a low titer and/or may produce a high background staining. For most histochemical staining, no particular pretreatment is necessary for frozen cartilage sections. For immunohistochemistry, however, depending on the antigen, pretreatments may be required, even in frozen sections. Thus, the close network of collagenous matrix molecules and large proteoglycans may require an unmasking of certain antigenic structures that may be achieved by enzymatic pretreatment. In addition, tissue to be cut frozen should not contain calcifications or bone-tissue segments, since these are very difficult to section. Remaining osseous tissue or focal calcifications may cause serious tissue disruption. Furthermore, the preparation of frozen sections is technically difficult and may lead to poor-quality sections, especially with relatively thick sections of more than 4-μm thickness. This in turn may lead to difficulties in the evaluation of tissue details, and the histochemical or immunohistochemical staining may give nonhomogenous distribution of the stain.

B. Paraffin Embedding

Of all the embedding procedures used in long-term preservation of tissues, fixation in formaldehyde (usually 4–6%) followed by embedding in paraffin wax is the commonly used method. The preparation of tissue blocks for long-term storage provides an opportunity to repeat or extend studies on archival material. Thus, embedding in wax has major technical advantages over the frozen section technique. Wax-embedded tissue can be sectioned much more easily than frozen tissue, and the resulting sections are much thinner (as thin as 2–3 μm). The preservation of tissue structures is also significantly better, and many morphological details that escape frozen section analysis may be detectable. On the other hand, during fixation and embedding, the tissue samples undergo various chemical alterations. Although there is little influence on almost all histochemical staining—except for lipid staining—there may be a significant influence on the antigen preservation, resulting in problems in immunohistochemistry. These can be overcome, at least for many antibodies, by adequate antigen retrieval. However, the application of new, untested antibodies may require extensive pretesting.

When cartilage tissue samples contain calcifications or if bone material adheres to the samples, a decalcification step is required. This decalcification can be performed by the use of chelating agents—in most instances by use of 0.1 M ethylenediaminetetraacetic acid (EDTA)—after fixation of the tissue. Chelating agents do not influence the structure of antigens, and thus do not alter methods for antigen retrieval. Using such a "mild" decalcification approach, specific information can be obtained for critical tissue regions, such as the cartilage-bone transition zone at joints or the cartilaginous end plate of the intervertebral discs. However, any decalcification step suppresses information about pathological calcifying processes in cartilage tissues, and because this information is often desirable, other embedding techniques may be used.

C. Resin Embedding

Tissue samples may be embedded in resin for the preparation of hard-tissue sections. This procedure is most often used for the histological investigation of bone-tissue samples. Its major advantage is that no decalcification is required. The resulting tissue blocks can be stored for long periods of time. The tissue sections are very thin (approx 1 μm), and the preservation of structural details is usually excellent. However, the commonly used embedding procedures, such as those using epoxy or acrylate resins, lead to severe chemical alterations of the tissue structure and thereby prevent the successful application of immunohistochemistry. Even histochemical staining such as the Prussian blue stain may not be successful on this material, because of alterations of the chemical structure of tissue components. However, stains for the localization of calcifications can be successfully performed (e.g., von Kossa's silver impregnation technique).

Recently, a modification of resin-embedding techniques has been established that allows the application of most of the usual histochemical staining techniques, and permits the use of immunohistochemistry.[4] This novel technique uses a low-temperature embedding procedure that does not destroy the antigenic structures in the tissue. Very recent applications of this technique to immunohistochemistry on cartilage tissue show that, for example, serial section staining for distinct antigens can be combined with the histochemical localization of calcifications within those tissues. However, this novel technique is more laborious, and the antibodies must be applied in higher concentrations than for other types of embedding. Thus, this technique is more costly, and its use should be limited.

IV. HISTOCHEMICAL STAINING OF CARTILAGE TISSUES

Although in most instances the application of routine stains, such as hematoxylin and eosin (H&E), provides sufficient information to properly evaluate most structural details of cartilage samples, specific histochemical stains may be necessary for further information. Most of these histochemical stains provide specific data on the structure and composition of the ECM. This is achieved by a more or less selective binding of certain chemical components to matrix constituents. Based on these observations, we can divide the most frequently used histochemical staining procedures into the following categories: stains for the localization of collagenous (e.g., van Gieson's, Masson's trichrome), elastic (e.g., orcein, Elastica), and reticular fibers (e.g., silver impregnation techniques); localization of proteoglycans and glycosaminoglycans (GAGs) (e.g., alcian blue and periodic acid-Schiff [PAS], safranin O); identification and localization of lipids (e.g., Sudan) and identification of abnormal tissue deposits, such as hemosiderin (Prussian blue) or calcifications (von Kossa). This list of stains and applications represents only a selection, with an overview of possible applications. Individual stains may be modified with respect to technical requirements or the scientific question.

A. Staining of Collagenous Connective Tissue

To selectively localize collagen fibers, the fairly selective binding of picric acid to those fibers can be used. Typical histochemical stains for the identification of collagen fibers are the van Gieson's and Masson's trichrome stains. The technical procedures are described in more detail in Section IV.A1,2. In the van Gieson's stain, collagen fibers are strongly stained red, and in the Masson's trichrome stain they are green or blue, depending on the chromogen used. It must to be taken into consideration that these collagen stains do not reveal very small, "reticular" collagen fibrils that can be visualized using silver impregnation techniques.

1. Van Gieson's Stain

- 10-min staining of nuclei with Weigert's iron hematoxylin.
- Wash in water.
- 1–5 min in picrofuchsin solution (5 mL 1% aqueous solution of acid fuchsin solution added to 95 mL aqueous picric acid).
- Remove excess solution.
- Dehydrate, clear, and mount sections.

2. Masson's Trichrome Stain

- 10-min staining of nuclei with Weigert's iron hematoxylin.
- Wash in water.
- 5 min in 1% ponceau-acetic acid solution (equal volumes of 0.5% ponceau 2R in 1% acetic acid and 0.5% acid fuchsin in 1% acetic acid).
- Wash in water.
- About 5 min differentiation in 1% phosphomolybdic acid.
- Counterstain with light green (2% light green in 2% citric acid diluted 1:10 with distilled water prior to use) or aniline blue (boil 97.5 mL distilled water, and add 2 g aniline blue while still hot; add 2.5 mL glacial acetic acid, cool, and filter).
- Dehydrate, clear, and mount.

B. Staining of Elastic Fibers

Besides the collagenous matrix, elastic fibers represent a further system of extracellular fibrillar proteins that are of particular interest for the skeletal system. They are also essential for the identification of elastic cartilage. The most frequently employed staining methods use either orcein or a modification of the van Gieson's stain, the so-called Elastica-van Gieson's stain. These reactions show a selective binding to the protein "elastin." This matrix protein is part of the elastic fibril complex that is composed of elastin and microfibrils. In both described methods, elastic fibers are outlined as dark brown to black fibers.

1. Orcein Stain (Unna 1891)[12]

- 30–60 min in orcein solution (1 g orcein in 100 mL 70% alcohol, add 1 mL 25% hydrochloric acid).
- Wash in water.
- Differentiate in 95% alcohol.
- Clear and mount.

2. Elastica-van Gieson's Stain

- Immerse section in water.
- 2 min in acidified potassium permanganate (95 mL 0.5% potassium permanganate and 5 mL 3% sulphuric acid).
- Wash in water.
- 1 min in 1% oxalic acid.
- Wash in water and 70% alcohol (optional).
- 45-min staining in Weigert's resorcin fuchsin (0.25 g acid fuchsin, 0.5 mL nitric acid, 10 mL glycerin, picric acid until saturation, 90 mL distilled water).
- Wash in water.
- Differentiation in alcohol.
- Wash in water.
- 5 min in van Gieson's stain.
- Wash in water.
- Dehydrate, clear, and mount.

C. Staining of Reticular Fibrils

Besides the bundles of collagen, "reticular" fibers can be selectively morphologically identified by impregnation of those fibrils with silver under distinct reaction conditions, as described in detail in Section IV, C1. Reticular fibrils represent a biochemically heterogeneous group of matrix proteins that comprise tiny collagen fibrils—such as small interstitial collagen fibrils and collagen microfibrils—as well as non-collagenous microfibrils. During the reaction with silver, these fibrils are stained black. Larger associations of collagen bundles remain unstained, as do proteoglycans or glycoproteins.

1. Reticulin Stain (Gömöri 1937)[4]

- 2 min in 0.25% potassium permanganate.
- Wash in water.
- 1 min 3% potassium bisulfite solution.
- Wash in water.
- 1 min in freshly prepared 2% iron ammonium sulfate solution.
- Wash in water.
- 1 min in silver solution (10 mL 10% silver nitrate solution, add about 2 mL 1 M NaOH, add ammonia until the solution clears, add distilled water to bring to 100 mL).
- Wash in water.
- 10 min in formaldehyde solution 1:9 (made using 35% formalin).
- Wash in water.
- 10 min in 1% gold chloride solution.
- Wash in water.
- 1 min in 3% potassium bisulfite solution.
- 1 min in 1% sodium thiosulfate solution.
- Wash in water.
- Dehydrate, clear, and mount.

D. Staining of the Extracellular Ground Substance

Further targets for selective histochemical localization are components of the extracellular ground substance. These can be stained by histochemical reaction, either as an overall reaction covering all proteoglycans and glycoproteins, or as selective stains for glycoproteins with acidic or neutral/alkaline pH. Although the base reaction (PAS reaction) alone couples the chromogen to all GAGs and glycoproteins more or less extensively, a combination of this staining with the alcian blue stain may allow a distinction between acidic (alcian blue-positive) and neutral/alkaline (PAS-positive) proteoglycans and GAGs. The alcian blue stain reacts strongly blue, and the PAS reaction provides a pink stain.

Alternatively, a fairly selective staining of GAGs and proteoglycans is also possible using the safranin O/fast green stain, which is also frequently used for the staining of cartilage tissue under normal as well as pathological conditions.

1. Alcian Blue/PAS Stain

- 5 min in 1% alcian blue in 3% acetic acid (pH 2.5).
- Wash in water.
- 5 min in 1% periodic acid.
- Wash in water (distilled and tap water).
- 15 min in Schiff's reagent.
- Wash in water.
- 1 min in Mayer's hematoxylin.
- Blue in tap water.
- Dehydrate, clear, and mount.

2. Safranin O/Fast Green Stain

- 3 min in Weigert's hematoxylin.
- Wash in water.
- 15 s differentiation in acid alcohol (1% hydrochloric acid in 70% alcohol).
- Wash in water.
- 3-min staining in 1:5000 aqueous fast green.
- Wash briefly in 1% acetic acid.
- 3 min (maximum) staining in 0.1% safranin O.
- Rinse in 95% alcohol.
- Dehydrate, clear, and mount.

E. Staining for Lipid Deposits

Another histochemical stain for skeletal tissue analysis may be lipid staining. There are several staining techniques with different reaction targets. They may react with the lipid component itself, or an attached lipoprotein. However, in most instances, only the reaction with the lipid component itself is useful in evaluating the presence or absence of lipid deposits.

For the detection of lipid material, some prerequisites must be taken into consideration, since embedding techniques using solvents such as alcohols or acetone usually rapidly remove all lipid substances. These embedding procedures are usually an integral part of paraffin and resin embedding, so tissue embedded using these methods is inappropriate for lipid analysis. Thus, in paraffin-embedded material, only the presence of lipoproteins can be analyzed, and the stains for lipids are usually restricted to frozen section techniques. The most frequently used method is the Sudan red stain, which provides a strongly red signal in frozen sections.

1. Sudan III Stain (frozen sections)

- 15–30 min in Sudan solution (0.3 g Sudan III in 100 mL hot 70% alcohol, for several hours at 60°C, cool to room temperature, add 2–3 mL distilled water to solution prior to use).
- Wash in 50% alcohol.
- 3–5 min counterstaining of nuclei.

- Wash in water.
- 10 min blueing in tap water.
- Clear and mount.

F. Stains for Abnormal Deposits

In addition to the above mentioned extracellular material (Sections A–D), the detection of the deposition/presence of substances resulting from certain pathological processes may be of interest. One of the most interesting deposits in a multitude of tissues is the (older) blood residues, which can be identified as hemosiderin deposits. The histochemical identification of hemosiderin within a tissue section is regarded as proof of blood residues, since the staining method (Prussian blue) specifically reacts with trivalent iron ions, which occur as a result of a chemical transformation process actively executed by phagocytic cells. Prussian blue does not react with the divalent iron ions that are widely distributed in the body—e.g., in hemoglobin. Thus, this stain is not influenced by any blood contamination or exogeneous additions of the usually divalent iron ions. This stain yields a strong blue color.

With respect to skeletal tissue, the deposition of tissue calcifications may also be of particular interest. The histochemical stain for calcifications is a silver stain technique originally described by von Kossa. This method uses the chemical reaction between calcium ions and the reagents, resulting in the development of a black to dark brown color. However, this staining technique can be applied only to non-decalcified tissue samples, since decalcification will remove the calcium more or less completely. Therefore, except for the localization of minor calcium deposits, more pronounced deposits can be identified only on undecalcified sections, which may be prepared by resin-embedding.

1. Prussian Blue Stain (Perls 1867)[10]
- 20 min in equal quantities of 2% potassium ferricyanide and 2% hydrochloric acid.
- Wash in water.
- Counterstain 5 min in 1% neutral red.
- Wash in water.
- Dehydrate, clear, and mount.

2. Von Kossa Stain
- 45 min in 1% silver nitrate solution under bright light (bright sunlight or 100-W incandescent bulb).
- Wash in water.
- 5 min 3% sodium thiosulfate.
- Wash in water.
- Counterstain 5 min with van Gieson's stain.
- Dehydrate, clear, and mount.

V. HISTOCHEMICAL FINDINGS IN NORMAL CARTILAGE TISSUES

Normal cartilage tissues differ in the presence and/or distribution of certain components of the ECM. Thus, normal hyaline cartilage (e.g., of the joint surface) contains a delicate, almost invisible network of collagen fibrils (composed of collagen types II, IX, XI), which stain light red with the van Gieson's stain (Fig. 1) or blue/green with Masson's trichrome stain. There are no elastic fibers or reticular fibers to be identified. The ground substance normally contains a mixture of GAGs and glycoproteins, showing significant staining with the PAS reaction as well as with alcian blue. Normally, there are no lipid or hemosiderin deposits. Calcification occurs exclusively in the zone of cartilage calcification, close to the

Figure 1. Normal hyaline cartilage, stained for connective tissue fibers (van Gieson's stain) reveals a slightly diffuse staining pattern indicative of the fine meshwork of collagen fibrils within the amorphous ground substance. Original magnification ×400. (*See* color plate 11 appearing in the insert following p. 270.)

subchondral bone. This area is well-delineated by the "tidemark," a basophilically stained line seen in routine H&E staining. In the growing skeleton, hypertrophic chondrocytes are additionally surrounded by calcified cartilage matrix, which can be distinguished by the von Kossa's stain.

In contrast, elastic cartilage contains large amounts of elastic fibers that can easily be identified by a positive orcein/Elastica stain (Fig. 2). This cartilage type also contains the other components seen in the hyaline cartilage with a comparable distribution.

Fibrocartilage is significantly different from the other cartilage types with respect to the content of fibrillar collagen (on the molecular level, mainly collagen types I and III together with some minor collagen types). Fibrocartilage shows a significantly more intense red staining with the van Gieson's stain (Fig. 3), as well as increased staining with the Masson's trichrome stain and less intense staining for the GAGs and proteoglycans. The PAS stain shows only minor pink staining, and the alcian blue stain is mostly almost completely negative. Normal elastic cartilage and fibrocartilage show no calcifications, no lipid deposition (except for fat cells that may occasionally be interspersed in fibrocartilaginous structures, such as the insertion zone of menisci), and no hemosiderin deposits.

A particular type of cartilage tissue is represented by the intervertebral disc, which contains fibrocartilage in the annulus fibrosus and hyaline cartilage in the end plate. The nucleus pulposus seems to be unique, since this type of cartilage combines hyaline and fibrocartilage properties with the residues of the notochord. Thus, the tissue composition of these three anatomical zones is significantly different, and this is also reflected by the presence of certain components of the ECM. Some differences can be detected by histochemical staining, such as the density of collagen fibers, which is high in the annulus

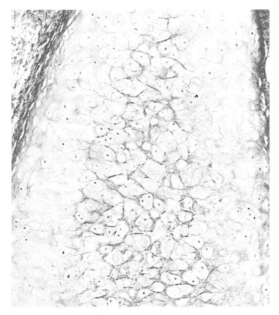

Figure 2. In normal elastic cartilage, the chondrocytes are surrounded by ring-like collagen fibers (red in van Gieson's stain) and tiny elastic fibers (black). Original magnification ×400. (*See* color plate 11 appearing in the insert following p. 270.)

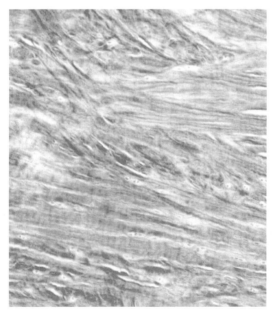

Figure 3. Fibrocartilage of the meniscus reveals a strong staining for the parallel thick collagen fiber bundles, which are characteristic of this type of cartilage. Elastica-van Gieson's stain; original magnification ×400. (*See* color plate 11 appearing in the insert following p. 270.)

fibrosus and far lower in the nucleus pulposus and the end plate. Elastic fibers are present in the annular regions—showing very delicate fibril structures—and the GAGs of the normal intervertebral disc are mainly non-charged, providing a positive PAS, but only minor alcian blue staining. Since tissue degeneration occurs very frequently in these discs, any change in the matrix is relevant for both the biomechanical properties of the disc tissue and the monitoring of tissue alterations, described in more detail in Section VI.

VI. HISTOCHEMICAL STAINING IN MAJOR PATHOLOGICAL CARTILAGE TISSUE CHANGES

A multitude of abnormal histochemical findings and patterns have been described in various pathological conditions of cartilage. Among those alterations, the cartilage degeneration in osteoarthrosis and that in degenerating intervertebral discopathy may represent the clinically most important and widespread diseases. In this section, we will discuss major changes in the histochemical staining pattern in these two diseases. Nevertheless, many other physiological or pathological conditions may occur in the cartilage system, and certain features may be monitored using histochemical staining such as trauma residues of the cartilage, changes of the matrix and cells in cartilage transplants, certain metabolic diseases (e.g., ochronosis, gout, and calcium arthropathy), and primary and secondary inflammatory diseases of the cartilage system (e.g., rheumatoid arthritis), and others. Because of space limitations, these will not be discussed here.

A. Osteoarthrosis

This condition occurs very frequently in weight-bearing joints because of mechanical overload. The resulting changes in the affected joint cartilage can be summarized by a loss of the cartilaginous surface until complete denudation of the joint surface occurs. During this process, the collagenous network undergoes an extensive change, which is reflected by a replacement of the collagen type II fibers by collagen type I- and III-containing fibers. This is also seen in histochemical staining for collagen fibrils by a so-called "fibrillar unmasking," which shows a significantly stronger staining with both van Gieson's and Masson's stains for collagen fibers. In parallel, the non-collagenous ground substance undergoes changes, a process that mostly precedes the collagen fiber changes. Thus, a very early sign of osteoarthrosis is the loss of proteoglycans at the joint surface (as evidenced by loss of safranin O staining; Fig. 4) and the change from a neutral to a predominantly acidic GAG staining pattern in the alcian blue-PAS stain.[5] More advanced stages are indicated by cartilage calcifications, which can be identified with the von Kossa stain. In the more advanced stages, the typical pattern of complete or near complete loss of the joint cartilage, significant new bone formation and focal islands of regenerative cartilage usually needs no histochemical confirmation (Fig. 5). However, in the very early stages, the loss of proteoglycans close to the joint surface and the fibrillar "unmasking" (e.g., the *de novo* synthesis of non-cartilage collagen types) may be of diagnostic significance. In experimental studies on osteoarthrosis, basic histochemical analysis should be included in order to identify the stages. The histochemical staining pattern may be used as a basis to define any type of cartilage tissue alteration.

B. Degeneration of the Intervertebral Disc

Although the pathological changes of the cartilage tissues in degenerative joint lesions affect only one type of cartilage tissue and therefore follow a certain line of alteration,

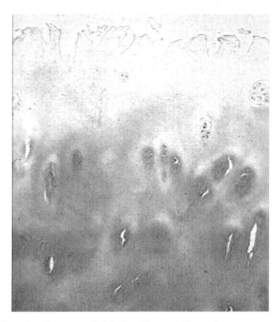

Figure 4. Safranin O stain of osteoarthritic hyaline cartilage shows a superficial loss of typical staining. This indicates a reduction of proteoglycans in the superficial layer of this cartilage. Original magnification ×400. (*See* color plate 11 appearing in the insert following p. 270.)

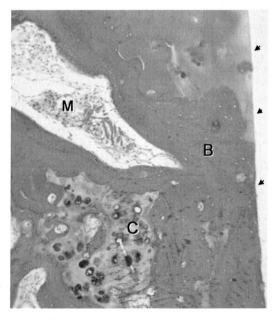

Figure 5. Advanced stages of osteoarthitis are characterized by a severe loss of the hyaline joint cartilage, regenerative islands of immature cartilage, and osteosclerosis. Original magnification ×250. (M) indicates marrow space; (C) indicates an isolated island of chondral tissue; (B) indicates sclerotic bone. Arrows at right depict cut surface of tissue. (*See* color plate 11 appearing in the insert following p. 270.)

the changes within the intervertebral discs associated with tissue degeneration are much more complex and variable.[7] This is at least in part because of the diversity of the cartilage tissue types. In addition, much less is known about the pathophysiology of disc degeneration, and therefore any type of "staging" pathological processes in the discs is much more uncertain.

When the histochemical changes of the degenerating intervertebral disc are examined, it is useful to have an individual view of each of the three histo-anatomic regions. In the nucleus pulposus, beginning with late adolescence and continuing into early adulthood, the tissue is disrupted with multiple clefts and tears, the chondrocytes react with cellular proliferation, and clusters of chondrocytes form.[7] In addition, chondrocyte necrosis can be seen, and a granular matrix transformation of as yet unknown molecular background develops. In this tissue, the histochemical collagen staining reveals an increase in the collagen-positive staining, which is comparable to the collagen fiber "unmasking" seen in osteoarthrotic joint cartilage. Here, a similar molecular mechanism is obvious, such as a loss of the cartilage collagen type II and an increase in non-cartilaginous collagen types I and III. In addition, the ground substance shows a change from neutral and alkaline GAGs to acidic types and an increased affinity for alcian blue staining. Minor focal calcifications can be monitored using the von Kossa's stain. In the annulus fibrosus, which represents a very compact collagenous network with relatively few GAGs, degeneration is similarly associated with an increase in acidic GAGs. Likewise, adjacent to clefts and tears, an enhanced and often strong staining is seen with alcian blue. Granular matrix alterations, which may occur in both the nuclear and the annular tissues, may stain strongly with alcian blue. However, this feature is not seen consistently, so it has been assumed that those granular matrix changes may be composed of debris from various proteins and glycosaminoglycans. In the cartilaginous end plate of the intervertebral disc, tissue degeneration that closely resembles osteoarthrosis is seen. Thus, a loss of proteoglycans and fibrillar unmasking with enhanced collagen staining are frequently seen, often associated with calcifications that may be so delicate that they are identified only by the use of histochemical staining. Peripheral lesions, mostly affecting the annulus fibrosus and presenting as tears, sometimes provide evidence for bleeding residues. These can be identified by the Prussian blue stain which shows strong blue deposits in those areas, often as small, round inclusions in macrophages.

VII. TECHNIQUES FOR IMMUNOHISTOCHEMICAL STAINING OF CARTILAGE TISSUE

The application of immunohistochemical staining has significantly expanded our knowledge of molecular changes at the tissue level. This technique may be applied, by use of specific antibodies, to an almost unlimited number of possible targets, since antibodies can be generated against every protein/peptide (including the protein core of proteoglycans). With respect to cartilage, a considerable number of antigens can be used in order to identify and localize specific structures. These can be used to identify cellular or extracellular targets.

In Section VIII, we will discuss a selection of potentially interesting antigens that may be helpful for studies of cartilage tissues. However, we must first take a closer look at the various immunohistochemical techniques in order to describe the advantages and disadvantages of those methods. This chapter provides only a brief overview of technical details. The more interested reader and the practical applicant are referred to more detailed descriptions in the literature.

In general, all immunostaining techniques are based on the binding of a specific antibody to a target antigen. This binding is mediated by the variable site of the antibody, and the invariable end of the antibody remains unbound. The complex of antigen and antibody can be visualized by binding of the antibody via its invariable end to a secondary antibody system. This is possible because species-specific protein structures serve as targets for the secondary system (e.g., primary antibodies generated in rabbits can be localized by an anti-rabbit secondary system). The resulting primary-secondary antibody complex is finally detected by the reaction of an enzyme (e.g., peroxidase, alkaline phosphatase), which is coupled to the secondary antibody and which provides a color reaction when appropriate substrates are added. Recent advances provide a significant amplification of the resulting signals by complexing the antibody system to large signals, thereby increasing the sensitivity of the immunoreaction.

A. The Peroxidase Techniques

The peroxidase techniques are widely used for the localization of a broad range of antigens. Within this group of techniques, there are certain variations that mainly affect the type and size of the resulting signal and influence the sensitivity of the signal. Recent developments have significantly reduced the concentration of antibodies required to immunostain an antigen, by use of methods such as enhancement of the signal by metal (e.g., silver) ions. A brief overview is provided here to describe the various peroxidase techniques.

The avidin-biotin-complex method uses the high affinity of avidin or streptavidin to biotin. Since the latter can be coupled covalently to the secondary antibody without affecting the structure of the secondary antibody, the addition of avidin to this system results in a multiplication of the signals, thus increasing signal intensity. The second technique (labeled avidin-biotin technique = LAB) also uses biotinylation of the secondary antibody, which is then coupled with avidin molecules that are already linked to the peroxidase so that even more enzyme molecules can be coupled to the reaction site. This also enhances immunostaining significantly, and recent investigations describe the LAB technique as being 4–8 times more sensitive than the avidin-biotin-complex technique. Therefore, in most laboratories the LAB, or the corresponding LSAB technique based on streptavidin, are used.

1. ABC Immunostaining Method

- Pretreat slide with buffer.
- Application of normal serum, 20–30 min incubation.
- Incubation with specific primary antibody (polyclonal) as pretested.
- Washing step.
- Application of biotinylated secondary antibody (as pretested), 20–30 min incubation.
- Washing step.
- 20–30 min incubation with avidin-biotin complex.
- Washing step.
- Incubation with chromogenic substance (e.g., diaminobenzidine) until color development (control of color development under the microscope).
- Counterstaining of nuclei.
- Mounting.

The LAB/LSAB-system uses a (ready-to-use) mixture of the biotinylated secondary antibody with the enzyme-linked avidin/streptavidin so that the procedure is abbreviated. All other steps are performed in a similar manner.

Very recently, further enhancement of the signal has been achieved by use of larger signal molecules, such as dextran. Using this method, polymer conjugates (e.g., En Vision, DAKO) provide multiple reaction sites for the peroxidase so that significantly more signals are generated.

B. The Alkaline Phosphatase-Anti-Alkaline Phosphatase Technique (APAAP)

The second most important system is the APAAP system, which also uses the binding of primary and secondary antibodies to the antigen and the resulting complex. However, this final complex is visualized by coupling of the complex to alkaline phosphatase (ALP) and is then enhanced by linkage to further ALP complexes using anti-alkaline phosphatase antibodies. The resulting signal is significantly amplified and also provides a strong staining with specific localization of the antigen. Various dyes can be used as chromogenic substances, so that various colors can be developed.

1. APAAP Method

- Pretreat slide with buffer.
- Incubation with monoclonal specific primary antibody.
- Washing step.
- Application of anti-mouse serum, 30-min incubation.
- Washing step.
- Application of APAAP complex, 30-min incubation (this step together with washing steps can be repeated up to three times).
- Washing step.
- Application of chromogenic substance.
- Washing step.
- Mounting.

When polyclonal antibodies are to be used, the APAAP staining must be modified. In this instance, following incubation with the primary antibody and subsequent washing, a secondary antibody produced in the mouse against the primary antibody is applied. This is followed by the secondary anti-mouse system, as described in Section VII, B1.

The selection of a method depends on each individual study design, and may require pretesting prior to the analysis. The peroxidase-dependent systems have the advantage of high sensitivity. The recent development of signal enhancement provides an even greater staining sensitivity than for the APAAP technique. In the case of double-staining experiments, both systems can be applied. In addition, there are several other systems that may be used (e.g., colloidal silver staining).

C. Section Pretreatment

For all immunostaining, the pretreatment of tissue sections is of particular importance. This is required in order to make antigens accessible to the antibodies. Previous studies have shown that particularly in cartilage tissue, an enzymatic pretreatment is necessary, since the presence of large amounts of GAGs and proteoglycans leads to masking of antigens. Thus, even frozen sections need some enzymatic unmasking. Although this enzymatic unmasking usually must be pretested for each antibody and

Table 1. List of Selected Relevant Antibodies and Their Targets

Antibody	Cellular targets
S 100-protein	Chondrocytes, adipocytes, melanocytes, nerve-sheath cells
CD 45	Leukocytes
CD 20/79a	B-lymphocytes
CD 3/4	T-lymphocytes
Myeloperoxidase	Granulocytes
CD 68	Histiocytes, macrophages
CD 31	Endothelial cells
Factor VIII-rel antigen	Endothelial cells
CD 34	Perivascular smooth-muscle cells
α-SMC-actin	Smooth-muscle cells
Ki-67/MIB-1	Sell proliferation marker

Antibody	Major extracellular targets
Collagen II/IX/XI	Cartilage
Collagen X	Hypertrophic cartilage
Collagen I/III/V	Ubiquitous interstitial matrix
Laminins/perlecans	Basement membranes

even for each batch, certain estimations can be provided in general. For the localization of ECM components, such as collagens, frozen sections of cartilage usually require a pretreatment with hyaluronidase (in most instances 5 mg/mL diluted in phosphate-buffered saline (PBS) 20–30 min at room temperature). When paraffin-embedded sections are used, this pretreatment is enhanced by the addition of other enzymes, such as 0.1% pronase and/or 0.1% trypsin (in 0.4% $CaCl_2$). Cellular targets may require pretreatment with proteinase XXIV (e.g., CD 68) or proteinase E. The use of acrylate sections following low-temperature embedding (*see* Section III, C) requires the use of much more concentrated primary antibodies, and may also make it necessary to increase incubation times of the enzymes or increase their concentration. Tests of the reaction conditions should always be performed prior to the analysis, and the parallel use of negative and positive controls is highly recommended.

VIII. TARGETS FOR IMMUNOHISTOCHEMICAL STAINING IN CARTILAGE TISSUES AND THEIR FINDINGS IN NORMAL TISSUES

Among the multitude of commercially and non-commercially available antibodies, several antibodies are of particular interest for cartilage tissue analysis (*see* Table 1). These can be divided into cellular antigens that provide information on the phenotype or functional status of cartilage cells and extracellular antigens, which may give insight into the composition of the ECM and its pathological alterations.

A. Common Cellular Antigens

The identification of cellular phenotypes within cartilage tissue covers the presence of local cells and the identification of cells that have invaded the cartilage from another origin, such as inflammatory cells. Table 1 provides a list of selected antibodies. Generally, chondrocytes of various locations can be identified by immunostaining with the S 100-protein, which is not specific for cartilage and also occurs in other tissue structures, such as fat cells, nerve-sheath cells, and the dendritic cells of lymph follicles. Since those structures are usually clearly identifiable by morphological characteristics, the S 100-protein staining may be useful in identifying chondrocytes under pathological conditions. However, it is important to consider that fibrocartilage chondrocytes often do not react or react only very weakly with the S 100-protein antibodies, and thus they may avoid immunodetection.

A broad application for the identification of cells under pathological conditions covers the typing of immune cells that may occur in cartilage—e.g., during primary or secondary inflammatory processes, such as rheumatoid arthritis. Here, markers for leukocytes (common leukocytic antigen, CD 45) and specific markers for B–cells (e.g., CD 20 or CD 79a) and T–cells (e.g., CD 3 or CD 4) may be useful. Histiocytes and macrophages can be identified using other antigens (mainly CD 68, a lysosomal protein, which is also present in granulocytes). The formation of blood vessels can be monitored by immunostaining of endothelia (CD 31 = PECAM or factor VIII-associated antigen) and smooth-muscle cells surrounding small blood vessels ("pericytes") can be stained using antibodies against CD 34.

Certain information can also be obtained on the cellular function. Of significance is the determination of the cell proliferation index (the antibody MIB-1 recognizes the Ki–67 antigen, which is only expressed in proliferating cells) and antigens involved in activation and suppression of cellular decay (e.g., bcl-2-antigen and others). Similarly, cytokines, such as TGF–βs, TNF–α and others, can be localized. In addition, a multitude of cellular enzymes and surface proteins may provide important information on tissue changes.

B. ECM Antigens

One important application of immunohistochemistry is the identification and localization of the various collagen isoforms in cartilage tissue. These have particular significance because the collagen isotype composition is important for the biomechanical tissue properties, and may also reflect pathological changes. Recently, several commercial antibodies have proven to be of sufficient technical quality for use in cartilage tissues. Likewise, the presence of collagen type II along with types IX and XI is specific for cartilage tissue, regardless of the site of the cartilage. In contrast, the occurrence of the non-cartilage collagen types I and III reflect either major pathological changes in hyaline cartilage or represent fibrocartilage in which a mixture of collagen I and III together with the cartilage-specific collagen types occurs. Of particular interest is collagen type X, which is exclusively associated with chondrocyte hypertrophy.[13] Since this hypertrophic status of chondrocytes is physiologically present only in the growing skeleton, where it is an essential feature of the growth plate, and since the closure of the epiphyses is closely associated with the disappearance of this particular collagen type, collagen type X has proved to monitor chondrocyte hypertrophy during degeneration and other pathological processes.[2,3]

In contrast to the collagens, much less is known about the various components of the non-collagenous cartilage matrix, which are made up mainly by proteoglycans. Thus, specific antibodies against proteoglycans may be of interest for studying the metabolism and pathophysiology of those cartilage constituents.

IX. IMMUNOHISTOCHEMICAL OBSERVATIONS IN VARIOUS PATHOLOGICAL CARTILAGE TISSUES

Among the multitude of pathological processes that affect cartilage tissues, the degenerative lesions previously discussed in the Section IV of this chapter are of interest for immunohistochemical analysis. Again, the high frequency of these lesions and the enormous sociomedical impact of these diseases render them highly interesting for studies.

A. Osteoarthrosis

As already indicated in the histochemical findings, osteoarthrotic cartilage is characterized by a loss of cartilage, fibrillar "unmasking," chondrocyte proliferation, and ultimately the complete loss of the cartilaginous surface. Immunohistochemical studies have confirmed and extended these observations. Thus, the "fibrillar unmasking" is associated by a switch in collagen types with a replacement of the cartilage-type collagens by ubiquitous interstitial collagens.[1,7] Thus, immunohistochemically, a loss of collagen type II staining is seen along with the presence of collagen types I and III within the cartilage (collagen type III even seems to precede the appearance of collagen type I). Interspersed in this change of collagen types seems to be the expression of collagen type X. Usually, this collagen type is exclusively found in hypertrophic cartilage; thus, the (re-)expression of collagen type X indicates hypertrophic chondrocytic phenotype.[3] At present, this expression of hypertrophic cartilage collagen type X is regarded as the earliest sign of tissue disarrangement. However, it is still unclear whether this expression remains reversible and represents just a reparative process, or if it is already an irreversible pathological process. With ongoing osteoarthrotic changes, the cartilage-specific collagens gradually disappear until the total denudation of the joint surface leads to a complete loss, except for areas with regenerating cartilage.

On the cellular level, no specific cellular marker has yet demonstrated changes in the cellular phenotype. Secondary inflammatory infiltrates may be identified by immunostaining. However, the presence of immune cells should always be suspicious for primary inflammation of osteoarthritis (rheumatoid arthritis). In those instances, the typing of immune cells may provide further information on the type of inflammation. Finally, the ingrowth of blood vessels into the cartilage residues may be monitored by CD 31 staining.

B. Degeneration of the Intervertebral Disc

Because of the complexity of the intervertebral disc, significantly less is known about the immunohistochemically detectable changes in pathological intervertebral disc tissues. The data gathered by histochemical staining support this conclusion, and much of the information available is based on isolated findings. However, several significant changes in the cellular phenotype as well as the extracellular matrix have been recorded.

The most extensive changes have been seen in the ECM of the nucleus pulposus, which normally contains no collagen type I.[8,11] The expression of this collagen type therefore indicates major tissue alteration. In the fibrocartilaginous anulus fibrosus, a loss of cartilage-specific collagens (types II, IX or XI) suggests "scarring," and the occurrence of non-cartilage collagens in the end plate with its hyaline cartilage parallels the changes seen in osteoarthrosis. Interestingly, in contrast to joint degeneration, the hypertrophic cartilage collagen type X is expressed in the discs only in very advanced stages, not in the "early" stages.[2] In addition, the aberrant expression of matrix constituents that are normally not present in disc tissues has been seen in less advanced lesions of disc degeneration. This holds particularly true for the pericellular occurrence of collagen type IV, which is otherwise restricted to basement membranes.[7]

On the cellular level, very recent investigations provide evidence that of distinct phenotypic changes in the disc-cell populations. Thus, we have shown that beginning in early adulthood, disc tissue contain cells with histiocytic phenotype (CD 68-positive cells), which are associated with tissue degeneration. These cells may originate from monocytes/macrophages that have migrated into the discs. However, it is even more likely that those cells have arisen from transformation of local cells, since their morphology is otherwise undistinguishable from surrounding chondrocytes. This finding seems to be of particular significance because phagocytic activity within the tissue may be an important prerequisite for the development of clefts and tears that in turn are the cause for herniation.[9] To date, very little is known of other, non-collagenous matrix components that await further investigation.

X. CONCLUDING REMARKS

The application of histochemical and immunohistochemical staining techniques is essential for the analysis of physiological and pathological changes of a large variety of tissues. With respect to cartilage, certain prerequisites must be taken into consideration. These mainly comprise the type of tissue embedding, the choice of histochemical staining techniques, and the selection of appropriate antibodies for immunohistochemistry, including pretreatment and type of detection system. Once these are taken into consideration, a multitude of staining applications can reliably be performed.

REFERENCES

1. Aigner T, Reichenberger E, Bertling W, et al: Type X collagen expression in osteoarthritic and rheumatoid articular cartilage. *Virchows Arch B Cell Pathol Incl Mol Pathol* 63:205–211, 1993.
2. Boos N, Nerlich A, Wiest I, et al: Immunolocalization of type X collagen in human lumbar intervertebral discs during ageing and degeneration. *Histochem Cell Biol* 108:471–480, 1998.
3. Boos N, Nerlich AG, Wiest I, et al: Immunohistochemical analysis of type X collagen expression in osteoarthritis of the hip joint. *J Orthop Res* 17:495–502, 1999.
4. Gömöri G: Silver impregnation of reticulum in parffin sections. *Am J Pathol* 13:993–1002, 1937.
5. Lebeau A, Muthmann H, Sendelhofert A, et al: Histochemistry and immunohistochemistry on bone marrow biopsies. A rapid procedure for methyl methacrylate embedding. *Pathol Res Pract* 191:121–129, 1995.
6. Mankin HJ, Dorfman H, Lippiello L, Zarins A: Biochemical and metabolic abnormalities in articular cartilage from osteoarthritic human hips. II. Correlation of morphology with biochemical and metabolic data. *J Bone Joint Surg [Am]* 53:523–537, 1971.
7. Nerlich AG, Wiest I, von der Mark K: Immunohistochemical analysis of interstitial collagens in cartilage of different stages of osteoarthrosis. *Virchows Arch B Cell Pathol Incl Mol Pathol* 63:249–255, 1993.
8. Nerlich AG, Schleicher ED, Boos N: Immunohistologic markers for age-related changes of human lumbar intervertebral discs. *Spine* 22:2781–2795, 1997.

9. Nerlich AG, Weiler C, Zipperer J, et al: Immunolocalization of phagocytic cells in normal and degenerated intervertebral discs. *Spine,* 27:2484–2490, 2002.

10. Perls M: Nachweis von Eisenoxyd in gewissen Pigmenten. *Virchows Arch* 39:42–53, 1867.

11. Roberts S, Menage J, Duance V, et al: Collagen types around the dells of the intervertebral disc and cartilage end plate: an immunolocalization study. *Spine* 16:1030–1038, 1991.

12. Unna PG: Notiz betreffend die Taenzer'sche Orceinfärbung des elastischen Gewebes. *Monatsh prakt Dermatol* 12:394–396, 1891.

13. von der Mark K, Kirsch T, Nerlich A, et al: Type X collagen synthesis in human osteoarthritic cartilage: indication of chondrocytic hypertrophy. *Arthritis Rheum* 35:806–811, 1992.

23

Staining Techniques for Plastic-Embedded Specimens

Antonio Scarano, Giovanna Petrone, and Adriano Piattelli

Dental School, University of Chieti, Chieti, Italy

I. INTRODUCTION

Analysis of the bone-implant interface has been conducted on decalcified, paraffin-embedded sections, after implant removal, or in methacrylate-embedded tissue prepared by cutting and grinding.[5,15] In resin-embedded specimens, it is necessary to use stains with a molecular weight (mol wt) that allows penetration into the resin without problems. Several useful staining methods are described in this chapter.

II. TOLUIDINE BLUE

Toluidine blue has a mol wt of 369 Daltons.[13,16] Toluidine blue staining is very easy to perform, and can be carried out in about 15 min. Before the staining procedure, it is necessary to do a 5-min pretreatment of the specimen with H_2O_2 to improve the staining. Toluidine blue stain is prepared in the following manner:

Borax	1 g
Toluidine blue	10 g
Distilled water	100 mL

The solution is then filtered, and 30 mL of ethanol are added. This alcohol usually evaporates, and thus it will be necessary to periodically add some drops to the solution. One or two drops of the staining solution are put on the histological slide and are left for 15 min; then the stain is removed and the slide is washed under running water.

The drops must be placed very carefully in the center of the slide. The periphery of the slide must absolutely be avoided because the alcoholic solution can infiltrate between the specimen and the slide, resulting in the detachment of the specimen. This infiltration may also result in the staining of the inferior part of the specimen, resulting in problems in specimen focusing.

If the toluidine blue solution does not stain the specimen, more alcohol must be added or the slide may be placed a container with hot (about 30°C) water for 10–15 min. If the water temperature is higher than 30°C, the specimen may detach. Toluidine blue stains the tissues with various blue hues (*see* Fig. 1).

From: *Handbook of Histology Methods for Bone and Cartilage*
Edited by: Y. H. An and K. L. Martin © Humana Press Inc., Totowa, NJ

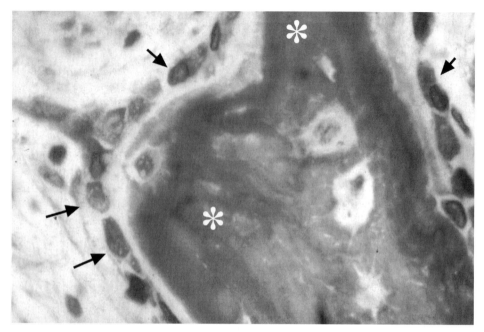

Figure 1. Staining with toluidine blue and acid fuchsin. Osteoblasts (black arrows) and woven bone areas (marked with *) are present.

III. SEVERAL SPECIAL STAINS

Acid fuchsin stains cementum, dentin, bone, and the soft tissues with various red hues. Sometimes it is used alone, but more often it is used to counterstain slides that have already been stained with toluidine blue (Fig. 1). Acid fuchsin has a good penetration in the resin, and it stains the tissues very strongly.

Von Kossa stain (silver nitrate) results in brownish-black color of the tissues that contain calcium carbonate and calcium phosphate (CaP) (Fig. 2). It is used as a aqueous solution of 0.9%. The solution must completely cover the resin-embedded tissues, and then the slides must be exposed to sunlight or bright light for 10–40 min.

Acid fuchsin and silver nitrate: This staining procedure is used to demonstate the presence of osteoid matrix. Silver nitrate is used first, and then the slides are counterstained with acid fuchsin.

Other stains such as periodic acid-Schiff (PAS), light green, and Masson's trichrome can be used, but these staining solutions have an acidic pH that can detach the specimen from the slide.

IV. HISTOCHEMICAL STAINING FOR ACP AND ALP

Enzyme histochemistry has become important in the study of bone tissue and the enzyme stains open a wide field for research of biological hard tissues such as bone and implants.[7] Acid phosphatase (ACP) and alkaline phosphatase (ALP) are enzymes responsible for the hydrolysis of phosphate esters, and are present in a wide variety of tissues,

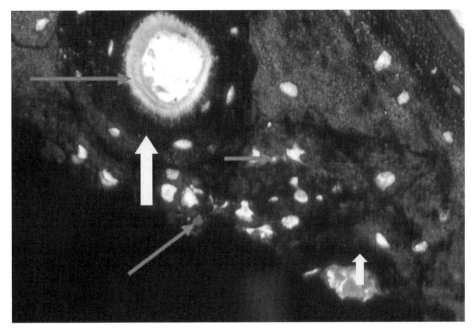

Figure 2. Silver nitrate (von Kossa) and acid fuchsin staining of mineralized bone that appears black. Mineralized bone is indicated by yellow arrows, and unmineralized areas are indicated by red arrows. (*See* color plate 12 appearing in the insert following p. 270.)

both mineralized and non-mineralized.[1-4] ACP activity is usually found in osteoclasts, although it can also occur to a lesser extent on some bone surfaces, presumably where resorption had occurred or where the enzyme had been released by the osteoclasts.

ALP activity (Fig. 3) is expressed early along the maturational pathway of bone cells, and is retained until the formation of early osteocytes and then lost.[10-12] ALP probably has a number of different functions:[9] i) it may serve as a calcium binding or transport protein; ii) it may serve as a generator of free phosphate; iii) it may degrade mineralization inhibitors.

Simultaneous demonstration of ALP and ACP in the same tissue section has been reported in paraffin or methacrylate-embedded tissues, but not on block sections with hard implant materials in bone (Fig. 4).[6,8] Bone ACP activity has been shown to be affected by demineralizing agents and also by fixatives.[14]

For the enzyme histological staining of acid phosphatase, the protocol is as follows:

1. Preparation of the following solutions:
   a. Dissolution of 2 g of pararosaniline in 40 mL of 2 N HCl; the solution is then moderately heated, filtered, and stored in the dark at 4°C;
   b. Solution of 4% sodium nitrite in distilled water;
   c. Michaelis Veronal-Acetate buffer solution, pH 5,5;
   d. Dissolution of 150 mg of naphthyl-phosphate AS-TR in 10 mL of N,N-dimethylformamide.
2. Staining: The sections are incubated for 4–5 h in 5 mL of solution C with 12 mL of distilled water + 1 mL of solution D. Then 0.8 mL of solution A and 0.8 mL of solution B are admixed and placed in the substrate-buffered solution. The specimens are then counterstained with toluidine blue.

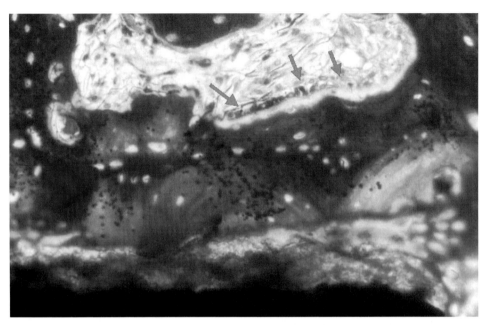

Figure 3. Silver nitrate (von Kossa) and alkaline phosphatase staining. Osteoblasts that are positive for ALP are present (arrows). (*See* color plate 13 appearing in the insert following p. 270.)

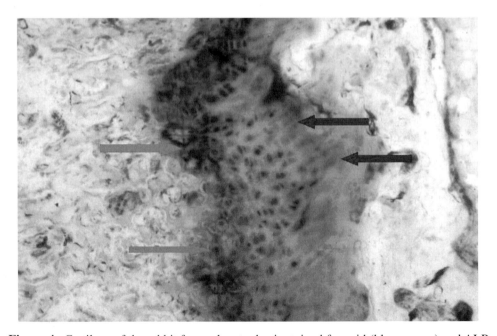

Figure 4. Cartilage of the rabbit femoral metaphysis stained for acid (blue arrows) and ALP (red arrows). (*See* color plate 14 appearing in the insert following p. 270.)

For the enzyme histological staining of ALP the protocol is as follows:

1. Preparation of the following solutions:
    a. Dissolution of 1 mg of 5-bromo-4-chloro-3-indolylphosphate-p-toluidine salt in 0.2 mL of N,N-dimethylformamide;
    b. Tris-maleate buffer, pH 8.9;
    c. Dissolution of diazonium salt in 1.5 mL of *N,N*-dimethylformamide;
    d. 10% solution of $MgCl_2$ in distilled water.
2. Staining:
    a. Slides are incubated for 24 h in 0.2 mL of solution A + 2 mL of solution B + 0.32 mL of solution D and a few drops of solution C. The enzyme activity is shown by the diazonium dye. When naphthyl-phosphate is used as a substrate, a black dye is formed using either fast blue RR or fast black B, and the color is brown when fast violet is used.
    b. The slides are then counterstained with toluidine blue or basic fuchsin.

REFERENCES

1. Anderson HC: Biology of disease. Mechanism of mineral formation in bone. *Lab Invest* 60:320–330, 1989.
2. Bianco P: Structure and mineralization of bone. In: Bonucci E, ed: *Calcification in Biological Systems.* CRC Press, Boca Raton, FL, 1992:243–268.
3. Bonucci E: Is there a calcification factor common to all calcifying matrices? *Scanning Microsc* 1:1089–1162, 1987.
4. Eanes ED: Dynamics of calcium phosphate precipitation. In: Bonucci E, ed: *Calcification in Biological Systems.* CRC Press, Boca Raton, FL, 1992:1–17.
5. Emmanual J, Hornbeck C, Bloeman RD: A polymethyl methacrylate method for large specimens of mineralized bone with implants. *Stain Technol* 62:401–410, 1987.
6. Gruber HE, Marshall GJ, Nolasco LM, et al: Alkaline and acid phosphatase demonstration in human bone and cartilage: effects of fixation internal and methacrylate embedments. *Stain Technol* 63:299–306, 1988.
7. Hillman G, Hillman B, Donath K: Enzyme, lectin and immunohistochemistry of plastic embedded undecalcified bone and other hard tissues for light microscopic investigations. *Biotech Histochem* 66:185–193, 1991.
8. Liu CC: A simplified technique for low temperature methyl-methacrylate embedding. *Stain Technol* 62:155–159, 1987.
9. Lo Storto S, Silvestrini G, Bonucci E: Ultrastructural localization of alkaline and acid phosphatase activities in dental plaque. *J Periodontal Res* 27:161–166, 1992.
10. Marks SC, Popoff SN: Bone cell biology: the regulation of development, structure and function in the skeleton. *Am J Anat* 183:1–44, 1988.
11. Morris DC, Masuhara K, Takaoka K, et al: Immunolocalization of alkaline phosphatase in osteoblasts and matrix vesicles of human fetal bone. *Bone Miner* 19:287–292, 1992.
12. Martin TJ, Ng KW, Suda T: Bone cell physiology. *Endocrinol Metab Clin North Am* 18:833–858, 1989.
13. Murice-Lambert E, Banford AB, Folger RL: Histological preparation of implanted biomaterials for light microscopic evaluation of the implant-tissue interaction. *Stain Technol* 64:19–24, 1989.
14. Popp W, Zwick A: Unfixed material embedded in a methacrylate resin (Technovit 7100) for immunofluorescent staining. *Stain Technol* 62:73–75, 198.
15. Steflik DE, McKinney RV, Mobley GL, et al: Simultaneous histological preparation of bone, soft tissue and implanted biomaterials for light microscopic observations. *Stain Technol* 57:91–98, 1982.
16. Van der Lubbe HBM, Klein CPAT, De Groot K: A simple method for preparing thin (10 microM) histological sections of undecalcified plastic embedded bone with implants. *Stain Technol* 63:171–176, 1988.

24

In Situ Hybridization of Bone and Cartilage

Shintaro Nomura and Seiichi Hirota

Department of Pathology, Osaka University Medical School, Suita, Osaka, Japan

I. INTRODUCTION

In situ hybridization is a technique that combines histology and molecular biology. *In situ* hybridization provides cell-type specific expression of genes along with their histological characteristics. This chapter is intended for beginners in either molecular biology or histology who want to begin *in situ* hybridization histochemistry. The chapter examines equipment and reagents that are specific for *in situ* hybridization; preparation of specimens (dissection, fixation, decalcification, embedding and sectioning); preparation of probes (design of probe, labeling, storage); hybridization (pretreatment of sections, hybridization, washing); and detection of the hybridized probe. In addition to the introduction of a general method used in the authors' laboratory, several optional or alternative protocols are described (*see* Table 1).

II. USES OF *IN SITU* HYBRIDIZATION

In situ hybridization allows us to determine the difference in expression pattern between homologous genes that belong to the same family. For example, the homology of amino acid sequence between BMP-2 and BMP-4 is more than 90%, and as a result it is very difficult to prepare antibodies that can distinguish between BMP-2 and BMP-4. However, the nucleotide homology in the mature protein region is approx 70%, and this difference is recognizable by hybridization.[5,9] Lower nucleotide homologies (50%) are reported in the precursor (pro-peptide) and noncoding (30%) region, which are easily recognizable even in low-stringency conditions. Therefore, *in situ* hybridization is far more useful for distinguishing cell-type-specific gene expression between highly homologous proteins than immunohistochemistry. In addition, we do not need to use full-length cDNA as a probe. A suitable probe size is between 300 and 600 nucleotides, which makes polymerase chain reaction (PCR) isolation possible. Finally, immunohistochemical analysis provides localization of gene products, but does not indicate which cell produced this, particularly when it is secreted extracellularly.[1,8] With *in situ* hybridization, researchers are no longer required to wait until a good-quality antibody appears on the market.

From: *Handbook of Histology Methods for Bone and Cartilage*
Edited by: Y. H. An and K. L. Martin © Humana Press Inc., Totowa, NJ

Table 1. Choices of *In Situ* Hybridization Methods

Fixation	**Paraformaldehyde,*** formalin, glutaraldehyde
Decalcification	**EDTA,** formic acid,[5]** (HCl),*** undecalcified[6]
Embedding	**Paraffin,** frozen, plastic[6]
Probe	**cRNA,** oligonucleotide, (cDNA), (PCR product)
Labeling	**Digoxigenin,** radioisotope,[7] (biotin)
Detection	**Immunohistochemistry,** autoradiography[7]
Signal developer	**APase,** POD, FITC,[8] rhodamine, silver grain[7]

* The standard method is indicated bold.[9]
** Alternative methods with references.
*** The methods in parentheses did not work in our laboratory.

III. EQUIPMENT AND REAGENTS

In addition to the use of ordinary equipment and reagents for molecular biology and histology, several specific ones are needed before starting this system. You should check those described in this section to determine whether or not they are in your laboratory.

A. Moisture Chamber

The moisture chamber is used for hybridization and immunoreaction. We usually use the "Incubation Chamber" (20CG Cosmo Bio., Tokyo, Japan. *http://www.cosmobio.co.jp*). Similar types of moisture chambers can be purchased from other companies, but you must ask the supplier if the chamber can be used at 60°C. Exposure to this temperature may bend the plastic lids on some chambers, and they will not retain moisture during hybridization.

B. Diethyl Pyrocarbonate (DEPC)

Diethyl pyrocarbonate (DEPC) quickly inactivates contaminating RNase. All glassware should be treated with DEPC-treated water to eliminate contaminating RNase. All water to be used for *in situ* hybridization should be treated by adding 0.02% DEPC for 60 min and autoclaved. All glassware is soaked in 0.02% DEPC-treated water for 60 min and baked at 65°C for 2 h.

C. 3-Triethoxylosilylpropylamine

3-Triethoxylosilylpropylamine is essential for coating glass slides. Without this silane-coating step, sections are easily detached from glass slides during the hybridization and washing steps. Glass slides are soaked in 2% 3-triethoxylosilylpropylamine in acetone for 10 s. Excess silane and acetone are rinsed off using acetone and DEPC-treated water, and then coated slides are air-dried and kept at room temperature. Silane-coated slides may be stored for 2–3 mo.

D. DIG RNA Labeling and Detection Kit

We usually use DIG-labeled cRNA probe (Roche Diagnostics) for hybridization. All reagents, buffers, antibodies, and enzymes required for labeling and detection are provided in the kit.

IV. PREPARATION OF SPECIMEN

A. Dissection and Fixation

Preparing a well-fixed specimen is essential to obtain satisfactory results of *in situ* hybridization. Bone and cartilage tissues from the femur, mandible, and rib of mice, rats, and guinea pigs can be analyzed by *in situ* hybridization without trimming. Larger samples must be trimmed to smaller than 1 cm cube, or the time needed for decalcification and dehydration will be too long. The conventional method is to cut tissues with a sharp razor blade or small scissors to expose bone marrow to fixative. Bone and cartilage are dissected with the surrounding soft tissues and fixed with 4% paraformaldehyde (electron microscopy grade) in 0.1 M phosphate buffer, pH 7.2 (this must be made up fresh before use and cooled on ice), at 4°C overnight. Perfusion is an excellent technique for fixation and gives better histology than immersion. However, it requires a longer time (more than 2 h for complete fixation of bone and cartilage in the rat femur). In addition to paraformaldehyde, we often use 10% neutral buffered formalin (NBF) or 2% glutaraldehyde in 0.1 M phosphate buffer, pH 7.2, for fixation. Other fixatives have not been tested comparatively.

B. Dehydration and Decalcification

Histological analysis of paraffin sections requires the following steps. Fixed samples are transferred to 0.1 M phosphate buffer, pH 7.2 (PB), and incubated at 4°C overnight to remove residual fixative. They are then dehydrated by a graded ethanol series (70%, 80%, 90%, and 3 changes of 100% for 6–12 h each at 4°C), and de-fatted in chloroform at 4°C overnight. After dehydration and defatting, samples are hydrated with a graded ethanol series (3 changes of 100% for 4 h followed by 1 change each of 90%, 80%, and 70% at 4°C overnight) and decalcified with 20% ethylenediaminetetraacetic acid (EDTA) (pH 7.4). Alternatively, decalcification can be carried out using Morse's solution (10% sodium citrate and 22.5% formic acid). We have found that hydrochloric acid (HCl) is not a good reagent for decalcification. We observed the disappearance of mRNA signals after overnight treatment with 10% HCl. Depurination and degradation of mRNA may occur with use of HCl. Ten to 14 days are needed for complete decalcification of rat femur. Slow shaking and agitation of the specimen during decalcification and a fresh change of EDTA every 3 d helps speed decalcification. At the end, the specimen becomes soft, and can be cut by a razor blade as easily as Cheddar cheese.

The protocol for preparing undecalcified sections is described in the following section.

C. Embedding and Sectioning

Decalcified specimens are dehydrated in a graded ethanol series, cleared in xylene or chloroform, and embedded in paraffin (m.p. 56–58°C). Sections of 3–6 μm are cut and mounted on silane-coated slides. Dried paraffin sections are stored at 4°C until use. Alternatively, decalcified specimens are rinsed in PBS (phosphate-buffered saline) and transferred to 0.5 M sucrose in PBS at 4°C for 24 h. After blotting off excess liquid, specimens are embedded in O.C.T Compound (Fisher Scientific) and frozen with liquid nitrogen to prepare frozen sections.

For preparing undecalcified sections, fixed specimens are dehydrated, cleared in xylene, and embedded in a 7:3 mixture of methylmethacrylate (MMA) and butylmethacrylate resins containing 3% benzoyl peroxide, 1:600 vol of N, N-dimethylaniline, and 1:20 vol of methanol and polymerized at 4°C for 24 h. Plastic sections are cut at 3 μm and mounted on silane-coated slides.

V. PREPARATION OF PROBE

We have learned that cRNA probes give us excellent results compared with oligonucleotide (low signal intensity), cDNA (often provide strong artificial signals) and PCR probes. Also, we usually use DIG (digoxigenin)-labeled probe for its sensitivity, resolution, stability, and safety. The suitable size of a cRNA probe is between 300 and 800 bases. The important problem is determining which part of cDNA will yield a good result. Our experience taught us that the result obtained changes dramatically, depending on which portion of the probe was used for hybridization. We found that we need to generate several probes and determine the optimal probe by using them one by one in hybridization experiments. Previous reports often indicate the best portion of cDNA for use for a probe. Often, the best way is to ask authors to provide the probe they used or subclone the same portion of cDNA by reverse-transcriptase polymerase chain reaction (RT-PCR) into the plasmid vector containing T3, T7, or SP6 RNA polymerase promoter. DIG-11-UTP is used as the transcription substrate. The important points for generating cRNA probes are:

1. Check the amount and size of the generated probe by agarose gel electrophoresis. Usually, more than 10 molecules of cRNA are transcribed from one molecule of template DNA, and the cRNA shows discrete bands after electrophoresis but the mobility of DIG-labeled cRNA is slower than expected.
2. DNase treatment after transcription is essential for obtaining a good result. Poor results obtained without DNase treatment are probably caused by the interaction of template DNA and cRNA product.
3. The probe must be stored at –20°C in the presence of 50% formamide because cRNA easily takes a secondary structure. In addition, the stored probe must be heat-denatured before use (85°C, 3 min). Alternatively, ^{35}S-UTP is also available for generating a radioisotope-labeled cRNA probe. The half-life of ^{35}S is approx 90 d. The freshly made ^{35}S probe should be used within 45 d. Oligonucleotide probe is labeled by a tailing reaction in which DIG-dUTP or ^{35}S-dTTP is used for substrate. The size of the tail is critical. The optimum length of the tail is less than one-half the size of the oligonucleotide (20 bases of DIG-dUTP or ^{35}S-dTTP for 40 bases of oligonucleotide). You should calculate the amount of substrate in addition to the enzymatic activity of terminal deoxynucleotidyl transferase.

VI. HYBRIDIZATION AND WASH

A. Pretreatment of Sections

Pretreatment is essential to prepare sections suitable for hybridization. Sections are dried with a blower (2–5 min), de-paraffinized in xylene (10 min, 3 changes), and rehydrated in graded ethanol series. After washing with twice with PB, sections are incubated in 1 μg/mL of proteinase K (Roche Diagnostics) in TE solution (10 mM Tris-HCl, pH 8.0, 1 mM EDTA) for 15 min at 37°C. Following proteinase K treatment, sections are re-fixed with 4% paraformaldehyde in PB for 10 min at room temperature to inactivate proteinase K. They are then washed once with PB and treated with 0.2 M HCl to inactivate the internal alkaline phosphatase (ALP), which is used for detection. HCl treatment is also effective in removing basic proteins. After washing once with PB, sections are equilibrated with 0.1 M triethanolamine-HCl buffer, pH 8.0, for 2 min. Acetylation of the sections is performed by incubating with freshly prepared 0.25% acetic anhydride in 0.1 M triethanolamine-HCl buffer, pH 8.0, for 10 min at room temperature. After acetylation, sections are dehydrated by graded ethanol series, air-dried, and used for hybridization the same day.

B. Hybridization and Wash

The hybridization solution contains 50% deionized formamide, 10% dextran sulfate, 1× Denhardt's solution, 600 mM NaCl, 0.25% SDS, 250 µg/ml of *E. coli* tRNA, 10 mM dithiothreitol (DTT), and 0.1 to 2.0 µg/mL of DIG-UTP or ^{35}S-UTP-labeled cRNA probe. The denatured probe is diluted with hybridization solution and incubated at 85°C for 3 min, then about 50 µl/cm^2 of hybridization solution is placed on the sections, and they are covered with Parafilm and incubated at 50°C for 16 h in a moisture chamber saturated with 50% formamide. For an oligonucleotide probe, the probe concentration used for hybridization is between 0.01 and 0.1 µg/mL, and the hybridization temperature is 35–45°C. The optimum conditions for hybridization using oligonucleotide probes should be determined critically.

After hybridization, the Parafilm is dislodged with pre-incubated 5× standard saline citrate (SSC) at 50°C, then the slides are incubated with 50% formamide in 2× SSC for 30 min at 50°C to remove excess probe. The slides are further incubated with TEN (10 mM Tris-HCl, pH 8.0, 1 mM EDTA, 500 mM NaCl) buffer for 10 min. RNase A treatment (10 µg/mL) is carried out at 37°C in TEN buffer for 30 min, and excess RNase A is removed by washing with TEN buffer. The slides are incubated with 2× SSC and 0.2× SSC for 15 min twice at 50°C. When an oligonucleotide probe is used for hybridization, the standard washing temperature is 37°C.

VII. DETECTION OF HYBRIDIZED PROBE

Washed slides are incubated with DIG-1 (100 mM Tris-HCl, pH 7.5, 150 mM NaCl) for 2 min, and then with 1.5% blocking reagent (supplied with DIG-labeling and detection kit, Roche Diagnostics) for 60 min at room temperature. 100 µg/cm^2 specimen of 1:500 diluted polyclonal sheep anti-digoxigenin Fab fragment (alkaline phosphatase conjugate) with DIG-1 is pipetted on to the section and incubated at room temperature for 30 min or 4°C overnight. After immunoreaction, slides are washed twice with DIG-1 for 15 min and equilibrated with DIG-2 (100 mM Tris-HCl, pH 9.5, 100 mM NaCl, 50 mM MgCl$_2$) for 3 min. Coloring solution containing 337.5 µg/mL of NBT (nitrotetrazolium blue chloride) and 165 µg/mL of BCIP (5–bromo-4-chloro-3-indolyl phosphate) in DIG-2 is applied to the sections and incubated at room temperature or 37°C until the signal-to-noise ratio becomes maximal (usually 3–24 h). The reaction is stopped by rinsing the slides with TE solution and the slides are mounted with Crystal Mount (Biomeda Corp., Foster City, CA) with or without counterstaining with methyl green. ALP conjugated anti-DIG antibody yields satisfactory results. POD-conjugate or fluorescence-conjugated antibody can also be used for detection (Fig. 1).

When the radioisotope ^{35}S-UTP is used for labeling, the washed slides are dehydrated and dipped in NTB-3 emulsion (Eastman Kodak, Rochester, NY) diluted 1:1 with 2%

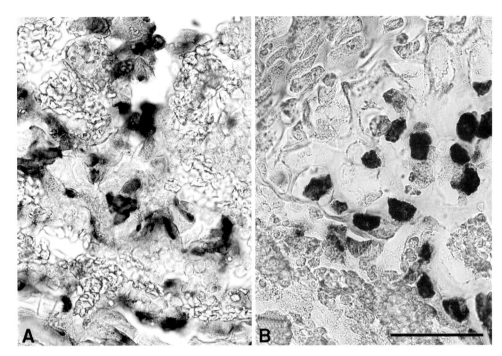

Figure 1. Cell-specific expression of osteopontin determined by *in situ* hybridization. Section prepared from 4-wk-old rat femur was hybridized with osteopontin cRNA probe labeled with DIG-11-UTP. (A) A population of osteoblasts surrounding the bone matrix express osteopontin. (B) Messenger RNA encoding osteopontin gene was detected in hypertrophic chondrocytes. Bar = 150 μm.

glycerol solution. The dipped slides are placed on an ice-cold plate for 15 min, dried at room temperature for 3 h, and exposed at 4°C in desiccated slide boxes. The exposed slides are developed in D-19 developer for 3 min at 20°C, fixed in F-5 fixative for 7 min, and finally washed with water for 30 min. They are counterstained with H&E and examined using a dark-field microscope.

REFERENCES

1. Hirakawa K, Ikeda T, Yamaguchi A, et al: Localization of the mRNA for bone matrix proteins during fracture healing as determined by in situ hybridization. *J Bone Miner Res* 9:1551–1557, 1994.
2. Ikeda T, Nomura S, Yamaguchi A, et al: In situ hybridization of bone matrix proteins in undecalcified adult rat bone sections. *J Histochem Cytochem* 40:1079–1088, 1992.
3. Kondo E, Nakamura S, Onoue H, et al: Detection of bcl-2 protein and bcl-2 messenger RNA in normal and neoplastic lymphoid tissues by immunohistochemistry and in situ hybridization. *Blood* 80:2044–2045, 1992.
4. Nakajima Y, Shimokawa H, Onoue H, et al: Identification of the cell type origin of odontoma-like clusters in microphthalmic (mi/mi) mice by in situ hybridization. *Pathol Int* 46:743–750, 1996.
5. Nakase T, Nomura S, Yoshikawa H, et al: Transient and localized expression of bone morphogenetic protein 4 messenger RNA during fracture healing. *J Bone Miner Res* 9:651–659, 1994.

6. Nomura S, Hirakawa K, Nagoshi J, et al: Method for detecting the expression of bone matrix proteins by in situ hybridization using decalcified mineralized tissue. *Acta Histochem Cytochem* 26:303–309, 1993.
7. Nomura S, Wills AJ, Edwards DR, et al: Developmental expression of 2ar (osteopontin) and SPARC (osteonectin) RNA as revealed by in situ hybridization. *J Cell Biol* 106:441–450, 1988.
8. Terai K, Takano-Yamamoto T, Ohba Y, et al: Role of osteopontin in bone remodeling caused by mechanical stress. *J Bone Miner Res* 14:839–849, 1999.
9. Yoshimura Y, Nomura S, Kawasaki S, et al: Colocalization of noggin and bone morphogenetic protein-4 during fracture healing. *J Bone Miner Res* 16:876–884, 2001.

VI Analysis Techniques

25

Bone Histomorphometry

Concepts and Common Techniques

Jean E. Aaron and Patricia A. Shore

School of Biomedical Sciences, University of Leeds, Leeds, UK

I. INTRODUCTION

The "quality" of bone, as well as its quantity, contributes to the biomechanical performance of the skeleton and encompasses aspects of both macromolecular composition and microarchitectural arrangement. Histology is usually at the forefront of analysis at this level, because noninvasive scanning methods lack the resolution and are often costly, and biochemical methods do not provide the topography. This chapter outlines some of the old and new microanatomical methods that our laboratory has found particularly useful when applied to undecalcified bone.

II. PHYSICAL METHODS

For those laboratories without hard-tissue histology facilities that require some form of microanalysis, there are two long-established methods.[11,22] The first provides a measure of the relative volume of bony tissue within a cancellous specimen based upon Archimedes' Principle. It requires that the cortical envelope and any adhering soft tissue be removed, and that the specimen should be trimmed into a regular shape. Blood is eliminated by a water or air jet, and fat is extracted either by immersion for 48 h in ethanol/acetone or by refluxing in petroleum ether at 35°C for 3 h for a typical bone biopsy specimen 8 mm in diameter × 10 mm in length. After drying in an oven overnight at 105°C and cooling in a desiccator, the marrow-free sample is weighed in air. Following evacuation in a flask of carbon tetrachloride to eliminate air pockets, the sample is reweighed in carbon tetrachloride, specific gravity 1.592. The dimensions of the specimen are taken with a micrometer to determine its total volume (TV). It follows that:

$$\text{Density of bony tissue} = \frac{\text{Wt}_{air} \times 1.592}{\text{Wt}_{air} - \text{Wt}_{CCl4}} \qquad (1)$$

$$\text{Relative volume bony tissue, BV/TV} = \frac{\text{Wt}_{air} - \text{Wt}_{CCl4}}{1.592 \times \text{TV}} \qquad (2)$$

The results can be used to evaluate osteopenia and are similar to those acquired by histology, for which BV/TV for cancellous bone at the iliac crest (the international standard

From: *Handbook of Histology Methods for Bone and Cartilage*
Edited by: Y. H. An and K. L. Martin © Humana Press Inc., Totowa, NJ

biopsy site; *see* Chapter 3) is generally 5–35%. The state of mineralization of the specimen and whether osteomalacia is present may be subsequently determined by ashing weighed fragments of the dried sample in platinum dishes for 24 h at 600°C and reweighing to determine the percentage ash content. Our normal range was 57–67%, compared with a range of 54–62%, as obtained by Vogt[61] and Dequecker et al.[23] The percentage ash is reduced in osteomalacia; however, the procedure is not as sensitive as histology in detecting mild cases.

III. HISTOLOGICAL METHODS

A. *Histomorphometry of Fresh Frozen and Plastic-Embedded Specimens*

Undecalcified bone histomorphometry is generally performed on thin plastic-embedded sections (*see* Chapters 11 and 20). However, there is a growing requirement for sections suitable for histochemistry and immunohistochemistry, and although cold-setting plastics have sometimes been used successfully,[24,28] the preparation of fresh frozen material is generally recognized as the gold standard for biochemical preservation. However, there is often dissatisfaction with the cellular morphology in frozen sections, particularly of hard tissues. It is possible to have the best of both worlds by cutting frozen sections, then plastic-embedded sections from the *same* block of tissue[13]—this process offers the added advantage of immediate results, since plastic-embedding alone requires a minimum of 12 d of processing.

The procedure begins with the routine preparation of sections of fresh frozen undecalcified bone by freezing the material immediately in a cardice/liquid *n*-hexane mixture (–75°C) or in liquid nitrogen and isopentane (–150°C) and attaching the frozen specimen to the microtome chuck with a layer of carboxymethylcellulose gel (CMC; 1.6% solution stored at 4°C to shorten the freezing time). Further CMC (BDH Chemicals, Poole, UK) is added to support the tissue, and the gel is contained until it freezes by a removable frame that surrounds the specimen. When frozen around the tissue by further immersion in the quenching fluid, the CMC gel becomes a block of reinforced ice.[2]

Specimens are sectioned on an LKB PMV 2258 or 450 MP heavy-duty cryomicrotome (Leica, Germany) using a hardened steel D-profile knife set at an angle of 2°. This equipment provides a robust system that is more effective for hard tissues than a regular cryostat. During the cutting process, the section is supported by a film of poly-vinylpyrrolidone, spread using the edge of a glass slide in two thin, consecutive layers over the surface of the block, and composed of equal volumes of 40% PVP_{10} and 20% PVP_{360}, a mixture that combines flexibility with strength. A square of cigarette paper is attached to the freshly applied film for additional support. Sections measuring 8 μm thick are cut at slow speed and pressed onto cooled glass slides previously coated with a pressure-sensitive adhesive (Durotak, Product No. 180–1197, National Adhesives and Resins Ltd, Slough, UK). The sections are allowed to thaw in 10% buffered formalin, pH 7.2, for 5 min, and during this time the paper detaches and the PVP dissolves, leaving sections that may be stained for morphology either by the von Kossa/eosin method (Table 1) or in 0.1% toluidine blue stain, pH 3.5 (Table 2);[13] alternatively, they are ideal for immunohistochemistry.[14,15]

The remainder of the frozen block will be undamaged and may be thawed in 10% buffered formalin, pH 7.2, dehydrated, and embedded in methylmethacrylate (MMA)[3] (Table 3) or

Table 1. The von Kossa/Eosin Method for Rapid Undecalcified Cryosections of Bone

Process	Method	Time
1. Preservation	Place the slide horizontally in a petri-dish and immerse in cold (4°C) neutral buffered formalin.	10 min
	Wash carefully in distilled water.	2×3 min
2. Staining	Immerse in 5% silver nitrate and illuminate 20 cm from a 100 watt bulb until the bone appears brown.	Approx 30 sec
	Wash carefully in distilled water.	2×3 min
3. Stain stabilization	Immerse in 3% sodium thiosulphate.	1 min
	Counterstain in 1% aqueous eosin.	10 min
	Wash carefully in tap water.	2×3 min
4. Mount	Hydromount (National Diagnostics, Aylesbury, Bucks, UK). Note: It is essential to use an aqueous mounting medium.	

(After Carter et al.[13])

Color of the tissue: Bone—brown; osteoid tissue—red; cells—yellow.

Table 2. Toluidine Blue-Staining Procedure for Bone Sections

Solutions	Method	Time
0.1% Toluidine blue, pH 3.5	1. Distilled water	3 min
	2. 0.1% toluidine blue	30 min
	3. Distilled water	5 min
	4. Dehydrate in absolute alcohol	3×3 min
	5. Clear in methylcyclohexane	2×3 min
	6. Mount in XAM (BDH Chemicals, Poole, UK) or other neutral medium	

Table 3. The Embedding of Undecalcified Bone in Methylmethacrylate

Process	Method	Time
1. Preservation		
	70% ethanol (or 10% buffered formalin for previously frozen material)	1 d
2. Dehydration		
	96% ethanol	1 d
	100% ethanol	1 d
	100% ethanol/chloroform 1:1	1 d
3. Impregnation with resin		
	Methylmethacrylate	3 d
	Methylmethacrylate/0.1% benzoyl peroxide	3 d
4. Embedding/polymerization		
	Methylmethacrylate/20% dibutylpthalate/2.0% benzoyl peroxide	3 d (30°C)

other resin of choice. Subsequent staining of the plastic sections (cut on a Jung K heavy-duty microtome or a Polycut microtome; Leica, Germany) with the Goldner's tetrachrome stain, for example (Table 4), shows all the regular remodeling features without any apparent detrimental effects. Moreover, any previous tetracycline labeling is not eluted by the process.

Table 4. Modified Goldner's Trichrome Method for Methylmethacrylate Embedded Sections

Solutions	Method	Time
1. Weigert's Hemotoxylin	1. Distilled water	3 min
• Sol'n A—1 g hematoxylin 100 mL 96% ethanol	2. Weigert's hematoxylin	20 min
• Sol'n B—1.1 g $FeCl_3 \cdot 6H_20$ + 1 mL 25% HCl	3. Rinse in running tap water	20 min
• Made up to 100 mL with distilled water	4. Distilled water	5 min
• Before use, mix A+B in 1:1 ratio	5. Ponceau/fuchsin/azophloxine	5 min
	6. Acetic acid 1%	15 sec
2. Masson-Ponceau de Xylidine	7. PTA/Orange II	20 min
• 0.75 g Ponceau de xylidine	8. Acetic acid 1%	15 sec
• 0.25 g Acid fuchsin	9. Light green	5 min
• 1 mL Glacial acetic acid	10. Acetic acid 1%	3 min
• Made up to 100 mL with distilled water	11. Distilled water	5 min
	12. Dehydrate in absolute alcohol	3×3 min
3. Azophloxine	13. Clear in methylcyclohexane	2×3 min
• 0.5 g Azophloxine (a.k.a. acid red)	14. Mount in XAM (BDH Chemicals,	
• 0.6 mL Glacial acetic acid	Poole, UK) or other neutral medium	
• Made up to 100 mL with distilled water		
4. Ponceau-Fuchsin-Azophloxine		
• 7.5 mL Panceau de xylidine		
• 2 mL Azoploxine		
• 88 mL 0.2% Glacial acetic acid		
5. Light Green		
• 1 g Light green		
• 1 mL Glacial acetic acid		
• Made up to 500 mL with distilled water		
6. Phosphotungstic Acid (PTA)/Orange II		
• 3 g Phosphotungstic acid		
• 2 g Orange II		
• Made up to 100 mL with distilled water		
7. 1% Acetic Acid		

B. Histomorphometry and Fluorochrome Staining of the Calcification Front

The customary procedure for tetracycline *labeling* has been described elsewhere (*see* Chapter 5). However, a useful adjunct for analysis is tetracycline *staining*,[1] whereby the fluorochrome marker is applied to the bone, not in vivo as is customary, but in vitro— i.e., the intact fresh biopsy is immersed for 48 h in a 1% neutral solution of tetracycline hydrochloride (achromycin) in 10% neutral buffered formalin (NBF). After washing in deionized water (3 times, 15 min each), followed by embedding and sectioning, differences in the pattern of normal and pathological states are apparent under the fluorescence microscope. In particular, the stain, like the label, is associated with the calcification front. The fluorochrome stain may be used alone or combined as a second marker with a single label for the determination of the apposition rate (Fig. 1). Since the problem of toxicity for the patient does not arise with the in vitro stain, a wider range of fluorochromes of contrasting colors, such as xylenol orange and calcein, may be used to aid interpretation.

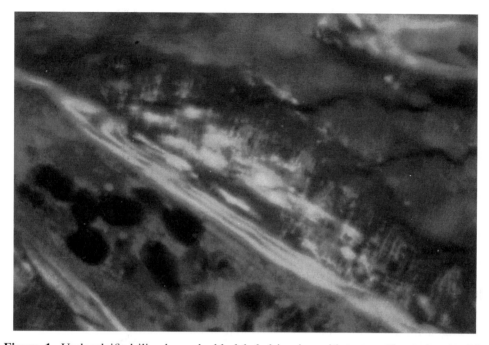

Figure 1. Undecalcified iliac bone double-labeled in vivo with tetracycline and stained in vitro with calcein. The position of the calcification front on the three successive occasions is indicated by the three parallel fluorescent bands. In addition, osteocytes associated with the calcifying region also contain mineral and fluoresce with calcein stain, indicative of their direct role in the calcification event. Epifluorescence microscope, UV light (magnification ×220). (*See* color plate 15 appearing in the insert following p. 270.)

C. Histomorphometry of Remodeling Variables

It is only when structural change is substantial that subjective appraisal is sufficient. More often, quantitative analysis is required for reliable comparison. For many years, this was accomplished using integrating eyepieces with patterns of parallel lines and regularly distributed points, applied to groups of about 16 sections per specimen. The introduction of computers was confined at first to only a few laboratories because the hardware was prohibitively expensive and the software was limited, requiring high-contrast preparations in particular. Computer-assisted methods are now widely familiar, encompassing structural and remodeling variables ranging from bone volume and trabecular width to osteoid borders, resorption cavities, and cell populations. However, analysis requires considerable expertise and remains time-consuming, despite the reduction in sections per specimen to 2–4 (*see* Birkenhager-Frenkel et al.,[12] who emphasize the need for adequate numbers of sections from different levels). The Goldner tetrachrome stain (Table 4) is widely applied to bone, despite misgivings expressed by some authors about its reliability in differentiating all osteoid tissue. We use the Goldner method in association with our semiautomated OsteoMeasure system. (Another semi-automated image analyzer is the Morphomat: Zeiss, Germany.)

1. The OsteoMeasure System

This semi-automated system (OsteoMetrics, Inc., Atlanta, GA) is attached to a digitizing pad, upon which the features to be measured are outlined. Detailed individual square fields are analyzed under the optical microscope in a sequence that commences in the top left-hand corner beneath the cortex, and traverses the section systematically to produce a continuous precisely matched image on the final color printout of the total area of interest (Fig. 2). On completion of the scan, a list of variables is automatically calculated, some measured directly and others derived indirectly. All are named according to the nomenclature recommended by Parfitt et al.,[49] which it is generally advisable to follow. The variables that we have used most frequently are indicated in Table 5. Most measurements are performed using plain light optical microscopy at a magnification sufficient to resolve cellular detail, about ×150. For a comprehensive analysis, attachments for the microscope include incident light fluorescence (epifluorescence) for measuring the distance between the fluorescent bands in tetracycline-labeled material (interlabel thickness, Ir.L.Th). From this, and knowing the time interval, the mineral apposition rate (MAR) is calculated; the extent of the calcification front is also determined (mineralizing surface, i.e., all double-labeled sites plus half the single-labeled sites expressed relative to the bone surface or the osteoid surface). A polarizer and analyzer are used for the display of cement lines and lamellation in order to identify and measure the mean wall thickness (WTh). Alternatively, the mineralization rate (μm or mcm/d) and WTh (μm or mcm) can be determined separately by manual methods using a calibrated eyepiece and taking four equidistant readings at each site, a procedure we have found to be convenient.

IV. MICROANATOMICAL METHODS

A. Trabecular Architecture—Two-Dimensional Image

The mass of cortical tissue is a major factor in determining skeletal strength and fracture predisposition. However, cancellous bone, although it occupies only 20% of the adult skeleton, tends to be prominent at the major sites of osteoporotic fracture, namely the wrist, spine and hip, and its biomechanical performance is influenced by its mass as well as other factors, particularly the microarchitecture. This varies from site to site in relation to the direction of mechanical stress. Until comparatively recently, little attention was paid to the trabecular architecture, because it was considered that any change was so closely related to the bone mass that its separate appraisal was unnecessary. Increasing evidence suggests that this is not the case, and that some subjects with a satisfactory bone mass suffer a minimum trauma fracture, while others with apparent skeletal atrophy do not. Although for many years the pursuit of remodeling imbalance was the primary concern of bone histologists, there has been an escalating interest in the associated microarchitecture since early descriptions by Atkinson[10] and Wakamatsu and Sissons.[62] At the same time, the development of computers has made image analysis accessible to all, and has allowed the previously limited range of variables to expand.

Trabecular bone loss may occur either as a result of generalized trabecular thinning or the total removal of individual trabeculae, or it may be a combination of the two. The pattern of loss determines biomechanical properties and also influences therapeutic prospects, because thinned bars can be thickened, yet the replacement of lost bars is problematic. Thus, diminished formation may lead to trabecular attenuation, as seems to be the case in aging men, in femoral fracture patients, and in patients treated with corticosteroid drugs. Increased resorption may lead to trabecular atrophy and disconnection—a weaker arrangement that probably contributes to the sex-related difference in fracture because it

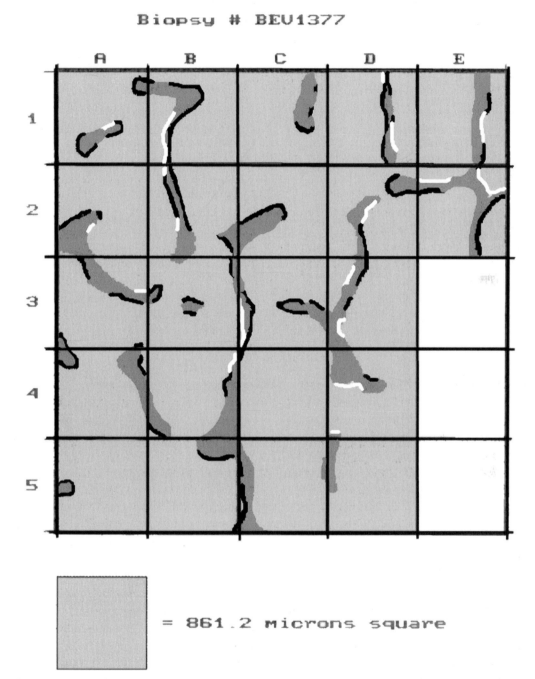

Figure 2. A typical OsteoMeasure printout (original in color) of cancellous bone following semi-automated image analysis, which commences in the top left-hand corner and proceeds horizontally. Each square represents a single field. The dark gray (color-coded blue) area is mineralized bone; the black (red) is osteoid tissue; white outlines resorption cavities. The surface extent of osteoclasts and osteoblasts can be similarly mapped. The three blank fields contained artifactual damage and were excluded.

**Table 5. Histomorphometric Variables Processed by the Semi-Automated Image
Analysis System (OsteoMeasure)**

Static indices	Abbreviation	Value	Units	Normals
Bone Volume	BV/TV	13.5243	(%)	23.19 (4.37)
Osteoid Volume (/TV)	OV/TV	0.0567	(%)	0.32 (0.19)
Osteoid Volume (/BV)	OV/BV	0.4194	(%)	1.48 (0.93)
Mineralized Volume	Md.V/TV	13.4676	(%)	
Bone Surf/Tissue Vol Index	BS/TV	2.6964	(mm^2/mm^3)	3.50 (0.46)
Bone Surface/Volume Index	BS/BV	19.9374	(mm^2/mm^3)	
Total Osteoid Surface	OS/BS	3.1533	(%)	12.10 (4.64)
Bone Interface (Total)	BI/BS	3.1261	(%)	
Osteoblast Surface	Ob.S/BS	0.1555	(%)	3.90 (1.94)
Eroded Surface	ES/BS	1.8423	(%)	4.09 (2.33)
Osteoclast Surface	Oc.S/BS	0.2435	(%)	0.69 (0.61)
Quiescent Surface	QS/BS	95.0044	(%)	
Reversal Surface	Rv.S/BS	1.5988	(%)	2.70 (2.96)
Remodelling Surface	Rm.S/BS	4.9956	(%)	
Active Eroded Surface	S1.S/BS	0.3554	(%)	
Trabecular Thickness	Tb.Th	100.3139	(μm)	133.0 (22.0)
Trabecular Profile Thickness	Tb.Pf.Th	0.0000	(μm)	
Osteoid Thickness	O.Th	6.5073	(μm)	10.34 (2.05)
Mineralized Thickness	Md.Th	*	(μm)	
Osteoblast Volume Density	N.Ob/T.Ar	0.0000	$(/mm^2)$	
Osteoblast Surface Density	N.Ob/B.Pm	0.1545	(/mm)	
Osteoblast Osteoid Surf. Den.	N.Ob/O.Pm (Lm)	4.8999	(/mm)	
Osteoblast Index	N.Ob/Ob.Pm	99.3769	(/mm)	
Osteoclast Volume Density	N.Oc/T.Ar	0.000	$(/mm^2)$	
Osteoclast Bone Surface Den.	N.Oc/B.Pm	0.0221	(/mm)	
Osteoclast Eroded Surf. Den.	N.Oc/E.Pm	1.1981	(/mm)	
Osteoclast Index	N.Oc/Oc.Pm	9.0644	(/mm)	
Structural indices	Abbreviation	Value	Units	Normals
Trabecular separation	Tb.Sp	641.4160	(μm)	570.6 (98.9)
Trabecular Number	Tb.N	1.3482	(/mm)	1.75 (0.23)
Kinetic indices	Abbreviation	Value	Units	Normals
Mineralizing Surface	MS/BS		(%)	76.4 (11.3)
Mineralizing Surface (Osteoid)	MS/OS		(%)	>60
Mineral Apposition Rate	MAR		(μm/d)	0.51 (0.04)
Adjusted Apposition Rate	Aj.Ar		(μm/d)	
Bone Formation Rate (Surface)	BFR/BS		$(μm^3/μm^2/y)$	35.8 (8.9)
Bone Formation Rate (Rel)	BFR/BV		(%/y)	
Bone Formation Rate	BFR/TV		(%/y)	
Mineralization Lag Time	Mlt		(d)	
Osteoid Maturation Time	Omt		(d)	
Total Period	Tt.P		(d)	
Formation Period	FP		(d)	
Active Formation Period	FP (a+)		(d)	
Resorption Period	Rs.P		(d)	
Reversal Period	Rv.P		(d)	
Remodelling Period	Rm.P		(d)	
Quiescent Period	QP		(d)	
Activation Frequency	Ac.f		(/y)	

Those variables we use most are underlined. (*See* Parfitt et al.[48] for details about individual indices.)

occurs in aging women and in crush fracture patients.[3,4] An example of a drug used to reverse these trends is fluoride, which has a long history in association with bone. At a microanatomical level, the atrophied spongiosa of osteoporotic women is consolidated by fluoride therapy. However, fractures have been reported to continue despite the restored bone mass, because the thickening of the trabecular remnants that provides increased resistance to compression forces is not accompanied by an improved capacity to withstand bending forces, since that is dependent upon more regular trabecular interconnection.[5] In other words, the bone mass is not the whole story.

Many authors consider it unlikely that treatment regimens will be developed that will be capable of reconnecting a disconnected trabecular system (*see* ref. 21 for review). However, a new spongiosa may be created from the remnants of the old one by a natural progression from trabecular thickening, which in due course stimulates angiogenesis within the widened bars. The proliferating blood vessels occupy newly created intratrabecular resorption channels, which perforate the expanding bone and transform it into a network.[6] Such a possibility for trabecular regeneration supports a continuing role for the measurement of trabecular architecture and new bone distribution in relation to fracture prevention.

Several semi-automated systems of computer-aided microscopy include microanatomical as well as histological variables on their menu. For example, the OsteoMeasure system calculates the trabecular width, number, and separation. Other systems reported in the literature include the Optomax V AMS (Optomax Inc, Hollos, NH)[52] and the Zeiss MOP 3 digitizer (Carl Zeiss Inc., New York).[48] Values are often derived indirectly from simple area and perimeter measurements[48] rather than by direct measurement.[3] Other methods are specific for one variable—for example, a direct computerized technique for the measurement of the trabecular width was derived by Garrahan et al.,[31] based upon generating expanding circles around the median axis of each trabecula until the circle was tangential to the two opposing boundaries, at which point the diameter of the circle is the width of the trabecula. A close correlation was described between this direct measure and the indirect calculation of the trabecular width derived from the area and perimeter, and was originally named the mean trabecular-plate thickness.[48] Similarly, another aspect of trabecular structural pattern was quantified by defining trabecular nodes (or junctions) and termini following the thinning of the binary image to a linear framework examined using an IBAS image analyzer (Kontron, West Germany).[30] Some authors have criticized these methods on the basis of inadequate mathematical veracity, and alternatives have appeared that include the trabecular pattern factor,[36] the marrow space (or bone) star volume,[60] fractal analysis,[63,68] ConnEuler,[35] and "fabric"/ anisotropy.[38,65]

The development of a dedicated and readily accessible system based upon the personal computer was prompted by the increasing diversity of these measurements, combined with the prohibitively expensive hardware employed and the necessity of using high-contrast stains that are often not the stains of choice for sections also intended for other histomorphometric purposes. To this end, techniques described in the literature were collated to produce a rapid unitary system of comprehensive shape analysis leading to the production of our automated Trabecular Analysis System (TAS).

1. The TAS System

This automated image analyser[7] (software available from SKPaxton@leeds.ac.uk or Charlie@osteometrics.com) enables the microarchitecture to be measured in cancellous

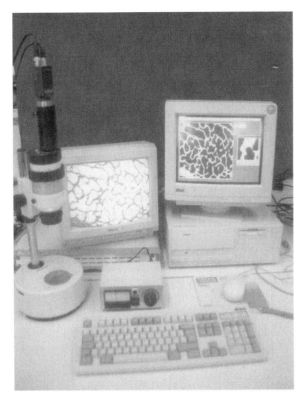

Figure 3. The automated trabecular analysis system TAS showing the microscope with closed-circuit TV camera, image analyzer and microcomputer. On the screen is a typical histological specimen.

bone sections, prepared routinely using the toluidine blue stain (0.1%, pH 3.5, for 30 min; Table 2) or the Goldner method (Table 4). The section is placed upon the microscope stage of a transmitted light dissecting microscope (for example, a Wild M7A) with a zoom lens (Fig. 3). A low magnification of about ×15 is generally suitable, and the area of interest is defined by an adjustable window. A closed circuit black-and-white television camera attached to the viewing tube of the microscope transmits the image for capture in a 256 × 256-pixel, 64 gray-level format by a VIP image analyzer (Sight Systems, Newbury, Berkshire, UK), connected to an IBM-compatible PC, programmed in Turbo Pascal v.5, with specific sections in Assembler for enhanced speed of computation.

i) Image thresholding (segmenting): This follows the initial calibration step and separates the trabecular network from any background features (for example, marrow tissue) in the original image, which is composed of individual pixels with a gray-level value between 0 (black) and 63 (white). The optimum threshold value is selected manually, and following this all pixels below it become white and all those above become black, creating a binary "bitmap" that may be compressed and stored on disk.

ii) Image editing: An algorithm removes "noise" in the form of single dissociated pixels, and an editing facility that includes erasure or addition enables minor artifacts, such as sectioning cracks, to be removed before analysis. Certain structural features also require attention (Fig. 4), because they will produce misleading configurations when the image is further processed. During editing, zoom magnification enables the binary area for amendment to be inspected

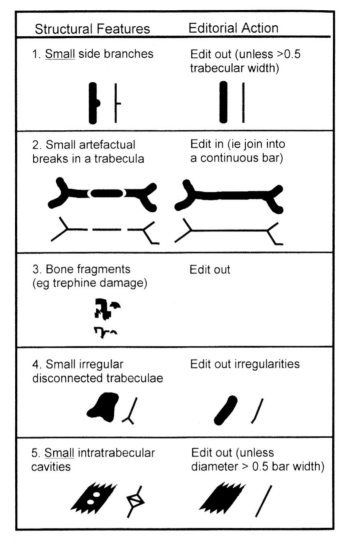

Structural Features	Editorial Action
1. Small side branches	Edit out (unless >0.5 trabecular width)
2. Small artefactual breaks in a trabecula	Edit in (ie join into a continuous bar)
3. Bone fragments (eg trephine damage)	Edit out
4. Small irregular disconnected trabeculae	Edit out irregularities
5. Small intratrabecular cavities	Edit out (unless diameter > 0.5 bar width)

Figure 4. Artifacts and histological features for attention when editing the image prior to an automated TAS analysis.

more closely for accuracy. Reference is also made when necessary to the original histological slide under the light microscope for clarification about structural detail.

iii) Image processing: After delineating the area of interest with a "rubber-banded box" function that allows considerable flexibility of shape, all outer features (such as the cortices and peripheral trephine damage) are removed to minimize subsequent processing. The selected image is thinned to its medial axis ("skeletonized") by a modification of Hilditch algorithm H,[45] whereby the trabeculae are reduced to strings of single pixels (Fig. 5). This process of systematically repeated passes and deletions generates the first microarchitectural variable, bone volume or area (BV/TV; % or mm^2) and the second variable, bone surface (BS; mm^2/mm^3 or mm). The ratio of these provides the trabecular width (TbWi; μm). The routine produces further analysis, including node number (joint points of three or more strings of pixels), terminus number (end points of a pixel string) and node: terminus ratio, together with the computation of individual trabeculae (strut number and character, e.g., node-node, node-terminus, termi-

TAS v2.09 Jan. 2001 Trabecular Analysis Report

Created 6 Feb 2001
Report Generated on 6 Feb 2001 19:40:21
File TimeStamp is undefined

Thresholds: 0,114
Pixels are 0.0109 x 0.0115mm
BV   12.1379%
BS   2.8687mm/mm2
TbTh 70.5786mcm
NNd 3
NTm 38
NNd:NTm ratio   0.0789

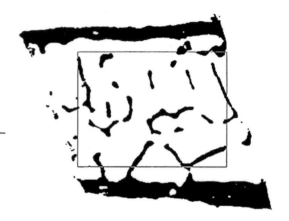

BAr 1.1528mm2
BPm 27.2451mm
TbWi 84.6238 mcm
TbN 1.7198
TbSp 510.8970 mcm
TbPF 3.5007
Tar 9.4975mm
BS3d 2.3925 mm2/mm3
SDn 19.7114mm
Total Strut Number 26

Cuts 0
Singles 2
Nd-Nd 1
Tm-Nd 7
Tm-Tm 12
Tm-Cut 6
Nd-Cut 0
Mean Nd-Nd 0.4835mm
Mean Tm-Tm 0.5519mm
Mean Tm-Nd 0.3315mm
Mean Tm-Cut 0.7734mm
Mean Nd-Cut 0.0000mm
TbLe 14.0670mm

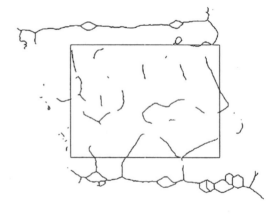

AOI used.
AOI Status
AOI information for new-5.tif
AOI area is 9.4975 mm2
AOI is Rectangular
Size: 3.4672 x 2.7393 mm
Pos: 2.2203, 1.2378 mm

Figure 5. A typical image and data printout from the automated trabecular image analysis system TAS. The binary intact and thinned images are reproduced, and the area of interest is defined by the rectangle.

Table 6. Mathematical Equations Applied to the Derivation of Trabecular Indices

Structural variable	Equation
Trabecular width (mcm)	= 2,000 * bone area mm²/trabecular perimeter mm
Trabecular thickness (mcm)	= Trabecular width/1.2[a]
Trabecular separation (mcm)	= Trabecular thickness ([100/% bone volume] − 1)
Trabecular number (/mm) (calculated)	= % bone volume × 10/trabecular thickness mcm
Trabecular pattern factor	= (Perimeter 1 − Perimeter 2)/(Area 1 − Area 2)[b]
Marrow space star volume (mm³)	= $(\pi/3) \times l_n^3$ where 1 is intercept length

[a] A correction factor for section obliquity.

[b] P1 and A1 are from the original image; P2 and A2 are from the dilated image.

(After Whitehouse,[65] Parfitt et al.,[48,49] Vesterby et al.,[59] Hahn et al.,[36] Croucher et al.[18])

nus-terminus), and isolated bone profiles.[49] The variables measured by the software program (Fig. 5) and the equations described in the literature for their determination are listed in Table 6. A general function is also available for the direct measurement of point-to-point distance using a mouse cursor and also for "radial" scans of path lengths through marrow spaces or through bony tissue,[58] using either a superimposed regular grid pattern[18] or a random point selector instructed to perform as many passes as the study requires. This indicates the star volume,[60] and another program produces a fractal analysis.[68]

One reason for the multiplicity of variables that has arisen in the literature is that removal of trabecular cross-bracing ties weakens the bone to an extent that is disproportionate to the mass of tissue lost. For example, if the distance between the cross-ties is doubled, the resistance to bending forces is reduced fourfold. A histological measure of trabecular interconnection would therefore seem to be essential. On the other hand, there are reports[17] that in normal bone the mechanical properties are almost entirely accounted for by the bone volume (bone mineral density) and structural anisotropy (orientation).[34,39] The fact that this is not invariably the case has generated a special impetus for those methods that inform about trabecular interconnection from the two-dimensional (2D) image of a histological section.

Topological properties such as trabecular interconnection are fundamental in characterizing the microstructural framework. For a network, the connectivity indicates the maximal number of branches that can be broken before the structure is separated into two parts, and it has been described as the number of trabeculae minus one.[47] If the junctions are conjoined by a single path, the arrangement is simply connected and vulnerable to fragmentation when one branch is broken, yet a multiply connected system is more stable[19] (*see* Section IV.B.2) and Fig. 7). Histological methods that relate to this aspect of trabecular bone are as follows.

i) Node: terminus ratio (NNd:NTm): The computer-generated thinned image of the trabecular network previously described provides a pattern that varies with age and pathology, which can be quantified.[43] Following descriptions by Garrahan et al.[30] of the NNd:NTm ratio as a measure of trabecular interconnection, the index has been applied by others[52,55,56] and has usefully differentiated between groups despite the fact that the majority of so-called termini are artifacts of the plane of sectioning and the mathematical basis is viewed by stereologists as insubstantial.

ii) Trabecular pattern factor (TbPF): This index of trabecular interconnection was proposed by Hahn et al.[36] on the basis that a highly connected structure presents mainly concave surfaces in a section, and a poorly connected structure presents convex surfaces. It is calculated by determining the trabecular area (A1) and perimeter (P1) before and after (A2, P2) dilatation (for example, corresponding to one pixel) of the binary image, a process that will cause the concave perimeter to decrease and the convex perimeter to increase, thereby distinguishing between the two. The quotient (P1-P2)/(A1-A2) is the TbPF. The results are apparently influenced by the magnification, and by whether or not computer-smoothing procedures are implemented.[27] They are also affected by the dimension of dilatation, which should be small enough to avoid the confluence of juxtaposed surfaces and large enough to accommodate trabecular arrangements with minimal curvature.[17]

iii) Marrow space star volume: The measurement of the star volume was applied to cancellous bone as an index of connectivity by Vesterby et al.[59] and Vesterby.[60] The marrow space star volume indicates the mean volume of marrow space that can be seen unobstructed in all directions from a random point within it, and is derived from the distance cubed between the point and its intercepting radius with the bone surface. It follows that in a regularly interconnected cancellous structure the value is low, and in a disconnected structure it is high. Another stereological method recently applied to connectivity is the ConnEuler method,[35] calculated from the number of holes and bridged components in two parallel sections separated by a distance of 10–40 μm.[19]

iv) Fractal analysis: Fractal analysis provides an index of the complexity of a structure[68] and was developed from similarities observed between nature (natural fractals) and certain types of mathematical objects (ideal fractals). Although ideal fractals have a profile that is unchanged whether it is observed by a low or high magnification (self-similarity[42]), natural fractals also possess self-similarity, but only within a limited range. The fractal dimension may be used in medicine as an independent measure to describe the structural changes associated with disease. A number of authors have applied this to the cancellous network[17,25] on the basis that an accurate measurement of the trabecular bone surface in histological sections is central to reliable spatial description. However, the problem is that estimation of the bone surface increases with magnification. As a result, it has been suggested that fractal analysis may provide an appropriate index because it presents a dimensionless constant derived from the surface extent at a range of magnifications. As such, it is reported to be a simple descriptor of bone structure that has been applied to both histological sections and radiographs to enable the identification of disease- or age-related change.

B. Trabecular Architecture—Three-Dimensional Image

Reconstruction by sequential thin sectioning and the use of thick slices are alternative histological approaches to recent advanced methods for the three-dimensional (3D) analysis of cancellous bone. These methods include: microcomputed tomography, which requires costly specialized equipment and substantial doses of X-rays to achieve a good signal-to-noise ratio;[26,41,44] magnetic resonance microimaging, which is the sub-millimeter resolution counterpart of MRI and which requires a lengthy acquisition time;[16,37] and radiography, which lacks resolution.[32]

1. Serial Section Techniques

To overcome the limitations presented by the 2D histological section when considering connectivity, reconstruction from serial sections is an option. However, it is only rarely attempted, particularly since the spacing between consecutive sections should be between one-third and one-tenth of the length of the feature of interest—i.e., 15–50 μm distant in the case of trabeculae 150 μm long.[20,47] This makes such studies prohibitively time-consuming for routine application, and unacceptably demanding of computer memory space and data storage capacity for many research purposes. On the other hand, a novel and relatively rapid approach is to photograph the 2D image of the surface of the bone embedded in plastic. The process is repeated at intervals as the block of tissue is sectioned on a heavy-duty microtome such as the Jung K. Gray-level images are recorded on magnetic VHS videotape using a good quality video-recorder attached to the output from a CCTV camera (MF Wilson and JE Aaron, unpublished results; Fig. 6) or by means of a PC attached to the camera using an 8-bit resolution 768 × 512 frame grabber with 256 gray shades (e.g., Data Translation Vision-EZ or PCVision Plus) to digitize and segment into a binary image for storage on a computer disc.[46] For this to be successful, there must be sufficient contrast between the bone tissue and the embedding medium. To achieve this, Odgaard et al.[46] removed the marrow tissue by means of an air jet followed by immersion for 48 h in ethanol/acetone before embedding in epoxy resin. Black araldite coloring paste (8.5 g in 85 mL of resin; Ciba-Geigy, Basel, Switzerland) was added to the resin, which was warmed to 30°C to reduce the viscosity before mixing. A few seconds under vacuum apparently improved the penetration of the resin. As an alternative, we left the marrow in place and after dehydration in alcohol and subsequent immersion in 1:1 absolute alcohol:chloroform for 1 d used MMA embedding medium, which permeates cancellous bone well. To this was added Trylon opaque black color paste (0.1 g in 3 mL resin; regularly stocked by model makers' shops). The procedure involved 3 d refrigeration of the specimen in MMA monomer, followed by the same period in fresh monomer containing the catalyst benzoyl peroxide (0.1 g in 100 mL of monomer), after which the specimen was transferred to the final embedding mixture consisting of 2.5 g benzoyl peroxide, 25 mL di-n-butylphthalate plasiticizer and 3.3 g Trylon coloring paste in 100 mL MMA monomer. An automatic shaking machine was used at room temperature until polymerization was complete, to prevent the Trylon paste from settling as a separate phase.

Modifications to the microtome were introduced by Odgaard et al.,[46] including the mounting of a video camera directly above the specimen with appropriate optics (55 mm Micro-Nikkor, f/2.8, a modified Novoflex bellows and a C-mount; or in our case by fitting a Wild M7A dissecting microscope) and ring light (essential for uniform illumination of the block; Volpi AG, Switzerland). Below the specimen, an optoelectronics interrupter was fitted to ensure precision of the carriage position at the time of photography. Without this facility, reference landmark features (e.g., three bristles) must be added to the embedding medium for accurate image alignment,[67] and corresponding markers on the carriage and runners may also be helpful. It was found that a thin film of low-viscosity mineral oil on the surface of the tissue block improved the contrast between the white bone and the black medium. The sections removed during the process may also be used for other histomorphometric purposes, because although the medium is black *en bloc*, in a typical section 5–30 μm thick it is translucent pale gray and completely unobtrusive under the optical microscope. Using their comprehensively automated system, Odgaard et al.[46] recorded ("image-grabbed") alternate sections and were able to produce, digitize, and store as many as 170 of these per h.

2. Thick-Slice Technique

As indicated previously, bone mass *per se*, when derived by either invasive or noninvasive methods, is not a precise predictor of skeletal failure. Comparison of the bone mass between minimum trauma fracture and non-fracture populations generally fails to separate the two groups,[29,40] and a substantial overlap remains between them.[8] The osteoporotic process is usually more extensive in cancellous bone than in cortical bone, which is less metabolically active. Elderly women in particular display a pattern of cancellous loss typified by a diminution in interconnectivity.[54] Elements become progressively detached from the main trabecular network, creating a discontinuous structure that is characterized by the appearance of termini (free ends) and isolated trabecular islands (Fig. 7).

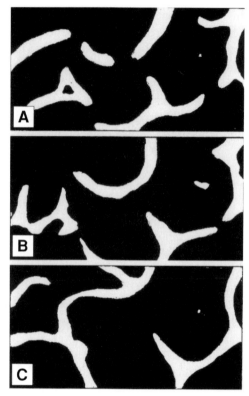

Figure 6. Three sequential tracings showing the appearance (middle) and disappearance (before and after) of an isolated island of bone taken from a VHS videorecording of 160 serial images of human iliac crest captured from the block surface during microtomy. Magnification ×30.

The number of termini may assist in the determination of fracture predisposition.[8,57] However, bone histomorphometry is generally performed upon sections that are approx 10 μm thick—essentially two-dimensional. This means that the appraisal of trabecular continuity by counting termini is inherently unreliable, as the majority of apparent termini will be artifacts of the plane of section as illustrated in Fig. 8.

Thick slices of material have been used by some authors in the past to study trabecular microarchitecture.[9,10,53,66] However, these methods generally involve the removal of the obscuring marrow tissue with the consequence for osteopenic tissue that portions of detached trabeculae may be lost with the extracted marrow, leading to the underestimation of true termini. We have recently reported a novel method for identifying real trabecular termini that uses dual-surface staining of thick slices (300 μm). It is both inexpensive and rapid, and the marrow tissue is retained.[57] The application of alizarin red stain to one surface and light green to the other allows the 2D image to be visualized, while at the same time the 3D trabecular image may be observed within the depth of the slice (*see* Table 7 for the staining procedure). In these preparations the apparent termini are stained red or green, and real termini (and also real islands of bone) are unstained and appear white, an image enhanced by viewing in partially polarized light (Fig. 9).

A Microslice 2 (Malvern Instruments, Ultra Tech Manufacturing Inc., Santa Ana, California) cuts the thick slices of previously embedded undecalcified bone (*see* Table 3 for

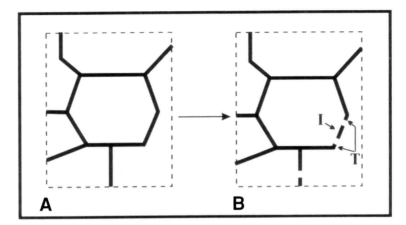

Figure 7. Diagram of a) a multiply connected trabecular system that is stable and b) a simply connected system that is less stable. The loss of connectivity in (b) results in the presence of trabecular termini (T) and isolated trabecular islands (I).

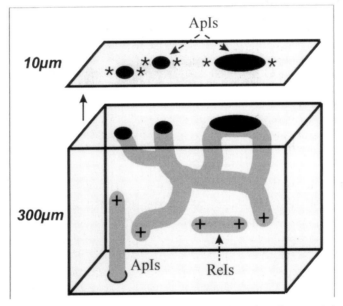

Figure 8. Diagram illustrating apparent (*) and real (+) trabecular termini and apparent (ApIs) and real (ReIs) islands (isolated trabeculae) in a 10-µm-thick histological section (2D image) and a 300-µm slice (3D image) of cancellous bone.

embedding details) by means of a rotating diamond-impregnated disc, cooled by a jet of water. Slice thickness may be subsequently measured accurately using a micrometer. A width of 300–400 µm was found to give optimum results (thickness in excess of this generally lacked structural clarity under the optical microscope), and we have now standardized our slices to 300 µm. Using a hand counter, the number of real (i.e., unstained) trabecular termini and real isolated islands of bone (unstained throughout) were counted within the depth of the slice (Fig. 9). The region of interest was defined within an area of recorded size

Table 7. Staining of 300 μm Thick Slices of Plastic-Embedded Bone

Solutions	Method
Stain A—1% Alizarin red S, pH 4.2 (pH adjusted with NH₄OH) Stain B—1% Light green, pH 2.7	1. Coat one side of the slice with a thin layer of petroleum jelly. 2. Immerse the slice in stain A until maximum staining is achieved (approx 5 min). 3. Wash the slice in tap water and blot dry. 4. Remove the petroleum jelly with methylcyclohexane (approx 5 min) and blot dry. 5. Immerse the slice in stain B for 5 min. 6. Wash in distilled water. 7. Dehydrate rapidly in 3 changes of absolute ethanol. 8. Clear in methylcyclohexane for 5 min. 9. Blot excess liquid and observe unmounted or, if preferred, mount in a neutral mounting medium which will clear any surface imperfections.

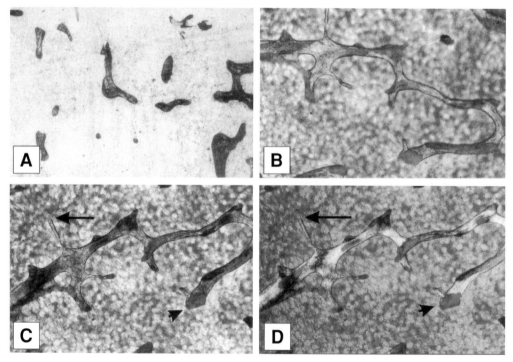

Figure 9. Photomicrographs of cancellous bone in a thin section and a thick slice. (A) A typical 10-μm section stained with toluidine blue contains many apparent termini. In contrast, (B–D) show a 300-μm slice where there are fewer apparent termini; (B) is stained with alizarin red on both surfaces; (C) is stained on one surface with alizarin red and on the other with light green, the color contrast improving separation; (D) is the same as (C) viewed in partially polarized light for clarity. The arrow indicates a real terminus (unstained) within the depth of the slice; these are relatively rare. The arrowhead indicates an apparent terminus (stained). Magnification ×20. (*See* color plate 16 appearing in the insert following p. 270.)

by placing a loose masked cover slip on top of the slice, arranged to exclude cortical bone and peripheral damage (as in Fig. 5). Our recent application of this technique to two groups of patients with and without vertebral fracture, but with the same bone mass, as measured by dual-energy X-ray absorptiometry (DEXA) showed a significant difference in the number of trabecular termini when all other histomorphometric methods failed to do so.[8] It is anticipated that this relatively simple aspect of bone "quality" will be joined by other suspected and unsuspected factors as the structural heterogeneity and internal modulation of the organic and inorganic components of the ECM are better understood.

Acknowledgment: The authors wish to thank Dr. RC Shore, Division of Oral Biology, Dental Institute, University of Leeds, for his most generous assistance with the illustrations.

REFERENCES

1. Aaron JE, Makins NB, Francis RM, et al: Staining of the calcification front in human bone using contrasting fluorochromes in vitro. *J Histochem Cytochem* 32:1251–1261, 1984.
2. Aaron JE, Carter DH: Rapid preparation of fresh-frozen undecalcified bone for histological and histochemical analysis. *J Histochem Cytochem* 35:361–369, 1987.
3. Aaron JE, Makins NB, Sagreiya K: The microanatomy of trabecular bone loss in normal aging men and women. *Clin Orthop* 215:260–271, 1987.
4. Aaron JE, Francis RM, Peacock M, et al: Contrasting microanatomy of idiopathic and corticosteroid-induced osteoporosis. *Clin Orthop* 243:294–305, 1989.
5. Aaron JE, de Vernejoul M-C, Kanis JA: The effect of sodium fluoride on trabecular architecture. *Bone* 12:307–310, 1991.
6. Aaron JE, de Vernejoul M-C, Kanis JA: Bone hypertrophy and trabecular generation in Paget's disease and in fluoride-treated osteoporosis. *J Bone Miner Res* 17:399–413, 1992.
7. Aaron JE, Johnson DR, Kanis JA, et al: An automated method for the analysis of trabecular bone structure. *Comput Biomed Res* 25:1–6, 1992.
8. Aaron JE, Shore PA, Shore RC, et al: Trabecular architecture in women and men of similar bone mass with and without fracture: II. Three-dimensional histology. *Bone* 27:277–282, 2000.
9. Amling M, Hahn M, Wening VJ, et al: The microarchitecture of the axis as the predisposing factor for fracture of the base of the odontoid process. *J Bone Joint Surg [Am]* 76:1840–1846, 1994.
10. Atkinson PJ: Variation of trabecular structure of vertebrae with age. *Calcif Tissue Res* 1:24–32, 1967.
11. Birkenhäger-Frenkel DH, Groen JJ, Bédier de Prairie JA, et al: A simple physico-chemical method of assessment of osteoporosis. *Voeding* 22:634–639, 1961.
12. Birkenhager-Frenkel DH, Schmitz PIM, Breuls PNWM, et al: Biological variation as compared to inter-observer variation and intrinsic error of measurement within bone biopsies. In: PJ Meunier, ed: *Bone Histomorphometry.* Second International Workshop, Société de la Nouvelle Imprimerie Foumié, Toulouse, France, 1977:63–67.
13. Carter DH, Barnes JM, Aaron JE: Histomorphometry of fresh-frozen iliac crest bone biopsies. *Calcif Tissue Int* 44:387–392, 1989.
14. Carter DH, Sloan P, Aaron JE: Immunolocalization of collagen types I and III, tenascin and fibronectin in intramembraneous bone. *J Histochem Cytochem* 39:599–606, 1991.
15. Carter DH, Sloan P, Aaron JE: Trabecular generation de novo. A morphological and immunohistochemical study of primary ossification in the human femoral anlagen. *Anat Embryol (Berl)* 186:229–240, 1992.
16. Chung HW, Wehrli FW, Williams JL, et al: NMR micro-imaging of trabecular bone. *J Bone Miner Res* 10:1452–1461, 1995.
17. Compston JE: Connectivity of cancellous bone: assessment and mechanical implications. *Bone* 15:463–466, 1994.

18. Croucher PI, Garrahan NJ, Compston JE: Assessment of cancellous bone structure: Comparison of strut analysis, trabecular pattern factor and marrow space star volume. *J Bone Miner Res* 11:955–961, 1996.
19. De Hoff RT, Aigeltinger E, Craig K: Experimental determination of the topological properties of 3-D microstructures. *J Microsc* 95:69–91, 1972.
20. De Hoff RT: Quantitative serial sectioning analysis. *J Microsc* 131:25–263, 1982.
21. Dempster DW: The contribution of trabecular architecture to cancellous bone quality. *J Bone Miner Res* 15:20–23, 2000.
22. Dequecker J, Remans J, Franssen R, et al: Aging patterns of trabecular and cortical bone and their relationship. *Calcif Tissue Int* 7:23–30, 1971.
23. Dequecker J: *Bone Loss in Normal and Pathological Conditions.* Leuven University Press, 1972.
24. Evans RA, Dunstan CR, Hills EE: Extent of resorbing surfaces based on histochemical identification of osteoclasts. *Metab Bone Dis* 25:29–34, 1980.
25. Fazzalari NL, Parkinson LH: Fractal properties of subchondral cancellous bone in severe osteoarthritis of the hip. *J Bone Miner Res* 12:632–639, 1997.
26. Feldkamp L, Goldstein S, Parfitt A, et al: The direct examination of 3-D bone architecture in vitro by computed tomography. *J Bone Miner Res* 1:3–11, 1989.
27. Flautre B, Hardouin P: Microradiographic aspect on iliac bone tissue in post-menopausal women with and without vertebral crush fractures. *Bone* 15:477–481, 1994.
28. Franklin RM, Martin MT: Staining and histochemistry of undecalcified bone embedded in a water soluble plastic. *Stain Technol* 55:313–321, 1980.
29. Gardsell P, Johnell O, Nielson B: Predicting fractures in women by using forearm densitometry. *Calcif Tissue Int* 44:235–242, 1989.
30. Garrahan NJ, Mellish RWE, Compston JE. A new method for the two-dimensional analysis of bone structure in human iliac crest biopsies. *J Microsc* 142:341–349, 1986.
31. Garrahan NJ, Mellish RW, Vedi S, et al: Measurement of mean trabecular plate thickness by a new computerized method. *Bone* 8:227–230, 1987.
32. Geraets WGM, van der Stelt PF, Netelenbos CJ, et al: A new method for automatic recognition of the radiographic trabecular pattern. *J Bone Miner Res* 5:227–233, 1990.
33. Goldstein SA: The mechanical properties of bone: dependence on the anatomical location and function. *J Biomech* 20:1055–1061, 1987.
34. Goldstein SA, Goulet R, McCubbrey D: Measurement and significance of three-dimensional architecture to the mechanical integrity of trabecular bone. *Calcif Tissue Int* 53:S127–S133, 1993.
35. Gundersen HJG, Boyce RW, Nyengaard JR, et al: The ConnEulor unbiased estimation of connectivity using physical disectors under projection. *Bone* 14:217–222, 1993.
36. Hahn M, Vogel M, Pompesins-Kempa M, et al: Trabecular bone pattern factor—a new parameter for simple quantification of bone microarchitecture. *Bone* 13:327–330, 1992.
37. Hipp JA, Janujwicz A, Simmons CA, et al: Trabecular bone morphology from micro-magnetic resonance imaging. *J Bone Miner Res* 11:286–292, 1996.
38. Hodgskinson R, Currey JD: The effects of structural variation on the Young's modulus of non-human cancellous bone. *Proc Inst Mech Eng* 204:43–52, 1990.
39. Hodgskinson R, Currey JD: The effect of variations in structure on the Young's modulus of cancellous bone: comparison of human and non-human material. *Proc Inst Mech Eng* 204:115–121, 1990.
40. Hordon LD, Raisi M, Aaron JE, et al: Trabecular architecture in women and men of similar bone mass with and without vertebral fracture. *Bone* 27:271–276, 2000.
41. Kinney JH, Lane NE, Haupt DL: In vivo, three-dimensional microscopy of trabecular bone. *J Bone Miner Res* 10:264–270, 1995.
42. Mandelbrot BB: *Fractals: Form Chance and Dimension.* WH Freeman, San Francisco, CA, 1977.
43. Mellish RWE, Ferguson-Pell MW, Cochran GVB, et al: A new manual method for assessing two-dimensional cancellous bone structure: comparison between iliac crest and lumbar vertebra. *J Bone Miner Res* 6:689–696, 1991.

44. Muller R, Hildebrand T, Hauselmann HJ, et al: In vivo reproducibility of three-dimensional structural properties of non-invasive bone biopsies using 3D-pQCT. *J Bone Miner Res* 11:1745–1750, 1996.
45. Naccache NJ, Shinghal R: An investigation into the skeletonization approach of Hilditch. *Pattern Recogn* 17:279, 1984.
46. Odgaard A, Anderson K, Melson F, et al: A direct method for fast three-dimensional serial reconstruction. *J Microsc* 159:335–342, 1990.
47. Odgaard A, Gundersen HJG: Quantification of connectivity in cancellous bone with special emphasis on 3-D reconstruction. *Bone* 14:173–182, 1993.
48. Parfitt A, Villanueva A, Kleerekoper M, et al: Relationship between surface volume and thickness of iliac crest trabecular bone in aging and in osteoporosis. *J Clinical Invest* 72:1396–1409, 1983.
49. Parfitt AM, Drezner MK, Glorieux FH, et al: Bone histomorphometry: standardization of nomenclature, symbols and units (Report of the ASBMR Histomorphometry Nomenclature Committee). *J Bone Miner Res* 2:595–610, 1987.
50. Parfitt AM: Implications of architecture for the pathogenesis and prevention of vertebral fracture. *Bone* 13:541–547, 1992.
51. Parfitt, AM: Overview of fracture pathogenesis. *Calcif Tissue Int* 53:S2, 1993.
52. Parisien M, Mellish RWE, Silverberg SJ, et al: Maintenance of cancellous bone connectivity in primary hyperparathyroidism: trabecular strut analysis. *J Bone Miner Res* 7:913–919, 1992.
53. Ritzel H, Amberg M, Posl M, et al: The thickness of human cortical bone and its changes in aging and osteoporosis: a histomorphometric analysis of the complete spinal column from thirty seven autopsy specimens. *J Bone Miner Res* 12:89–95, 1997.
54. Schnitzler CM, Pettifor JM, Mesquita JM, et al: Histomorphometry of iliac crest in 346 normal black and white South African adults. *Bone Miner* 10:183–199, 1990.
55. Shahtaheri SM, Aaron JE, Johnson DR, et al: The impact of mammalian reproduction on cancellous bone architecture. *J Anat* 194:407–421, 1999.
56. Shahtaheri SM, Aaron JE, Johnson DR, et al: Changes in trabecular bone architecture in women during pregnancy. *Br J Obstet Gynaecol* 106:432–438, 1999.
57. Shore PA, Shore RC, Aaron JE: A three-dimensional histological method for direct determination of the number of trabecular termini in cancellous bone. *Biotechnic Histochem* 75:183–192, 2000.
58. Spiers FW, Beddoe AH: "Radial" scanning of trabecular bone: consideration of the probability distribution of path lengths through cavities and trabeculae. *Phys Med Biol* 22:670–680, 1977.
59. Vesterby A, Gundersen H, Melson F: Star volume of bone marrow space and trabeculae of the first lumbar vertebra: sampling efficiency and biological variation. *Bone* 10:7–13, 1989.
60. Vesterby A: Star volume of marrow space and trabeculae in iliac crest: sampling procedure and correlation to star volume of first lumbar vertebrae. *Bone* 11:149–155, 1990.
61. Vogt JH: Investigations on the bone chemistry of man. I. Ash content of the spongy substance of the iliac crest. *Acta Med Scand* 135:221–230, 1949.
62. Wakamatsu E, Sissons H: The cancellous bone of the iliac crest. *Calcif Tissue Res* 4:147–161, 1969.
63. Weinstein RS, Majumdar S, Genant HK: Fractal geometry applied to the architecture of cancellous bone biopsy specimens. *Bone* 13:A38, 1992.
64. Whitehouse WJ, Dyson E, Jackson C: The scanning electron microscope in studies of trabecular bone from a human vertebral body. *J Anat* 103:481–496, 1971.
65. Whitehouse WJ: The quantitative morphology of anisotropic trabecular bone. *J Microsc* 101:153–168, 1974.
66. Whitehouse WJ: Irregularities and asymmetries in trabecular bone in the inominate and elsewhere. *Metab Bone Dis* 2S:271–278, 1980.
67. Yanuka M, Dullien FAL, Elrick DE: Serial sectioning and digitization of porous media for two and three dimensional analysis and reconstruction. *J Microsc* 135:159–168, 1984.
68. *http://math.bu.edu/DYSYS/chaos-game/node6.html.*

Table 1. Schedule for the Subcutaneous Administration of a Sequential Range of Fluorochromes

Weeks before sacrifice	Fluorochrome	Color	Dose
11	Tetracycline	Yellow	25 mg/kg
9	Calcein	Green	25 mg/kg
6	Alizarin complexon	Red	25 mg/kg
1	Tetracycline	Yellow	25 mg/kg

Total implantation time is 12 wk.

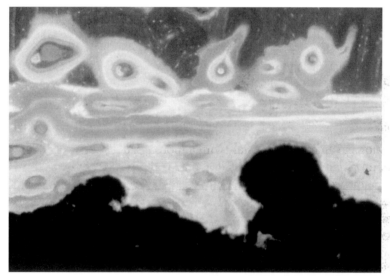

Figure 1. Fluorescence micrograph of bone response to a rough titanium-implant surface. Three labels were administered subcutaneously, i.e., tetracycline (yellow, at 1 wk post-implantation), calcein (green, at 3 wk post-implantation), and alizarin complexon (red, at 6 wk post-implantation). (*See* color plate 17 appearing in the insert following p. 270.)

tetracycline antibiotics are toxic for certain experimental animal species. An example of a fluorochrome sequential labeling schedule is provided in Table 1. Fig. 1 shows an example of a fluorochrome-labeled light microscopy section. By measuring the distance between the bands, which represent the mineralization front, additional information about the bone formation rate can be obtained.

C. Microradiography

Microradiography is a method in which a light microscopy section is examined using X-rays instead of visible light. This noninvasive method provides information about the progress of the repair process and remodeling activity of the bone surrounding the implant. Old, highly mineralized bone will appear in light tones in the microradiograph. Grayer tones represent the newly formed, incompletely mineralized bone. For an extensive description of the microradiograph procedure, *see* reviews by Eschberger[7] and Plenk.[12] Unfortunately, the level of resolution of microradiographs is rather low. This hinders accurate evaluation of the interfacial implant-bone response. In view of this, it can be theorized that because of recent improvements in microcomputer-assisted tomography, microradiographs will become obsolete.[18]

IV. HISTOMORPHOMETRIC ANALYSIS

For the accurate evaluation of an implant, quantitative histomorphometry must be used in addition to subjective histological analysis. The following areas are of interest for the quantitative evaluation of hard-tissue implants:

1. The implant: Using presently available techniques, *in situ* light microscopic sections of the implant can be made.[6,17] The histological appearance of an implant can provide information about the stability or degradation behavior of a material.
2. The surrounding tissue: The zone of remodeled bone or soft-tissue capsule surrounding the implant is considered to be the inflammatory and healing reaction in response to the surgical trauma and the continued presence of the implant.
3. The interface: This type of tissue is directly adjacent to the implant surface. The nature of this tissue is determined by the chemical, physical, and biologic properties of the biomaterial.
4. The interstitial tissue: This is the tissue that has grown into the pores of a porous implant. The degree of ingrowth will, in addition to the chemical and physical properties of the material, also depend upon the biomechanical conditions of the implantation model.[8]

Considering these areas of interest, various parameters can be used to describe the structure of the bone that is in contact with the implant.

A. Histologic Grading Scales

On the basis of the areas of interest described in Section IV, the use of a histological grading scale should be the first histomorphometric evaluation. In such a scale, the histological characteristics of the bone-implant reaction are evaluated by assigning scoring points. An example of a grading scale is outlined in Table 2.[10] The concepts and reasons for their design are described here.

The quality and quantity of the reaction of the tissues surrounding an implant are determined by the surgical technique (implant fit, drilling parameters, vascular and periosteal damage), implant characteristics (bulk and surface properties), implant site (cortical or trabecular bone, loading condition), and implantation time (short- or long-term studies).[15] Considering these parameters, the grading scale in Table 2 for the surrounding tissue reactions is based on semi-quantitative and qualitative classifications. Although it is always possible that the implant will evoke no reaction in the surrounding tissues, in most situations the surrounding tissue will show a reaction. The quality and quantity of this reaction can range from minimal to severe. For bone implants, the quantity of the tissue reaction can be characterized by the width in micrometers of the zone next to the implant, where other tissue has replaced the original bone tissue. The quality of this tissue can vary between original compact bone, new lamellar bone (usually with a changed osteon orientation), woven bone, and inflammatory tissue (Fig. 2).

The interface represents the tissue that is in close contact with the implant surface. As mentioned earlier, this local tissue reaction is determined by the physicochemical properties of the implant material. For bone implants, the optimal situation arises when there

Table 2. Histologic Grading Scale for Bone Implants

Reaction zone	Response	Score
Bone reaction semi-quantitative	Thickness rating (mm):	
	0–50	4
	51–250	3
	251–500	2
	>501	1
	Not applicable.	0
Bone reaction qualitative	Similar to original cortical bone.	4
	Lamellar or woven bone with bone-forming activity.	3
	Lamellar or woven bone with bone-forming activity and osteoclastic activity.	2
	Tissue other than bone (e.g., fibrous tissue).	1
	Inflammation.	0
Interface qualitative	Direct bone-to-implant contact without soft-tissue interlayer.	4
	Remodeling lacuna with osteoblasts and/or osteoclasts at surface.	3
	Localized fibrous tissue not arranged as a capsule.	2
	Fibrous tissue capsule.	1
	Inflammation.	0
Interstitium qualitative	Mature bone and differentiation of bone marrow can be observed in the interstitium.	4
	Bone formation can be observed in the interstitium.	3
	Tissue in interstitium consists of fibrous connective tissue characterized by condensation of collagen fibers at the implant interface.	2
	Tissue in interstitium consists of fibrous connective tissue with a pronounced cellular and vascular component.	1
	Implant cannot be evaluated because of problems that may not be related to the material to be tested.	0

Adapted from reference[10].

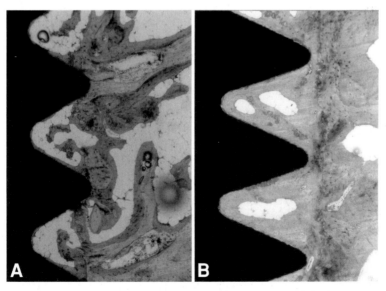

Figure 2. Light micrograph showing the histological appearance of the bone response to (A) titanium implant provided with 1-μm-thick calcium phosphate coating. After 6 wk of implantation, bone ingrowth proceeded over the implant surface. (B) A similar implant provided with a 4-μm-thick coating after 12 wk of implantation. The screw's threads are almost completely filled with new bone.

is direct bone-to-implant contact. In the grading scale, as depicted in Table 2, the bone-implant interface is classified principally according to its morphologic appearance. If required, this scale can be further differentiated by additional specification of the observed tissues.[5]

Occasionally, for very specific clinical applications, porous implant materials are used. Examples include porous ceramic, metallic, and polymeric materials, as used for scaffold material in bone reconstruction and tissue engineering. The tissue that grows into these porous materials can show widely variable stages of organization. In a bony environment, the tissue within the interstice or porosity may consist of connective tissue with a pronounced cellular and vascular component; connective tissue characterized by condensation of collagen fibers at the interface of the implant material; remodeling bone; and remodeled bone, lamellar bone, and/or differentiating marrow.[4] The interstitial tissue classification, as shown in Table 2, is based on these histologic patterns.

Before using grading scales, consensus must be reached about the histological appearance of the various situations. For this purpose, a series of photographs representing the various situations can be used as a reference. It must also be noted that the various evaluation parameters must be scored at several points along the implant interface. For example, depending on the total length of the implant, the evaluation can be performed at regular 100–250-µm intervals along the implant surface. Also, the measurements must begin some distance from the implant margins in order to prevent non-implant-related side effects. Subsequently, for the final score, the means of all measurements for each section can be calculated.

B. Quantitative Interfacial Analysis

In addition to qualitative analysis using histologic grading scales, a quantitative assessment of the bone response can be performed. However, it should be noted that many of the procedures are typically very time-consuming. In addition, they frequently provide information that is difficult to understand for the general reader, and which causes more confusion than insight. In general, the following parameters are of major interest in evaluating the bone response close to the implant surface:

1. Percentage of bone contact: The percentage of implant length at which there is direct bone-to-implant contact, without intervening tissue. These measurements are performed along the total length of the implant.
2. Bone density: The percentage of bone fill in predetermined areas around the implant.

The percentage of bone contact provides information about the fixation of the implant in the bone. In follow-up studies, it provides insight on the effect of the physicochemical properties of an implant material and loading mode of an implant on bone repair.[9,15,19]

The bone density around the implant reflects the degree of compatibility and integration of the inserted implant under certain defined conditions. A less than ideal bone biocompatibility will result in reduced integration of the implant in the stress-transferring system of the surrounding bone. This implies that the implant will act as a constant mechanical stimulus, reflected in increased bone turnover around the implant.[3,14]

It should also be noted that for specific types of implants, additional parameters can be evaluated. For example, for perimucosal oral implants the first screw thread that shows direct bone contact can be determined, and information about the gingival response can be obtained.[2] The same is true for specific types of implants such as calcium phosphate

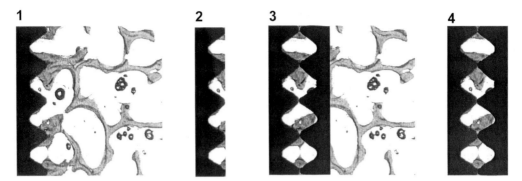

Figure 3. Illustration of computer-based image analysis measurements to determine bone density inside and outside a threaded implant. First, the area of interest is determined. Subsequently, the bone density inside the screw threads is determined. Then, the implant surface is flipped over, resulting in the total region of interest. The bone density in this area is measured. Finally, using subtraction, the bone density outside the screw threads is measured.

(CaP)-coated implants, for which thickness of the coating that remains at the end of the implantation period can be measured.[2]

To perform the quantitative evaluation, an automatic or semi-automatic computer-assisted image-analysis system is used. The required software is commercially available, and can be very simple to operate. An example of computer-based image analysis measurements of the bone density around an implant is given in Fig. 3.

V. FINAL REMARKS

Histomorphometry can be very valuable in measuring the changes in the tissues that surround an implant. However, parameters used are often complex and the procedures for quantifying them are usually time-consuming. Recent improvements in computer-assisted image-analysis systems have made some of the procedures more efficient, which may help save time. Nevertheless, the parameters as used in the evaluation procedure must be as simple as possible, yet still provide the required information. Besides sophisticated quantification of the implant-tissue response, histomorphometric-grading scales can be used. Usually, they can be designed to be sensitive enough to reveal differences in tissue response to implanted materials. Therefore, they must be considered a useful addition to the armamentarium of analytic methods for evaluating the structural changes in the implant-surrounding tissue.

REFERENCES

1. Black J: *Biological Performance of Materials.* Marcel Dekker, Inc., New York, NY, 1992.
2. Caulier H, Van der Waerden JPCM, Wolke JGC, et al: A histological and histomorphometrical evaluation of the application of screw-designed calcium phosphate (Ca-P) coated implants in the cancellous maxillary bone of the goat. *J Biomed Mater Res* 35:19–30, 1997.
3. Corten FGA, Caulier H, Vand der Waerden JPCM, et al: Assessment of bone surrounding implants in goats: ex vivo measurements by dual X-ray absorptiometry. *Biomaterials* 18:495–501, 1997.
4. Damien CJ, Parsons JR: Bone graft and bone graft substitutes: a review of current technology and applications. *J Appl Biomater* 2:187–208, 1991.

5. Dhert WJA, Thomsen P, Blomgren AK, et al: Integration of press-fit implants in cortical bone: a study on interface kinetics. *J Biomed Mater Res* 41:574–583, 1998.

6. Donath K, Breuner GA: A method for the study of undecalcified bones and teeth with attached soft tissue. *J Oral Pathol* 11:318–326, 1982.

7. Eschberger DG, Eschberger J: Microradiography. In: von Recum AF, ed: *Handbook of Biomaterials Evaluation.* Taylor and Francis, Philadelphia, PA, 1999:743–754.

8. Heimke G: The aspects and modes of fixation of bone replacements. In: Heimke G, ed: *Osseointegrated Implants Volume 1.* CRC Press, Boca Raton, FL, 1990:1–30.

9. Hulshoff JEG, Jansen JA: Initial interfacial healing events around calcium phosphate (Ca-P) coated oral implants. *Clin Oral Implants Res* 8:393–400, 1997.

10. Jansen JA, Dhert WJA, van der Waerden JPCM, et al: A semi-quantitative and semi-qualitative histologic analysis method for the evaluation of implants. *J Invest Surg* 7:123–134, 1994.

11. Osborn JS, Newesly H: Dynamic aspects of the implant-bone interface. In: Heimke G, ed: *Dental Implants: Materials and Systems.* Carl Hanser Verlag, Munich, Germany, 1980:111–23.

12. Plenk H: Microscopic evaluation of hard tissue implants. In: Williams DF, ed: *Techniques of Biocompatibility Testing Volume 1.* CRC Press, Boca Raton, FL, 1986:35–82.

13. Rahn BA: Intra vitam staining techniques. In: von Recum AF, ed: *Handbook of Biomaterials Evaluation.* Taylor and Francis, Philadelphia, PA, 1999:727–738.

14. Søballe K: Hydroxyapatite ceramic coating for bone implant fixation. Mechanical and histological studies in dogs. *Acta Orthop Scand Suppl* 255:1–58, 1993.

15. Szmukler-Moncler S, Salama H, Reingewirtz Y, et al: Timing of loading and effect of micromotion on bone-dental implant interface: review of experimental literature. *J Biomed Mater Res (Appl Biomater)* 43:192–203, 1998.

16. Tencer AF: Osteocompatibility. In: von Recum AF, ed: *Handbook of Biomaterials Evaluation.* Taylor and Francis, Philadelphia, PA, 1999:539–566.

17. Van der Lubbe HBM, Klein CPAT, de Groot K: A simple method for preparing thin histological sections of undecalcified plastic embedded bone with implants. *Stain Technol* 63:171–177, 1988.

18. Van Oosterwijck H, Duyck J, Vander Sloten J, et al: The use of microfocus computerized tomography as a new technique for characterizing bone tissue around oral implants. *J Oral Implantol* 26:5–12, 2000.

19. Vercaigne S, Wolke JGC, Naert I, et al: A histological evaluation of TiO_2 grit-blasted and Ca-P magnetron sputter coated implants placed into the trabecular bone of the goat: part 2. *Clin Oral Implants Res* 11:314–324, 2000.

27

Histomorphometric Analysis of Bone–Cement and Cement–Metal Interface

Jian-Sheng Wang,[1] Gonzalo G. Valdivia,[2] Michael J. Dunbar,[3] Cecil H. Rorabeck,[2] Robert B. Bourne,[2] and Suzanne Maher[4]

[1]Biomaterials and Biomechanics Laboratory, Department of Orthopaedics, Lund University Hospital, Lund, Sweden
[2]Division of Orthopaedic Surgery, London Health Sciences Centre, University of Western Ontario, London, Ontario, Canada
[3]Division of Orthopaedics, QE II Health Sciences Centre, Dalhousie University, Halifax, Nova Scotia, Canada
[4]Laboratory for Biomedical Mechanics and Materials, The Hospital for Special Surgery, New York, NY, USA

I. INTRODUCTION

Bone cement primarily functions by filling the free space between the prosthesis and the bone. The connection between the cement and the bone and between the cement and the prosthesis has been repeatedly and intensively studied since cement was introduced for use with hip arthroplasty. The irregularities of the bone surface and the penetration of the cement into the trabecular spongiosa are an important prerequisite for long-term survival of the implant.[16] Loosening of cemented femoral components occurs either at the cement-prosthesis interface—and eventually at the bone-cement interface—or directly at the bone-cement interface, which is basically a biomechanical and biological phenomenon. Identification of the sequence of events that initiate and lead to loosening is important in the effort to improve the survivorship of prosthetic components. In this respect, morphological evaluations of cemented femoral components are essential for the evaluation of the biological and mechanical responses to the prosthesis.[14,22]

Several investigators have reported hypotheses regarding the factors that influence the failure of the cement-prosthesis interface. Possible causes of loosening at the bone-cement interface have been related to thermal injury, cement shrinkage, monomer toxicity, creep, and inappropriate viscosity. Biological causes of loosening at the interface include local vascular injury, infection, and reaction to wear particles. Biomechanical reasons include the design of the prosthesis, micromotion, stress shielding, stress concentration, and cement interface porosity. All these factors may eventually result in

From: *Handbook of Histology Methods for Bone and Cartilage*
Edited by: Y. H. An and K. L. Martin © Humana Press Inc., Totowa, NJ

damage accumulation in the cement mantle, debonding at the cement-prosthesis interface, and osteolysis.

In order to comment on prosthetic survival within a cement mantle, it is important to know the orientation of the cement at the cement-bone and cement-stem interface and to observe the details of the processes of skeletal remodeling and the effects of these processes on the stability of the prosthetic components. A useful and direct method for the evaluation of the integration of cemented implants is histomorphometric analysis. This chapter will introduce three methods for quantitative analysis at the bone-cement and cement-prosthesis interfaces as well as cement-mantle thickness.

II. METHOD 1: INTERFACE CONTACT STUDY

A. Introduction

Bone cement is subject to volumetric shrinkage in the range of 1–5%.[5] The shrinkage of cement could compromise the integrity of the cement-bone or cement-prosthesis interface. Wang et al.[22] demonstrated that most cemented implants are associated with small gaps that are less than 100 µm and occupy about 10–15% of the surrounding bone-cement and cement-stem interface. These gaps may reduce the bonding strength and initiate the debonding when loading the prostheses.[19] Jasty et al.[7] investigated several femora with cemented implants harvested at autopsy. They found cement-metal interface debonding to some degree in all of the femora that had been functioning for more than 4 yr. However, quantification of the histomorphometric interface changes was not reported. Improving interface integrity is essential to prolong the longevity of cemented femoral components. Therefore, it is important to determine the nature of—and changes in—the interface integrity for cemented prosthesis.

B. Materials and Methods

Cemented implants with bone should be prepared through immersion-fixation in phosphate-buffered 4% formalin for about 2 mo. The specimens can be sectioned transversely by using either a water-cooled diamond saw or a high-pressure water cutter.[14,22] Before cutting, bone specimens should be marked longitudinally on the bone surface with a sharp cut that will help to find the gap position of the consecutive sections from proximal to distal. Ten-millimeter-thick sections are obtained at 10-mm intervals over an axial distance of approx 200 mm. Usually, about five sections can be obtained per implant (Fig. 1). These sections are used to evaluate the morphology. All specimens are investigated blindly in random order. The integrity of the interfaces between bone and cement and between the cement and stem interfaces is examined using a microscope with a computerized imaging system (analySIS, Soft Imaging System, Germany).

When the interfaces show a separation between bone and cement, or between cement and stem, the separation is known as an interface gap (Fig. 2). The circumferences of the bone-cement and cement-stem interfaces are measured. The length and width of all the gaps between bone and cement and between cement and stem on the cross-section are measured by the imaging system. The width of the gaps is graded as follows: Grade I <100 µm, Grade II 101–500 µm and Grade III more than 501 µm. The percentage of the circumference of the interface occupied by the gap is calculated by dividing the distance of the gap part of the circumference by the total distance of the interface circumference in each section, and multiplying by 100. The percentage of the

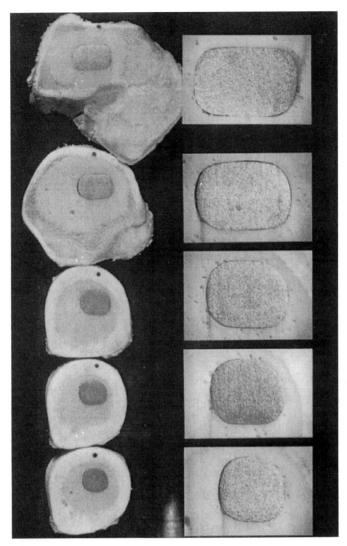

Figure 1. Consecutive sections from cemented implant with pig femur (cut by a high-pressure water cutter). The black marks above the edge of each sample indicate the position of the implanted prosthesis. There are many pores and gaps surrounding the prosthesis. Magnification: left ×1, right ×2.5.

circumference of the interface contact can also be calculated by dividing the distance of the contact circumference by the total distance of the interface circumference in each section and multiplying by 100. Using this method, the parameter of interface contact can be easily obtained.

III. METHOD 2: INTERFACE POROSITY STUDY

A. Introduction

Several studies have revealed that extensive porosity is aggregated at the cement-stem interface in retrieved cement-mantle and laboratory-prepared specimens.[2,6,8] This aggre-

A

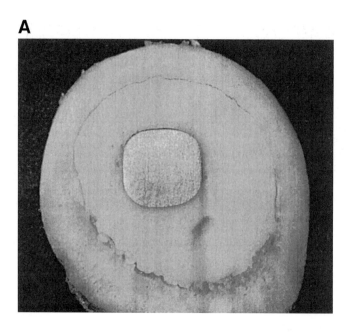

B

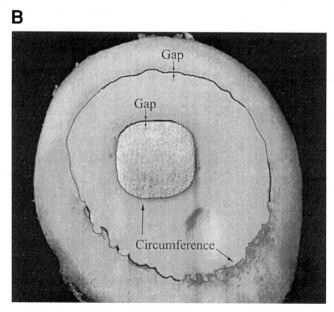

Figure 2. (A) A cross-section of cemented stem shows gaps surrounding the stem and bone. (B) This picture is same as (A); it shows measurement of circumferences (thinner line) and gaps (thicker line). Magnification ×2.

gation of pores could influence the interface bonding between the stem and the cement.[4,6,23] Interfacial porosity between cement and prosthesis can be formed during the preparation of bone cement (Fig. 3), stem insertion and polymerization of bone cement. Examination of the interface porosity is important in determining the integration of cemented implants.

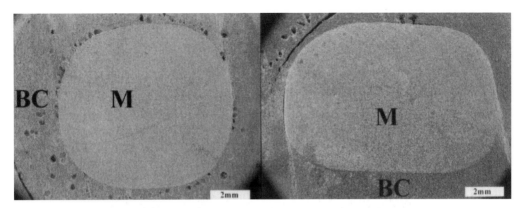

Figure 3. The photos show many pores on the interface between bone cement (BC) and stem (M = metal). In the left photo, the cement was mixed at atmospheric pressure; in the right photo, the cement was mixed under vacuum.

B. Materials and Methods

Transverse sections of cemented implants with bone can be obtained by using either a water-cooled diamond saw or a high-pressure water cutter. Consecutive sections are used to evaluate the interface porosity. All specimens are investigated blindly in random order. The porosity between bone and cement and between the cement and stem interfaces is examined using a microscope. When the specimens need a better contrast, the surface of each section is stained using black oil (Fig. 4). A microscope with a direct light examines the specimens. The pores in bone cement at a distance of 0.5 mm from the bone or prosthesis are defined as interface pores (Fig. 4). The pores at the interface are counted, and the circumferences of the cement-bone and cement-prosthesis interfaces are measured using a microscope with a computerized imaging system (analySIS, Soft Imaging System, Germany). The percentage of the interface porosity is calculated by dividing the number of pores at the interface by the circumference.

IV. METHOD 3: CEMENT THICKNESS STUDY

A. Introduction

The adequacy of femoral cement mantles after hip arthroplasty are usually assessed using conventional radiographs. However, concern has been raised regarding the adequacy of plain radiographs for the evaluation of the cement mantle. In their study of eight retrieved femurs from clinically successful total hip arthroplasty, Kawate et al.[9] noted that plain X-rays missed areas of the cement thinner than 1 mm. In addition, they reported that thin areas showed the greatest number (92%) of cement micro-fractures. In their 18-yr follow-up of 161 cemented total hips, Smith et al.[20] noted that the use of slightly different projections made their grading of the cement mantle more accurate because it allowed them to observe voids and areas of thin cement not identified in the original postoperative films. In an experimental analysis, Reading et al.[17] found that plain X-rays failed to account for several defects in the cement when compared to direct visualization of cross-sections.

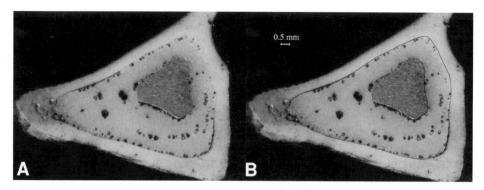

Figure 4. (A) This is a section from the cemented prosthesis of a rabbit tibia. The bone cement was mixed at atmospheric pressure. There are many pores along the cement-bone and cement-stem interfaces. (B) This photo is identical to (A), except the scale bar used for measurement of circumference is shown.

A tool has been developed for the accurate in vitro assessment of cement-mantle thickness. Central to the design of this new method was the use of resin replicas of femoral stems in order to avoid image degradation caused by scatter; the use of a high-definition computed tomography (CT) scanner and the computerized analysis of cement-mantle thickness.

B. Materials and Methods

Exact plastic replicas are made of the cemented femoral stems chosen for study. The replicas are manufactured by first making silicone rubber molds of each required size. The RTV silicone base is measured and placed into a disposable container that is approximately four times the volume of the rubber. The activator is accurately measured by weight comparison and then added to the rubber. The mixture is then thoroughly mixed utilizing a flat-blade spatula. The mixture is stirred slowly until the mixture reaches a uniform color. The mixed RTV silicone rubber is then placed into a deaeration chamber capable of 28–29 inches of mercury vacuum. The rubber must be allowed to expand and collapse back to its original volume. The vacuum is maintained for an additional 1–2 min. The vacuum is then released. Each stem is placed inside a plastic container. The mixture is then poured slowly over the entire stem. The rubber is allowed to cure for a minimum of 16 h at room temperature (21°C). Lower temperatures and/or low humidity will cause the cure-time to lengthen; conversely, higher temperatures and/or high humidity will cause the cure-time to shorten. Once cured, the block of silicone is removed from the plastic container. The stem is then ready to be carefully removed from the container, and the silicone mold is ready for producing replica stems. The material used to make the stem replicas was Easy-Cast BN-72 (Gersan Industries, Inc., High Point, NC). This is a two-part urethane that mixes at a 1:1 ratio by weight. It has a gel time of 2–5 min and a demold time of 6–10 min. It is a low viscosity and can be poured easily into small or intricate molds, giving excellent air release with little to no shrinkage.

The stem replicas are cemented into a predetermined number of cadaver femora. Fresh or thawed femora are best, but embalmed cadaver femora can also be used. Preparation of the femurs must be done according to the manufacturer's instructions and instrumentation. Third-generation cementing techniques are usually employed, which include brushing, pressure-water lavage, use of a distal cement restrictor, vacuum mixing of two units of radio-opaque bone cement, retrograde filling with a gun, and pressurization. The final stem size is chosen according to the largest broach that can be seated easily. If employed, the recommended distal and/or proximal stem centralizers are chosen.

Radio-opaque bone cement usually contains about 10% barium sulfate. Unfortunately, this gives cement a radio-opacity almost equal to that of bone. In order to enhance the contrast and facilitate automated analysis of the images, we add 1 g of barium sulfate per 10 g of bone cement.

Following implantation, the specimens can be imaged using a clinical CT scanner (HiSpeed Advantage™ helical scanner, General Electric). Thin slices (1 mm) should be acquired at predetermined intervals (1–5 mm) over the axial distance of the stems. The X-ray parameters used were of 80-kVp tube potential and 200 mA per CT slice. Retrospective acquisition of a 100×100 mm field of view in a 512×512 reconstruction matrix was performed. This provided for a pixel spacing of 0.1953 mm. One-millimeter-thick slices were acquired at 5-mm intervals over an axial distance of approx 150 mm. Typically, approx 25 axial images were obtained per implant (Fig. 5).

The axial images are next transferred to a computer workstation, where they are analyzed using proprietary and custom-made algorithms. The cement-prosthesis interface is determined using a software tool based on the Geometrically Deformable Model (GDM).[12] The obtained implant contour is sampled with a vertex spacing of two pixels (0.39 mm) (Fig. 6A). A single operator traces the cement-bone interface in each axial image. The tracing is then fitted with a B-spline contour (Fig. 6B). The obtained outer cement B-spline contour is interpolated to a constant number of vertices (400). Using a customized computer program, the cement-mantle thickness is determined at each implant contour vertex as the distance from this point to the closest vertex in the outer cement contour (Fig. 6C). Using the long axis of the proximal stem cross-section geometry as a reference, the thickness measurements are grouped into twelve 30-degree annular segments for the purpose of the comparative analysis (Fig. 6D). Minimum, maximum, and mean cement-thickness values are computed for each 30-degree region in each axial slice. Cement-mantle thickness is compared overall and by axial regions: proximal, middle, and distal thirds; and annular regions: anterior (segments 3 and 4), posterior (segments 9 and 10), medial (segments 6 and 7), lateral (segments 1 and 12), medial corners (segments 5 and 8), and lateral corners (segments 2 and 11). Statistical analysis is carried out using ANOVA and the Student's t-test. Finally, using the acquired data, three-dimensional (3D) reconstructions of the stem geometry can be performed. After applying four-point interpolation algorithms, the thickness measurements are then mapped on the surface of the stem, offering a visual representation of the cement-mantle-thickness distribution (Fig. 7).

V. METHOD 4: CEMENT PENETRATION STUDY

A. Introduction

When bone cement is inserted into a prepared cancellous bed and further pressurized through implant insertion, it extrudes through porous cancellous bone and forms cement *pedicles* of varying depths, widths, and profile, which subsequently polymerize into a

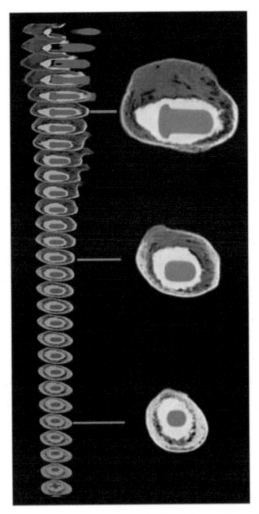

Figure 5. Typical axial images obtained for each specimen.

fixed shape (Fig. 8A). Cement pedicle characteristics vary with cancellous bone morphology,[18] quality and strength of bone,[10] canal preparation techniques,[15] cementing mixing and insertion techniques,[1] and the distribution of pressure during prosthesis insertion.[10] Traditionally, the depth of cement penetration has been the only feature of interlock used to quantify the cement/bone interface morphology. However, it is clear that the interface is more complex than can be captured by a single geometric value.

To more fully characterize the morphological state of the interface, a method has been developed that i) measures the depth and width of the cement pedicles, ii) explores the regional variation in features, and iii) defines a parameter that combines multiple pedicle features into one characteristic value. A clearer description of the cement/bone interface morphology may allow for a closer understanding of the distribution in its mechanical properties, as reported throughout the literature.[8,14,15]

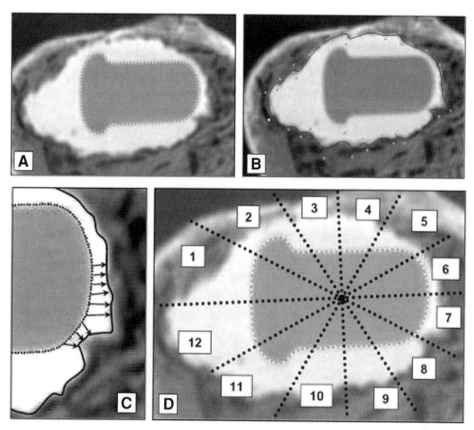

Figure 6. Computerized analysis of the cement mantle. (A) GDM contour of the stem (cement-prosthesis interface). (B) B-spline of the outer cement boundary (cement-bone interface) with control points. (C) Measurement of cement thickness every second pixel along the stem contour. (D) Twelve 30-degree annular segments used in the analysis (1–6 anterior, 7–12 posterior).

B. Methods and Materials

A femur is cast into a rectangular wooden mold using Potter's Plaster. After setting, the plaster block is removed and transversely sectioned using a Buehler Abrasive Cutting machine with an oil-based coolant. The surfaces of each slice are polished, scanned, and imported into National Institutes of Health (NIH) image software for analysis.

The image is magnified, and the material interfaces of each slice are manually contoured (Fig. 8B). A two-dimensional (2D) coordinate system is defined, with its origin at the center of the prosthesis cross-section. The threshold level of the image is decreased so that only the black outline of the cement/bone interface contour is visible. Image-analysis software constructs lines through the image. The (x,y) coordinates of each point that intersects a line are recorded (Fig. 8C). The coordinate values are imported to an Excel spreadsheet. The angular position of each point relative to the anterior/posterior axis (Fig. 8B), and its distance from the center of the prosthesis are computed. The data is ordered according to the increasing relative angular position. In this way, the cement/bone inter-

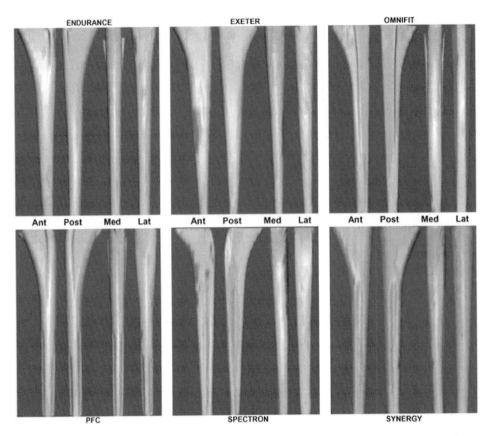

Figure 7. Surface mapping of the cement-mantle thickness. Red <1 mm; yellow 1–2 mm; white 2–4 mm and blue >4 mm. (*See* color plate 18 appearing in the insert following p. 270.)

face is now geometrically represented by a series of 2D coordinates, the origin of which lies at the center of the prosthesis. Excel custom-written programs[13] identify cement pedicles on the basis of relative changes in the distance between the center of the prosthesis and adjacent perimeter coordinate data. Pedicle depth and width are measured automatically (Fig. 8D). To prevent data distortion, a threshold of 0.5 mm was defined, below which the waviness of the interface was not considered to be a pedicle.

A single parameter, called the *random undulating parameter (RUP)* was designed, which combined the waviness of the interface into a single value. Because the cement mantle is not perfectly cylindrical in shape, the RUP was computed in 10-degree increments around the interface (Fig. 9). This parameter combines all features of the interface into a single parameter, as graphically and numerically illustrated in Fig. 9.

VI. SUMMARY

The definition of a cement pedicle, although rarely quoted in the literature,[1,3] determines reported cemented penetration depths. This could, in part, explain the ranges of pedicle depths that are quoted in the literature.[11,21] The semi-automated methods described here are

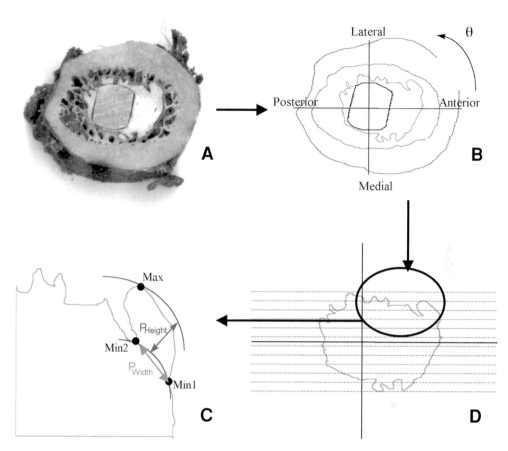

Figure 8. (A) Even in a single transverse slice through a cemented femoral implant, the variations in pedicle morphology are evident. (B) The interfaces are outlined. The center of the prosthesis cross-section is computed and used as the origin for a 2D coordinate system. (C) Lines parallel to the anterior/posterior axis are constructed, and the coordinates of the points of intersection between the cement/bone contour and the parallel lines are recorded. Note: the lines are separated in this figure for clarity. (D) Cement pedicle height (P_{height}) and width (P_{width}) are computed by identifying local minimum points (Min1 and Min2) and a local maximum point (Max). Reproduced in part with permission from: Professional Engineering Publishing Limited—the Proceedings of the Institute of Engineers.

advantageous because interobserver variability are minimized. However, in automating pedicle measurements, the width and depths of the individual pedicles are dependent on the mathematical "instructions" given to the custom programs, which define how to identify a pedicle. A parameter, such as the RUP, which includes all undulations of the interface, and avoids the identification of individual pedicles, would appear to be a more ideal approach to describing the complex morphology of the cement/bone interface.

Acknowledgment: We thank Water Jet Sweden AB, Ronneby, Sweden, Herman Anderssons Platt AB, Hörby, Sweden. Financial support was provided by the Swedish Medical Research Council (09509), Stiftelsen for bistand at rorelsehindrade i skane and Medical Faculty, Lund University.

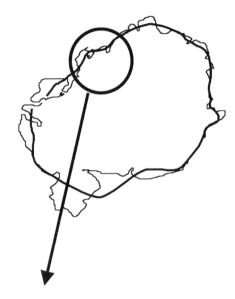

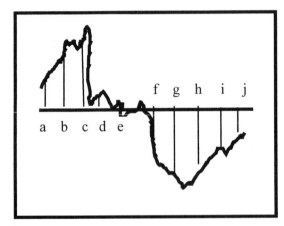

$$RUP = \frac{a + b + c + \dots}{n}$$

Figure 9. The method by which the RUP is computed is illustrated. Note: a,b,c are the heights of points along the cement/bone interface, and n is the total number of heights measured. Reproduced with permission from: Professional Engineering Publishing Limited—the Proceedings of the Institute of Engineers.

REFERENCES

1. Bannister GC, Miles AW: The influence of cementing technique and blood on the strength of the bone-cement interface. *Eng Med* 17:131–133, 1988.
2. Bishop NE, Ferguson S, Tepic S: Porosity reduction in bone cement at the stem-cement interface. *J Bone Joint Surg [Br]* 78:349–356, 1996.
3. Bugbee WD, Barrera DL, Lee AC, et al: Bone-cement interface strength in the proximal femur: the effect of cementing technique. *Proc 38th Orthop Res Soc* 1992:376.
4. Davies JP, Kawate K, Harris WH: Effect of interfacial porosity on the torsional strength of the cement-metal interface. *Transactions 41st Annual Meeting Orthop Res Soc* 1995:713.

5. Haas SS, Brauer GM, Dickson GM: A characterization of polymethylmethacrylate bone cement. *J Bone Joint Surg [Am]* 57:380–391, 1975.

6. James SP, Schmalzried TP, McGarry FJ, et al: Extensive porosity at the cement-femoral prosthesis interface: a preliminary study. *J Biomed Mater Res* 27:71–78, 1993.

7. Jasty M, Maloney W, Bragdon CR, et al: Histomorphological studies of the long-term skeletal responses to well fixed cemented femoral components. *J Bone Joint Surg [Am]* 72:1220–1229, 1990.

8. Jasty M, Maloney W, Bragdon CR, et al: The initiation of failure in cemented femoral components of hip arthroplasties. *J Bone Joint Surg [Br]* 73:551–558, 1991.

9. Kawate K, Maloney WJ, Bragdon CR, et al: Importance of a thin cement mantle. Autopsy studies of eight hips. *Clin Orthop* 355:70–76, 1998.

10. Krause WR, Krug WR, Miller J: Strength of the cement-bone interface. *Clin Orthop* 163:290–299, 1980.

11. Kusleika R, Stupp SI: Mechanical strength of PMMA cement—human bone interfaces. *J Biomed Mater Res* 17:441–458, 1983.

12. Lobregt S, Viergever MA: A discrete dynamic contour model. *IEEE Trans Med Imaging* 14:12–23, 1995.

13. Maher SA: Modelling the morphological features of the cement/bone interface in hip replacements. Master of Engineering Science Thesis, National University of Ireland, Dublin, Ireland, 1996.

14. Maher SA, McCormack BAO: Quantification of interdigitation at bone cement/cancellous bone interfaces in cemented femoral reconstructions. *Proc Inst Mech Eng* 213:347–354, 1999.

15. Majowski RS, Miles AW, Bannister GC, et al: Bone surface preparation in cemented joint replacement. *J Bone Joint Surg [Br]* 75:459–463, 1993.

16. Reading AD, McCaskie AW, Barnes MR, et al: A comparison of 2 modern femoral cementing techniques: analysis by cement-bone interface pressure measurements, computerized image analysis, and static mechanical testing. *J Arthroplasty* 15:479–487, 2000.

17. Reading AD, McCaskie AW, Gregg PJ: The inadequacy of standard radiographs in detecting flaws in the cement mantle. *J Bone Joint Surg [Br]* 81:167–170, 1999.

18. Rosenstein A, MacDonald W, Iliadis A, McLardy-Smith: Revision of cemented fixation and cement-bone interface strength. *Proc Inst Mech Eng* 206:47–49, 1992.

19. Shepard MF, Kabo JM, Lieberman JR: Influence of cement technique on the interface strength of femoral components. *Clin Orthop* 381:26–35, 2000.

20. Smith SW, Estok DM, 2nd, Harris WH: Total hip arthroplasty with use of second-generation cementing techniques. An eighteen-year-average follow-up study. *J Bone Joint Surg [Am]* 80:1632–1640, 1998.

21. Steege JW, Polizos T, Lewis JL, et al: Failure mechanisms in PMMA around loaded tibial components: *Proc 32nd Orthop Res Soc* 1986:355.

22. Wang J-S, Franzen H, Lidgren L: Interface gap after implantation of a cemented femoral stem in pigs. *Acta Orthop Scand* 70:234–239, 1999.

23. Wang J-S, Kjellsson F, Tanner KE, et al: Influence of stem insertion time on the static shear strength and interface integrity of the stem-cement interface. *Transactions 46th Annual Meeting Orthop Res Soc* 2000:255.

28

Histologic Analysis of Bone Healing

Ryland B. Edwards, III, Mandi J. Lopez, and Mark D. Markel

Comparative Orthopaedic Research Laboratory, Department of Medical Sciences, School of Veterinary Medicine, University of Wisconsin-Madison, Madison, WI, USA

I. INTRODUCTION

The histologic analysis of fracture healing can be accomplished through a combination of techniques, including determination of callus area, grading of fracture union, fracture-gap tissue type, new bone formation, cell kinetics, immunohistochemistry, and tissue vascularity. Previous chapters have presented details on techniques related to bone labeling, tissue collection and fixation, embedding, sectioning, staining, and basic histomorphometry. This chapter focuses on measurements that determine the stage and quality of fracture healing.

II. SPECIMEN PREPARATION

Specimens are placed in 70% ethanol for histologic fixation immediately after euthanasia, or after mechanical testing or other sampling procedures if these are to be performed. The bones are processed for calcified histologic analysis as previously described.[8,13,36] The tissue is dehydrated in increasing concentrations of ethanol followed by acetone. Infiltration and embedding are performed with methylmethacrylate (MMA) under vacuum, and slow polymerization is completed in a 36° C oven.[30] In general, three sections from each block are cut coronally to a width of 200–400 μm using a diamond-wafering blade (Isomet 2000 Precision Saw; Buehler, Lake Bluff, IL). If the cranial and caudal aspects of the bone are to be examined, the coronally divided cortices are glued with cyanoacrylate, and subsequently are sectioned sagittally. In addition, transverse sections can be made by gluing the divided sections. Each section is subsequently ground to 100 μm ± 2 μm using a speed-lapping machine (ML-521D; Maruto Instrument, Tokyo, Japan) set at 80 rpm and a pressure of 0.7 kg/cm^2 and then selectively used for fine-detail microradiography, fluorescent microscopy, and staining techniques.

III. MICRORADIOGRAPHY

Microradiographs provide detailed images of the mineralized architecture of bone cortices, the endosteal and periosteal callus, and the fracture gap. Microradiographs are most commonly used to determine total bone content or percent porosity, and to analyze

From: *Handbook of Histology Methods for Bone and Cartilage*
Edited by: Y. H. An and K. L. Martin © Humana Press Inc., Totowa, NJ

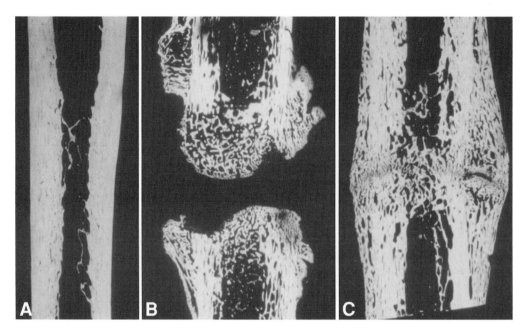

Figure 1. High-detail microradiographic images of intact bone and fracture healing. (A) Intact canine tibia, diaphysis. (B) Mid-diaphyseal tibial osteotomy demonstrating delayed union. (C) Mid-diaphyseal tibial osteotomy with bridging endosteal and periosteal callus in addition to reformation of bone within the cortical fracture gap.

trabecular and callus architecture, orientation, and maturity. During secondary fracture healing, endosteal and periosteal callus mineralization proceed across the fracture gap, perpendicular to the osteonal axes of the cortical bone. Woven bone within the fracture gap is more porous and less organized, and over time, is remodeled by secondary osteons crossing the fracture gap from the bone ends. Mineralization of the callus, porosity of the fracture gap, orientation of the woven bone, and secondary osteonal remodeling will all depend on the fracture stabilization technique, fracture-gap width, soft-tissue trauma around the fracture, fracture location, and time period from fracture to analysis.

High-quality microradiographs provide images with resolution less than 1 μm, and are produced using a modification of the procedure described by Jowsey et al. (Fig. 1).[17] The 200–400-μm methacrylate-sliced sections are ground to 100 μm ± 2 μm thickness using diamond-plated lapping disks (grit 170/200 to 200/230) on a speed-lapping machine (ML-521D; Maruto Instrument). The specimen thickness is confirmed with a micrometer (Peacock Micrometer, Ozaki Manufacturing Company, LTD., Tokyo, Japan). For optimal X-ray technique, the resolution and quality of the image depend on having a small target focal spot at as great a distance as possible between the target and the specimen without lengthening exposure time excessively, and as short a distance as possible between the specimen and film. Fine-detail contact microradiography, with use of a vacuum technique, is performed (18 kVp, 2 min) (model 43855A; Hewlett-Packard Faxitron, McMinnville, OR) using Kodak film (LPF-7, Kodak Professional, Precision Line, Eastman Kodak Company, Professional Division, Rochester, NY) in a standard film sleeve. The target-to-specimen distance is 20 cm, with a 2-min exposure time, and the film is developed using an automated processor.

A. Porosity

There are several methods to determine the porosity of cortical and newly formed bone. The microradiographs may be digitized using a digital camera (Sony DXC-390, 3CCD-Color Video Camera, Sony Corporation, Tokyo, Japan) attached to a light microscope, and software such as NIH Image (NIH Image, National Institutes of Health, Bethesda, MD) or Scion Image (Scion Image for Windows [Version 4.0.1], Scion Corporation, Fredrick, MD). The threshold level of the images is manually adjusted, creating a binary image to distinguish bone and pore space. Porosity, defined as void area per unit area of tissue, can then be calculated as the number of pixels representing void space within the tissue area of interest and expressed as a percentage.[13,42,43] A point-counting method originally described by Harris and Weinberg[14] also has been used by numerous authors.[20,21,39] A superimposed eyepiece grid with five intersecting lines is used with a magnification of ×40. Each line intersection is counted as a point, and the presence of bone or pore is determined for each intersection and recorded. Measurements are made for each area of interest. For fracture healing, these regions include the endosteal callus, periosteal callus, cortical bone adjacent to the fracture gap, and the gap between the cortical bone ends. An example of such an evaluation scheme resulted in 18 areas of interest (Fig. 2). Porosity of the endosteal callus, periosteal callus, and gap tissue is expressed as a percentage of new bone area, and the porosity of the cortical bone is expressed as a percentage of total bone area.

IV. STAINING AND NEW BONE FORMATION IN FLUORESCENT MICROSCOPY

The determination of new bone formation and bone formation rates may be accomplished by the administration of fluorochrome labels on a continuous or intermittent schedule during the period of fracture healing. Continuous bone labeling allows the determination of total new bone formation, and intermittent labeling allows the determination of the mineral apposition rate (MAR). Descriptions of specific bone labeling techniques may be found in Chapter 5. Briefly, fluorochromes such as alizarin complexone, calcein, calcein blue, tetracycline, or xylenol orange may be administered as markers of new bone formation. Continous bone labeling is usually accomplished by the administration of tetracycline at 20–25 mg/kg to avoid deleterious effects on osteogenesis that can be seen at dosages exceeding 50 mg/kg (Fig. 3).[9] However, even at dosages of 10–15-mg/kg/d, investigators have demonstrated a 10–30% reversible decrease in osteoblastic activity.[9] Tetracycline has the attributes of the ideal bone label, as defined by Frost.[9] It is minimally toxic, inexpensive, simple to administer, widely available, stable, detectable through the use of fluorescence microscopy, labels new bone formation, and may be used as a tissue time marker. Tetracycline is incorporated into new bone along the initial plane of mineralization. Because the center of a tetracycline band can be localized 20 times more accurately than the edges, a common practice is to administer tetracycline for a short period followed by a drug-free interval, and then use a second brief administration period. Measurements are then made from the center of the resulting bands to determine bone formation rates. Bone biopsies should be obtained several days after the last tetracycline administration to allow cementation of the tetracycline and prevent storage escape.

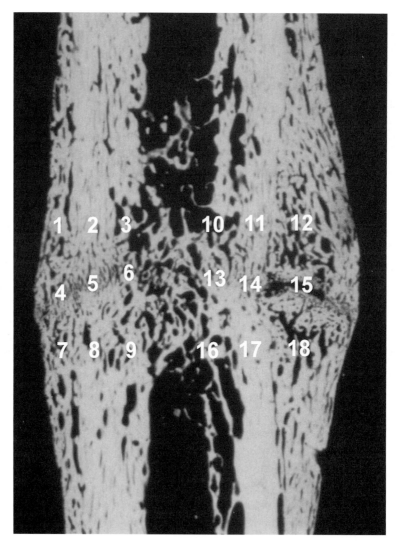

Figure 2. Fracture gap demonstrating the 18 regions of interest within the periosteal callus, the endosteal callus, the fracture gap, and the cortex adjacent to the fracture.

A. Total New Bone Determination

Unstained sections, 100 μm thick, are cover slipped with #1 coverglasses (refractive index nD = 1.5220 ± 0.001) on microscope slides for fluorochrome label analysis using dark-field microscopy. Two techniques may be used to determine total new bone formation following continuous tetracycline labeling. A point-counting method described by Harris and Weinberg[14] may be used, or fluorescent new bone and void areas can be traced using commercially available software (OsteoMeasure, OsteoMetrics Inc., Atlanta, GA), as described by Hanson et al.[13]

Using the point-counting method, a superimposed eyepiece grid with five intersecting lines is used with a magnification of ×40. Each line intersection is counted as a point, and the presence of fluorescent-labeled bone or unlabeled bone is determined for each intersec-

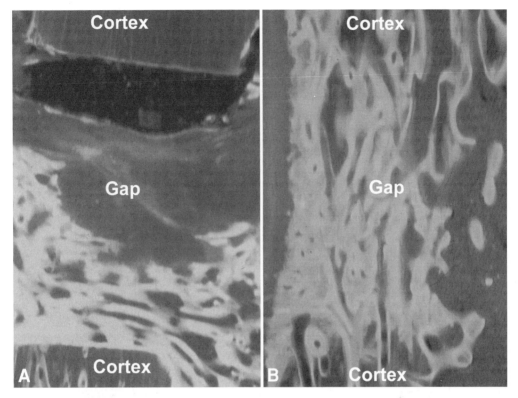

Figure 3. Healing fracture demonstrating continuous bone-labeling with oral tetracycline at a dose of 20 mg/kg daily at (A) 4 wk, and (B) 12 wk after osteotomy. (*See* color plate 19 appearing in the insert following p. 270.)

tion and recorded. The measurements are made within the endosteal callus, periosteal callus, cortical bone adjacent to the fracture gap, and the fracture gap between the cortical bone ends. All bone formed in the fracture gap and in the periosteal callus is new bone, whereas new bone within the cortex is expressed as a percentage of total bone (labeled and unlabeled bone). Depending on the location within the bone, endosteal bone may or may not be new bone, and should be compared to control specimens to determine new bone percentages.

Using the OsteoMeasure software (OsteoMeasure, OsteoMetrics Inc.), fluorescent new bone areas are manually traced. If the same regions of interest are used from which the porosity was calculated using microradiographs, the percentage fluorescence of the field is converted to the percentage of total bone surface area. Otherwise, fluorescent-labeled bone, unlabeled bone, and pore space can be traced individually and newly formed bone is expressed as a percentage of total bone area.

Intermittent bone labeling allows determination of the MAR. Fluorescent labels must be administered at a marker interval (time between labels) that allows differentiation of the administration time-points (Fig. 4). Fluorescent labels of differing colors may also be administered at different stages of treatment protocols to determine the effect of treatment on the bone formation rate. The distance between the centers of bands in double-labeled osteons is determined, and the mean distance is calculated. The MAR (µm/d) is calculated from these data.

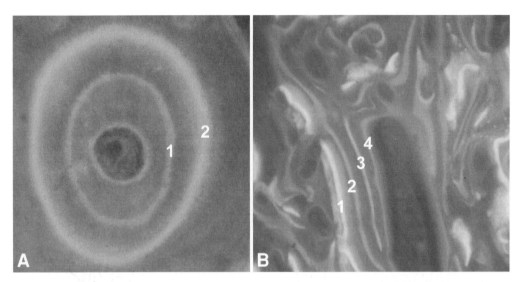

Figure 4. New bone formation demonstrated with (A-1) xylenol orange, and (A-2) tetracycline. (B) Section demonstrates quadruple labeling with (1) tetracycline, (2) xylenol orange, (3) calcein red, and (4) calcein blue. (*See* color plate 20 appearing in the insert following p. 270.)

V. CALLUS AREA

The determination of the fracture callus area provides a means of monitoring healing noninvasively by radiography, and can provide insight into the response to techniques used to augment or accelerate fracture healing. Serial radiographs taken over a period of time can document callus maturation through remodeling (altered size and density), and callus area will allow the prediction of bending and torsional strengths of the healing fracture by calculation of the area and polar moments of inertia of the fractured bone.

Several techniques have been described for determining callus area from radiographs and histologic sections.[2,13,20] The radiographs can be digitized, or the callus area can be traced directly from the radiographs to paper. The callus area is determined with software such as NIH Image (NIH Image, National Institutes of Health) by tracing the margins of the callus (Fig. 5).[13,20] The area can be normalized to bone size when variability exists among animals in different treatment groups.[20] Magnification of the callus is corrected by placing a magnification marker (Custom Protheses Magnification Marker, Techmedica, Camarillo, CA) within the collimated field during radiography. Aro et al. described the use of an automated planimeter (9864A Digitizer with 9821A calculator, Hewlett Packard, Loveland, CO) to determine radiographic and histologic callus size and composition.[2] Histologic callus size may differ significantly from radiographic callus size, particularly if the callus is composed of a higher percentage of cartilage than bone.

VI. TISSUE TYPE

The tissue types within the fracture gap and callus can be determined in their entirety of for selected predetermined locations. Gap-tissue analysis allows determination of the maturity of the fracture and its progression through the normal healing process. The tissue types are usually divided into undifferentiated fibrous or granulation tissue (repair tissue),

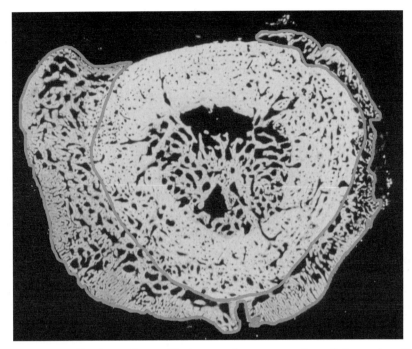

Figure 5. High-detail microradiographic image of a cross-section of the canine tibia. The periosteal callus has been traced, demonstrating the region from which the cross-sectional area would be calculated.

cartilage, and bone. To determine the tissue type of the entire section, two basic techniques can be employed. Historically, the histologic sections were projected and traced on paper, and using simultaneous microscopic examination of sequential sections stained with Goldner's trichrome and toluidine blue, the tissue type was identified and the area quantified with a planimeter.[2,20] A second indirect method is to digitize the microscopic images (Sony DXC-390, 3CCD-Color Video Camera, Sony Corporation) and use software such as NIH Image (NIH Image, National Institutes of Health), Scion Image (Scion Image for Windows [Version 4.0.1], Scion Corporation), or Adobe Photoshop (Adobe Photoshop 5.5, Adobe Systems Incorporated, San Jose, CA) to quantify the area of each tissue type present within the gap. Image-analysis software is available that allows tracing of the tissue type during microscopic visualization and direct determination of the area (OsteoMeasure, OsteoMetrics Inc.). Typically, tissue-type analysis is reported as a percentage of the total gap area (Fig. 6). The gap is initially filled with undifferentiated repair tissue shortly after injury, which progresses over time either directly to bone or to bone through a cartilage analog via endochondral ossification.

VII. FRACTURE UNION

Fracture union may be graded with the use of radiographs,[10] fine-detail radiography, or by histology.[13] Radiographic union is based on a modification of the International Symposium on Limb Salvage (ISOLS).[10] The radiographs are graded on a scale from 1 to 4 (poor = 1, fair = 2, good = 3, excellent = 4) (Table 1). The cortex fracture-gap junctions are examined for the presence of endosteal bridging callus, periosteal bridging callus, and

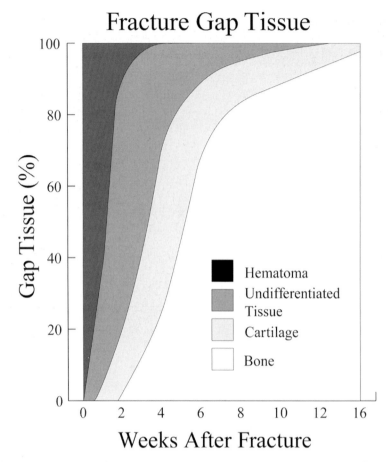

Figure 6. Graph demonstrating the relative area occupied by hematoma, undifferentiated tissue, cartilage, and bone during fracture healing from time 0 until 14 wk after fracture.

Table 1. Radiographic Union Score

Grade	Description
1. Excellent	Fracture line no longer visible.
2. Good	Osteotomy line still visible. Fusion greater than or equal to 75% of cortical thickness.
3. Fair	Osteotomy line still visible. Fusion 25–75% of cortical thickness.
4. Poor	No evidence of callus. Fusion less than 25% of the cortical thickness.

Grading scale adapted from Glasser D, Langlais F: The ISOLS radiological implants evaluation system. In: Langlais F, Tomeno B, eds: *Limb Salvage: Major Reconstructions in Oncologic and Nontumoral Conditions.* 5th International Symposium St. Malo, Springer-Verlag, Berlin, Germany, 1991: xxiii–xxxi.

bony union of the cortices within the fracture gap. Hanson et al.[13] described a technique to evaluate union based on microradiographs. The fracture gap was evaluated at the medial, lateral, cranial, and caudal surfaces, and graded 1 if united and 0 if union was absent. If union was present on all four cortices, it was considered complete, and it was reported as partial if only 1–3 junctions had formed a bony union.

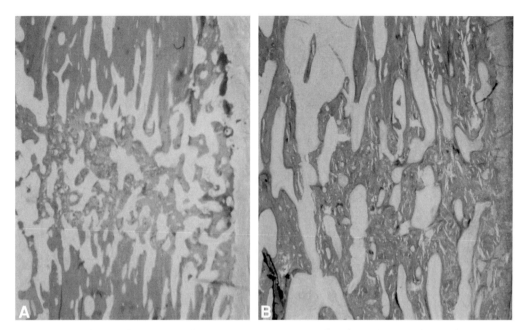

Figure 7. Light microscopy of the osteotomy at (A) 8 wk, and (B) 12 wk following osteotomy. Images demonstrate a decrease in the anisotropy over time as the woven bone within the fracture gap is remodeled. (Goldner's trichrome staining, ×4). (*See* color plate 21 appearing in the insert following p. 270.)

VIII. TRABECULAR BONE ORIENTATION WITHIN FRACTURE GAP

The anisotropy of the trabecular bone within the fracture gap may be evaluated to determine maturation and remodeling of newly formed bone. Woven bone demonstrates high anisotropy (Fig. 7), but osteonal remodeling leads to decreased anisotropy. Microradiographs are digitized into images 512×512 pixels, with 256 levels of gray. This may be accomplished with image-analysis software such as NIH Image (NIH Image, National Institutes of Health). Scion Image (Scion Image for Windows (Version 4.0.1, Scion Corporation), or Adobe Photoshop (Adobe Photoshop 5.5, Adobe Systems Incorporated). The gray-scale threshold is set to create a binary image so that bone and marrow space can be distinguished.

Quantitative analysis is performed using principles based on Saltykov's method of directed secants.[7,20,37,42,43] A circular region is scanned with an array of equidistant parallel lines, and a count of the number of intersections between the bone structural elements and the test array is produced. The test array is incrementally rotated through 180°, and counts are generated by measuring the number of intersections between the test array and the structural elements of bone. The mean intercept length is determined from the density and length of intersections per unit-scan line length in a measured direction. A polar plot of the mean intercept lengths yields a circle for random isotropic sections and an ellipse for partially oriented structures.[37] The direction and extent of orientation of trabecular bone within the fracture gap can then be calculated. This stereology program has been validated and used to characterize remodeling of cancellous bone in humans,[15] equine patella,[7] proximal sesamoid,[42] and third carpal bones,[43] and the fracture gap in the canine tibia.[20] If the trabecular bone orientation is independent of the analysis direction, it is termed isotropic; otherwise, it is termed anisotropic.

IX. MICROANGIOGRAPHIC ANALYSIS OF FRACTURE HEALING

Bone vasularity and vascular patterns during fracture healing have been well-described by Rhinelander and Wilson,[18,28,29] and are based on work originally described by Trueta and Barclay.[4,34,35] The afferent blood supply to long bones is from the nutrient artery, metaphyseal arteries, and the periosteal arterioles. The nutrient artery terminates in the medullary canal as the ascending and descending medullary arteries and anastomoses with the terminal branches of the metaphyseal arteries. The nutrient and metaphyseal arteries create the medullary arterial supply and provide the majority of the afferent blood supply to the bone marrow and the cortex. Periosteal arteries join long bones at fascial attachments, and therefore their distribution is variable among bones. Medullary arterioles supply the inner two-thirds of the cortex, and the periosteal arterioles supply the outer third and anastomose with the terminal branches of the medullary arterioles. However, in regions with little periosteal blood supply, because of an absence of fascial attachments the medullary arterioles supply the entire cortex.[29]

The three primary afferent blood systems are enhanced at the site of the injury. In addition, an extra-osseous blood supply derived from surrounding soft tissues contributes to initial fracture healing and vascularization of the periosteal callus. In stable fracture fixation, the medullary blood supply rapidly vascularizes the medullary callus, the healing porotic cortical bone, and the periosteal callus. The extra-osseous blood supply persists in delayed healing, complex fractures with cortical fragmentation, or when the medullary cavity is obstructed with tight-fitting nails.

The techniques described by Rhinelander and Wilson may be utilized in isolated limb preparations or by central vessel cannulation.[23–28,38] Perfusion of a single limb produces better results than central perfusion techniques. The vascularity of the fracture callus and gap may be evaluated with the use of barium sulfate suspended in formalin. The region containing the bone or fracture gap of interest can be isolated by vascular ligation. For example, perfusion of the hind limb of the dog is best accomplished by femoral artery and vein cannulation. The femoral artery and vein are cannulated after the animal is anesthetized, and the animal then is heparinized by injecting 330 U/kg body wt intravenously. Five minutes after injection of heparin, the animal is euthanized with an overdose of barbiturate. Perfusion is initiated with 50% micropulverized barium sulfate in 0.9% saline. Infusion pressure is maintained at 120 mmHg (normal arterial pressure for the dog) and continued until the efferent fluid is nearly free of blood. At this time, the perfusion is continued with a 30% barium sulfate solution suspended in 10% neutral buffered formalin (NBF) to produce partial internal fixation of the perfused tissues. Infusion with barium sulfate-formalin mixture is continued until the venous effluent produces a strong formalin odor. After the infusion is completed, the cannulated limb is placed in a 1:2 mixture of 10% NBF and 95% alcohol for 24 h. The cannulas are maintained for 24 h to allow preliminary fixation of tissues and stabilization of the barium sulfate within the vascular tree. The cannulas and the skin are removed 24 h after perfusion to allow complete fixation of tissues.

If the proximal limb, such as the coxofemoral joint, is to be evaluated, central catheterization of the abdominal aorta and caudal vena cava is performed. Central catheterization

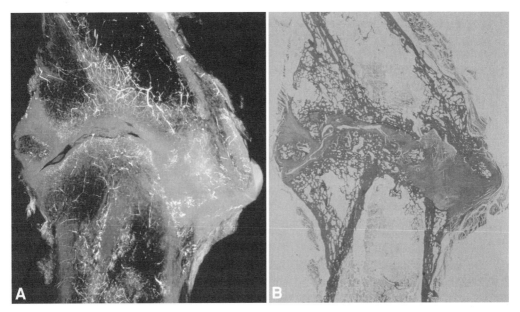

Figure 8. High-detail microradiographic image demonstrating microangiographic perfusion of fracture healing (A) and light microscopy of a serial section (B).

requires larger volumes of barium sulfate in saline and formalin to clear the venous pools. Perfusion of small animals such as rats is best performed by cannulation of the left ventricle or the aortic arch.

Typically, vascularity is evaluated subjectively and analyzed descriptively (Fig. 8). The technique is particularly useful for evaluation of impaired fracture healing, such as delayed union, atrophic vs hypertrophic non-union, and healing of open fractures.

X. CELL KINETICS

Fracture healing involves a complex cellular response from soft tissues, periosteum endosteum and marrow space, and the adjacent cortical bone. Fracture signals cell proliferation and differentiation in each of these regions at the time of fracture and during the repair process. Cell kinetic studies provide a means of identifying actively dividing cells, and help to characterize the normal fracture healing response, and the effect of therapeutic interventions on the cellular response during repair. Historically, tritiated thymidine ([^{3}H]-TdR) was considered the classic cell kinetic marker, but it has the disadvantage of being time-consuming and expensive. It also necessitates the precautions and inconvenience associated with use of radioactive materials.[3,6,11,16,19,22,32,41] The use of an immunohistochemical technique with 5-bromo-2′-deoxyuridine (bromodeoxyuridine or BrdU) provides a more rapid and nonradioactive technique for cell kinetic studies.[5,12,31,33,40,41] Bromodeoxyuridine is a halogenated analog of thymidine and is incorporated into newly synthesized DNA by proliferating cells via the same pyrimidine salvage pathway as thymidine.[12,41] The immunohistochemical techniques for calcified bone during fracture healing have been described by Xiang and Markel.[41]

A. Bromodeoxyuridine Injections and Tissue Processing

Based on this work,[41] ethanol-fixed, epon-embedded, calcified bone sections provide the best results when employing BrdU to study cell kinetics in fracture healing. One hour before euthanasia, BrdU (Sigma, St. Louis, MO) is dissolved in saline and injected intravenously (100 mg/kg). Immediately after euthanasia, the bone of interest is dissected from the surrounding soft tissues and placed in 70% ethanol. A 40-cm section of bone encompassing the fracture site is cut transversely, and 2-mm sections are cut either coronally or sagittally and embedded in epon. The epon is prepared from a commercially available kit (Araldite/Embed-812; Electron Microscopy Sciences, Ft. Washington, PA) by mixing Embed-812 (12.6 g), araldite 502 (11.8 g), DMP-30 (0.5 g), and DDSA (22.7 g). The tissue sample is dehydrated at room temperature with graded ethanol (80% ethanol, 1 h; 95% ethanol, twice for 1.5 h; 100% ethanol, twice for 1.5 h). The tissue then is cleared with propylene oxide and infiltrated with increasing epon concentrations at room temperature (25% epon for 16 h; 50% epon for 24 h; 75% epon for 24 h; and 100% epon for 3 d). Vacuum of 380 mm Hg is applied while the sample is embedded in 100% epon. The sample then is embedded for 2 additional days in 100% epon under 380 mmHg at room temperature. Finally the embedded block is polymerized at 60°C for 2 d.

B. Section Preparation and DNA Denaturation

The embedded sections are trimmed and then sectioned and surfaced with a precision saw and polisher/grinder (Ecomet III, Buehler, Evanston, IL) to expose the tissue. Next, 3-μm sections are cut on a motorized sledge microtome (Polycut E 5000; Reichert-Jung, Nussloch, Germany) with a tungsten carbide blade (Reichert-Jung 16-cm 50° T.C. knife, Cambridge, Nussloch, Germany), floated on a preheated 50°C distilled water bath, and mounted on chrome alum gelatin solution-coated glass slides. The slides are placed on a slide plate at 56°C for 2 h, clamped in a slide press and placed in an oven at 56°C overnight to promote adhesion.[1,41] For BrdU immunohistochemical staining, the slides are submerged in 1:1 saturated sodium ethoxide and 100% ethanol for 20 min to remove epon and denature DNA. The slides then are rinsed in two changes of 100% ethanol for 5 min each to remove the sodium ethoxide, and rehydrated in graded ethanols (100%, 90%, and 70%) and rinsed in two changes of phosphate-buffered saline (PBS) for 5 min each.

C. Immunohistochemical Staining

The immunohistochemical protocol described here uses a commercially available mouse anti-BrdU monoclonal antibody (MAb) (Becton Dickinson, San Jose, CA) and a commercial kit (Histostain-SP mouse universal kit; Zymed, San Francisco, CA).[41] The anti-BrdU antibody is supplied at a concentration of 25 μg/mL and diluted with Tween 20/PBS (pH 7.4) and tested in dilutions of 1:30 and 1:50. Staining with 3,3′ diaminobenzidine tetrahydrochloride (DAB; Zymed) provided better results than 3-amino-9-ethylcarbazole (AEC; Zymed). In addition, AEC stain diffused from the nuclei when slides were stored for long periods of time. This protocol employs sodium ethoxide for DNA denaturation as described by Apte and Puddle.[1] Acid thermal denaturation has been reported to be detrimental to cell morphology, and results in detachment of calcified bone sections from the glass slides.[1,41]

1. Submerge slides in 0.3% methanolic acid H_2O_2, twice for 15 min.
2. Rinse slides in 0.05 M PBS, pH 7.4, twice for 3 min.
3. Rinse sections in 1% Tween 20 in 0.05 M PBS, pH 7.4 (polyoxyethylensorbitan monolaurate, Tween 20; Sigma), for 1 min.
4. Encircle sections with a hydrophobic PAP pen (Newcomer Supply, Oak Park, IL).
5. Add 10% non-immune goat serum for 10 min and then blot off.
6. Incubate the sections in a moist petri dish at 4°C overnight with the primary antibody (anti-BrdU) at a dilution of 1:50, and then rinse slides in 0.05 M PBS, pH 7.4, twice for 3 min.
7. Incubate sections with biotinylated goat anti-mouse IgG for 10 min and then rinse in 0.05 M PBS, pH 7.4, twice for 3 min.
8. Incubate with streptavidin-peroxidase conjugate for 10 min, and then incubate with a substrate-chromogen mixture for 5 min. Rinse slides in 0.05 M PBS, pH 7.4, twice for 3 min.
9. The sections are then rinsed well with distilled deionized water and cover slipped.

D. Control Tissues

Reagent controls are run on sections cut from the same embedded samples with non-immune mouse serum or PBS substituted for the primary antibody (anti-BrdU). Negative controls come from tissues, bone and small intestine, processed from an animal not injected with BrdU. Positive control tissues are small intestine (jejunum) of the individual animals injected with BrdU.

Acknowledgment: The authors would like to thank Paul A. Manley, DVM, MSc, DACVS, Peter Muir, BVSc, MVetClinStud, PhD, DACVS, and Vicki L. Kalscheur, HT, of the Comparative Orthopaedic Research Laboratory and the Department of Surgical Sciences, and Yan Lu, MD, of the Comparative Orthopaedic Research Laboratory and the Department of Medical Sciences, School of Veterinary Medicine, University of Wisconsin-Madison for assistance in preparation of this manuscript.

REFERENCES

1. Apte SS, Puddle B: Bromodeoxyuridine (BrdUrd) immunohistochemistry in undecalcified plastic-embedded tissue. Elimination of the DNA denaturation step. *Histochemistry* 93:631–635, 1990.
2. Aro H, Eerola E, Aho AJ: Determination of callus quantity in 4-week-old fractures of the rat tibia. *J Orthop Res* 3:101–108, 1985.
3. Aronson J, Shen XC, Gao GG, et al: Sustained proliferation accompanies distraction osteogenesis in the rat. *J Orthop Res* 15:563–569, 1997.
4. Barclay AE: *Micro-arteriography and Other Radiological Techniques Employed in Biological Research.* Blackwell Scientific Publications, Oxford, UK, 1951.
5. Boswald M, Harasim S, Maurer-Schultze B: Tracer dose and availability time of thymidine and bromodeoxyuridine: application of bromodeoxyuridine in cell kinetic studies. *Cell Tissue Kinet* 23:169–181, 1990.
6. Chai BF, Tang XM: Electron radioautographic study of experimental fracture healing. *Chin Med J* 102:851–856, 1989.
7. Cheal EJ, Snyder BD, Nunamaker DM, et al: Trabecular bone remodeling around smooth and porous implants in an equine patellar model. *J Biomech* 20:1121–1134, 1987.
8. Dickson GF: *Methods of Calcified Tissue Preparation.* Elsevier, Amsterdam, The Netherlands, 1984: pp. 1–54.
9. Frost HM: Bone histomorphometry: Choice of marking agent and labeling schedule. In: Recker RR, ed: *Bone Histomorphometry: Techniques and Interpretation.* CRC Press, Inc., Boca Raton, FL, 1983:37–52.

10. Glasser D, Langlais F: The ISOLS Radiologic Implant Evaluation System. In: Langlais F, Tomeno B, eds: *Limb Salvage: Major Reconstructions in Oncologic and Nontumoral Conditions.* Berlin, Germany, Springer-Verlag, 1991:xxiii–xxxi.

11. Gothlin G, Ericsson JLE: On the histiogenesis of the cells in fracture callus. Electron microscopic autoradiographic observations in parabiotic rats and studies on labeled monocytes. *Virchows B Cell Pathol* 12:318–329, 1973.

12. Gratzner HG: Monoclonal antibody to 5-bromo- and 5-iododeoxyuridine: a new reagent for detection of DNA replication. *Science* 218:474–475, 1982.

13. Hanson PD, Warner C, Kofroth R, et al: The effect of intramedullary polymethylmethacrylate and autogenous cancellous bone on the healing of frozen segmental allografts. *J Orthop Res* 16:285–292, 1998.

14. Harris WH, Weinberg EH: Microscopic method of measuring increases in cortical bone volume and mass. *Calcif Tissue Res* 8:190–196, 1972.

15. Hayes WC, Snyder B: Toward a quantitative formulation of Wolff's law in trabecular bone. In: Cowin SC, ed: *Mechanical Properties of Bone, Vol 45.* American Society of Mechanical Engineers, New York, NY, 1981:43–68.

16. Hyldebrandt N, Damholt W, Mordentoft EL: Investigation of the cellular response to fracture assessed by autoradiography of the periosteum. *Acta Orthop Scand* 45:175–181, 1974.

17. Jowsey J, Kelly PJ, Riggs BL, et al: Quantitative microradiographic studies of normal and osteoporotic bone. *J Bone Joint Surg [Am]* 47:785–806, 1965.

18. Kirby BM, Wilson JW: Effect of circumferential bands on cortical vascularity and viability. *J Orthop Res* 9:174–179, 1991.

19. Manabe S, Shima I, Yamauchi S: Cytokinetic analysis of osteogenic cells in the healing process after fracture. *Acta Orthop Scand* 46:161–176, 1975.

20. Markel MD, Wikenheiser MA, Chao EY: Formation of bone in tibial defects in a canine model. Histomorphometric and biomechanical studies. *J Bone Joint Surg [Am]* 73:914–923, 1991.

21. Meadows TH, Bronk JT, Chao EYS, et al: Effect of weight-bearing on healing of cortical defects in the canine tibia. *J Bone Joint Surg [Am]* 72:1074–1080, 1990.

22. Nichols JT, Toto PD, Choukas NC: The proliferative capacity and DNA synthesis of osteoblasts during fracture repair in normal and hypophysized rats. *Oral Surg Oral Med Oral Pathol* 25:418–426, 1968.

23. Rhinelander FW: The normal microcirculation of diaphyseal cortex and its response to fracture. *J Bone Joint Surg [Am]* 50:784–800, 1968.

24. Rhinelander FW: The normal circulation of bone and its response to surgical intervention. *J Biomed Mater Res* 8:87–90, 1974.

25. Rhinelander FW: Effects of medullary nailing on the normal blood supply of diaphyseal cortex. *Clin Orthop* 350:5–17, 1998.

26. Rhinelander FW, Nelson CL, Stewart RD, et al: Experimental reaming of the proximal femur and acrylic cement implantation: vascular and histologic effects. *Clin Orthop* 141:74–89, 1979.

27. Rhinelander FW, Rouweyha M, Milner JC: Microvascular and histogenic responses to implantation of a porous ceramic into bone. *J Biomed Mater Res* 5:81–112, 1971.

28. Rhinelander FW, Stewart CL, Wilson JW: Bone vascular supply. In: Simmons DJ, Kunin AS, eds: *Skeletal Research.* Academic Press, New York, NY, 1979:367–396.

29. Rhinelander FW, Wilson JW: Blood supply to developing, mature, and healing bone. In: Sumner-Smith G, ed: *Bone in Clinical Orthopaedics.* Saunders, Philadelphia, PA, 1982:81–158.

30. Schenk RK, Olah AJ, Herrman W: Preparation of calcified tissues for light microscopy. In: Dickson GR, ed: *Methods of Calcified Tissue Preparation.* Elsevier, Amsterdam, The Netherlands, 1984:1–56.

31. Silvestrini R, Costa A, Veneroni S, et al: Comparative analysis of different approaches to investigate cell kinetics. *Cell Tissue Kinet* 21:123–131, 1988.

32. Tonna EA, Cronkite EP: Cellular response to fracture studied with tritiated thymidine. *J Bone Joint Surg [Am]* 43:352–362, 1961.

33. Trent JM, Gerner E, Broderick R, et al: Cell cycle analysis using bromodeoxyuridine: comparison of methods for analysis of total cell transit time. *Cancer Genet Cytogenet* 19:43–50, 1986.

34. Trueta J, Barclay AE, Daniel PM, et al: *Studies of the Renal Circulation.* Blackwell, Oxford, UK, 1947:pp. 1–7.

35. Trueta J, Harrison MHM: The normal vascular anatomy of the femoral head in man. *J Bone Joint Surg [Br]* 35:442–461, 1953.

36. Villanueva AR: Bone. In: Sheehan DC, Hrapchak BB, eds: *Theory and Practice of Histotechnology.* Battelle Press, Columbus, OH, 1980:89–117.

37. Whitehouse WJ: The quantitative morphology of anisotropic trabecular bone. *J Microsc* 101:153–168, 1974.

38. Wilson JW, Rhinelander FW, Stewart CL: Vascularization of cancellous chip bone grafts. *Am J Vet Res* 46:1691–1697, 1985.

39. Wu J, Shyr HS, Chao EYS, et al: Comparison of osteotomy healing under external fixation devices with different stiffness characteristics. *J Bone Joint Surg [Am]* 66:1258–1264, 1984.

40. Wynford-Thomas D, Williams ED: Use of bromodeoxyuridine for cell kinetic studies in intact animals. *Cell Tissue Kinet* 19:179–182, 1986.

41. Xiang Z, Markel MD: Bromodeoxyuridine immunohistochemistry of epon-embedded undecalcified bone in a canine fracture healing model. *J Histochem Cytochem* 43:629–635, 1995.

42. Young DR, Nunamaker DM, Markel MD: Quantitative evaluation of the remodeling response of the proximal sesamoid bones to training-related stimuli in thoroughbreds. *Am J Vet Res* 52:1350–1356, 1991.

43. Young DR, Richardson DW, Markel MD, et al: Mechanical and morphometric analysis of the third carpal bone of thoroughbreds. *Am J Vet Res* 52:402–409, 1991.

29

Histomorphometry of Metabolic Bone Conditions

Ellen M. Hauge,[1] Torben Steiniche,[1] and Troels T. Andreassen[2]

[1]*Institute of Pathology, Aarhus University Hospital, Aarhus, Denmark*
[2]*Institute of Anatomy, University of Aarhus, Aarhus, Denmark*

I. INTRODUCTION

Changes in bone metabolism and bone structure occur in various metabolic conditions. This chapter discusses the histomorphometric findings in osteoporosis, hyperparathyroidism, osteomalacia, acromegaly/growth hormone (GH) deficiency, and hyper/hypothyroidism. Although osteoporosis is characterized by major changes in bone structure, the disturbances of bone remodeling are still debated. However, the histomorphometric indices that describe the mechanisms of bone loss are important in the understanding of the usefulness and limitations of the histomorphometric method. Using osteoporosis as an example, this chapter presents the methodological aspects of bone histomorphometry in more detail.

II. POSTMENOPAUSAL OSTEOPOROSIS

Aging is responsible for a considerable increase in the incidence of fractures at the spine, hip, and wrist, and decreased biomechanical competence is directly related to the loss of bone mass and loss of bone structure.[83] The loss of ovarian function induces an accelerated loss of bone mass and deterioration of cancellous bone structure.

A. Disintegration of the Cancellous Bone Structure

Bone mass, which is measured by bone-mineral density and by histomorphometry, decreases with age, as observed in cross-sectional studies. The greater the age, the lower the cancellous bone volume of the iliac crest.[113] However, age affects bone structure as well. Trabeculae are thinned,[94] and entire trabecular elements are removed[25,46,79,94] with age. The removal of trabecular elements apparently occurs in both sexes, but makes a greater contribution to the age-related bone loss in women.[25,46,79] It has been hypothesized that preferentially thin trabeculae are removed—and that those that remain are only slightly reduced in thickness[94]—or that a compensatory thickening of existing trabeculae occurs following removal.[115] In postmenopausal osteoporosis, this effect of age is accentuated. Bone mass is lower in osteoporotic subjects, but the trabecular network is also less interconnected compared with age-matched normal subjects.[62,70,88,108]

From: *Handbook of Histology Methods for Bone and Cartilage*
Edited by: Y. H. An and K. L. Martin © Humana Press Inc., Totowa, NJ

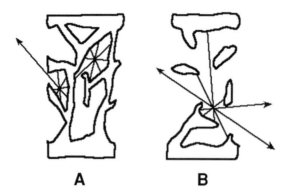

Figure 1. The principle of measuring star volume of the marrow space is shown. Using randomly located points inside the marrow space, the mean intercept length is measured. In normal cancellous bone (A), only a few intercepts are undefined (arrows). Reduced interconnectedness of osteoporotic cancellous bone (B) results in an increased number of undefined intercepts.

The need for quantification of the cancellous bone structure and the destructive process accompanying bone loss has generated methods for the study of bone structure observed in two-dimensional (2D) sections of iliac crest bone biopsies.

1. Two-Dimensional Methods

In young subjects, the cancellous bone structure resembles interconnected parallel plates. Based on this model assumption, Parfitt et al.[94] devised a method that provides indirect measurements of the bone structure by estimating the mean trabecular-plate thickness, plate density (number of plates per unit of length), and plate separation (mean intertrabecular distance). However, the assumption that trabeculae are parallel plates is not always fulfilled in osteopenic conditions, which may be characterized by a more rod-like structure[67] arising from extensive perforation of the trabecular plates.

Various computerized methods have been applied. In strut analysis,[42] the number of trabecular branchings and free endings in two dimensions are counted, and the trabecular bone-pattern factor[46] assesses changes in trabecular curvature. The methods represent 2D approaches to the quantification of cancellous bone structure. They are well-intercorrelated, and reflect aspects of the changes in bone structure. However, the results cannot in any way be transformed to three-dimensional (3D) terms. The course of the architectural disintegration during bone loss is a three-dimensional question that requires three-dimensional answers to be understood in detail.

2. Three-Dimensional Methods

The architectural organization of structural elements in cancellous bone is characterized by anisotropy—i.e., a preferential orientation of trabeculae. Most stereological methods require the use of isotropy and uniform random sampling. Star volume is a stereologically unbiased estimator, which returns the volume-weighted mean size of the structure (Fig. 1).[114] However, intercepts that are not delimited by trabeculae are not informative, and these are numerous in iliac crest biopsies of severe osteoporosis.

The trabecular star volume has been shown to be largely insensitive to changes in trabecular volume and thickness.[114] On the other hand, the star volume of the marrow space

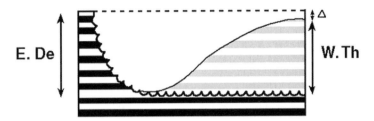

Figure 2. Schematic drawing of the cancellous bone remodeling, including evolving a complete cycle in one location on the bone surface. The erosion depth (E.De) can be estimated when the bone resorption has reached its final depth. The thickness of the rebuilt wall (W.Th) can be measured, and a net bone balance (Δ) can be calculated from the linear processes of resorption and formation. The cement line is depicted as the horizontal irregular line (∪∪).

is a highly sensitive estimator of changes in size, which could be caused by loss of trabecular elements. The difficulty in measuring marrow-space star volume in iliac crest biopsies involves the cut edges and the risk of non-informative intercepts that point outward from the specimen (Fig. 1).

Using a topological approach to cancellous bone connectivity, the problem of bias in the 2D approaches can be solved. Three-dimensional (3D) connectivity is defined as the maximal number of bridges that may be cut without separating the structure. A strict mathematical definition such as that proposed by Euler describes this approach and allows it to be estimated in bone samples using pairs of neighboring histological sections and, as such, is a very powerful tool.[45] The Euler connectivity discriminates better between a normal structure and a disintegrated structure than the star volume.[9]

B. Bone Loss Mechanisms in Cancellous Bone

Although the cancellous bone structure measured in iliac crest biopsies obtained in postmenopausal osteoporosis is more open and less well-connected than that of age-matched controls,[88,94,108] it appears that the processes leading to postmenopausal bone loss are caused either by i) events occurring earlier in life, ii) premature aging and not by specific disease mechanisms, iii) insufficient peak bone mass determined by several factors working within the constraints of genetic predisposition, or iv) by a combination of these factors.

1. Permanent Changes in Bone Mass

A. REMODELING BALANCE AND TRABECULAR PERFORATIONS

Permanent reduction in bone mass is the result of a disturbed bone-remodeling process. The net balance between resorption and formation is negative, leading to a loss of bone in every remodeling cycle (Fig. 2). Bone remodeling occurs as a process of coupled bone resorption and formation; bone resorption in one location is always followed by bone formation in the same location. Thus, bone resorption is spatially and temporally coupled to bone formation. Histomorphometrically, the net balance between resorption and formation can be evaluated at the level of the bone multicellular unit—i.e., the osteon level. The final depth of resorption lacunae (erosion depth) is an estimate of bone resorption, the thickness of rebuilt walls (wall thickness) an estimate of bone formation, and the remodeling balance is the difference between wall thickness and erosion depth.

Wall thickness is reported to be lower in postmenopausal vertebral osteoporotics compared with normals.[4,61,93] Since wall thickness is known to decrease with age,[65] age is a possible confounder in two studies,[61,93] but not in a study by Arlot et al.[4] that compared age-matched normal subjects with osteoporotic subjects. In established osteoporosis, the erosion depth is not higher,[108] but it appears to be the case during the perimenopausal period.[34]

In an ideal situation, the amount of bone formed within a resorption cavity completely repairs the defect. With age, both erosion depth[36] and wall thickness[65] decrease, but not to the same extent, since an incomplete filling in of resorption cavities leads to a slight balance deficit (–2 μm) between wall thickness and erosion depth in every remodeling cycle[108]—the cause of the slow age-related bone loss. A similarly negative remodeling balance of –2 μm is found in postmenopausal osteoporosis,[108] which concurs with the rate of bone loss observed densitometrically.[92]

The imbalance between bone resorption and formation leads to thinning of the trabeculae. This further increases the risk of bone loss, since resorptive cells may erode through the thin trabeculae, leaving a perforated structure behind.[94] The perforated and unloaded trabeculae are removed by osteoclastic resorption,[84] and the trabecular elements become more widely separated and less well-connected.[108] Biomechanical competence then deteriorates, and the risk of fracture increases.

During menopause, permanent bone loss is accentuated[78] because of an increased bone turnover[105] and increased bone-resorption depth.[34] More remodeling cycles with a more pronounced negative net balance are initiated, leading to a more rapid thinning of trabeculae with an increased risk of perforation. The increased number of remodeling sites also increases the risk of trabecular perforations by increasing the frequency by which any point on the surface runs through a remodeling cycle (activation frequency), and by increasing the risk of opposite resorption lacunae that meet each other from each side of the trabecula. Considering the risk of perforations, a random activation of remodeling is assumed, which may not be the case.

B. ESTIMATING EROSION DEPTH AND WALL THICKNESS

The quantification of the bone remodeling balance implies that bone resorption and bone formation can be quantified. In cancellous bone, bone resorption and formation occur in three dimensions. The translocating, 2D aspect of bone resorption and formation is estimated from the erosion surface, osteoid surface, and mineralizing surface. In an attempt to evaluate the third dimension, the linear advancement (Fig. 2) of bone resorption (downward movement) and formation (upward movement) is estimated at random surface points that are orthogonal to the cancellous bone surface. The linear movement of the remodeling process is measured as the final erosion depth, and the final wall thickness, making it possible to calculate a net balance between the downward and the upward movement.

It is more difficult to study bone resorption than bone formation because of sampling problems. The process is rapid—there is no tissue marker of bone resorption, and it leaves no traces except for a hole, so it must be studied from what has been removed (Fig. 2).

One suggestion is to measure erosion depth as the number of eroded double lamellae at intersection points between a test line and erosion surface covered by pre-osteoblast-like cells or an early osteoid seam and multiply by the lamellar thickness,[35] which appears to be fairly constant. The validity of the erosion depth relies on the identification of surface points that have reached the final resorption depth and the identification of the quiescent surface at which resorption began.

A tracing procedure estimating the depth of resorption lacunae from a "reconstruction" of the entire resorbed cancellous surface is also suggested.[16] However, the estimate is prone to serious uncertainties, because the missing bone surface cannot be reconstructed reliably in two dimensions. Furthermore, some resorption lacunae may be abortive, and some lacunae may not have reached the final depth.

The reluctant implementation of the lamellae count measurement of final erosion depth introduced by Eriksen et al.[35] most likely reflects its technical challenge. The surface tracing methods[16] attempt to circumvent the technical difficulties. However, the final erosion depth may be estimated without the identification of resorptive cell types on the bone surface. The cell-specific resorption depths are not needed for the final erosion depth. It is only necessary to identify osteoid seams or incomplete walls on the surface and count the number of eroded lamellae below these structures. This approach increases the precision of the lamellar count method and eases its measuring procedure.

Wall thickness is often measured as the distance from the cement line to the bone surface of complete osteons (Fig. 2). In normal individuals, a point on the cancellous bone surface is renewed every 2–3 yr.[90] The wall width of complete walls therefore represents the accumulative changes over these years. In patients with very slow turnover rates— e.g., bisphosphonate-treated patients—one must wait several years for a given challenge to exert its effects on all osteons. If one measures only the growing osteons, all the measured osteons have been under the influence of the intervention.[32] This method—the 3D reconstruction of the formative site—is based on the flat-plate model for cancellous osteons. Using orthogonal intercepts, the measurements may be easily performed as pairs of osteoid and wall thickness according to the method by Steiniche et al.[107] Sampling by intersections between grid lines and bone surface in a uniform random manner ensures that the measurements of wall thickness are weighted according to its surface extent.[63] Using a given number of equidistantly spaced measurements introduces bias because individual profiles are given equal weight, despite their unequal length.

2. Reversible Changes in Bone Mass

A. ACTIVATION FREQUENCY

In cancellous bone, activation frequency estimates the rate by which any point on a bone surface is activated and evolves through a complete remodeling cycle. A change in activation frequency induces a shift from one steady state to another steady state, during which the bone remodeling is in a transient state where bone mass may be lost or gained. These losses or gains in bone mass are reversible. Bone is removed during resorption, and is not replaced until the subsequent bone formation is completed. This "lacking" bone is called the remodeling space.[89] Following a sudden increase in activation frequency, more remodeling sites are initiated, thus increasing the remodeling space. This is measured densitometrically as a decrease in bone mass. However, a sudden decrease in activation frequency is followed by an increase in bone mass, which is caused by a reduction of the remodeling space.[53] Apart from the activation frequency, the remodeling space is dependent on the duration of the remodeling period and the depth of the resorption cavities. Given a normal bone turnover of 8% per yr in the entire skeleton, a theoretical complete closure of the remodeling space would lead to a 1% increase in total cortical and cancellous mineralized bone volume, whereas recently formed osteoid and less mineralized bone would account for another 4%.[89] Thus, the reversible turnover-related deficit in mineralized bone mass amounts to 5% of total bone volume in normal adult bone. If bone turnover doubled, the reversible bone mass would increase in the same proportion. At sites of predominantly cancellous bone, such as the spine, the increase may be 10–15% of total cancellous bone volume, since the normal turnover in cancellous bone is 25–30% per yr.[89] In high-turnover disease, the increase may be even greater.

The menopause-related increase in bone turnover seems to be almost reversed by a late-postmenopausal fall.[54] Comparing normal postmenopausal women with osteoporotic women, bone turnover is reported to be lower in the osteoporotic individuals,[41,93] but others have found equal[61,108] or higher[33] bone turnover. The calculation of bone turnover is dependent on wall thickness, mineral apposition rate (MAR) and mineralizing surface. MAR[101] and wall thickness[65] decrease with age, whereas mineralizing surface may[101] or may not[26] decline with age, which could explain the varying results. Although several studies have addressed bone remodeling in relation to aging in normal subjects, no studies have focused on the age-related changes in postmenopausal osteoporotics.

C. Anti-Resorptive Treatment

1. Bisphosphonates

Bisphosphonates are analogs of inorganic pyrophosphate that possess a high affinity for the hydroxyapatite crystals in bone. They have the ability to inhibit bone resorption, and this has prompted their use in osteoporosis treatment. Bisphosphonates effectively reduce the risk of osteoporotic fractures in postmenopausal osteoporosis.[49] The early bisphosphonates, such as etidronate, may impair bone mineralization, but this does not seem to be the case for the newer ones such as alendronate and risedronate. Etidronate[111] and alendronate[16] reduce the activation frequency by 50–90% in postmenopausal osteoporosis. The MAR and wall thickness are unchanged by the treatment.[16,111] Etidronate decreases the final erosion depth and appears to improve the remodeling balance.[111] The dramatic decrease in activation frequency has led to concerns about an increase in mean bone age resulting in reduced bone quality, since microfractures may not be removed by the remodeling. Recently, this concern has been substantiated.[77]

2. Estrogens and Selective Estrogen Receptor Modulators

Replacement of estrogen in postmenopausal women slows down the activation frequency[109] and increases bone-mineral mass.[19] Loss of the increased bone-mineral mass resumes immediately if estrogen treatment is abandoned.[19] Estrogen replacement therapy is associated with several adverse effects, including reinitiation of endometrial bleeding and increased risk of breast cancer. Studies are therefore made of the possible separation of beneficial effects on postmenopausal bone remodeling from the harmful effects on the endometrium and mammary glands by the different response of the estrogen receptors *a* and *b* to estradiol and selective estrogen-receptor modulators. Raloxifene increases bone-mineral density by 2–3% in the hip and spine and reduces biochemical markers of bone turnover by 15–30%.[72,98] Estrogen increases spine and hip bone-mineral density by 3–5% and reduces markers of bone turnover by 30–50%.[100] In established osteoporosis, activation frequency is reduced by 50% following estrogen treatment, whereas no change is seen in final resorption depth.[58,109] On the other hand, in early postmenopausal women, the final erosion depth increases, leading to a negative remodeling balance,[34] but hormone replacement therapy prevents this increase in erosion depth.[34]

3. Remodeling Transients Caused by Changes in Activation Frequency

The coupling of bone resorption to bone formation is an important basis for interpreting the indices of bone remodeling. Anti-resorptive treatments inhibit bone remodeling. Initially, this is measured as a decrease in resorption surface, and no change is seen in bone-formation surface. A new steady state is present when a complete remodeling cycle has passed. Until then, the system is in a transient state, which temporarily shifts the equilibrium toward bone formation, and conclusions about the resulting response on bone cannot be drawn.[53,89] Transients also induce changes in the MAR, thickness of osteoid seams, and mineralization lag time. A sudden decrease in activation frequency shifts the cross-sectional population of osteons toward older osteons. A higher fraction of formative sites will be in the late states, when the MAR is lower and the osteoid seams are thinner.[90]

D. Missing Data and Potential Bias

Tetracycline-based indices are particularly prone to loss of information caused by non-compliance during labeling, very low bone mass, or low bone turnover, resulting in the presence of single labels only or insufficient sampling of double labels.[51] Bisphosphonates reduce bone turnover markedly and thus increase the risk of missing data on mineralizing surface and MAR. The unbalanced exclusion of cases between bisphosphonate and placebo treatment is likely to bias the results on bone turnover. This can be handled by assigning minimum values of the MAR to those who present with single labels only or insufficient double labels for a valid estimate.[51] Applying a sampling scheme with more than one level of biopsy sectioning may reduce the number of sections without identified label profiles,[18] and may also reduce the incidence of missing data when sections are sampled uniformly at random.

E. Sample Size and Design

Histomorphometric studies are often designed as follow-up studies, obtaining biopsies at baseline and at post-treatment (paired biopsy design). In experimental animals, however, bone samples are often obtained at the end of intervention only, although a start control group is included (single biopsy design). For the paired biopsy design to be optimal, the variation within subjects must be smaller than the variation between them. This has been confirmed for structural indices in a study in which two iliac crest biopsies were obtained from contralateral sides at the same time.[96] However, in a study of remodeling indices, the opposite was found on analysis of contralateral biopsies obtained at different time-points.[52] The discrepancy may be explained by the different indices studied or by the effect of time, with important implications for the variation within individuals. If the variation within subjects is greater than the variation between them, the optimal design is to compare biopsies obtained at the end of treatment only. Recently, two histomorphometric studies were conducted as single biopsy studies.[16,18] In some cases, conditions such as osteomalacia may not be discovered at the beginning of the study, but this could be avoided by obtaining a small-needle biopsy instead.

III. GLUCOCORTICOID-INDUCED OSTEOPOROSIS

Low-energy fractures occur with endogenous as well as exogenous glucocorticoid excess. The loss of bone mass, as evidenced by reduced bone-mineral density, is rapid during the first year and thereafter continues at a slower rate. Cancellous bone loss occurs more rapidly than cortical loss. The risk of fracture is related to the cumulated dose, duration of exposure, the initial bone mineral density, the underlying disease, and women's menopausal state. The effects of glucocorticoids on bone formation apparently relate to direct effects on osteoblasts inhibiting the synthesis of collagen type I[73] and osteocalcin,[82] and increasing osteoblast apoptosis.[117] The effects of glucocorticoids on bone resorption surfaces are less clear. Whether there is a direct effect on bone resorption is not presently known. However, glucocorticoid treatment induces secondary hyperparathyroidism as a result of impaired intestinal absorption[47] and reduced renal reabsorption[112] of calcium.

The inhibitory effects of glucocorticoids on bone formation are indicated by changes in biochemical markers and by histomorphometric findings. Histomorphometrically, consistent reductions are seen in the MAR,[12,17,99,110] bone formation rate and bone formation period,[17,99,110] and in wall thickness.[17,27,99,110] In patients who are on long-term glucocorticoid treatment, bisphosphonates do not induce increases in wall thickness, although this could theoretically be expected, since bisphosphonates inhibit[97] osteoblast apoptosis and glucocorticoids promote[117] apoptosis of osteoblasts.

Wall thickness decreases 20–33% and raises the question as to whether the final resorption depth also changes. There are no data on final resorption depth, but one study suggests that it is decreased, since the mean trabecular-plate thickness is lower and mean interstitial bone thickness is unchanged in patients treated with glucocorticoids.[110] Studies suggest that the erosion surface is increased,[12] decreased,[110] or unchanged.[99] These discrepancies may be explained by different study conditions and a relatively large variation in erosion surface.

Bone densitometry and bone-marker studies of glucocorticoid withdrawal[66] or surgical cure of Cushing's syndrome[55] suggest that at least part of the bone loss is reversible. This could be explained by a decrease in bone turnover followed by a reduced remodeling space. The rapid initial decrease in bone mass could also be explained by changes in bone turnover expanding the remodeling space, whereas the slow continued loss is most likely caused by impaired bone formation. In patients who are receiving chronic glucocorticoid treatment, bisphosphonates induce a small increase in bone mass, which is also explained by a decrease in bone turnover as indicated by the reduced activation frequency.[18]

IV. PRIMARY HYPERPARATHYROIDISM

Primary hyperparathyroidism is caused by an increased continuous secretion of parathyroid hormone as a result of adenomas or hyperplasic glands.[23] Because of the development of easy and reliable biochemical tests for determining the concentration of ionized serum calcium and intact parathyroid hormone, the disease is now diagnosed earlier and with an increased frequency. This explains the dramatic change in the clinical presentation. The classical bone disease of primary hyperparathyroidism, described by Friedrich von Recklinghausen in the 1890s, was characterized by pain, pathological fractures, and deformity. Today, most patients have only mild symptoms or no symptoms at all.[102] However, treatment is still recommended, because primary hyperparathyroidism leads to osteopenia[20,44,104] and may increase the risk of cardiovascular disease.[74]

A. Bone Mass and Structure

Densitometric studies show a slight loss of bone-mineral density of 5–8% at locations dominated by cancellous bone,[20,104] whereas a more substantial bone loss of 10–20% is seen in skeletal parts dominated by cortical bone.[44,104] Following surgical cure, bone density in the lumbar spine (predominantly cancellous bone) is restored.[21,103] On the other hand, an irreversible bone loss of 5–6% occurs at the distal forearm (predominantly cortical bone).[21] These findings indicate that different parts of the skeleton may react differently upon stimulation by parathyroid hormone, which is also observed following parathyroid hormone treatment of osteoporosis. In histomorphometric studies of iliac crest bone, a 20% reduction in cortical width is found in primary hyperparathyroidism.[95] However, in cancellous bone, primary hyperparathyroidism inhibits age-dependent bone loss and structural disintegration.[23,95,116] How does this influence the fracture rate in primary hyperparathyroidism? Recent studies show an overall increase in fracture risk.[60,69,81]

B. Bone Remodeling and the Effect on Bone Mass and Structure

The main effect of primary hyperparathyroidism on the skeleton is an increase in bone remodeling.[28,95] In iliac crest biopsies, erosion surfaces, osteoid surfaces, and mineralizing surfaces increase endocortically,[22] and an increase in intracortical porosity is seen.[14,22] The observed cortical thinning may be explained by a trabecularization of the endocortex. This occurs where endocortical resorption cavities perforate into Haversian canals. Since the scaffold for subsequent bone formation disappears, an irreversible bone loss occurs. In cancellous bone, an increase in the extent of erosion surfaces, osteoid surfaces, and mineralizing surfaces is also observed (Fig. 3), and the activation frequency is increased by more than 50%.[23] The resorption and formation periods are normal, whereas the quiescent period is shortened.[23] Conflicting data exist regarding the effect of primary hyperparathyroidism on the MAR, erosion depth, and wall thickness.[38] Studies have found a decrease in the MAR, and have proposed that this may be caused by a direct effect of the high calcium level on the osteoblasts.[38,85] However, other studies have shown a normal MAR.[23,95] Wall thickness and erosion depth are reported to be reduced in younger patients with primary hyperparathyroidism,[38] but in older patients these reductions are not found.[23] Although the bone formation rate at the tissue level is greatly increased in primary hyperparathyroidism, the adjusted appositional rate is normal or even slightly reduced.[23]

The main effect of primary hyperparathyroidism on bone tissue may be a downregulation of the set point for initiating bone remodeling, thereby shortening the quiescent period and thus leading to an increased activation frequency.

The effect of a high activation frequency on bone density, mass, and structure depends to a large extent on the bone balance per remodeling cycle (wall thickness minus resorption depth).[106] A negative bone balance per remodeling cycle and an increased bone turnover will lead to an accelerated thinning of the trabeculae.[106] In primary hyperparathyroidism, a bone balance not different from zero is observed, and explains why no trabecular thinning occurs.[23]

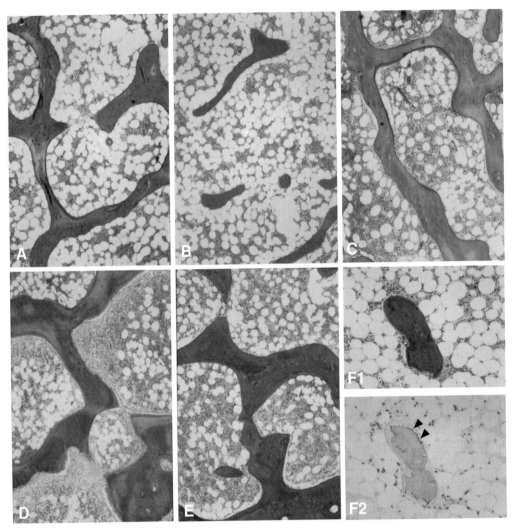

Figure 3. Goldner's trichrome-stained sections from iliac crest biopsies showing (A) Bone mass, bone turnover, and osteoid thickness from a normal middle-aged person. (B) Osteoporosis with decreased bone mass and disintegrated bone structure. (C) Primary hyperparathyroidism with increased bone turnover, as judged from the increased erosion and osteoid surfaces. Bone mass and osteoid thickness are within the normal ranges. (D) Secondary hyperparathyroidism with grossly increased bone turnover, foci of increased osteoid thickness, and mineralization defects. The bone marrow shows marked paratrabecular fibrosis. (E) Osteomalacia with very thick osteoid seams covering the entire surface, leaving no bone surfaces for osteoclastic resorption. The interface between mineralized bone and osteoid appears to be irregular. (F1) Aluminum intoxication with normal to low thickness of osteoid seams and an irregular osteoid-bone interface. (F2) Aluminum staining showing deposits of aluminum at the mineralization front (arrow heads). (*See* color plate 22 appearing in the insert following p. 270.)

An increase in activation frequency is one of the risk factors for the loss of entire trabecular elements (perforations).[106] Perforations can occur without an increase in erosion depth if bone remodeling by chance is initiated on two sides of a trabecula. The basis for the subsequent bone formation is lost, and irreversible bone loss occurs with disintegration of the cancellous lattice. Although the activation frequency is high in primary hyperparathyroidism, there are no signs of destruction of the cancellous network.[23,95,116] On the contrary, several investigators find that primary hyperparathyroidism may even protect the cancellous bone from the disintegration of the cancellous lattice, which normally occurs with age.[23,95,116] A reduced resorption depth may explain this positive effect of primary hyperparathyroidism. However, a reduction in resorption depth was only found in one study of younger patients with primary hyperparathyroidism.[38] Thick trabeculae will also reduce the risk of perforations, but the trabecular thickness appears normal.[95] Although an increase in trabecular perforations should be expected in primary hyperparathyroidism, because of the increased activation frequency, the opposite appears to occur.[23,95,116]

C. Reversible and Irreversible Bone Loss

In normal individuals, the remodeling space is 6–8% of the skeletal volume. The increased activation frequency seen in primary hyperparathyroidism leads to an increase in the number of ongoing remodeling cycles. This increases the remodeling space, and thus decreases the amount of bone. Furthermore, an increased bone turnover leads to a decrease in mean bone age, and since newly formed bone is not fully mineralized, this adds to the decreased bone mass measured by densitometric methods.

The observed decrease in bone-mineral density in the lumbar spine at around 8% in primary hyperparathyroidism[21] can be explained by an expansion in the remodeling space and a lower mean bone age. After surgical cure, a normalization of bone turnover occurs. The remodeling space is thereby reduced, leading to the rapid increase in bone-mineral density of the lumbar spine seen during the first 6 mo postoperatively. During the next 2.5 yr, a slow increase in bone-mineral density is observed, reflecting the increasing mean bone age (secondary mineralization). Three years after surgery, the bone-mineral density in the lumbar spine has returned to normal.[21] A slightly different picture is observed in the distal forearm. During the first 6 mo, a rapid increase in bone-mineral density is observed, reflecting a reduction in the remodeling space. During the next 2.5 yr, no measurable increase in bone-mineral density is observed,[21] because the effect of secondary mineralization is much less in cortical bone. The bone-mineral density is not totally regained, and irreversible bone loss has occurred. This process may be explained by the mechanism of cortical trabecularization.

V. OSTEOMALACIA

In pathophysiological terms, osteomalacia is characterized by defective mineralization of the osteoid matrix. The term "osteomalacia" has usually been used for diseases that result from a lack of vitamin D or a disturbance of its metabolism.[91] However, other conditions, such as inherited hypophosphatemia and a number of other renal tubular disorders, may cause osteomalacia without evidence of abnormal vitamin D metabolism. In renal osteodystrophy, a term that encompasses all of the disorders of bone and mineral metabolism associated with chronic renal disease, osteomalacia is often observed.[76] Many drugs induce osteomalacia by inhibiting vitamin D absorption, interfering with vitamin metabolism, or inhibiting phosphate absorption.[6] At least the first generations of bisphos-phonates used in the treatment of Paget's disease, hypercalcemia of malignancy, and osteoporosis may also cause osteomalacia by a direct effect on the bone cells.[5] Aluminum-related osteomalacia can develop in patients with chronic renal disease (Fig. 3), if they are exposed to high concentrations of aluminum, either in dialysate or from antacids containing aluminum—and used to treat hyperphosphatemia.

In many patients, osteomalacia is preceded for many years by clinically silent secondary hyperparathyroidism (Fig. 3), which accelerates the irreversible age-related loss.[91] If the compensatory mechanisms of calcium mobilization from bone are unable to maintain the calcium levels, a mixed state of secondary hyperparathyroidism and osteomalacia develops, which will later lead to frank osteomalacia.

In adults, the biochemical and radiological evidence of osteomalacia is often minimal, and the clinical diagnosis is therefore difficult. In many cases, a bone biopsy is needed to make the diagnosis.[7]

A. Mineralization Defect

Histological osteomalacia is usually characterized by an accumulation of osteoid tissue (Fig. 3). However, an increase in osteoid volume, osteoid surface, or osteoid thickness cannot be used alone or together as the histological criteria for the diagnosis.[39]

Osteoid volume (osteoid volume per bone volume) increases simply as a result of normal aging with trabecular thinning.[91] Increased osteoid surfaces are also seen in diseases with low or high bone turnover, although there is no mineralization defect. In the low bone-turnover disease myxedema, an increase in the extent of osteoid surfaces is caused by a prolongation of the formative period.[37] In primary hyperparathyroidism, an increase in osteoid surface and osteoid volume are seen simply as a result of the high activation frequency.[23] Thus, the histological diagnosis of osteomalacia cannot be based on these static osteoid parameters alone. Dynamic fluorochrome-based parameters must be included in the evaluation.[39] One key index for the diagnosis of osteomalacia is the mineralization lag time. Mineralization lag time is the mean time between matrix deposition and subsequent mineralization averaged over the entire formation period. It is given by the osteoid thickness divided by the adjusted appositional rate.[91]

The diagnosis of osteomalacia should therefore include an increased mineralization lag time and an increased osteoid-seam thickness.[39,91] In addition, a number of qualitative changes characterize osteomalacia. An increasing fraction of bone surfaces will be covered with osteoid seams of increased thickness. The border between mineralized bone and the overlying osteoid is blurred, and scattered areas of hypomineralized bone are often seen in the newly formed osteons. Tetracycline fluorescent bands are frequently wider and blurred. If there is any risk of aluminum intoxication, an aluminum stain must be performed.[75]

VI. INTERMITTENT PARATHYROID HORMONE TREATMENT

Animal experiments have clearly demonstrated an anabolic effect of intermittent parathyroid hormone (PTH) treatment; however, at present only few clinical trials have been published. In 1970, Kalu et al. showed that the PTH itself caused the anabolic bone effect.[59] When PTH is secreted from the parathyroid glands, it consists of 84 amino acids (PTH(1–84)). The PTH (1–34) fragment is also fully bioactive and subsequent animal experiments and human trials have been using PTH(1–34) and PTH(1–84) as well as other bioactive fragments and analogs.

In studies of anabolic effects, labeling with fluorochromes and measuring of dynamic histomorphometric parameters prove useful. In PTH-treated rats, a substantial increase in cancellous bone-mineralizing surface, the MAR, and the bone formation rate has been found.[29,30,68] The new bone deposition proceeds rapidly on the surfaces of the trabeculae by the activation of bone-lining cells,[29] and is not initiated by resorption evolving into formation in the coupled process of remodeling. The treatment also augments cancellous bone volume, trabecular thickness, and indices of interconnectedness.[30,68] The interconnectedness does not appear to be affected in severely osteopenic rats,[68] indicating that no new trabeculae are formed by the treatment. In cortical bone, PTH treatment induces a substantial endocortical bone deposition, which can be demonstrated by fluorochrome labeling and measuring of measurement of the MAR and bone formation rate.[3,30] Although a substantial increase in periosteal mineralizing surface is seen, only a small amount of new bone is deposited as shown by the low MAR and bone formation rate.[3] Along with the increased bone mass, a corresponding increase is found in the mechanical strength of the bones.[3,30] When the treatment is discontinued, the new bone is removed quickly and the mechanical strength returns to initial values.[30] This removal of newly deposited bone has clearly been demonstrated by sequential fluorochrome labeling of the animals during the treatment period, followed by subsequent resorption measurements of the labeling lines.[30] The anabolic effects of PTH have also been observed in ferrets, rabbits, and dogs, and the results correspond with the findings in rats.

PTH treatment of osteoporotic patients primarily shows an anabolic effect in vertebrae, where bone-mineral density enhances rapidly after onset of treatment.[40,71] Histomorphometric investigations have been performed using iliac crest biopsies, and substantial increases were found in cancellous bone volume, trabecular thickness, and activation frequency.[10,56] Early histomorphometric investigations in response to PTH treatment show that new bone formation takes place on quiescent cancellous bone surfaces.[57] In predominantly cortical bone, changes including both decline and increase in bone mass have been reported;[40,71] however, most investigations have found a loss of cortical bone. At present, we do not know to what extent such a decline in cortical bone mass influences the strength of the bone. Ovariectomized cynomolgus monkeys have been treated with PTH, and their cortical bone has been analyzed.[15] PTH dose dependently increases intracortical porosity. However, most porosity is concentrated near the endocortical surface, where its effect on bending and torsion strength is small. Correspondingly, no detrimental effect on the mechanical properties of the cortical bone is found. The authors estimated the strength of the cortical bone, assuming that porosity was uniformly distributed throughout the cross-section, and concluded that such a distribution significantly decreases the strength of the bone. In human trials, therefore, a nonhomogeneous distribution of porosity must be considered when evaluating to what extent the decline in cortical bone mass induced by PTH treatment influences bone strength.

The studies have primarily investigated effects of PTH treatment on intact bones. However, very recent animal experiments show that PTH treatment promotes mechanical strength development in healing fractures by enhancing the amount of callus.[1,8] The ability of PTH to increase the amount of callus is particularly interesting in relation to delayed fracture healing, and further experiments are needed to elucidate these healing aspects.

VII. GROWTH HORMONE

Growth hormone (GH) exerts a profound effect on the skeleton by inducing linear growth, modeling and remodeling.[87] There is an interplay between GH and insulin-like growth factor I (IGF-I), as GH induces local production of IGF-I (autocrine/paracrine acting) and enhances circulating levels of IGF-I (endocrine acting), secreted by the liver.[87] In this section, however, only the effect of GH on bone metabolism and bone mass will be discussed. In 1972, Harris and colleagues used histomorphometric assessments to show that GH administration enhanced femoral and tibial cortical bone mass in dogs.[50] Their data also showed that GH administration increased both periosteal and endocortical bone deposition and augmented intracortical bone resorption. When GH is given to rats, a substantial periosteal bone deposition takes place, both at the diaphyseal bones and vertebrae.[2,3] Interestingly, GH adminstration does not deposit new bone at the periosteal vertebral surface toward the vertebral canal, whereas bone is deposited at the endocortical surface at this location.[2] When GH treatment induces linear growth, an increase in cancellous bone volume, mineralizing surface, osteoblast surface, and osteoclast surface is observed,[87] whereas no change in bone volume is found in old rats without linear growth.[2] Along with the increased bone mass, a corresponding increase is found in the mechanical strength of the bones.[2,3] GH administered to monkeys has resulted in increased mineralizing surface, bone formation rate, and osteoclast surface in vertebrae, the femur, and the tibia.[87]

Iliac crest biopsies from patients with acromegaly have shown increased cortical and trabecular bone mass as well as an increased resorption surface and mineralizing surface.[48] This indicates an increased bone turnover, which has been confirmed by measuring biochemical markers for bone resorption and formation.[87]

In patients with GH deficiency, a decreased bone-mineral density, bone-mineral content,[87] and increased fracture frequency are reported.[87] When treating the patients with GH, an initial decline is found in lumbar spine and femoral neck bone-mineral density and bone-mineral content.[87] Continuous treatment for 2 yr or more, however, results in increased lumbar spine and femoral neck bone-mineral density and bone-mineral content.[87] GH treatment of patients with GH deficiency has been shown to cause an increase in osteoid surface, mineralizing surface, and erosion surface; consequently, the quiescent surface is decreased.[11,13] The investigators found no changes in cancellous bone volume, whereas there was an increase in cortical thickness.

VIII. THYROID HORMONES

Increased bone metabolism and decreased bone mass are found in patients with hyperthyroidism.[43] This condition induces an increased risk of fractures.[43] Cross-sectional histomorphometric investigations show the formative and resorptive surfaces to be extended.[80] The complete remodeling period is decreased, caused by a substantial shortening of both the resorption and formation periods.[31] No difference in resorption depth is observed,[31] but the wall thickness is lower in hyperthyroid patients, resulting in a negative bone balance. Therefore, hyperthyroidism causes a substantial bone loss, since both the remodeling space increases and a net negative bone balance appears. However, when measuring the trabecular thickness, no changes are found.[31,64]

Hypothyroidism decreases activation frequency, and both the resorption period and the formation period are prolonged substantially.[31] Furthermore, a decreased osteoid seam and a decreased MAR are demonstrated.[24,64,86] The resorption depth is decreased and the wall thickness is increased, leading to a positive remodeling bone balance.[31] Correspondingly, the trabecular thickness is found to increase.[24,64,86] The positive bone balance, however, does not result in a detectable increase in cancellous bone volume, which might be caused by the decreased activation frequency.[31]

REFERENCES

1. Andreassen TT, Ejersted C, Oxlund H: Intermittent parathyroid hormone (1–34) treatment increases callus formation and mechanical strength of healing rat fractures. *J Bone Miner Res* 14:960–968, 1999.
2. Andreassen TT, Melsen F, Oxlund H: The influence of growth hormone on cancellous and cortical bone of the vertebral body in aged rats. *J Bone Miner Res* 11:1094–1102, 1996.
3. Andreassen TT, Oxlund H: The influence of combined parathyroid hormone and growth hormone treatment on cortical bone in aged ovariectomized rats. *J Bone Miner Res* 15:2266–2275, 2000.
4. Arlot ME, Delmas PD, Chappard D, et al: Trabecular and endocortical bone remodeling in postmenopausal osteoporosis: comparison with normal postmenopausal women. *Osteoporos Int* 1:41–49, 1990.
5. Bell NH, Johnson RH: Bisphosphonates in the treatment of osteoporosis. *Endocrine* 6:203–206, 1997.
6. Bikle DD: Drug-induced osteomalacia. In: Favus ed: *Primer on the Metabolic Bone Diseases and Disorders of Mineral Metabolism.* Lippincott Williams and Wilkins, Philadelphia, PA, 1999:343–346.
7. Bingham CT, Fitzpatrick LA: Noninvasive testing in the diagnosis of osteomalacia. *Am J Med* 95:519–523, 1993.
8. Bostrom MPG, Gamradt SC, Asnis P, et al: Parathyroid hormone-related protein analog RS-66271 is an effective therapy for impaired bone healing in rabbits on corticosteroid therapy. *Bone* 26:437–442, 2000.
9. Boyce RW, Ebert DC, Youngs TA, et al: Unbiased estimation of vertebral connectivity in calcium-restricted ovariectomized minipigs. *Bone* 16:637–642, 1995.
10. Bradbeer JN, Arlot ME, Meunier PJ, et al: Treatment of osteoporosis with parathyroid peptide (hPTH 1–34) and oestrogen: increase in volumetric density of iliac cancellous bone may depend on reduced trabecular spacing as well as increased thickness of packets of newly formed bone. *Clin Endocrinol (Oxf)* 37:282–289, 1992.
11. Bravenboer N, Holzmann P, de Boer H, et al: The effect of growth hormone (GH) on histomorphometric indices of bone structure and bone turnover in GH-deficient men. *J Clin Endocrinol Metab* 82:1818–1822, 1997.
12. Bressot C, Meunier PJ, Chapuy MC, et al: Histomorphometric profile, pathophysiology and reversibility of corticosteroid-induced osteoporosis. *Metab Bone Dis Relat Res* 1:303–311, 1979.
13. Brixen K, Hansen TB, Hauge E, et al: Growth hormone treatment in adults with adult-onset growth hormone deficiency increases iliac crest trabecular bone turnover: a 1-year, double-blind, placebo-controlled study. *J Bone Miner Res* 15:293–300, 2000.
14. Brockstedt H, Christiansen P, Mosekilde L, et al: Reconstruction of cortical bone remodeling in untreated primary hyperparathyroidism and following surgery. *Bone* 16:109–117, 1995.
15. Burr DB, Hirano T, Turner CH, et al: Intermittently administered human parathyroid hormone(1–34) treatment increases intracortical bone turnover and porosity without reducing bone strength in the humerus of ovariectomized cynomolgus monkeys. *J Bone Miner Res* 16:157–165, 2001.
16. Chavassieux P, Arlot ME, Reda C, et al: Histomorphometric assessment of the long-term effects of alendronate on bone quality and remodeling in patients with osteoporosis. *J Clin Invest* 100:1475–1480, 1997.

17. Chavassieux P, Pastoureau P, Chapuy MC, et al: Glucocorticoid-induced inhibition of osteoblastic bone formation in ewes: a biochemical and histomorphometric study. *Osteoporos Int* 3:97–102, 1993.

18. Chavassieux PM, Arlot ME, Roux JP, et al: Effects of alendronate on bone quality and remodeling in glucocorticoid-induced osteoporosis: a histomorphometric analysis of transiliac biopsies. *J Bone Miner Res* 15:754–762, 2000.

19. Christiansen C, Christensen MS, Transbøl I: Bone mass in postmenopausal women after withdrawal of oestrogen/gestagen replacement therapy. *Lancet* 1:459–461, 1981.

20. Christiansen P, Steiniche T, Brixen K, et al: Primary hyperparathyroidism: biochemical markers and bone mineral density at multiple skeletal sites in Danish patients. *Bone* 21:93–99, 1997.

21. Christiansen P, Steiniche T, Brixen K, et al: Primary hyperparathyroidism: effect of parathyroidectomy on regional bone mineral density in Danish patients: a three-year follow-up study. *Bone* 25:589–595, 1999.

22. Christiansen P, Steiniche T, Brockstedt H, et al: Primary hyperparathyroidism: iliac crest cortical thickness, structure, and remodeling evaluated by histomorphometric methods. *Bone* 14:755–762, 1993.

23. Christiansen P, Steiniche T, Vesterby A, et al: Primary hyperparathyroidism: iliac crest trabecular bone volume, structure, remodeling, and balance evaluated by histomorphometric methods. *Bone* 13:41–49, 1992.

24. Coindre JM, David JP, Riviere L, et al: Bone loss in hypothyroidism with hormone replacement. A histomorphometric study. *Arch Intern Med* 146:48–53, 1986.

25. Compston JE, Mellish RWE, Garrahan NJ: Age-related changes in iliac crest trabecular microanatomic bone structure in man. *Bone* 8:289–292, 1987.

26. Dahl E, Nordal KP, Halse J, et al: Histomorphometric analysis of normal bone from iliac crest of Norwegian subjects. *Bone Miner* 3:369–377, 1988.

27. Dempster DW, Arlot MA, Meunier PJ: Mean wall thickness and formation periods of trabecular bone packets in corticosteroid-induced osteoporosis. *Calcif Tissue Int* 35:410–417, 1983.

28. Dempster DW, Parisien M, Silverberg SJ, et al: On the mechanism of cancellous bone preservation in postmenopausal women with mild primary hyperparathyroidism. *J Clin Endocrinol Metab* 84:1562–1566, 1999.

29. Dobnig H: Evidence that intermittent treatment with parathyroid hormone increases bone formation in adult rats by activaiton of bone lining cells. *Endocrinology* 136:3632–3639, 1995.

30. Ejersted C, Oxlund H, Eriksen EF, et al: Withdrawal of parathyroid hormone treatment causes rapid resorption of newly formed vertebral cancellous and endocortical bone in old rats. *Bone* 23:43–52, 1998.

31. Eriksen EF: Normal and pathological remodeling of human trabecular bone: three dimensional reconstruction. *Endocr Rev* 7:379–408, 1986.

32. Eriksen EF, Gundersen HJG, Melsen F, et al: Reconstruction of the formative site in iliac trabecular bone in 20 normal individuals employing a kinetic model for matrix and mineral apposition. *Metab Bone Dis Relat Res* 5:243–252, 1984.

33. Eriksen EF, Hodgson SF, Eastell R, et al: Cancellous bone remodeling in type I (postmenopausal) osteoporosis: quantitative assessment of rates of formation, resorption, and bone loss at tissue and cellular levels. *J Bone Miner Res* 5:311–319, 1990.

34. Eriksen EF, Langdahl B, Vesterby A, et al: Hormone replacement therapy prevents osteoclastic hyperactivity: a histomorphometric study in early postmenopausal women. *J Bone Miner Res* 14:1217–1221, 1999.

35. Eriksen EF, Melsen F, Mosekilde L: Reconstruction of the resorptive site in iliac trabecular bone: a kinetic model for bone resorption in 20 normal individuals. *Metab Bone Dis Relat Res* 5:235–242, 1984.

36. Eriksen EF, Mosekilde L, Melsen F: Trabecular bone resorption depth decreases with age: differences between normal males and females. *Bone* 6:141–146, 1985.

37. Eriksen EF, Mosekilde L, Melsen F: Kinetics of trabecular bone resorption and formation in hypothyroidism: evidence for a positive balance per remodeling cycle. *Bone* 7:101–108, 1986.

38. Eriksen EF, Mosekilde L, Melsen F: Trabecular bone remodeling and balance in primary hyperparathyroidism. *Bone* 7:213–221, 1986.

39. Eriksen EF, Steiniche T, Mosekilde L, et al: Histomorphometric analysis of bone in metabolic bone disease. In: Tiegs ed: *Endocrinology and Metabolism Clinics of North America Vol 18. Part I. Metabolic Bone Disease.* W.B. Saunders Company, Philadelphia, PA, 1989:919–954.

40. Finkelstein JS, Klibanski A, Arnold AL, et al: Prevention of estrogen deficiency-related bone loss with human parathyroid hormone-(1–34): a randomized controlled trial. *JAMA* 280:1067–1073, 1998.

41. Garcia Carasco M, de-Vernejoul MC, Sterkers Y, et al: Decreased bone formation in osteoporotic patients compared with age-matched controls. *Calcif Tissue Int* 44:173–175, 1989.

42. Garrahan NJ, Mellish RWE, Compston JE: A new method for the two-dimensional analysis of bone structure in human iliac crest biopsies. *J Microsc* 142:341–349, 1986.

43. Greenspan SL, Greenspan FS: The effect of thyroid hormone on skeletal integrity. *Ann Intern Med* 130:750–758, 1999.

44. Grey AB: The skeletal effects of primary hyperparathyroidism. *Bailliere's Clin Endocrinol Metab* 11:101–116, 1997.

45. Gundersen HJG, Boyce R, Nyengaard JR, et al: The ConnEulor: unbiased estimation of connectivity using physical disectors under projection. *Bone* 14:217–222, 1993.

46. Hahn M: Trabecular bone pattern factor—A new parameter for simple quantification of bone micro-architecture. *Bone* 13:327–330, 1992.

47. Hahn TJ, Halstead, Baran: Effects of short term glucocorticoid administration on intestinal calcium absorption and circulating vitamin D metabolite concentrations in man. *J Clin Endocrinol Metab* 52:111–115, 1981.

48. Halse J, Melsen F, Mosekilde L: Iliac crest bone mass and remodelling in acromegaly. *Acta Endocrinol* 97:18–22, 1981.

49. Harris ST, Watts NB, Genant HK, et al: Effects of risedronate treatment on vertebral and non-vertebral fractures in women with postmenopausal osteoporosis: a randomized controlled trial. Vertebral Efficacy With Risedronate Therapy (VERT) Study Group. *JAMA* 282:1344–1352, 1999.

50. Harris WH, Heaney RP, Jowsey J, et al: Growth hormone: the effect on skeletal renewal in the adult dog. *Calcif Tissue Res* 10:1–13, 1972.

51. Hauge E, Mosekilde L, Melsen F: Missing observations in bone histomorphometry on osteoporosis. Implications and suggestions for an approach. *Bone* 25:389–395, 1999.

52. Hauge EM, Mosekilde L, Melsen F, et al: How many patients do we need? Variation and design considerations in bone histomorphometry. *Bone* 28:556–562, 2001.

53. Heaney RP: The bone remodeling transient: Implications for the interpretation of clinical studies of bone mass change. *J Bone Miner Res* 9:1515–1523, 1994.

54. Heaney RP, Recker RR, Saville PD: Menopausal changes in bone remodeling. *J Lab Clin Med* 92:964–970, 1978.

55. Hermus AR, Smals AG, Swinkels LM, et al: Bone mineral density and bone turnover before and after surgical cure of Cushing's syndrome. *J Clin Endocrinol Metab* 80:2859–2865, 1995.

56. Hodsman AB, Kisiel M, Adachi JD, et al: Histomorphometric evidence for increased bone turnover without change in cortical thickness or porosity after 2 years of cyclical hPTH(1–34) therapy in women with severe osteoporosis. *Bone* 27:311–318, 2000.

57. Hodsman AB, Steer BM: Early histomorphometric changes in response to parathyroid hormone therapy in osteoporosis: evidence for de novo bone formation on quiescent cancellous surfaces. *Bone* 14:523–527, 1993.

58. Jerome CP, Carlson CS, Register TC, et al: Bone functional changes in intact, ovariectomized, and ovariectomized, hormone-supplemented adult cynomolgus monkeys (Macaca fascicu-

laris) evaluated by serum markers and dynamic histomorphometry. *J Bone Miner Res* 9:527–540, 1994.

59. Kalu DN, Pennock J, Doyle FH, et al: Parathyroid hormone and experimental osteosclerosis. *Lancet* 1:1363–1366, 1970.

60. Kenny AM, MacGillivray DC, Pilbeam CC, et al: Fracture incidence in postmenopausal women with primary hyperparathyroidism. *Surgery* 118:109–114, 1995.

61. Kimmel DB, Recker RR, Gallagher JC, et al: A comparison of iliac histomorphometry in post-menopausal osteoporotic and normal subjects. *Bone Miner* 11:217–235, 1990.

62. Kleerekoper M, Villanueva AR, Staniciu J, et al: The role of three-dimensional microstructure in the pathogenesis of vertebral compression fractures. *Calcif Tissue Int* 37:594–597, 1985.

63. Kragstrup J, Gundersen HJG, Melsen F, et al: Estimation of the three-dimensional wall thickness of completed remodeling sites in iliac trabecular bone. *Metab Bone Dis Relat Res* 4:113–119, 1982.

64. Kragstrup J, Melsen F, Mosekilde L: Effects of thyroid hormone(s) on mean wall thickness of trabecular bone packets. *Metab Bone Dis Relat Res* 3:181–185, 1981.

65. Kragstrup J, Melsen F, Mosekilde L: Thickness of bone formed at remodeling sites in normal human iliac trabecular bone: variations with age and sex. *Metab Bone Dis Relat Res* 5:17–21, 1983.

66. Laan RF, van Riel PL, van de Putte LB, et al: Low-dose prednisone induces rapid reversible axial bone loss in patients with rheumatoid arthritis. A randomized, controlled study. *Ann Intern Med* 119:963–968, 1993.

67. Laib A, Barou O, Vico L, et al: 3D micro-computed tomography of trabecular and cortical bone architecture with application to a rat model of immobilisation osteoporosis. *Med Biol Eng Comput* 38:326–332, 2000.

68. Lane NE, Thompson JM, Strewler GJ, et al: Intermittent treatment with human parathyroid hormone (hPTH[1–34]) increased trabecular bone volume but not connectivity in osteopenic rats. *J Bone Miner Res* 10:1470–1477, 1995.

69. Larsson K, Lindh E, Lind L, et al: Increased fracture risk in hypercalcemia. Bone mineral content measured in hyperparathyroidism. *Acta Orthop Scand* 60:268–270, 1989.

70. Legrand E, Chappard D, Pascaretti C, et al: Trabecular bone microarchitecture, bone mineral density, and vertebral fractures in male osteoporosis. *J Bone Miner Res* 15:13–19, 2000.

71. Lindsay R, Nieves J, Formica C, et al: Randomised controlled study of effect of parathyroid hormone on vertebral-bone mass and fracture incidence among postmenopausal women on oestrogen with osteoporosis. *Lancet* 350:550–555, 1997.

72. Lufkin EG, Whitaker MD, Nickelsen T, et al: Treatment of established postmenopausal osteoporosis with raloxifene: a randomized trial. *J Bone Miner Res* 13:1747–1754, 1998.

73. Lukert BP, Mador A, Raisz LG, et al: The role of DNA synthesis in the responses of fetal calvariae to cortisol. *J Bone Miner Res* 6:453–460, 1991.

74. Lundgren E, Ljunghall S, Akerstrom G, et al: Case-control study on symptoms and signs of "asymptomatic" primary hyperparathyroidism. *Surgery* 124:980–985, 1998.

75. Malluche HH, Langub MC, Monier-Faugere MC: The role of bone biopsy in clinical practice and research. *Kidney Int Suppl* 73:S20–S25, 1999.

76. Malluche HH, Monier-Faugere MC: The role of bone biopsy in the management of patients with renal osteodystrophy [editorial]. *J Am Soc Nephrol* 4:1631–1642, 1994.

77. Mashiba T, Hirano T, Turner CH, et al: Suppressed bone turnover by bisphosphonates increases microdamage accumulation and reduces some biomechanical properties in dog rib. *J Bone Miner Res* 15:613–620, 2000.

78. Meema HE: Menopausal and aging changes in muscle mass and bone mineral content. *J Bone Joint Surg [Am]* 48:1138–1144, 1966.

79. Mellish RWE, Garrahan NJ, Compston JE: Age-related changes in trabecular width and spacing in human iliac crest biopsies. *Bone Miner* 6:331–338, 1989.

80. Melsen F, Mosekilde L: Morphometric and dynamic studies of bone changes in hyperthyroidism. *Acta Pathol Microbiol Scand [A]* 85A:141–150, 1977.

81. Melton LJ, III, Atkinson EJ, O'Fallon WM, et al: Risk of age-related fractures in patients with primary hyperparathyroidism. *Arch Intern Med* 152:2269–2273, 1992.

82. Morrison NA, Shine J, Fragonas JC, et al: 1,25-dihydroxyvitamin D-responsive element and glucocorticoid repression in the osteocalcin gene. *Science* 246:1158–1161, 1989.

83. Mosekilde L: Sex differences in age-related loss of vertebral trabecular bone mass and structure—biomechanical consequences. *Bone* 10:425–432, 1989.

84. Mosekilde L: Consequences of the remodelling process for vertebral trabecular bone structure: a scanning electron microscopy study (uncoupling and unloaded structures). *Bone Miner* 10:13–35, 1990.

85. Mosekilde L, Melsen F: A tetracycline-based histomorphometric evaluation of bone resorption and bone turnover in hyperthyroidism and hyperparathyroidism. *Acta Med Scand* 204:97–102, 1978.

86. Mosekilde L, Melsen F: Morphometric and dynamic studies of bone changes in hypothyroidism. *Acta Pathol Microbiol Scand [A]* 86:56–62, 1978.

87. Ohlsson C, Bengtsson BA, Isaksson OG, et al: Growth hormone and bone. *Endocr Rev* 19:55–79, 1998.

88. Oleksik A, Ott SM, Vedi S, et al: Bone structure in patients with low bone mineral density with or without vertebral fractures. *J Bone Miner Res* 15:1368–1375, 2000.

89. Parfitt AM: Morphological basis of bone mineral measurements: transient and steady state effects of treatment in osteoporosis. *Miner Electrolyte Metab* 4:273–287, 1980.

90. Parfitt AM: The physiologic and clinical significance of bone histomorphometric data. In: Recker ed. *Bone Histomorphometry: Techniques and Interpretation.* CRC Press, Boca Raton, FL 1983:143–221.

91. Parfitt AM: Osteomalacia and related disorders. In: Avioli, Krane, ed: *Metabolic Bone Disease and Clinically Related Disorders.* W.B. Saunders Company, Philadelphia, PA, 1990:329–396.

92. Parfitt AM: Bone remodeling in type I osteoporosis. *J Bone Miner Res* 6:95–97, 1991.

93. Parfitt AM: Relations between histologic indices of bone formation: Implications for the pathogenesis of spinal osteoporosis. *J Bone Miner Res* 10:466–474, 1995.

94. Parfitt AM, Mathews CHE, Villanueva AR, et al: Relationships between surface, volume and thickness of iliac bone in ageing and in osteoporosis. Implications for the microanatomic and cellular mechanism of bone loss. *J Clin Invest* 72:1396–1409, 1983.

95. Parisien M, Mellish RW, Silverberg SJ, et al: Maintenance of cancellous bone connectivity in primary hyperparathyroidism: trabecular strut analysis. *J Bone Miner Res* 7:913–919, 1992.

96. Parisien MV, McMahon D, Pushparaj N, et al: Trabecular architecture in iliac crest bone biopsies: intra-individual variability in structural parameters and changes with age. *Bone* 9:289–295, 1988.

97. Plotkin LI, Weinstein RS, Parfitt AM, et al: Prevention of osteocyte and osteoblast apoptosis by bisphosphonates and calcitonin. *J Clin Invest* 104:1363–1374, 1999.

98. Prestwood KM, Gunness M, Muchmore DB, et al: A comparison of the effects of raloxifene and estrogen on bone in postmenopausal women. *J Clin Endocrinol Metab* 85:2197–2203, 2000.

99. Quarles LD: Prednisone-induced osteopenia in beagles: variable effects mediated by differential suppression of bone formation. *Am J Physiol* 263:E136–E141, 1992.

100. Recker RR, Davies KM, Dowd RM, et al: The effect of low-dose continuous estrogen and progesterone therapy with calcium and vitamin D on bone in elderly women. A randomized, controlled trial. *Ann Intern Med* 130:897–904, 1999.

101. Recker RR, Kimmel DB, Parfitt AM, et al: Static and tetracycline-based bone histomorphometric data from 34 normal postmenopausal females. *J Bone Miner Res* 3:133–144, 1988.

102. Rude RK: Hyperparathyroidism. *Otolaryngol Clin North Am* 29:663–679, 1996.

103. Silverberg SJ, Gartenberg F, Jacobs TP, et al: Increased bone mineral density after parathyroidectomy in primary hyperparathyroidism. *J Clin Endocrinol Metab* 80:729–734, 1995.

104. Silverberg SJ, Shane E, de la CL, et al: Skeletal disease in primary hyperparathyroidism. *J Bone Miner Res* 4:283–291, 1989.

105. Slemenda CW, Longcope C, Peacock M, et al: Sex steroids, bone mass, and bone loss. A prospective study of pre-, peri-, and postmenopausal women. *J Clin Invest* 97:14–22, 1996.

106. Steiniche T: Bone histomorphometry in the pathophysiological evaluation of primary and secondary osteoporosis and various treatment modalities. *APMIS* 103, 1995.

107. Steiniche T, Christiansen P, Vesterby A, et al: Reconstruction of the formative site in trabecular bone by a new, quick, and easy method. *Bone* 13:147–152, 1992.

108. Steiniche T, Christiansen P, Vesterby A, et al: Marked changes in iliac crest bone structure in postmenopausal osteoporotic patients without any signs of disturbed bone remodeling or balance. *Bone* 15:73–79, 1994.

109. Steiniche T, Hasling C, Charles P, et al: A randomized study on the effects of estrogen/gestagen or high dose oral calcium on trabecular bone remodeling in postmenopausal osteoporosis. *Bone* 10:313–320, 1989.

110. Stellon AJ, Webb A, Compston, JE: Bone histomorphometry and structure in corticosteroid-treated active hepatitis. *Gut* 29:378–384, 1988.

111. Storm T, Steiniche T, Thamsborg G, et al: Changes in bone histomorphometry after long-term treatment with intermittent, cyclic etidronate for postmenopausal osteoporosis. *J Bone Miner Res* 8:199–207, 1993.

112. Suzuki Y, Ichikawa Y, Saito E, et al: Importance of increased urinary calcium excretion in the development of secondary hyperthyroidism of patients under glucocorticoid therapy. *Metabolism* 32:151–156, 1983.

113. Vedi S, Compston JE, Webb A, et al: Histomorphometric analysis of bone biopsies from the iliac crest of normal British subjects. *Metab Bone Dis Relat Res* 4:2316–2321, 1982.

114. Vesterby A: Star volume of marrow space and trabeculae in iliac crest: sampling procedure and correlation to star volume of first lumbar vertebra. *Bone* 11:149–155, 1990.

115. Vesterby A, Gundersen HGJ, Melsen F, et al: Normal postmenopausal women show iliac crest trabecular thickening on vertical sections. *Bone* 10:333–339, 1989.

116. Vogel M, Hahn M, Delling G: Trabecular bone structure in patients with primary hyperparathyroidism. *Virchows Arch* 426:127–134, 1995.

117. Weinstein RS, Jilka RL, Parfitt AM, et al: Inhibition of osteoblastogenesis and promotion of apoptosis of osteoblasts and osteocytes by glucocorticoids. Potential mechanisms of their deleterious effects on bone. *J Clin Invest* 102:274–282, 1998.

30

Histology of Articular Cartilage Repair

Stefan Nehrer[1] and Myron Spector[2]

[1]Department of Orthopaedic Surgery, University of Vienna, Vienna, Austria
[2]Department of Orthopaedic Surgery, Brigham and Women's Hospital
Harvard Medical School, Boston, MA, USA

I. INTRODUCTION

The avascular nature of articular cartilage and its relatively low density of chondrocytes with low mitotic activity are a disadvantage to healing. Defects resulting from trauma or surgery may remain indefinitely (i.e., no healing), or fill with reparative tissue comprising fibrocartilage and fibrous tissue and perhaps some hyaline cartilage—but rarely with tissue that has the composition and architecture of articular cartilage. This is the process of "repair." "Regeneration" of such lesions—i.e., complete filling with articular cartilage—has never been found in the postnatal mammal.

Articular cartilage is a specialized subset of hyaline cartilage (cartilage in which type II collagen, hyaluronic acid, and aggrecan predominate) that displays a distinctively organized structure including: an arcuate collagen fiber structure originating with thick fibers rising perpendicularly from the calcified cartilage through a middle zone and bending near the superficial zone to form fibers oriented parallel to the surface; and an associated columnar arrangement of spherical cells perpendicular to the base, with more flattened cells aligned parallel to the surface. These histological features, as well as cell density and the pattern of proteoglycan staining, distinguish articular cartilage from other forms of hyaline cartilage, such as nasal and tracheal cartilage. Attachment of articular cartilage to a calcified cartilage base can be considered another distinguishing feature of this tissue type. The biomechanical function of articular cartilage is markedly different from the other hyaline cartilages—an indication of the importance of its distinctive and essential architecture to its performance. Thus, one reason to critically distinguish the cartilage forms that comprise reparative tissue that fill an articular cartilage defect involves their widely divergent mechanical properties, and thus the variations in performance and serviceable life that can be expected as they support joint loading.

II. METHODS OF EVALUATING ARTICULAR CARTILAGE REPAIR

There are three primary methods for evaluating the outcome of healing in cartilage defects in an animal model: histology, biochemistry, and mechanical properties. Interestingly, none

From: *Handbook of Histology Methods for Bone and Cartilage*
Edited by: Y. H. An and K. L. Martin © Humana Press Inc., Totowa, NJ

of these are the same criteria used to evaluate success clinically—pain relief, then function. Other clinical assessments can be made through arthroscopic procedures, including viewing or probing the surface. However, these results do not always correlate with patient symptoms, and thus are not used as reliable indicators of the success of healing.

In experimental work, most authors use histological methods of evaluating cartilage repair. This allows the evaluation of many important factors in the reparative process: the types of tissues filling the defect—including both cell and extracellular matrix (ECM) characteristics—attachment to adjacent structures (cartilage, calcified cartilage, or bone), and the health of the adjacent tissues. The method of staining may also be useful in eliciting biochemical information. For example, several staining methods are specific to sulfated glycosaminoglycans (GAGs) such as safranin O and alcian blue, yet immunohistochemical stains can be used to demonstrate collagen type and cartilage-specific proteins. Finally, histology can reveal structural information—primarily collagen organization—that may give a general idea of the functionality of the reparative tissue.

A semi-quantitative schema for evaluating the degree of degradation of articular cartilage—the Mankin scale[8]—has recently been adapted to provide a quantitative assessment of the success of cartilage healing in reparative procedures.[1,11–13] However, this approach must be exercised with caution. The use of an ordinal semi-quantitative scale precludes the accurate use of parametric statistics. Still, in many studies the ordinal data are used as parametric input for the reporting of statistical comparisons.[1,5] The meaning of these statistics should be considered only approximate. Furthermore, a composite score of many categories is often reported and used for comparison between groups. This comparison is therefore made under the assumption that the highest score possible in each category accurately reflects its relative importance in healing. This is most certainly not the case, as the "importance" in healing is at this time at best a subjective judgment of the experimenter.

More recently, quantitative histological methods have been used for the evaluation of the reparative tissue in defects in animal models[4,7] In one approach, formerly applied to rabbit investigations employing osteochondral defects, the strategy has been to obtain a quantitative description of the degree of cartilage restoration: repair dimensions, degree of attachment, surface roughness, and repair location.[7] The other approach[4] used to analyze the reparative tissue in chondral defects in a canine model has been to determine the areal percentage of selected tissue types in the defect and the percentage bonding to the adjacent articular cartilage and underlying calcified cartilage.

Other methods of analysis are more specialized, and may complement histological analysis. The measurement of mechanical properties on reparative tissue may indicate the degree to which the tissue functionally replaces normal cartilage. The major variables examined include modulus of elasticity and permeability. Biochemical analysis is normally focused on synthesis of the major components of the cartilage ECM: collagen and proteoglycans. Both of these methods have had limited use partly because of the destructive nature of the typical ex vivo testing procedures that prevent histological analysis of the same tissue.

It would be desirable to have information from all of these outcomes. However, practical limitations, including the limited size of defects and the expense of animal models, often make this impossible. For a preliminary investigation of healing, histology provides the widest range of information and is widely accepted. Mechanical and biochemical evaluations are more appropriate for more specialized follow-up studies. Advances in the technology of mechanical testing, including non-destructive probes that may be used in situ, promise to expand the use of mechanical testing in the analysis of cartilage repair.

This chapter primarily focuses on a method to quantitatively evaluate the areal percentage of cartilage defects occupied by selected tissue types.

III. METHODS

A. Histology, Histochemistry, and Immunohistochemistry

For samples obtained from animal studies and from block-resected human specimens (as may come from joint arthroplasty or at autopsy), the reparative tissue site can be cut from the bone, fixed in 10% formalin, and dehydrated in ethanol solutions.[4] The amount of fixative and fixation time must be adjusted to the volume of the tissue sample. Decalcification may be necessary for the preparation of microtomed sections of paraffin-embedded tissue. The use of techniques for the preparation of non-decalcified sections using plastic-embedding techniques is beyond the scope of this chapter. The time in the decalcification solution will be related to the amount of mineralized tissue in the sample. After decalcification, the samples can be embedded in paraffin. Microtomed sections of paraffin-embedded tissue can be stained with hematoxylin and eosin (H & E) and safranin O and immunohistochemically labeled with monoclonal antibodies (MAbs) to type I, type II, and type X collagen.

B. Method of Histomorphometric Evaluation

Areal analysis of the various tissue types[6] can be performed on sections from the middle portion of each defect, as described previously.[4,14] A 10×10-eyepiece grid can be used in the eyepiece of a microscope for manual determination of the areas of repair tissues for quantitative analysis. Alternatively, an automated method has been described,[10] using the intensity of the safranin O stain to define areas of cartilage. The variation in the content of proteoglycan in cartilage is a disadvantage of this technique.

Tissue filling of a defect site can be categorized as fibrous tissue, fibrocartilage, hyaline cartilage, articular cartilage, matrix "flow," or bone, according to criteria specified in Sections III. B.1–6 (Fig. 1).[4,14]

1. Fibrous Tissue

Fibrous tissue consists of spindle-shaped cells with bipolar, tapered ends and elongated nuclei. The cells are intimately associated with the surrounding collagenous matrix, and do not reside in lacunae. The matrix contains type I collagen fibers, oriented parallel to each other, which form bundles that are roughly parallel to the surface. The collagen fibers are clearly visible at low power under polarized light, and the matrix does not stain positively for GAGs (i.e., safranin O-negative). The collagen fibers often display a crimped pattern with a period of 10–20 μm.

2. Fibrocartilage

The characteristics of fibrocartilage are intermediate between those of fibrous tissue and hyaline cartilage. Cells are rounded and reside in lacunae surrounded by a pericellular matrix, thus distinguishing fibrocartilage from fibrous tissue. The matrix is principally comprised of type I collagen, with fibers visible microscopically, distinguishing this tissue from hyaline cartilage. Some matrix domains may stain for GAGs.

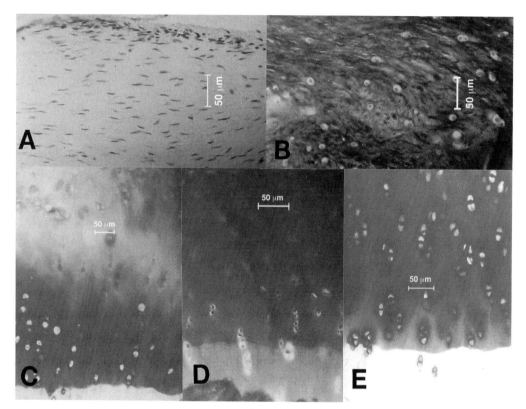

Figure 1. Light micrographs of tissue types found in articular cartilage and healing defects. The micrographs have been oriented with the articulating surface at the top and the tidemark at the bottom. Scale bars are provided in each of the panels. (A) Fibrous tissue, hematoxylin and eosin (H & E) stain. The collagen fibers and elongated cells are aligned parallel to the tissue and joint surface. Untreated control after 1.5 mo. (B) Fibrocartilage stained with Masson's trichrome. Note the fibrous nature of the matrix and chondrocytic appearance of the cells. Defect treated with an autologous periosteal flap alone with the cambium cell layer facing into the defect after 1 yr. (C) A mixture of hyaline cartilage (bottom of panel) and fibrocartilage (top of panel). This fibrocartilage is nearly hyaline in appearance. Safranin O/fast green stain. Defect treated with autologous chondrocytes expanded in monolayer culture and injected under a periosteal flap, 6 mo postoperative. (D) Hyaline cartilage stained with safranin O/fast green. Note the complete absence of red safranin O staining for GAGs. Defect treated with autologous chondrocytes expanded in monolayer culture and injected under a periosteal flap at 1 yr. (E) Normal articular cartilage stained with safranin O/fast green. (*See* color plate 23 appearing in the insert following p. 270.)

3. Hyaline Cartilage

Hyaline cartilage is identified primarily by the characteristic appearance of its type II collagen matrix. No individual collagen fibers or bundles are visible in the matrix. The hyaline matrix also has a distinctive appearance under polarized light, with diffuse transmission through the matrix except where the large collagen bundles are seen inserting into the calcified cartilage at the tidemark. Cells display a spherical morphology (except near the surface, where they are usually elongated, as in normal articular cartilage). Normally, the cells in hyaline cartilage have well-developed lacunae, and pericellular staining by safranin O is more intense than interterritorial matrix staining. However, tissue lacking normal safranin O stain or cellular appearance can be seen, and may be graded as hyaline. Portions of hyaline cartilage that meet the histological criteria of articular cartilage, including complete matrix staining and columnar arrangement of cells, are recorded as a subset of hyaline cartilage.

4. Articular Cartilage

Articular cartilage can be defined as a specialized subset of hyaline tissue that displays the distinctive organized articular structure, including: columnar arrangement of cells at the base rising through a middle zone; an arcuate collagen-fiber structure originating with thick fibers rising perpendicular from the calcified cartilage through the middle zone; and a distinct surface zone with fibers oriented parallel to the surface and more flattened cells also aligned parallel to the surface. These histological features, as well as cell density, matrix staining, and appearance under polarized light, should be required to be near normal, as made by comparison with adjacent healthy cartilage. Because of the variations of articular cartilage with depth, reparative tissue should be judged according to its position relative to the base of the defect. Although attachment to the calcified cartilage is required for tissue to be judged as basal articular cartilage, continuity with other adjacent tissues may not always be considered normal basal-, middle-, or superficial-zone articular cartilage. An area of reparative tissue may be considered to be normal basal-, middle-, or superficial-zone articular cartilage, even if the other zones normally found in articular cartilage are not present.

5. Matrix "Flow"

Matrix flow can also be evaluated. It is believed to represent a mechanical bulging of adjacent tissue into the defect (as opposed to proliferation of this adjacent tissue). This flow does not normally extend laterally into the defect beyond a distance approximately equal to the thickness of the cartilage layer. The flowing matrix occupies space in the defect, but does not represent newly synthesized repair tissue. Matrix-flow material can usually be readily identified in areas at the periphery of the defect. Areas of flow appear as hyaline tissue continuous with the adjacent cartilage. This flowing material often displays a variety of changes such as cloning and loss of matrix staining. The extent of these changes can be reflected in the grading of adjacent cartilage (*see* Section II.5.D.) Under polarized light, the collagen fibers and the columnar architecture appear to be continuous adjacent cartilage, but bent over, leaning into the defect. The collagen fibers bend as much as 90°, with some parts touching the base of the defect, but they do not attach to the calcified cartilage. Matrix flow can be recorded separately in grading of tissue types within a defect.

6. Bone

Bone formation may be observed in cartilage defects. These areas stain intensively for type I collagen and display histological features of normal bone tissue. The area occupied by these tissues can be expressed as a percentage of the original defect cross-sectional area. In addition, the areal percentage of the tissue type can be normalized by the total percentage of defect filling for the group. Areal percentages of tissue types may be determined in multiple randomly selected sections in the direction of the longer diameter through the center of the retrieved tissue. Additionally, staining with antibodies for collagen types and safranin O for proteoglycans can be graded as none, weak, moderate, and intensive in each specimen.

C. Evaluation of the Calcified Cartilage and Subchondral Bone

The percentage of the length of the calcified cartilage to which the reparative tissue has bonded can also be evaluated. For reparative tissue to be bonded to the base of the defect, the calcified cartilage layer must be intact. Bonding criteria should be based on collagen fiber continuity from the reparative tissue to calcified cartilage, not simply by apposition of the two surfaces.

Attachment of reparative tissue to adjacent cartilage can also be determined as a percentage of the length of both edges of the defect. Integration can be based primarily on the appearance of at least some collagen fibers integrated at the interface, as viewed with polarized light.

D. Evaluation of Articular Cartilage Surrounding the Defect

Semi-quantitative grading of changes to surrounding structures can be based on a qualitative assessment.[8] Scores can range from 0 to 3, with 3 representing normal tissue. A score of 0 represents excessive change; 1, moderate change; and 2, slight change. Categories examined can include the state of the subchondral bone and the effects on the adjacent cartilage using the methods of safranin O staining, cloning, and the integrity of the surface and deeper tissues. For subchondral bone, a grade of 0 can indicate active remodeling of most of subchondral bone underlying the defect, as reflected in active osteoclastic and osteoblastic activity. A grade of 1 may indicate such changes in the subchondral bone underlying approx 50% of the lesion. A grade of 0 for safranin O staining indicates a complete absence of such staining, and a grade of 1 is assigned to regions with faint staining or no staining over approx 50% of the area. For cloning, a grade of 0 can be assigned to areas with approx 50–100% of the cells present in clones, and a grade of 1 to regions with 10–50% of the cells in clones. For surface and deep tissue integrity, a grade of 0 may mean that there are many ruptures and surface irregularities throughout most of the region, and a grade of 1 indicates that such features are found in approximately one-half of the area. For all of the these, a grade of 2 reflects trace indications of changes in the features noted.

E. Assessment of Inter-Observer Error During Histomorphometric Grading

An experiment was recently conducted to evaluate the inter-observer error in grading of tissue types[3] using the schema described in Section IID. Three observers took part in this study: a frequent user of the method; a graduate student, previously unskilled in histology/pathology who was intensively trained on how to use the scale, and a pathologist given minimal training on the scale. Ten histological sections from 10 subjects were selected to provide a broad range of defect appearance with respect to tissue types, filling, geometry, integrity of surrounding tissues, and perceived ease of grading. Each defect was graded blindly for geometry and tissue types by each of the three investigators. Inter-observer agreement was evaluated by computing the mean, standard deviation, and coefficients of variation (COVs) among the three observers for each category on each sample.

COVs for recorded measurements of defect geometry (base and heights) were all under 5%, indicating that the geometry of the defect could be accurately determined by a single observer. The COV among the observers for identification of tissue types varied somewhat from tissue to tissue, and was related to the absolute value of the quantity recorded. In general, the higher the value measured, the lower the COV.

As might have been expected, there was an inverse relationship between the COV and the absolute value of the measurement. The inter-observer error could be compared to the inter-subject error for a given mean value of measurement. In total repair tissue, all values for inter-observer error, as measured by the inter-observer COV, were below those for inter-subject error. For hyaline cartilage, the result was similar, with all but one inter-observer value less than all of the inter-subject values. In the case of fibrocartilage, there was slightly more overlap; however, the inter-observer values were generally lower than the intersubject values.

IV. HISTOLOGICAL AND IMMUNOHISTOCHEMICAL FINDINGS IN A CANINE MODEL

There can be wide variability in the tissue types comprising the reparative tissue in the cartilage defects that undergo treatment with a variety of cartilage repair procedures. Of particular importance is the amount and composition of tissue that forms as a result of spontaneous healing, which must be considered as a control for the investigation of new procedures. Animal models can be of value in providing information about the reparative processes induced by selected procedures, particularly on a comparative basis. In this respect, the depth and extent of the lesion must be standardized because these factors can profoundly influence the course of healing. One such animal model has employed 4-mm-diameter defects down to the tidemark as the lesion in which to evaluate selected reparative procedures.[2] Using this model, it was possible to distinguish specific tissue types within the reparative tissue, based on the cellular morphology and ECM staining for the presence of type I and II collagen and proteoglycan. Notably, some untreated defects were found to be partially filled with tissue that met the criteria for articular cartilage (Fig. 2A–D). These criteria included the attachment of the articular cartilage to the calcified cartilage layer, as reflected in the continuity of collagen fibers across the tidemark (Fig. 2A). The attachment of the reparative tissue to the adjacent articular cartialge was variable—some areas displayed an indistinguishable interface and others showed a clear separation between the reparative tissue and the adjacent cartilage (Fig. 2A).

Certain trends were noted in the distribution of selected tissue types throughout the lesion.[2] Hyaline cartilage was always found to be superficial to intact calcified cartilage, and damaged calcified cartilage was covered only by fibrous tissue or fibrocartilage. When found, articular cartilage was superficial to an intact calcified cartilage layer, and appeared to form more frequently in the corners of the defects. Fibrous tissue was usually found at the surface of the reparative tissue, and was generally superficial to fibrocartilage.

Also of interest was that some of the articular chondrocytes in the cartilage surrounding the defects stained positive for smooth-muscle actin (SMA) (Fig. 3A, B).[14] This positive labeling was found in the specimens from the untreated knees as well as in defects that underwent the cartilage repair procedures. Chondrocytic as well as fibroblastic cells within the reparative tissue also were found to contain this muscle actin isoform. In some

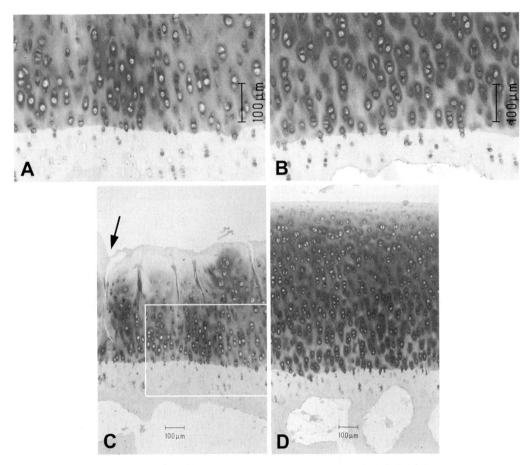

Figure 2. Histological micrographs showing an untreated chondral defect, 6 mo postoperative (A and C) and a normal articular cartilage control (B and D). The arrow in C shows the interface between the reparative tissue on the right and the adjacent articular cartilage on the left. The white box in C shows the area presented at higher magnification in (A). H&E stain.

cases, the cells that stained positive for SMA displayed the typical elongated appearance of myofibroblasts (Fig. 3B). These cells were found in the untreated defects as well as those treated with the periosteal and collagen flaps. In some areas, the large majority of cells (greater than 90%) were SMA-positive (Fig. 3B).

V. HISTOLOGICAL EVALUATION OF TISSUE RETRIEVED AFTER FAILED ARTICULAR CARTILAGE REPAIR PROCEDURES IN HUMAN SUBJECTS

The types of tissue-filling lesions in the human articular surface as a result of selected reparative procedures remains in question because of the understandable limitations in procuring such material for study, particularly for the asymptomatic treatments. The make-up of tissue in defects that are symptomatic and require revision may be of value in informing future studies of biopsies taken from asymptomatic lesions and evaluation of material from animal models. One such study evaluated tissue types in lesions treated with three methods and that required a revision surgical procedure:[9] abrasion arthroplasty

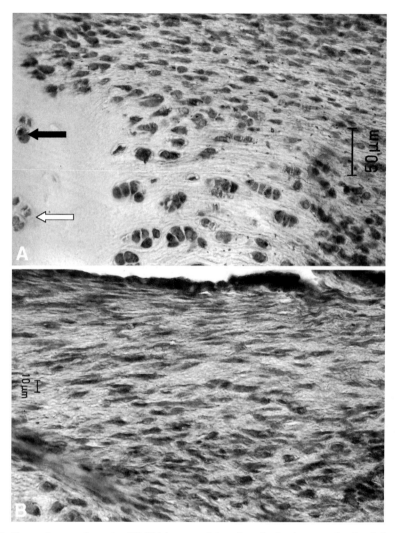

Figure 3. Smooth-muscle actin (SMA) immunohistochemical micrograph of a defect treated with an autologous periosteal cover alone, 6 wk postoperatively. The reddish chromogen labels the SMA. (A) demonstrates the presence of in chondrocytic cells in the articular cartilage adjacent to the defect (black arrow). Chondrocytes lacking this actin isoform are noted by the white arrow. Chondrocytic as well as fibroblastic cells that comprise the reparative tissue in A and B can be seen to contain SMA. Many of the SMA-containing elongated cells in the reparative tissue were consistent in appearance with myofibroblasts. (*See* color plate 24 appearing in the insert following p. 270.)

(AAP), perichondrial grafting (PCH), and autologous chondrocyte implantation (ACI). AAP was performed by removing 1–2 mm of the sclerotic subchondral bone and was always combined with debridement of flaps or fibrillation at the border of the defect. PCH was carried out by resecting rib perichondrium from one or two ribs and attaching the graft to the defect site with fibrin glue after a debridement of the borders of the defect. ACI was performed by injecting chondrocytes prepared by Genzyme Biosurgery (Cambridge, MA) under an autologous periosteal flap.

Histology of the retrieved specimens revealed a great variety of tissue types. In the specimens from AAP, fibrous spongiform tissue with fibroblastic cells and matrix with randomly orientated fibril bundles was seen in approx 20% of the cross-sectional area. Hyaline cartilage and fibrocartilaginous tissue that showed cell clustering and matrix fissuring and fibrillation were found in 30% and 28%, respectively; only 2% of the cross-sectional area was consistent with normal articular cartilage. Safranin O staining varied, with some moderate staining in fibrocartilaginous areas and depletion of proteoglycans in hyaline regions.

In the PCH samples, histology demonstrated an elevation of the subchondral bone, causing thinning of the cartilage to 20% of the depth of the adjacent cartilage. The cartilage layer showed no tidemark in the graft area, and fibrillation, clefts, and disruption of tissue were seen in the overlying reparative tissue. Some chondrocytes were arranged in columns, and others were organized into clusters. The matrix displayed a fibrous appearance with coarse collagen bundles in random orientation, alternating with hyaline-like tissue. The analysis of the areal percentage of tissue types of the retrieved specimens revealed about 20% bone. About 50% of the cross-sectional area was consistent in appearance with hyaline cartilage. However, most of this cartilage-like tissue showed signs of degeneration, such as clustering of chondrocytes and fissures or depletion of proteoglycan in the matrix, indicating a degenerative process. Only 3% of the cross-sectional area had the morphology of healthy normal articular cartilage. Immunohistochemistry confirmed weak type I and moderate type II collagen staining in the repair tissue. Chondrocytes near the advancing subchondral bone revealed moderate staining for type X collagen in the pericellular matrix, indicating that they were hypertrophic cells, and that the tissue was undergoing endochondral ossification.

Tissue retrieved after ACI demonstrated a fibrous appearance toward the joint and a more firm, whitish layer toward the defect surface. Histomorphometric analysis of the retrieved tissue at 3 mo (range; 1.5–6) after implantation revealed hyaline-like tissue in 2% of the cross-sectional area with chondrocytes in lacunae. These areas showed moderate staining with safranin O and type II collagen. The predominant tissue of the retrieved specimens after ACI was fibrous (60% of the cross-sectional area). The distribution of the tissue types in the cross-sections represented a continuous spectrum, with hyaline cartilage attached to the subchondral plate and fibrous tissue at the joint surface, consistent with the remaining fibrous layer of a periosteal graft. The retrieved detached periosteal flaps of the grafts revealed only small area of fibrocartilage, and about one-third of the cross-sectional area was filled with transition tissue (e.g., between fibrocartilage and hyaline cartilage). Compared to the histomorphometry of periosteum prior to the implantation, a remarkable remodeling process had taken place, and no distinct fibrous and cambium layers could be identified in the retrieved tissue.

The results of this study demonstrate that specific histological features may be associated with the failure of selected cartilage repair procedures. The findings also demonstrate that a quantitative histological procedure used for the evaluation of tissue types in experimental defects in animal models can also be employed for assessing tissue types in specimens obtained from human subjects. Comparison of sections stained with safranin O, and for type I and type II collagen facilitated the determination of tissue types. Notably in this study, computer-assisted histomorphometric systems that automatically analyzed areal percentages based on color scales did not adequately account for the complexity of composition and structure of tissue types.

REFERENCES

1. Ben-Yishay A, Grande DA, Schwartz RE, et al: Repair of articular cartilage defects with collagen-chondrocyte allografts. *Tissue Eng* 1:119–133, 1995.
2. Breinan HA, Hsu H-P, Spector M: Chondral defects in animal models: effects of selected repair procedures in canines. *Clin Orthop* 391:S219–230, 2001.
3. Breinan HA, Minas T, Hsu H-P, et al: Autologous chondrocyte implantation in a canine model: change in composition of reparative tissue with time. *J Orthop Res* 19:482–492, 2001.
4. Breinan HA, Minas T, Hsu H-P, et al: Effect of cultured autologous chondrocytes on repair of chondral defects in a canine model. *J Bone Joint Surg [Am]* 79:1439–1451, 1997.
5. Frenkel SR, Toolan B, Menche D, et al: Chondrocyte transplantation using a collagen bilayer matrix for cartilage repair. *J Bone Joint Surg [Br]* 79:831–836, 1997.
6. Grande DA, Pitman MI, Peterson L, et al: the repair of experimentally produced defects in rabbit articular cartilage by autologous chondrocyte transplantation. *J Orthop Res* 7:208–218, 1989.
7. Hacker SA, Healey RM, Yoshioka M, et al: A methodology for the quantitative assessment of articular cartilage histomorphometry. *Osteoarthritis Cartilage* 5:343–355, 1997.
8. Mankin HJ, Dorfman H, Lippiello L, et al: Biomechanical and metabolic abnormalities in articular cartilage from osteo-arthritic human hips. *J Bone Joint Surg [Am]* 53:523–537, 1971.
9. Nehrer S, Spector M, Minas T: Histologic analysis of tissue after failed cartilage repair procedures. *Clin Orthop* 365:149–162, 1999.
10. O'Driscoll SW, Marx R, Fitzsimmons J, et al: A method for automated cartilage histomorphometry. *Tissue Eng* 5:13–23, 1999.
11. O'Driscoll SW, Salter RB: The repair of major osteochondral defects in joint surfaces by neochondrogenesis with autogenous osteoperiosteal grafts stimulated by continuous passive motion. An experimental investigation in the rabbit. *Clin Orthop* 208:131–140, 1986.
12. Pineda S, Pollack A, Stevenson S, et al: A semiquantitative scale for histologic grading of articular cartilage repair. *Acta Anat* 143:335–340, 1992.
13. Wakitani S, Goto T, Pineda SJ, et al: Mesenchymal cell-based repair of large, full-thickness defects of articular cartilage. *J Bone Joint Surg [Am]* 76:579–592, 1994.
14. Wang Q, Breinan HA, Hsu HP, et al: Healing of defects in canine articular cartilage: Distribution of nonvascular alpha-smooth muscle actin-containing cells. *Wound Repair Regen* 8:145–158, 2000.

31

Histological Analysis of Cartilage Conditions

Theodore R. Oegema, Jr.,[1] Cathy S. Carlson,[2] and Ada A. Cole[3]

[1]*Departments of Orthopaedic Surgery and Biochemistry, University of Minnesota, Minneapolis, MN, USA*
[2]*Department of Veterinary Diagnostic Medicine, University of Minnesota, Minneapolis, MN, USA*
[3]*Department of Biochemistry, Rush Medical College, Chicago, IL, USA*

I. INTRODUCTION

Cartilage can lose structure and function as a result of a gradual disease process such as osteoarthritis or precipitously after an acute insult such as trauma. In this chapter, histological methods are reviewed for evaluating cartilage damage with an emphasis on three areas: human osteoarthritic tissue recovered from autopsy or surgery, joints from surgical or natural animal models of osteoarthritis, and cartilage damaged by acute trauma. There is a focus on primary references to well-established methods and recent developments and their applications. The basic methodology for sample preparation and staining is presented in other chapters. In many cases, it is especially informative to couple the observation of the gross specimen and histologic examination with biochemical and biomechanical analyses.

II. ANALYSIS OF HUMAN ARTICULAR CARTILAGE

A. Rationale for Evaluation

In contrast to the relative uniformity of animal joints (prior to experimental manipulations), human joints available for study are highly variable. If normal articular cartilages from human donors are to be used for study, care must be taken to ensure that the cartilage and joints are normal. Not all cartilages obtained from donors with no known history of joint disease, no apparent signs of surgery, and intact ligamentous components can be assumed to be normal. Not all cartilages from normal donors are normal even in joints that traditionally are not known to develop osteoarthritis. For example, out of 470 donors and a total of 1,033 joints obtained through the Regional Organ Bank of Illinois with no history of joint disease, only 38% of the ankles (talocrural joints) and 4% of the knees displayed no detectable degeneration.[32] These degenerative changes do not appear to be a component only of aging, especially in the ankle, as they are found in younger

From: *Handbook of Histology Methods for Bone and Cartilage*
Edited by: Y. H. An and K. L. Martin © Humana Press Inc., Totowa, NJ

donor cartilages and joints as well. Full-thickness defects can be found even in donors with no history of joint pain or disability. Of 470 donors, full-thickness defects were present in 7% of the ankle joints and 18% of the knee joints; in some cases the full-thickness defects in the knee joints involved more than 30% of the cartilage surface. The defects were more common in males than in females; 12% of the defects involving the ankle and 49% of the defects involving the knee were bilateral.

The cartilage evaluation should be based on both macroscopic and microscopic assessment. If normal cartilage is to be studied, then it should be normal at both macroscopic and microscopic levels. Sufficient variations already exist between human articular cartilage from different donors, different sites within the joint, and different joints, so that cartilage that is not entirely normal should be excluded from a study unless the study is designed to include cartilage with degenerative changes, and those changes should be included in the description of the joints and cartilages.

B. Joint Grading Scale

The same consideration described under Section III, A for acquiring samples of cartilage from animal models should be given to acquiring samples of human cartilage. The cartilage surface, color, and contour should be assessed, and it is also helpful to include a macroscopic grading scale, such as that of Collins,[16] as modified by Muehleman et al.[40] This 5-point scale includes normal–grade 0: no signs of cartilage degeneration; grade 1: limited fibrillation of the articular surface; grade 2: deep fibrillation and fissuring of any portion of the articular surface (Fig. 1) and possible osteophyte formation; grade 3: extensive fibrillation and fissuring of 30% or less of the articular surface eroded to the subchondral bone with osteophytes present; grade 4: greater than 30% of the articular surface eroded to bone with gross geometric changes including osteophytes. The application of India ink to the surface of the cartilage can be used to help define fibrillations. However, if the cartilage is to be used for chondrocyte metabolic or cartilage histological evaluations, it is advisable to avoid the use of ink and rely on the appearance of the surface of the cartilage to assign a grade.

C. Histological Cartilage Assessment

The Mankin score,[38] used originally to describe the histopathology of human hip OA, can be adapted with slight modifications to the changes seen in human cartilage from asymptomatic organ donors.[14] Although there are drawbacks to the use of this scale (*see* Section III, D) the Mankin score is a useful grading scale for confirming that there are no degenerative changes in the cartilage because the histology of the sections may indicate changes that are not apparent with macroscopic assessment. The Mankin grading scale takes into consideration three criteria: structural integrity, cellularity, and cartilage staining with safranin O as an indicator of proteoglycan and with fast green as an indicator for proteins.[51]

The Mankin score as originally published also includes an evaluation of the tidemark and subchondral bone. If these cartilage and bone layers are to be included in the study, the tissue must be decalcified prior to embedding and sectioning unless special knives are available for sectioning calcified cartilage and bone. Proteoglycan will be removed during the decalcification process, even when a gentler agent such as ethylenediaminetetraacetic acid (EDTA) is employed (Fig. 2; *see* Section III, B). If the study includes proteoglycan assessment, an agent such as cetylpyridinium chloride should be included in the fixative.

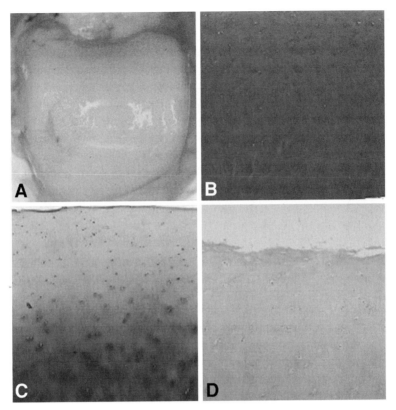

Figure 1. (A) Gross photograph of the superior surface of a talus from a woman (48 yr of age). The Collins grade for this talus was 2 because of the fibrillation. Outside this area, the remainder of the cartilage appears normal. Panels B-D are photomicrographs of safranin O-stained sections from the same talus. However, histological evaluation of the normal-appearing region outside the fibrillated area ranged from normal (Mankin grade O; B) to Mankin grade 3 (C) and finally to Mankin grade 5 (D).

The histopathological scores of the donor cartilages can range over the entire grading scale. "Normal" human articular cartilage can be characterized by a histopathological score of 0–5 and a Collins score 0–1. The previously examined human cartilages that received a histopathological score of 0 had three distinct zones (superficial, middle and deep) with no safranin O staining of the superficial zone but strong uniform safranin O staining in the middle and deep zones.[40] Some cartilages that also were considered normal (with Collins score 0–1 and Mankin score 4–5) had a disrupted superficial layer and reduced safranin O staining in either the middle layer, in the territorial matrix (matrix surrounding the chondrocyte lacunae), or in the interterritorial matrix. Where the cartilages had been eroded to the subchondral bone, samples from an area adjacent to the exposed bone and from an area a few centimeters distant from the lesion will typically receive a histopathology score from 9–13. These cartilages have no superficial or middle zones, fissures into the deep zone, large clusters of chondrocytes, and reduced staining in the remaining cartilage. Cartilages further removed from the lesions often have signs of degenerative morphological changes, such as a disrupted

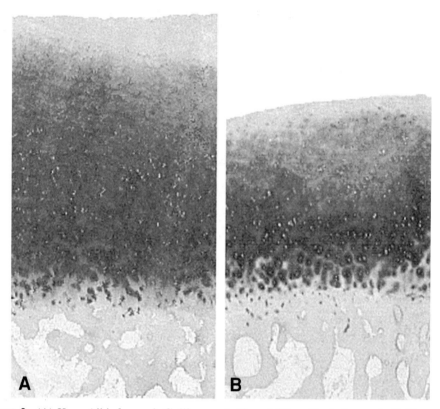

Figure 2. (A) Knee (tibiofemoral; Collins grade 0) and (B) ankle (talocrural; Collins grade 0) cartilages from the same limb of a 42-yr-old woman. The cartilage plugs, including sub-chondral, were removed from the joints and fixed in 4% paraformaldehyde, decalcified in 10% EDTA, embedded in paraffin, sectioned, and stained with safranin O. With the decalcifying procedure, proteoglycan loss is evident from both the knee and ankle, especially in the middle and upper deep zones.

superficial zone, loss of safranin O staining in the interterritorial matrix, and reduced territorial staining in the middle and deep zones. Although the cartilages from normal donors may have histopathology grades similar to those of cartilages from patients with osteoarthritis, the donor cartilages should be distinguished from the patient cartilages. Conversely, cartilage that is removed from the patient should not be considered normal, although it may be "normal-looking."

D. Assessment of Gene Expression— **In Situ** *Hybridization*

If the cartilages are obtained within 24 h of donor death and there is little evidence of chondrocyte death or loss of mRNA, they can be used for detection of gene expression using *in situ* hybridization. These tissues should be exposed to only RNase-free solutions and glass- or plasticware. The cartilage can be fixed in 4% paraformaldehyde and embedded in paraffin using routine histological procedures. Sections should be placed on coated slides to prevent loss during the prolonged processing. Sections are acetylated

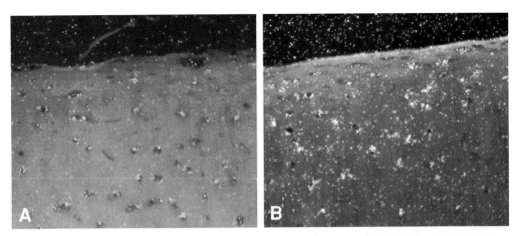

Figure 3. Autoradiographs of ankle cartilage from a 53-yr-old man (Collins grade 0; Mankin grade 3) that has been processed for *in situ* hybridization and incubated with a radiolabeled oligonucleotide probe specific for type IIB collagen (A) and aggrecan (B). The silver grains visible after autoradiography identifies the probe hybridized to mRNA within chondrocytes and appear as white dots with dark-field microscopy.

in acetic anhydride in triethanolamine and delipidated in chloroform and dehydrated prior to incubation with the *in situ* hybridization probes.

One procedure[13–15] is based on that of Sandell et al.[52] and uses short oligonucleotide probes approx 25-mer in length. Cartilage was analyzed for expression of type IIB collagen and aggrecan (Fig. 3) and showed specific labeling in different regions. The oligonucleotide probes are 3′-end labeled with 5′-[α-thiol-^{35}S]-dCTP using terminal deoxynucleotidyl transferase and hybridized under conditions of highest stringency corrected for each probe. Following hybridization and washing, autoradiography is performed by dipping the slides in Kodak NTB2 emulsion at 42°C. After drying, the slides are generally exposed (3–7 d at 4°C). The emulsion is developed with Kodak D19 and fixed with Kodak fix. The sections are then counterstained with cresyl violet to visualize the cells and matrix. To enhance the visualization of the bound radiolabeled oligonucleotide probes to mRNA within the cells, the tissue sections can be viewed with dark-field microscopy. We have found that this technique using the oligonucleotide probes with radiolabeling and autoradiography, provides the greatest sensitivity in detecting expression of low levels of mRNA.

III. EVALUATION OF ANIMAL MODELS

Appropriate evaluation of the histological changes occurring in animal models of cartilage conditions requires some degree of specialization/adaptation depending on the animal used, the condition evaluated, and the site to be examined.[59] The majority of animal models of cartilage conditions are those modeling osteoarthrosis, and the site most often examined is the knee joint.[1,3,12,43] Therefore, osteoarthrosis of the knee joint will be the specific example used in this chapter. It will be assumed that the entire joint is available for study.

A. Tissue Collection and Fixation

Because histological evaluations usually focus on a very specific site and because osteoarthrosis is a topographically variable condition, it is ideal to evaluate the joints radiographically or using magnetic resonance imaging (MRI) prior to collection of tissue for histological evaluation. These methods provide an overall evaluation of the joint and may influence the selection of the site to be evaluated.[11,64] A synovial fluid sample may be obtained prior to opening the joint, and this usually is done by lavage, in which a volume (amount depending on size of the joint, but typically 1–3 cc) of sterile saline is injected into each knee joint and, after repeated flexion and extension of the joint, is retrieved.[10,35,58] This must be done with care to avoid needle injury artifacts in the articular cartilage. Both knee joints may be processed and examined identically in the case of a surgical intervention model, in which the experimental knee is compared to the opposite knee. Alternatively, if the model is one of spontaneous disease and both knees are radiographically similar, one may be frozen at −70°C for future biochemical or biomechanical studies.[10]

The knee joint should be opened carefully, by transection of the quadriceps tendon, anterior reflection of the patella, and transection of the collateral and cruciate ligaments. Menisci may be removed or left intact. It is easiest to collect a sample of synovial membrane at the time the knee joint is opened, and this sample should be taken from similar location in each joint. A small scalpel should be used in opening the joint, and care should be taken not to incise or shave off areas of articular cartilage, as it may be difficult to distinguish real from artifactual (scalpel-induced) lesions once the tissues are processed. If the animal has been administered fluorochrome labels and these will be evaluated in the tissue to be collected, the opened knee joint or dissected bones (femur and tibia) should be fixed in 70% ethanol to preserve the labels.[29] Improved fixation of articular cartilage, however, is achieved using 4% phosphate-buffered paraformaldehyde at 4°C.[11] Paraformaldehyde-lysine-periodate has also been used with good results.[50] The paraformaldehyde fixative solution should be made fresh (within two weeks of use), stored at 4°C, and tissues should be transferred to 70% ethanol after 24 h. Prolonged fixation with paraformaldehyde will result in hard and brittle tissue. Alternatively, a simpler and also effective approach is to fix the tissues routinely in 10% neutral buffered formalin (NBF) at room temperature. Tissues can remain in formalin for long periods of time; however, optimal storage after fixation is in 70% ethanol. The disadvantage of this latter fixation technique is that tissues may not be ideally fixed for immunohistochemistry or *in situ* hybridization studies. Joint tissues that have been frozen after collection may be evaluated histologically with excellent results. These tissues should be thawed for up to 24 h at 4°C and then placed in the fixative of choice.

B. Decalcification

After gross evaluation of the tissues, the entire specimen may be decalcified, assuming that bony tissue is present. Although acid decalcification is rapid, superior morphological results are achieved using a chelating agent such as 10% disodium EDTA.[54] Decalcifying tissues in disodium EDTA is a relatively slow process, particularly when the tissues to be decalcified are large. The process may be accelerated by sectioning the tissue into slabs prior to decalcification. Specimens from monkeys and small laboratory animals may be precisely sectioned using an Isomet saw (Buehler, Lake Bluff, IL) fitted with a diamond saw blade.[9] In studies of OA, the tibia is usually sectioned midcoronally and the femur is sectioned in a frontal plane so that the section through the center of the femoral condyles is perpendicular to the articular surface and includes the trochlear groove. When evaluating a new model, all gross specimens should be evaluated before any sectioning is done. The chosen plane of section should include the center of the lesion in the most severely involved specimen, and all specimens should be sectioned in an identical manner to avoid variability caused by section location. Sections that are 2–3 mm thick may take several weeks to decalcify in disodium EDTA, with a change in decalcification solution every 3–4 d. Completely decalcified tissues will be pliable and will section easily with a scalpel blade. Although acid decalcification methods may severely alter histological morphology if overdecalcification occurs, 10% EDTA poses a minimal risk to tissues. EDTA decalcification is also the method of choice if immunostaining or *in situ* hybridization studies will be done on the tissues. After decalcification is complete, tissues should be rinsed in running water for at least 1 h and placed in 70% ethanol for paraffin processing.

In some cases, it may be necessary to fix and section the joints intact. However, it is nearly impossible to obtain a consistent plane of section through multiple bones in the joint. Thus, the resulting histological sections represent different tissue topography and are difficult to compare.

C. Sectioning and Staining

Samples of synovial membrane and slabs of decalcified joint tissue embedded in paraffin generally are sectioned at approx 6 μm in thickness and may be stained routinely. Toluidine blue and safranin O stains are used commonly for the evaluation of morphological features and assessment of matrix proteoglycan content.[31,55] Toluidine blue offers some advantages over safranin O with respect to fidelity of metachromasy and in its ability to distinguish qualitatively between sulfated glycosaminoglycans of the pericellular and interterritorial cartilage matrix.[21] When assessing matrix proteoglycan content, all sections from a study should be stained at the same time to prevent artifactual differences in staining intensity. It is sometimes helpful to include a reference cartilage as part of the quality control. If the intervention has resulted in the formation of fibrocartilage, additional sections may be stained with trichrome stain in order to distinguish hyaline cartilage from fibrocartilage or fibrous connective tissue.

D. Evaluation of Lesion Severity

The Mankin grading scheme traditionally has been used for the histological evaluation of lesions of osteoarthritis.[38] In this scheme, several histological variables are scored and a final joint score is calculated based on addition of the individual variable scores. Although this scheme is useful in some cases, it has several drawbacks. Firstly, it weights ranked variables (e.g., increasing grades of articular cartilage structural damage) more heavily than nominal variables (e.g., the presence or absence of a feature). Secondly, potential correlations among different variables are not taken into account. Third, although the scheme may allow one to differentiate normal from severely osteoarthritic cartilage, it is not sensitive enough to differentiate between mild and moderate lesions.[44] Finally, the resulting data are not continuous, eliminating the possibility of using analyses of variance or correlation analyses to compare these data with continuous variables such as body wt, age, or synovial fluid biomarker concentrations. A modification of the Mankin scheme for evaluating lesions of osteoarthritis using principal components analysis has recently been described in which these drawbacks are eliminated.[11] Other modifications have been proposed (compare Carlson et al.[11] with Chubinskaya et al.[14]). Principal component analysis is a type of multivariate analysis where derived variables (factors) are calculated based on linear functions of the individual variables.[56] Each variable contributes equally in the analysis and highly correlated grading variables (measurements as well as semiquantitative grades from a modified Mankin scheme) are grouped into factors that summarize the data. This method of analysis allows one to determine the combinations of variables that account for the greatest, second greatest, and successively smaller amounts of variation. The resulting factor scores represent continuous data and may be used as dependent variables in analyses of variance or covariance and in correlation analyses.

Using principal components analysis to evaluate histological data allows wide flexibility in the grading scheme used to evaluate lesions. Because histological changes may vary among species and with the particular interventions used, a scheme that includes all changes that may reproducibly be evaluated should be developed for each individual model. For example, in guinea pigs and hamsters, clefts at the tidemark are quite common, may be extensive, and should be included in the scheme, whereas these are not seen in monkey tissues and do not need to be included.[4,11,46] One way in which to generate such a scheme is to first examine and describe in detail the changes present in the set of histological sections. When all the sections have been described, a scheme can be created that includes all of the described changes. The scheme may be tested for reproducibility by having two or more observers independently evaluate it on the same set of sections, and calculating the intra- and interobserver variability.[45]

An example of the use of this type of scheme to characterize articular cartilage structure changes follows: **0,** articular cartilage smooth, uninterrupted; **1,** minimal/mild superficial fibrillation ($\leq 1/10$ of the articular cartilage thickness) involving <half of the plateau, condyle, or groove; **2,** minimal/mild superficial fibrillation ($\leq 1/10$ of the articular cartilage thickness) involving $\geq$half of the plateau, condyle, or groove; **3,** fibrillation/clefts/loss of articular cartilage involving superficial one-third of articular cartilage in <half of the plateau, condyle, or groove; **4,** fibrillation/clefts/loss of articular cartilage involving superficial one-third of articular cartilage in $\geq$half of the plateau, condyle, or groove; **5,** fibrillation/clefts/loss of articular cartilage involving superficial one-third to two-thirds of articular cartilage in <half of the plateau, condyle, or groove; **6,** fibrillation/clefts/loss of articular cartilage involving superficial one-third to two-thirds of articular cartilage in $\geq$half of the plateau, condyle, or groove; **7,** fibrillation/clefts/loss of articular cartilage involving >two-thirds depth of articular cartilage in <half of the plateau, condyle, or groove; **8,** fibrillation/clefts/loss of articular cartilage involving >two-thirds depth of articular cartilage in $\geq$half of the plateau, condyle, or groove; **9,** fibrillation/clefts/loss of articular cartilage to subchondral bone involving <half of the plateau, condyle, or groove; **10,** fibrillation/clefts/loss of articular cartilage to subchondral bone involving $\geq$half of the plateau, condyle, or groove.

A similar scheme may be generated to evaluate the degree and extent of loss of staining with toluidine blue and/or safranin O. The scheme should include all variables that may be evaluated, regardless of their perceived importance. It is preferable to collect these data separately from each site that will be evaluated (e.g., medial and lateral tibial plateau).

The data included in the principal components analysis may also include continuous data such as thickness and area measurements of articular cartilage, calcified cartilage, and subchondral bone. In addition, data from the evaluation of serial sections that have been immunostained (e.g., area of positive matrix immunostaining as a percentage of total articular cartilage area in the section or the number of immunopositive chondrocytes as a percentage of the total number of chondrocytes) may be included. The resulting factor compositions will reveal whether or not these variables are highly correlated with the graded variables. Alternatively, these data may be excluded from the principal components analysis, and their relationships may be examined with the factors using correlation or regression analyses. If the data are collected and evaluated separately for each site, quantitative comparisons of osteoarthritis severity may be made among the sites. Effects of treatment on factor scores and on individual variables may be evaluated by analyses of variance, using factor scores or individual variables as the dependent variables.

This type of evaluation has worked well with several models of spontaneous and induced osteoarthritis.[7,8,11] In general, grades for articular cartilage structure, loss of toluidine blue or safranin O staining, and chondrocyte clones are highly correlated and are included in Factor 1, which explains the largest amount of variation in the data.

IV. EVALUATION OF TRAUMA

Evaluating the consequences of acute or chronic trauma on articular cartilage structure and chondrocyte function is a daunting task. The histologic methodologies used for these studies have been largely adopted from those used to study osteoarthritis.

A. Evaluation of Early Matrix Damage

After acute trauma, all the available methods can be utilized to evaluate the chronic damage seen in osteoarthritis. After high-velocity, rapid-impact trauma, the swelling of the articular cartilage matrix has been taken as an indication of damage to the collagenous matrix.[62] This has been traditionally measured as change in wet wt with increases on the order of at least 3–6%, which is similar to that seen in models of early osteoarthritis. For the high-resolution imaging of changes of this type, magnetic resonance imaging (MRI) using proton with contrasting agents[63] and without[17,22,65] or [23]Na MRI[6,53] are almost sensitive enough. Images of this type are very informative since they can be done sequentially and have good spatial resolution. Rapid advances in imaging instrumentation and methods for acquiring, processing, and quantitating the data have made the method more attractive. The cost and limited access to instruments with the large magnets needed to get optimal resolution are still drawbacks.

Bone bruises indicative of damage to the subchondral plate or altered blood flow in the marrow space can also be followed by MRI.[61] As with osteoarthritis, surface damage has been evaluated by surface staining with diluted India ink and photographing the surface for quantitation of the length and width of the cracks.[30] Crack depth has been measured by standard histology.[30] To detect artifactual cracking, which occurs during processing, prestaining of damaged bone surface and the zone of calcified cartilage has been suggested,[26,39] but this method has not been used for cartilage cracks.

B. Evaluation of Calc[...]

Damage to the zone [...] chondral bone has been mapped by microradiography of pl[...] by regular light-level microscopy of fixed, undecalcified,[39]

Methods for examinati[...]idemark and the remodeling of the damaged subchondral bon[...]pted from those used for bone morphology. These have included [...]e thickness of subchondral plates and evaluation of the standard bon[...] parameters.[41] The use of tetracycline analogs to follow bone remodeling has been successfully used with single- and double-label combinations.[41,57] It has been more difficult to uniformly label the tidemark to follow rates of movement. There are two technical problems. One is that the labels given intravenously poorly penetrate the joint, and the label ends up largely near the tips of the few capillaries that penetrate to the tidemark from the marrow space.[42] The second is the loss of label at the tidemark because of dissolution and reformation at the mineralizing interface.

For example, in young rabbits, the tidemark moves at several or more microns per wk. Thus, the label at tidemark will move into the zone of calcified cartilage and can be followed for most of the 60–80 μm, which is the average thickness of the zone of calcified cartilage. However, in older rabbits, if the rate is too slow, the mineral at the interface will slowly exchange and the label will be lost. One practical solution is that if the experimental protocol is not harmed by exposure to bisphosphonates,[41] 2 d of oral disodium etidronate (20 mg/kg/d)[42] will allow movement as slow as 1 μm per wk to be detected.

Uniform labeling of the tidemark can be obtained by utilizing intra-articular injection. For both canines and rabbits, intra-articular injection of a fluorochrome gives uniform labeling of the tidemark. For example, 2,4 bis (N,N'-dicarboxy-methyl-amino ethyl fluorescein) made up in 1% $NaHCO_3$ and injected at a dose of 9.25 mg/kg as a single injection, followed by moving the joint 10–15 times will result in uniform labeling of the tidemark throughout most of the joint. These samples are processed by fixation in ethanol, followed by embedding in plastic and cutting and polishing if needed.[42] It should be noted that prolonged storage in alcohol will cause a loss of label.

If the sample is viewed microscopically with both partially polarized and fluorescent light, the distance of movement of the fluorescent band can be readily measured. Multiple labeling is possible, but since the bands are relatively wide, the proper combination of dyes with good spectral separation is needed. Because of the strong yellow-green autofluorescence of older cartilage, dyes that fluoresce in that region should be used only if other options are not available.

C. Evaluation of Cell Viability

In traumatized cartilage, chondrocytes can die by either necrosis or apoptosis. The measurement of live and dead cells in cartilage has largely used methods adapted from other tissues or cell-culture techniques, which use general principles of biology and usually have not been independently validated in cartilage. In many methods, the absence of a positive reaction for metabolic activity with histologically identifiable chondrocyte lacunae is taken as evidence of cell death. Some new methods measure a specific loss of function as a measure of death—i.e., staining of unfixed cells with propidium iodide, which indicates a loss of plasma membrane integrity, but the presence of DNA.[62]

Incorporation of a radioisotope precursor into protein (^{3}H and ^{14}C amino acids),[48,49] ^{35}SO$_4$$^{2-}$ into proteoglycan,[5] and ^{3}H-cytidine into RNA,[18] together with autoradiography are all established protocols for measuring cell viability. Although electron microscopy and examination of cells with the well-established changes in membrane morphology have also been used,[23] the method is laborious.

The use of commercially available live vs dead fluorescent assays frequently used on enzymatically released cells[2,28] or cells in culture has been adopted to cartilage slices.[62] In this methodology, a membrane-permeable nonfluorescent component moves into the cell and is modified by enzymes into a fluorescent compound that is retained in living cells. Dead cells are detected by using a membrane-impermeable fluorescent DNA dye that is excluded by living cells, but will stain the DNA of cells with compromised plasma membranes. Originally, fluorescein diacetate was used to detect the living cells, but the product has a pH-sensitive fluorescence and is not well-retained in the cell. Other substrates such as calcein AM[27] and Syto 13[66] have been substituted. In cartilage, propidium iodide has been the main living cell-impermeable, dead-cell-permanent DNA dye,[62] but ethidium bromide dimer is also useful.[66] The use of analogs that are retained after fixation has not yet been reported for cartilage.

To utilize this methodology, cartilage is cut into defined slices (0.4–2 mm) perpendicular to the surface, incubated in media at 37°C for a short period of time, the data captured and analyzed, and the percentage of dead vs live cells is calculated. This method used in combination with confocal microscopy is especially powerful. For each cartilage sample, it is important to determine how long the sample must be incubated in media with the reagents to achieve good penetration and enough reaction product. The samples must be processed in real time, since the product is retained only if the cells are alive. Cutting while preparing the sample may also damage cells near the newly cut surface,[60] so the appropriate controls must be included.

Reduction of tetrazolium salts to insoluble formazan products by living cells has been used extensively to determine cell viability in cell cultures or tissues, but has been used only to a limited extent to assess cell viability in damaged cartilage. MTT (3-[4,5-dimethylthiazol-zyl]-2,5-diphenyl tetrazolium bromide) forms a purple formazan product that is retained in a frozen section.[66] Nitroblue tetrazolium forms a dark blue, alcohol-insoluble precipitate that is stable during decalcification and processing through paraffin. In both cases, nonviable cells are identified as formazan-negative.[42]

Understanding how cells die in response to trauma is also important in planning interventions. Since chondrocytes are responsible for maintaining the surrounding matrix areas, if no chondrocytes are available, matrix integrity will eventually be lost.

Two pathways can be seen in cartilage cells: one is necrosis where basically the cell is so damaged it cannot function; the second is apoptosis where a cell is able to initiate and carry out a programmed cell death.[24,25,36]

The histological signature of cell death by necrosis at the light microscopic level is less clear than the signature of cell death by apoptosis. Although there are a number of initiation points that can start the apoptosis process, common early and late steps are used to detect death by apoptosis. A wide variety of commercial reagents and anti-sera are available, but many have not been validated in cartilage. An early step includes loss of membrane phospholipid asymmetry, which can be detected by annexin V binding to cell-surface phosphotidyl serine, but this method has not been used in cartilage. Intermediate steps, such as early and late capsases[34,47] are used for detection of apoptosis and have been employed in cartilage. The late step of DNA fragmentation is most frequently used and is commonly localized by the detection of the small DNA using an amplification system and TUNEL (terminal deoxynucleotidyl transferase-mediated d-UTP-rich end labeling) assays.

Because of the presence of extracellular matrix (ECM) and the possible presence of bone in the sample, the detection of apoptosis in cartilage has offered some challenges, including the overestimation of the number of apoptotic cells caused by the methods for unmasking. The TUNEL method has been generally applied in cartilage with bone from human[19,23] and rabbit joints,[58] and in vitro young and mature bovine cartilages.[60] Apoptosis is generally assayed with fairly standard fixation, proteolytic unmasking, and detection with commercially available TUNEL kits. Because apoptotic cells in cartilage are not phagocytosed by macrophages, the time frame for the detection post-apoptotic by DNA fragmentation may be longer than in other tissue.

Fixation is usually in neutral buffered formalin (NBF), occasionally with cetylpyridinium chloride.[58] The fixation time should be long enough for good fixation, but not prolonged because this makes unmasking more difficult.[25] If decalcification is needed, disodium EDTA[58] is preferred over formic acid,[25] since prolonged exposure to acid may cause breaks in DNA.

Cartilage sections—especially from larger, older samples—are difficult to keep adhered to slides, particularly during the unmasking step, so activated slides (coated with poly-L-lysine or amino-activated) are frequently used. Before unmasking, pretreatment of the sections with hypertonic salt solution[25] or heating in a microwave has sometimes been found to improve results.[33]

DNA fragments are typically unmasked with proteinase K.[58] This is sometimes followed with further removal of matrix proteoglycans with testicular hyaluronidase.[58] The fragments are then labeled with modified deoxynucleotides, usually biotin or digoxigenin.[25,58] The most popular method for labeling is elongation from the 3' OH of DNA fragments with terminal deoxynucleotidyl transferase. This will detect 5' recessed or blunt-ended fragments. 3' Recessed fragment strand breaks can be detected by ISEL using DNA polymerase Klenow fragments. Both enzymes have been used to evaluate human osteoarthritic cartilage, and both types of cleavages occur in the same cells.[19]

Final amplification in cartilage has been with horseradish peroxidase, hydrogen peroxide and diaminobenzidine[19] or alkaline phosphatase with nitroblue tetrazolium and 5-bromo-4-chloro-3'-indoly phosphate p-toluidine.[25] For the formal detection system, blocking endogenous peroxidase activity is not recommended because it can inhibit terminal deoxynucleotide transferase and cause breaks in DNA.[25] Positive controls can be generated by brief exposure to micrococcal nuclease or DNase I can be used as a positive control.[20] Alternatively, treatment with reagents that induce apoptosis, such as nitric oxide,[37] can be used as a positive biologic control. If sufficient cartilage is available (containing 10^5–10^6 cells), the percent of apoptotic cell numbers can be confirmed by enzymatically releasing the cells (usually sequential trypsin or Pronase and collagenase), staining the cells for DNA and fractionating the cells on a fluorescent-activated cell sorter where apoptotic cells have a low DNA content because of fragmentation.[58] Two caveats are: possible loss of damaged cells during enzymatic digestion and loss of spatial resolution.

REFERENCES

1. Altman RD, Dean DD: Osteoarthritis research. Animal models. *Semin Arthritis Rheum* 19 (Suppl 1):21–25, 1990.
2. Bell R, Bourret L, Bell D, et al: Evaluation of fluorescein diacetate for flow cytometric determination of cell viability in orthopaedic research. *J Orthop Res* 6:467–474, 1988.
3. Bendele A, McComb J, Gould T, et al: Animal models of arthritis: relevance to human disease. *Toxicol Pathol* 27:134–142, 1999.
4. Bendele AM, White SL, Hulman JF: Osteoarthrosis in guinea pigs: histopathologic and scanning electron microscopic features. *Lab Anim Sci* 39:115–121, 1989.
5. Bloebaum RD, Rubman MH, Merrell M, et al: Hyaluronan solution as a cartilage antidesiccant. *J Biomed Mater Res* 26:303–317, 1992.
6. Borthakur A, Shapiro EM, Beers S, et al: Sensitivity of MRI to proteoglycan depletion in cartilage: comparison of sodium and proton MRI. *Osteoarthritis Cartilage* 8:288–293, 2000.
7. Carlson CS, Jerome CP, Dodds RA, et al: Progression of knee joint osteoarthritis with age in guinea pigs. *Osteoarthritis Cartilage* 18(Suppl 13):528, 2000.
8. Carlson CS, Kraus VB, Vail TP, et al: Articular cartilage damage following complete medial meniscectomy in dogs is predicted by synovial fluid biomarker levels. *Trans ORS* 24:194 (abstract), 1999.
9. Carlson CS, Loeser RF, Jayo MJ, et al: Osteoarthritis in cynomolgus macaques: a primate model of naturally occurring disease. *J Orthop Res* 12:331–339, 1994.
10. Carlson CS, Loeser RF, Johnstone B, et al: Osteoarthritis in cynomolgus macaques. II. Detection of modulated proteoglycan epitopes in cartilage and synovial fluid. *J Orthop Res* 13:399–409, 1995.
11. Carlson CS, Loeser RF, Purser CB, et al: Osteoarthritis in cynomolgus macaques. III: Effects of age, gender, and subchondral bone thickness on the severity of disease. *J Bone Miner Res* 11:1209–1217, 1996.
12. Carney SL: Cartilage research, biochemical, histologic, and immunohistochemical markers in cartilage, and animal models of osteoarthritis. *Curr Opin Rheumatol* 3:669–675, 1991.
13. Chubinskaya S, Huch K, Mikecz K, et al: Chondrocyte matrix metalloproteinase-8: Up-regulation of neutrophil collagenase by interleukin-1β in human cartilage from knee and ankle joints. *Lab Invest* 74:232–240, 1996.
14. Chubinskaya S, Kuettner KE, Cole AA: Expression of matrix metalloproteinases in normal and damaged articular cartilage from human knee and ankle joints. *Lab Invest* 79:1669–1677, 1999.
15. Cole AA, Chubinskaya S, Schumacher B, et al: Chondrocyte MMP-8: Human articular chondrocytes express neutrophil collagenase. *J Biol Chem* 271:11,023–11,026, 1996.
16. Collins DH: *The Pathology of Articular and Spinal Diseases.* Edward Arnold and Co., London, 1949:76–79.
17. Cova M, Toffanin R, Szomolanyi P, et al: Short-TE projection reconstruction MR microscopy in the evaluation of articular cartilage thickness. *Eur Radiol* 10:1222–1226, 2000.
18. Czitrom AA, Keating S, Gross AE: The viability of articular cartilage in fresh osteochondral allografts after clinical tranplantation. *J Bone Joint Surg [Am]* 72:574–581, 1990.
19. Fischer BA, Mundle S, Cole AA: Tumor necrosis factor-alpha induced DNA cleavage in human articular chondrocytes may involve multiple endonucleolytic activities during apoptosis. *Microsc Res Tech* 50:236–242, 2000.
20. Gavrieli Y, Sherman Y, Ben-Susson SA: Identification of programmed cell death in situ via specific labeling of nuclear DNA fragmentation. *J Cell Biol* 119:493–501, 1992.
21. Getzy LL, Malemud CJ, Goldberg VM, et al: Factors influencing metachromatic staining in paraffin-embedded sections of rabbit and human articular cartilage: a comparison of the Safranin O and toluidine blue O techniques. *J Histotech* 5:111–116, 1982.

22. Grunder W, Wagner M, Werner A: MR-microscopic visualization of anisotropic internal carti-
    lage structures using the magic angle technique. *Magn Reson Med* 39:376–382, 1998.
23. Hashimoto S, Ochs RL, Komiya S, et al: Linkage of chondrocyte apoptosis and cartilage
    degradation in human osteoarthritis. *Arthritis Rheum* 41:1632–1638, 1998.
24. Horton WE, Feng L, Adams C: Chondrocyte apoptosis in development, aging and disease.
    Matrix Biol 17:107–115, 1998.
25. Horton WE, Tillman SF: Analysis of apoptosis in culture models and intact tissues. *Muscle
    Nerve Suppl* 5:S79–S82, 1997.
26. Huja SS, Hasan MS, Pidaparti R, et al: Development of a fluorescent light technique for
    evaluating microdamage in bone subjected to fatigue loading. *J Biomech* 32:1243–1249,
    1999.
27. Imbert D, Cullander C: Assessment of cornea viability by confocal laser scanning microscopy
    and MTT assay. *Cornea* 16:666–674, 1997.
28. Jeffrey J, Gregory D, Aspden R: Matrix damage and chondrocyte viability following a single
    impact load on articular cartilage. *Arch Biochem Biophys* 322:87–96, 1995.
29. Jerome CP, Carlson CS, Register TC, et al: Bone functional changes in intact, ovariectomized,
    and ovariectomized, hormone-supplemented adult cynomolgus monkeys (Macaca fascicularis)
    evaluated by serum markers and dynamic histomorphometry. *J Bone Miner Res* 9:527–540, 1994.
30. Kerin AJ, Wisnom MR, Adams MA: The compressive strength of articular cartilage. *Proc Inst
    Mech Eng [H]* 212:273–280, 1998.
31. Kiviranta I, Jurvelin J, Tammi M, et al: Microspectrophotometric quantitation of glycosamino-
    glycans in articular cartilage sections stained with Safranin O. *Histochemistry* 82:249–255,
    1985.
32. Koepp H, Eger W, Muehleman C, et al: Prevalence of articular cartilage degeneration in the
    ankle and knee joints of human organ donors. *J Orthop Sci* 4:407–412, 1999.
33. Labat-Moleur F, Guillermet C, Lorimier P, et al: TUNEL apoptotic cell detection in tissue sec-
    tions: Critical evaluation and improvement. *J Histochem Cytochem* 46:327–334, 1998.
34. Lee D, Long SA, Adams JL, et al: Potent and selective nonpeptide inhibitors of caspases 3
    and 7 inhibit apoptosis and maintain cell functionality. *J Biol Chem* 275:16,007–16,014,
    2000.
35. Lindhorst E, Vail TP, Guilak F, et al: Longitudinal characterization of synovial fluid biomarkers
    in the canine meniscectomy model of osteoarthritis. *J Orthop Res* 18:269–280, 2000.
36. Lotz M, Hashimoto S, Kuhn K: Mechanisms of chondrocyte apoptosis. *Osteoarthritis Carti-
    lage* 7:389–391, 1999.
37. Lotz M: The role of nitric oxide in articular cartilage damage. *Rheum Dis Clin North Am*
    25:269–282, 1999.
38. Mankin HJ, Dorfman H, Lippiello L, et al: Biochemical and metabolic abnormalities in articu-
    lar cartilage from osteoarthritis human hips. II. Correlation of morphology with biochemical
    and metabolic data. *J Bone Joint Surg [Am]* 53:523–537, 1971.
39. Mori S, Harruff R, Burr DB: Microcracks in articular calcified cartilage of human femoral
    heads. *Arch Pathol Lab Med* 117:196–198, 1993.
40. Muehleman C, Bareither DJ, Huch K, et al: Prevalence of degenerative morphological changes
    in the joints of the lower extremity. *Osteoarthritis Cartilage* 5:23–37, 1997.
41. Myers SL, Brandt KD, Burr DB, et al: Effects of a bisphosphonate on bone histomorphometry
    and dynamics in the canine cruciate deficiency model of osteoarthritis. *J Rheumatol*
    26:2645–2653, 1999.
42. Oegema TR Jr, Carpenter RJ, Hofmeister F, et al: The interaction of the zone of calcified carti-
    lage and subchondral bone in osteoarthritis. *Microsc Res Tech* 37:324–332, 1997.
43. Oegema TR Jr, Visco D: Animal models of osteoarthritis. In: An YH, Friedman RJ, eds: *Animal
    Models in Orthopaedic Research.* CRC Press, Boca Raton, FL, 1999:349–367.
44. Ostergaard K, Andersen CB, Petersen J, et al: Validity of histopathological grading of articular
    cartilage from osteoarthritic knee joints. *Ann Rheum Dis* 58:208–213, 1999.

45. Ostergaard K, Petersen J, Andersen CB, et al: Histologic/histochemical grading system for osteoarthritic articular cartilage: reproducibility and validity. *Arthritis Rheum* 40:1766–1771, 1997.

46. Otterness IG, Chang M, Burkhardt JE, et al: Histology and tissue chemistry of tidemark separation in hamsters. *Matrix Biol* 18:331–341, 1999.

47. Pelletier JP, Jovanovic DV, Lascau-Coman V, et al: Selective inhibition of inducible nitric oxide synthase reduces progression of experimental osteoarthritis *in vivo:* possible link with the reduction in chondrocyte apoptosis and caspase 3 level. *Arthritis Rheum* 43:1290–1299, 2000.

48. Quinn TM, Gordzinsky AJ, Hunziker EB, et al: Effects of injurious compression on matrix turnover around individual cells in calf articular cartilage explants. *J Orthop Res* 16:490–499, 1998.

49. Repo RU, Finlay JB: Survival of articular cartilage after controlled impact. *J Bone Joint Surg [Am]* 59:1068–1076, 1977.

50. Roach HI: Association of matrix acid and alkaline phosphatases with mineralization of cartilage and endochondral bone. *Histochem J* 31:53–61, 1999.

51. Rosenberg L: Chemical basis for the histological use of Safranin O in the study of articular cartilage. *J Bone Joint Surg [Am]* 53:69–82, 1971.

52. Sandell LJ, Morris N, Robbins JR, et al: Alternatively spliced type II procollagen mRNAs define distinct populations of cells during vertebral development: differential expression of the amino-propeptide. *J Cell Biol* 114:1307–1319, 1991.

53. Shapiro EM, Borthakur A, Dandora R, et al: Sodium visibility and quantitation in intact bovine articular cartilage using high field ^{23}Na MRI and MRS. *J Magn Res* 142:23–31, 2000.

54. Sheehan DC, Hrapchak BB: *Theory and Practice of Histotechnology, 2nd ed.* Battelle Press, Columbus, OH, 1980:94–96.

55. Shepard N, Mitchell N: Simultaneous localization of proteoglycan by light and electron microscopy using toluidine blue O. A study of epiphyseal cartilage. *J Histochem Cytochem* 24:621–629, 1976.

56. Sokal RR, Rohlf FJ: *Biometry, 2nd ed.* W.H. Freeman & Co., New York, NY, 1981:683–687.

57. Sun TC, Mori S, Roper J, et al: Do different fluorochrome labels give equivalent histomorphometric information? *Bone* 13:443–446, 1992.

58. Takahashi K, Hashimoto S, Kubo T, et al: Effect of hyaluronan on chondrocyte apoptosis and nitric oxide production in experimentally induced osteoarthritis. *J Rheumatol* 27:1713–1720, 2000.

59. Tenenbaum J: Experimental models of osteoarthritis: A reappraisal [editorial]. *J Rheumatol* 11:120–122, 1984.

60. Tew SR, Kwan AP, Hann A, et al: The reactions of articular cartilage to experimental wounding: role of apoptosis. *Arthritis Rheum* 43:215–225, 2000.

61. Thompson RC, Vener M, Griffiths H, et al: Scanning electron microscopic and magnetic resonance imaging studies of injuries to the patellofemoral joint after acute transarticular loading. *J Bone Joint Surg [Am]* 75:704–713, 1993.

62. Torzilli PA, Grigiene R, Borrelli Jr., J, et al: Effect of impact load on articular cartilage: cell metabolism and viability, and matrix water content. *J Biomech Eng* 121:433–441, 1999.

63. Wagner M, Werner A, Grunder W: Visualization of collagenase-induced cartilage degradation using NMR microscopy. *Invest Radiol* 34:607–614, 1999.

64. Watson PJ, Carpenter TA, Hall LD, et al: MR protocols for imaging the guinea pig knee. *J Magn Reson Imaging* 15:957–970, 1997.

65. Xia Y: Relaxation anisotrophy in cartilage by NMR microscopy (muM) at 14-micron resolution. *Magn Reson Med* 39:941–949, 1998.

66. Yang H, Acker J, Chen A, McGann L: In situ assessment of cell viability. *Cell Transplant* 7:443–451, 1998.

32

Histological Analysis of Soft-Tissues Biomaterial Interface

Relevance to Dental Implants

Antonio Scarano, Gian Antonio Favero, Elisabetta Fiera, and Adriano Piattelli

Dental School, University of Chieti, Chieti, Italy

I. INTRODUCTION

Histological analysis of soft-tissue specimens containing biomaterials is performed using the same techniques used for bone specimens containing implants. The reason for this is that routine histological microtomes cannot be used to section biomaterials and hard tissues, which have a hard-elastic texture. During histological preparation, this texture can lead to a fracture (gap) between the biomaterial and tissue. For this reason, specimens containing biomaterials and/or implants are embedded in hard plastic resins instead of paraffin. After fixing and embedding the specimen in hard resin, the procedure follows guidelines described in Chapters 18 and 23 for hard-tissue processing.

II. THE SOFT-TISSUE-IMPLANT INTERFACE

One of the factors that appears to influence the success of an implant is its relationship to the soft tissues, as in natural teeth.[1,4,7] These soft tissues separate the bone from the oral cavity, and also act as a barrier between the endosteal portion of the implant and the bacteria present in the mouth. The prognosis for an implant is related not only to the percentage of bone-implant contact, but also to the implant's relationship with the peri-implant soft tissues. Histological studies using both animal or human biopsies have demonstrated that in the vast majority of cases, an inflammatory infiltrate is absent in the soft tissues around osseointegrated implants. Often, a mucosa of normal appearance is present. Moreover, it is believed that the presence of gingivitis or a slight increase in pocket depth are not associated with an accelerated loss of the marginal bone, and do not represent an unfavorable long-term prognosis for the implants.

The mucosal tissue around osseointegrated implants is composed of epithelium and supracrestal fibers.[9] In the free mucosa, there is a sulcular epithelium and a junctional epithelium. The sulcular epithelium is composed of a keratinized, stratified squamous epithelium that covers the peri-implant sulcus as in the natural dentition, and it is continuous with the junctional epithelium. It is probable that the formation of a seal

From: *Handbook of Histology Methods for Bone and Cartilage*
Edited by: Y. H. An and K. L. Martin © Humana Press Inc., Totowa, NJ

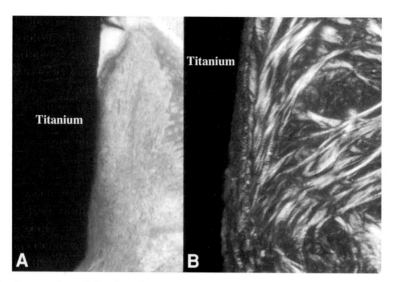

Figure 1. A root-shaped titanium implant was implanted in the mandible of a monkey for the evaluation of peri-implant soft tissues. (A) Peri-implant soft tissues stained with toluidine blue and acid fuchsin. (B) Under polarized light, it is possible to observe connective tissue fibers running parallel to the machined implant surface.

consisting of collagenous tissue prevents the apical proliferation of epithelium. The junctional epithelium consists of a layer of basal cells, three to four cells deep, which is adherent to the titanium surface. The apical limit of the junctional epithelium in healthy mucosa may be found at different levels, and is related to the connection of the abutment to the implant.

Ultrastructural studies have demonstrated that the cells of the junctional epithelium adhere to titanium, using desmosomes similar to those seen in natural teeth.[7] The precise mechanism by which the connection occurs has not yet been fully elucidated, but it seems that glycoproteins within the lamina densa may react with the superficial titanium oxide layer. It is important to remember that hemidesmosomes are often found in contact with biomaterials in cell cultures. In the most superior portion of the junctional epithelium, it is possible to observe many cellular strata, yet in the more apical portion, the epithelium presents completely different characteristics, probably because of plaque accumulation.

In some cases, the peri-implant epithelium is similar to that of a pocket epithelium, showing inflammatory cells in both the epithelial and connective tissue. In other cases, a modest inflammatory-cell infiltrate was found in the sulcular epithelium.

The supracrestal connective tissues around the implants have a width of approx 1–2 mm.[9] The collagen fibers do not insert directly onto the implant surface, but instead run parallel to the implant surface (Fig. 1) in an arrangement similar to the circular fibers of the periodontal ligament. The orientation of these fibers seems to be related to the implant surface—in fact, a porous implant surface seems to be associated with a perpendicular fiber arrangement, and the fibers run in a parallel manner around implants with a smooth surface texture.

III. HISTOLOGICAL ANALYSIS OF IMPLANT BIOCOMPATIBILITY IN SOFT TISSUES

A number of composites made from biopolymeric materials have been studied in an attempt to develop biodegradable artificial-bone substitutes. Materials presently used for bony reconstruction are autografts and allografts, metals, synthetic polymers such as polyurethane (PU) and poly(L-lactic acid) (PLLA), and ceramics such as hydroxyapatite [$Ca_{10}(PO_4)_6(OH)_2$]), carbonate apatite (CAp, [$Ca_{10}(PO_4)_6CO_3$]), or tricalcium phosphate (TCP). These all can cause problems. Commonly used biomaterials may trigger an array of iatrogenic effects, including inflammation, fibrosis, coagulation, and infection. In view of the inert and nontoxic nature of most biomaterials, it is puzzling that tissue-contact implants very often acquire an extensive overlay of phagocytic cells.[6] Only a few hours after implantation, most biomaterial implants trigger some degree of acute inflammatory responses, as reflected by the accumulation of inflammatory cells. The mechanism of such foreign body-mediated inflammatory responses is probably related to the histamine release from mast cells.[2]

Based on earlier observations, the mechanisms involved in these responses can be arbitrarily divided into three consecutive events: phagocyte transmigration through the endothelial barrier, chemotaxis toward the implant, and adherence to the biomaterial.

The biological reaction to these biomaterials is often studied using human biopsies and animal models. Retrieved nonresorbable barrier membranes or other types of biomaterials used in guided tissue or bone regeneration are good materials for biocompatibility evaluation.

Human specimens can be useful in obtaining information that is anectodal, and thus animal experiments are needed to obtain a time-course evaluation of the tissue responses. Most soft-tissue biocompatibility studies are done in rats and rabbits, and the materials to be tested are inserted in the subcutaneous (sc) tissues, in such a way as to avoid the action of the surrounding muscles. For studies in animal models, the size and shape of biomaterial samples is important, and it is possible to use sheets, blocks, and cylinders. After a skin incision, several pouches are created in the sc tissue with blunt dissection; it is important that the biomaterials do not touch each other. The authors use at least three animals and 10 specimens for each biomaterial to evaluate. We make both short-term and long-term observations, as it is important to evaluate both the acute and chronic effects of biomaterials. The specimens used in these studies are usually small, and are more easily infiltrated with methyl methacrylate (MMA) resins than specimens containing bone tissue. Also, the steps leading to the preparation of the slides are more rapid. The technical procedure is similar to that already reported. It is important to evaluate the presence of inflammatory or multinucleated cells, as well as areas of tissue necrosis or tissue alterations.

Commercially pure titanium samples inserted into subgingival tissue are more likely to be surrounded by a dense connective tissue with limited inflammatory cell infiltration (Fig. 2). No significant differences have been observed around implants with varying surface morphologies. In the case of contaminated titanium implants it is possible to observe an inflammatory infiltrate composed mainly of multinucleated giant cells that are in close contact with the surface of the implant.

Test samples made from PLLA are often surrounded by a large number of multinucleated giant cells that contain fragments of the PLLA inside their cytoplasm. The multinucleated cells are present until the material is completely resorbed (Fig. 3).

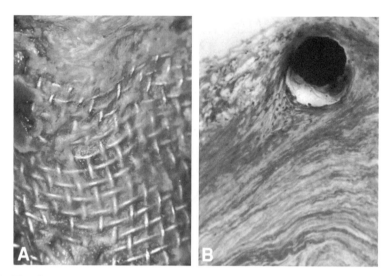

Figure 2. Titanium mesh removed 6 mo after implantation in the mandible of a patient; the titanium mesh was inserted sub-periosteally (A). Dense connective tissue surrounds a titanium wire (B). The titanium mesh was implanted in a man, along with a resorbable membrane to stimulate bone regeneration.

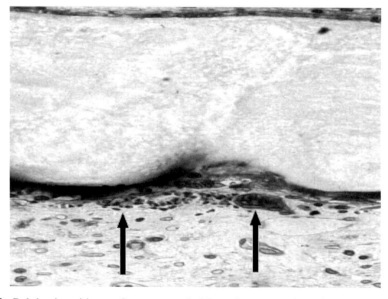

Figure 3. Polylactic acid are often surrounded by a large quantity of multinucleated giant cells (arrows). Toluidine blue and acid fuchsin. Magnification ×400.

In the case of retrieved expanded polytetrafluoroethylene (ePTFE) membranes, no multinucleated or other types of inflammatory cells are present around the nodules that constitute this material. The internal portion of this biomaterial is colonized by mesenchymal cells, fibroblasts, and capillaries (Fig. 4). The cells surrounding ePTFE are

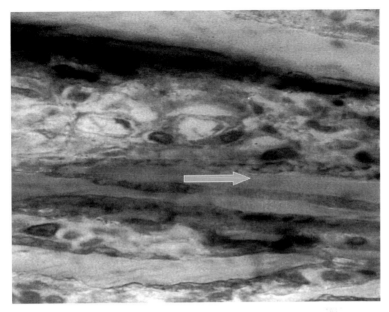

Figure 4. The internal portion of expanded polytetrafluoroethylene (ePTFE) (arrow) is colonized by mesenchymal cells, fibroblasts, and capillaries. Toluidine blue and acid fuchsin. Magnification ×1000.

fibroblasts, forming a five- to six-layer structure, and in this cell structure it is possible to observe a normal cell population.

Teflon is usually surrounded by dense connective tissue, yet in some cases monolayer multinucleated cells can be observed in close contact of the material. The Teflon internal area is never colonized by cells.

When hydroxyapatite is implanted into the soft tissues, it is rapidly resorbed by multinucleated cells. Hydroxyapatite particles, inserted subcutaneously in rabbits, can be resorbed within a period of 8 wk. The resorption process is mediated by mono- or multi-layered multinucleated cells, and in the cytoplasm of the same cells it is possible to observe hydroxyapatite particles. The internal part of these particles is colonized by mesenchymal cells and biological fluid.

IV. CELL CULTURES AND BIOCOMPATIBILITY TESTS

Surface roughness has been shown to affect cell proliferation and differentiation.[2,4] Osteoblasts grown on rougher surfaces (Fig. 5) have been demonstrated to produce a higher quantity of alkaline phosphatase (ALP), prostaglandin E_2, osteocalcin, and transforming growth factor β.[8] Cell cultures can, moreover, be used to evaluate the cytotoxicity of the test material with microscopic examination and the use of quantitative analysis. Cell morphology and characteristics during the adhesion process are evaluated to determine the cytotoxic cellular effects, alterations in the adhesion mechanisms, cell atypia, or cell damage. Also important is the tropism for various types of surfaces.

Chemical and physical characterizations are performed on biomaterials, and qualitative surface analysis of the same samples is obtained using XPS (X-ray Photoelectron Spec-

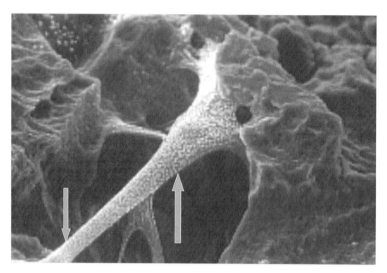

Figure 5. SEM image shows an osteoblast-like cell attachment on a rough implant surface (arrows).

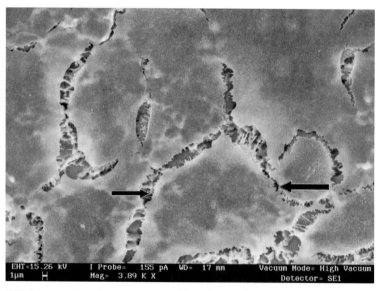

Figure 6. SEM image showing presence of keratinocytes on the titanium surface (arrows). The cells occupy almost the total surface of the implant.

troscopy) or ESCA (Electron Spectroscopy for Chemical Analysis), which can examine an implant surface area of 400 µm in diameter and 5 nm in depth, using a Perkin-Elmer PHI 5500 ESCA System instrument (Perkin-Elmer, Shelton, CT).

Roughness measurements are made of biomaterials surfaces using a Mitutoyo Surftest 211 Profilometer (Mitutoyo Instruments, Tokyo, Japan): an average of three readings is performed for each surface.

Common cell types for in vitro testing of biocompatibility are fibroblasts (such as gingival fibroblasts or V79 cells) and osteoblasts. In this laboratory, MG63 osteoblast-like cells (obtained from the American Type Culture Collection, Rockville, MD), originally isolated from a human osteosarcoma, are commonly used. A culture of 3×10^5 osteoblast-like cells in Modified Eagle's Medium (Biochrom HG, Berlin, Germany), 10% fetal bovine serum (FBS), with added L-glutamine and 1% penicillin and streptomycin is seeded in six-well plates (Corning). Cells are incubated at 37°C, with 5% CO_2 and 98% saturated atmosphere for 24 h. The cells grown on the sample surface can be dislodged using trypsin and the number of cells can be counted. Cells on a biomaterial surface can observed with an inverted microscope if the materials are translucent. Cell morphology can be examined using scanning electron microcopy (SEM) (Figs. 5, 6). The percentage of surface of biomaterials occupied by the cells can be evaluated.

Osteoblast-like cellular responses to different clinical implant surfaces may provide information relevant to the healing of bone in various implant surfaces. Several histomorphometrical studies have demonstrated a higher percentage of bone implant contact for roughened titanium surfaces than for smooth or machined surfaces. In general, osteoblasts have been found to proliferate, and subsequently to express a more differentiated phenotype on rougher surfaces.[10,11]

REFERENCES

1. Albrektsson T, Sennerby L: State of the art in oral implants. *J Clin Periodontol* 18:474–481, 1991.
2. Asako H, Kurose I, Wolf R, et al: Role of H1 receptors and P-selectin in histamine-induced leukocyte rolling and adhesion in postcapillary venules. *J Clin Invest* 93:1508–1515, 1994.
3. Donley TG, Gillette WB: Titanium endosseous implant-soft tissue interface: a literature review. *J Periodontol* 62:153–160, 1991.
4. Fartash B, Arvidson K, Ericsson I: Histology of tissues surrounding single crystal sapphire endosseous dental implants: an experimental study in the beagle dog. *Clin Oral Implants Res* 1:13–21, 1990.
5. Gould TRL, Westbury L, Brunette D: Ultrastructural study of the attachment of human gingiva to titanium in vivo. *J Prosthet Dent* 52:418–420, 1984.
6. Jiranek WA, Machado M, Jasty L, et al: Production of cytokines around loosened cemented acetabular components. Analysis with immunohistochemical techniques and in situ hybridization. *J Bone Joint Surg [Am]* 75:863–879, 1993.
7. Klinge B: Implants in relation to natural teeth. *J Clin Periodontol* 18:482–487, 1991.
8. Lincks J, Boyan BD, Blanchard CR, et al: Response of MG63 osteoblast-like cells to titanium and titanium alloy is dependent on surface roughness and composition. *Biomaterials* 19:2219–2232, 1998.
9. Listgarten MA, Lang NP, Schroeder HE, et al: Periodontal tissues and their counterparts around endosseous implants. *Clin Oral Implants Res* 2:1–19, 1991.
10. Mustafa K, Wennerberg A, Wroblewski J, et al: Determining optimal surface roughness of TiO(2) blasted titanium implant material for attachment, proliferation and differentiation of cells derived from human mandibular alveolar bone. *Clin Oral Implants Res* 12:515–525, 2001.
11. Mustafa K, Wroblewski J, Hultenby K, et al: Effects of titanium surfaces blasted with TiO_2 particles on the initial attachment of cells derived from human mandibular bone. *Clin Oral Implants Res* 11:116–128, 2000.

33

Pathological Diagnosis of Common Tumors of Bone and Cartilage

Jasvir S. Khurana[1] and Krishnan K. Unni[2]

[1]Department of Pathology, Temple Univsersity Hospital, Philadelphia, PA, USA
[2]Mayo Clinic & Mayo Medical Laboratories, Rochester, MN, USA

I. INTRODUCTION

Although primary bone tumors are relatively rare, they are usually concentrated in and referred to specialized centers that deal with them. Because of this, the general surgical pathologist is generally unfamiliar with these entities, and therefore a perceived increase in difficulty in their diagnosis and classification results.

Modern approaches (including advances in surgery, endoprosthetic design and manufacture, anesthesia, chemotherapy, imaging, pathology, and a team approach) have improved the outcome of patients with these tumors, from dismal to a level that allows most patients a low mortality and morbidity. Secondary tumors (metastatic to the skeleton) are far more common in adults, and here too an improved outcome is seen, although not as dramatic as in primary tumors. Tumors of the bone marrow (hematological malignancies such as lymphomas and leukemias) are traditionally treated as separate from primary and secondary bone tumors.

Knowledge of the roentgenographic features of a lesion is very helpful in diagnosing the tumor, especially in certain low-grade cartilaginous tumors, where the histologic appearances by themselves may not be straightforward. Other laboratory techniques (serum studies, immunohistochemistry, and genetic alterations) contribute little to the diagnosis at present. This situation may change in the future as our knowledge about these tumors increases.

II. APPROACH TO HANDLING BONE TUMORS IN THE LABORATORY

Successful therapy for tumors requires an accurate and timely diagnosis. Diagnosis may be made by means of a fine-needle aspiration smear, or more often, by Tru-cut or Craig-type closed needle or by open incisional biopsy. These can be processed by either frozen section or routine processing. Fine-needle aspirations alone may be enough to establish the presence of metastatic disease.

If early diagnosis is required, frozen sections can be performed on most bone tumors, unless they are extremely heavily ossified. The latter situation is rare, since even ossified

From: *Handbook of Histology Methods for Bone and Cartilage*
Edited by: Y. H. An and K. L. Martin © Humana Press Inc., Totowa, NJ

tumors have areas that are soft and can be amenable to frozen sections. As usual, the correlation between the gross and microscopic findings is critical. Rapid diagnosis is especially helpful in benign or low-grade tumors where pre-operative (also called neoadjuvant) chemotherapy is not employed.

In instances in which a delayed diagnosis is decided upon, brief fixation in formalin followed by decalcification (or combined fixation/decalcification) can be performed if needed. Weak acids (formic acid, hydrochloric acid, or nitric acid) or chelaters such as ethylenediaminetetraacetic acid (EDTA) are used, either alone or in commercial mixtures. It is advisable to monitor this process closely to prevent over-decalcification and loss of cellular detail.

On many occasions (for primary malignant bone tumors) biopsy is followed by systemic or combined regional/systemic pre-operative chemotherapy, and then by definitive resection or amputation. At the time of resection, it may be important to evaluate margins and confirm the biopsy diagnosis (mostly possible by frozen sections) and assess the degree of necrosis of the tumor in response to the chemotherapy. The latter is generally done by submitting a 3–5-mm slice of the tumor, taken on a band saw, to fixation, decalcification, and histologic analysis. The slice should include a representation of the entire tumor as much as possible. A percentage of the tumor showing necrosis is reported, and if this value is low, it may result in a change or modification of the postoperative (also known as adjuvant) chemotherapy regimen.

III. GRADING AND STAGING OF BONE TUMORS

Many systems are available for grading bone tumors. We follow the system established by Dr. A. C. Broders, which divides tumors into four grades (Grades 1–4) based on their similarity to the putative cell of origin (differentiation), the cellularity, and the cytological features of the neoplastic cells. We divide cartilaginous tumors into three rather than four grades. Necrosis, although common in high-grade tumors, is not used as a criterion. Only tumors that show variation from one to the other can be graded—for example, Ewing's sarcoma, which shows no variation from one example to the other, need not be graded or can be considered uniformly high-grade.

The musculoskeletal tumor society divides tumors into benign (grade zero) or malignant; and further divides malignant tumors into low- and high-grades (G1 and G2 respectively). This group uses a staging system (also called the Enneking, GTM, or the MSTS system).[28] Non-metastatic malignant, low-grade tumors are considered Stage I, and high-grade tumors are considered Stage II. Tumors that are confined to the bone (or, in the case of soft-tissue tumors if they are confined to a compartment bounded by fascial planes) are referred to as T1 tumors and are Stage A. If they have broken through the bone or compartment, they are considered T2 and Stage B. All tumors with metastatic disease (called M1) are considered MSTS Stage III. Thus, for example, a high-grade osteosarcoma that has broken through the bone but has not metastasized would, in the MSTS system, be G2T2M0 and be given the designation of Stage IIB.

Margins: Orthopedic oncologists in the United States use the term "intra-lesional excision" to refer to procedures such as curretting, in which a complete excision of the tumor may not be done. Wide margins refer to a tumor removed with a cuff of normal tissue around it, and radical margins involve a tumor removed along with the entire bone or

Table 1. Primary Bone Tumors

Cartilage-forming tumors
Osteochondroma
Chondroma
Chondroblastoma
Chondromyxoid fibroma
Chondrosarcoma (and its subtypes)
Mesenchymal chondrosarcoma

Bone-forming tumors
Osteoma
Osteoid osteoma
Osteoblastoma
Osteosarcoma
Parosteal osteosarcoma

Fibrogenic tumors
Desmoplastic fibroma
Fibrosarcoma
Benign and malignant fibrous histocytoma

Myeloma and lymphoma

Ewing's sarcoma

Giant cell tumor (osteoclastoma)

Chordoma

Vaso-formative tumors
Benign vascular tumors
Hemangioendothelioma

Adamantinoma

Neurogenic tumors

Lipogenic tumors

Conditions simulating bone tumors

compartment that it arose in. Europeans use the term "wide" to indicate the latter situation (i.e., equivalent to radical).

IV. CLASSIFICATION

Traditionally, the classification of primary bone tumors has been based on the putative origin or the matrix produced. Thus, classification could include benign or malignant bone-forming, cartilage-forming, vascular, fibrogenic, notochordal, lipogenic, neurogenic, or other tumors. We follow the system listed in Table 1.

V. RADIOLOGY OF BONE TUMORS

Although modern cross-sectional imaging studies (computerized tomography [CT] scans and magnetic resonance imaging [MRI]) have contributed enormously to delineating the extent and staging of tumors, their contribution to diagnosis has been less impressive. For the surgical pathologist, therefore, plain X-rays continue to be an important adjunct to the microscope in the study of bone tumors.

Analysis of the plain film follows a logical course.[53,54] One identifies whether one or multiple bones are involved—if a single bone, whether it is from the axial (skull, vertebral, or craniofacial) or appendicular skeleton, and if appendicular, whether it is proximal (limb girdles, hip, and shoulders) or distal appendicular (hands and feet). Furthermore, the portion of the bone that is principally involved (epiphysis, metaphysis, diaphysis, cortex, medulla, or periosteum) must be determined. It is important to determine if the lesion is well-defined (also called a geographic pattern), or whether it fades off imperceptibly into the surrounding bone (moth-eaten and permeative patterns). It is important to determine whether geographic lesions are surrounded by a sclerotic zone (rind of bone) or whether they are more punched out but without sclerosis. Finally, one should try to evaluate the reaction of the bone to the tumor by the type of periosteal reaction (solid, buttress, and sunburst) and the type of matrix produced by the tumor (chondroid or osteoid) (Table 2).

Certain contributions to the diagnosis are made by additional information gained by cross-sectional imaging. For example, the zonation phenomenon of myositis ossificans and the continuity of the marrow into an osteochondroma are highlighted by CT scans. Fluid (edema or cysts) is dark on T1, and bright on T2-weighted images on MRI scans. Sometimes fluid levels are seen by CT or MRI scans, and can be helpful. Similarly, fibrous tissue (fibromatosis) is dark on both T1- and T2-weighted images. Fat has a low density (about –80 Hounsfield units) by CT scans. Low signal intensity on T2-weighted images in the correct context (peri-articular lesion) may indicate hemosiderin and provide a clue to the diagnosis of pigmented villonodular synovitis. These scanning techniques are also helpful in the pre-operative assessment of response of tumor to therapy. Radionuclide imaging (usually in the form of Technetium scans) has been very useful as a screening method for metastatic bone disease.

VI. CARTILAGE-FORMING TUMORS

A. Osteochondroma

Osteochondromas are relatively common benign outgrowths of the bone that contain bone with bone marrow and capped by a layer of cartilage. The cortices and marrow cavity of the osteochondroma are continuous with the cortex and medulla of the bone, respectively. They usually develop on bones formed from endochondral ossification and are generally present in the metaphyseal region (there is a rare epiphyseal variant that may actually be a separate entity—a form of a physeal dysplasia).

Grossly, there is a stalk that is continous with the bone that the lesion arises on and is capped by a thin layer of cartilage. A thick cap (thicker than 1.5 cm) should raise the possibility of a secondary chondrosarcoma arising upon an osteochondroma. Microscopically, the lesion is bounded by a capsule (continuous with the periosteum of the bone). The stalk contains hematopoietic or fatty marrow. A proliferation of spindle cells within the stalk is never seen in an osteochondroma, and should raise the concern of the lesion being a parosteal osteosarcoma.

There is a hereditary autosomal dominant form of osteochondroma (hereditary multiple osteochondromatosis, diaphyseal aclasis), which is generally associated with remodeling

Table 2. Some Common Associations for Bone Tumors

Epiphyseal lesions
Chondroblastoma
Giant-cell tumor
Clear-cell chondrosarcoma
(Langerhans' cell histiocytosis)

Metaphyseal lesions
Chondromyxoid fibroma
Chondrosarcoma
Fibrosarcoma
Osteomyelitis
Osteochondroma
Osteosarcoma
Malignant fibrous histiocytoma
Non-ossifying fibroma or metaphyseal cortical defect
(Metastatic disease)
(Lymphoma/Myeloma)
(Langerhans cell histiocytosis)
(Paget's disease)
(Unicameral bone cyst)
(Hemangioma)
(Enchondroma)
(Fibrous dysplasia)

Diaphyseal lesions
Adamantinoma
Campanacci's disease or osteofibrous dysplasia
Ewing's tumor
Osteoid osteoma
Osteoblastoma
(Metastatic disease)
(Lymphoma/Myeloma)
(Langerhans cell histiocytosis)
(Paget's disease)
(Hemangioma)
(Fibrous dysplasia)
(Enchondroma)
(Chondrosarcoma)

Note: Although no entity is entirely specific to an area, those in parentheses have a greater tendency to have no particular affinity to a single location.

defects of the metaphysis. Whether osteochondromas are true neoplasms or growth aberrations of the physeal plate is controversial, but the finding of a relatively consistent gene mutation in the lesional tissue (EXT genes) seems to favor the idea that they are true neoplasms.[39]

Osteochondromas grow with the growth of the patient and become quiescent at skeletal maturity. In some cases, regression of the osteochondroma may occur. There is a small risk of secondary tumors (chondrosarcomas) developing upon osteochondromas.

Other bumps of the bone such as bunions, subungual exostosis, tori, bizarre parosteal osteochondromatous proliferations (Nora's lesion), and post-radiation bony nodules,

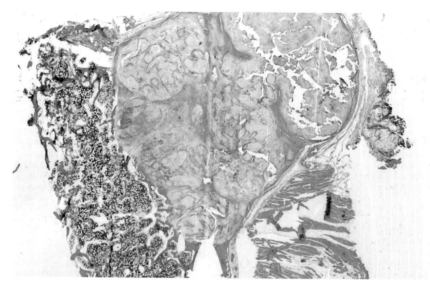

Figure 1. Periosteal chondroma. The lesion is small and superficial, and shows a lobular, hypocellular chondroid neoplasm. The chondroma is sharply circumscribed, and no permeative growth is seen.

should be differentiated from true osteochondromas because they do not have the same genetic defect, familial predisposition, or risk of secondary malignancy.

B. Chondroma

Chondromas are benign, usually asymptomatic tumors of mature hyaline cartilage. When located intra-osseously, they may be called enchondromas. When the location is periosteal, they have been called periosteal chondromas (Fig. 1). When they are large and occupy both these locations, some authors have referred to them as "enchondroma protuberens." Multiple chondromas represent a bone dysplasia, and may affect a few or multiple bones. When this condition occurs in a widespread but unilateral fashion, the term "Ollier's disease" has been used. In some cases, the lesions may be associated with angiomas of the soft tissue in the so-called "Maffucci's syndrome." The association of secondary chondrosarcomas arising on solitary chondromas is exceedingly small, but increases to approx 25% in Ollier's disease. Chondromas are fairly evenly distributed throughout all decades of life, with a slight female predominance. Almost one-half of the chondromas in the Mayo Clinic series occurred in the bones of the hands and feet. It is extremely rare to find chondromas in the flat girdle bones, the sternum, or the base of the skull (where chondrosarcomas or other tumors such as chordomas usually predominate).

Chondromas are usually asymptomatic lesions, and are often discovered incidentally on a skeletal survey (X-rays) or by virtue of being "hot" on a bone scan done for other reasons such as work-up for metastatic carcinoma. Chondromas of the small bones of the hands and feet may be painful because of cortical thinning or fracture, but fracture or painful chondromas of other long or flat bones is most unusual and should raise the suspicion of malignancy.

Grossly, chondromas are circumscribed cartilaginous lesions, which often show lobulations. Microscopically, they are mostly hypocellular, and show no permeation of the cortices or entrapment of trabecular bone. Myxoid change is unusual, and when prominent it should raise the possibility of chondrosarcoma. Chondrocytes may be clustered, or multiple chondrocytes may be present in a lacuna (true binucleation or multinucleation is not generally seen). Chondromas of the hands and feet are somewhat different, and may show some thinning of the overlying cortex. Microscopically, these lesions tend to be more cellular than chondromas of the long tubular bones and may show some myxoid change (mimicking grade 1 chondrosarcomas). Occasional nuclear enlargement or double-nucleation can be seen. In these instances, correlating the radiograms with the morphology can be helpful and if the X-rays are typical of a benign lesion, the overdiagnosis of chondrosarcoma can be avoided. Periosteal chondromas are usually somewhat more cellular, and may show some atypia. In cases of multiple chondromatosis, the lesions tend to be moderately hypercellular and have a tendency to show some spindling. Finally, synovial chondromatosis (sometimes called synovial chondrometaplasia) is composed of multiple lobulated masses of cartilage, which show clustering. They may be attached to the synovium or lie loose in the joint (and must be distinguished from osteocartilaginous loose bodies as a result of trauma or ostechondritis dissecans).

C. Chondroblastoma

Chondroblastoma is a benign cartilaginous neoplasm, showing predilection for the epiphysis of the long tubular bones. Lesions also occur in secondary epiphyses and apophyses such as the greater trochanter of the femur, or the tuburosity of the humerus. The majority of these neoplasms occur in patients under 25 yr of age. Chondroblastomas in unusual locations (such as flat bones or the short tubular bones) may occur in older age groups.

Some chondroblastomas can metastasize, and in these cases, resection of the metastases usually produces positive results.[34,77]

Radiologically, chondroblastomas are well-defined geographic lesions centered in the epiphysis. In about one-third of cases, fine matrix calcifications or trabeculations may be seen. Penetration into the joint is unusual; a secondary aneurysmal bone cyst (ABC) component is sometimes seen.

Grossly, they are circumscribed gray/pink lesions and may be calcified. A secondary ABC component may be seen.

Microscopically, the tumors exhibit a spectrum of histologic appearances. This is because of the inconstant amounts of matrix, secondary changes (ABC–like), and cytological variability. The chondroblast is typically a polygonal epitheloid cell with a sharp cytoplasmic border, lightly staining or clear cytoplasm. The nucleus of the chondroblast is round to oval with a prominent nuclear groove. Mitotic figures may be seen, but are not very common. Atypical mitoses are absent. Some chondroblastomas have cells with abundant pink cytoplasm (referred to as epitheloid variants). In still other examples, either a sprinkling or focal aggregates of spindle cells may be seen. Scattered osteoclast-type giant cells may be seen in many chondroblastomas. Pigmented cells (hemosiderin-laden macrophages as well as pigmented chondroblasts) are sometimes prominent (especially in lesions of the craniofacial skeleton). Calcification, chondroid formation, or ossification may occur. Calcification may be found focally, or more typically surrounding the chondroblast. The latter is especially true in the foci of necrotic chondroblasts. The result is a characteristic "chicken wire" pattern of calcium deposition. This feature is present in some but not all cases of chondroblastoma. The matrix in chondroblastomas is often pink-staining rather than blue. Mature chondrocytes are unusual. In some cases, features that are suggestive of a chondromyxoid fibroma may be seen. Focal cellular atypia or necrosis can be seen in up to 10% of cases. Vascular invasion is rare but is sometimes seen, especially in lesions of the skull bones.

The differential diagnosis includes the related lesion of chondromyxoid fibroma as well as epiphyseal lesions such as giant-cell tumor (GCT) and clear-cell chondrosarcoma. Most chondroblastomas occur in an age group when the epiphyses are open. Chondromyxoid fibromas are usually metaphyseal. GCT and clear-cell chondrosarcomas are typically neoplasms of an older age group. The presence of chondroblasts, chondroid differentiation, and calcific deposits should differentiate chondroblastoma from GCTs. Clear-cell chondrosarcomas are composed of broad sheets of cells with a voluminous clear cytoplasm. Although cells that are indistinguishable from chondroblasts may be found in clear-cell chondrosarcoma, these are a very minor component. Some osteosarcomas can resemble chondroblastomas.[5] These lesions often have a spindle-cell stromal component with significant cellular atypia.

Chondroblastomas are benign lesions that respond to local measures. Recurrences and even metastases can usually be managed by complete excision. In rare cases with multiple metastases, the outcome may be fatal.

D. Chondromyxoid Fibroma

This is a rare, benign lesion with a propensity to the metaphyses of the long bones and the short tubular bones of the hands and feet. Rarely, flat bone and craniofacial involvement is seen.

Radiographically, the lesions are geographic and are often eccentric, with sharp borders and centered about the metaphysis. Slight epiphyseal extension may be seen. Chondromyxoid fibromas of the hands and feet are often central, and cause expansion of the short tubular bones. Those in the flat bones are often irregularly lobulated. Some surface lesions have extensive mineralization.[80]

Grossly, the lesions are small, firm, and semi-translucent, and a minority may resemble cartilage. Microscopically, they are well-circumscribed and lobulated, and the center of the lobule is relatively hypocellular, with the periphery showing relative hypercellularity and some spindling (Fig. 2). Giant cells may be found at the periphery of the lobules. Myxoid foci may be seen but they are generally more uniform and less liquefactive than the myxoid change observed in chondrosarcomas. Secondary changes such as calcification, necrosis, and ABC-type change may occasionally be present.

Chondromyxoid fibromas must be differentiated from the related entity of chondroblastoma, chondrosarcoma, myxoid change occurring in fibrous dysplasia, and rarely, other myxoid tumors.[20,36,43,47,72,83,97] Chondrosarcomas can have a myxoid and lobulated appearance with peripheral hypercellularity, but there is usually evidence of a permeative growth pattern as well as more cytological atypia. Roentgenograms are often very helpful in this distinction. Lobulated growth patterns are not generally found in either fibrous dysplasia or chondroblastoma, and should be helpful in differentiating these two entities.

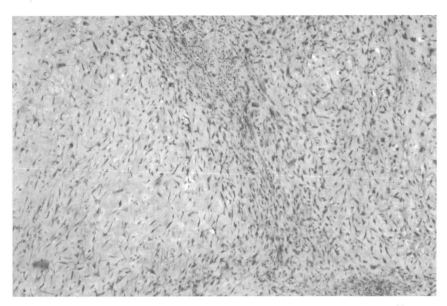

Figure 2. Chondromyxoid fibroma. This high-power microphotograph illustrates the hypocellular center and the hypercellularity at the periphery of a lobule.

Chondromyxoid fibromas are benign lesions, and have an excellent outcome. Curettage is generally curative, but occasionally recurrences and soft-tissue implants have been seen, which are amenable to surgical excision.

E. Chondrosarcoma

Chondrosarcomas are malignant tumors in which there is differentiation of the neoplastic cells to form chondroid but not osteoid.[13,15,22,25,30,52,57,66,98] They comprised about 9% of all malignant bone tumors in the Mayo Clinic series.

The term "conventional chondrosarcoma" is used for the most common variant, composed of hyaline cartilage, with a tendency to involve the larger bones of adult patients. These tumors are referred to as *primary* when they arise in a previously normal bone and *secondary* when they arise in underlying benign, usually cartilaginous neoplasma, such as osteochondromas.[31,38,52,75,87]

Depending on their location within the bone, they can be considered as *central* or intramedullary, and *peripheral* or having an epicenter in the cortex. Peripheral chondrosarcomas must be differentiated from periosteal osteosarcomas. In addition to these, a minority of chondrosarcomas gives rise to highly malignant tumors such as osteos^r mas, malignant fibrous histiocytomas, or fibrosarcomas. Such chondrosarco known as *dedifferentiated*.

Primary chondrosarcomas have a peak incidence in the fifth to seventh de' secondary chondrosarcomas in the fourth and fifth decades.

Chondrosarcomas are often centered around the trunk and proximal limb' of the pelvis as well as the long tubular bones of the proximal appendicula most frequently involved. Involvement of the bones of the hands and feet i<

Compared to osteosarcomas, chondrosarcomas have a slow biologic evolution. Metastases are rare by comparison, and occur late in the course of disease. Recurrent chondrosarcomas have been found to behave with a greater degree of malignancy, and may dedifferentiate.

Radiologically, chondrosarcomas tend to be large lesions. Central chondrosarcomas arise in either the diaphysis or the metaphysis. Epiphyseal origin (and joint involvement) is rare, except in the clear-cell variant of chondrosarcoma. Intramedullary spread is common, and can be extensive. Matrix calcifications are common and may take the form of "C's and O's." The margins of the lesion can vary from irregular geographic to permeated. Areas of increased lucency or inhomogeneity within the lesion should raise the suspicion of dedifferentiation.

Grossly, chondrosarcomas are composed of pearly white or light blue lobules of glistening hyaline cartilage, often with cystic or myxoid areas (Fig. 3A). Foci of hemorrhage and necrosis may be present (such areas as well as firm fleshy areas should be sampled to exclude dedifferentiation). The matrix of chondrosarcomas can vary in consistency from firm hyaline cartilage to a thin mucus resembling watery material.

Microscopically, chondrosarcomas are composed of hyaline cartilage, and may be lobular. Myxoid change leading to secondary liquefaction and cystic change is common (Fig. 3B). Necrotic foci may be present, and can later calcify. A low-power view suggestive of infiltration or entrapment of native bone is one of the most helpful clues in the diagnosis, and can differentiate these from benign chondromas. This entrapped bone can often be seen as islands of bone that may be necrotic. Chondrosarcomas also tend to be more cellular than chondromas. Spindling is not a feature of chondrosarcomas, and when present should suggest the alternative diagnosis of chondroblastic osteosarcoma. Reactive woven bone may be present, but malignant osteoid would require the lesion to be re-classified as an osteosarcoma.

Peripheral/secondary chondrosarcomas may lack an infiltrative quality. When chondrosarcomas supervene on a previous osteochondroma, the thickness of the cartilage cap increases along with wide fibrous septae formation, and the normal columnar arrangement of chondrocyte columns is lost. Nodules of cartilage can sometimes be found lying in the adjacent soft tissues in such instances.

1. Grading of Chondrosarcomas

We classify chondrosarcomas into three grades based upon the cellularity and nuclear atypia. Since mitotic activity is rare in chondrosarcomas, it is not used. Grade 1 chondrosarcomas are relatively hypercellular as compared to enchondromas, and have moderate atypia. Grade 2 chondrosarcomas are more cellular, with more pronounced atypia. Grade 3 chondrosarcomas are extremely rare, and are characterized by extreme cellularity, large bizarre nuclei, and small foci of spindling at the periphery of the lobules. About two-thirds of the lesions seen there corresponded to Grade 1 in one study, about one-third were Grade 2, and Grade 3 represented only a very small fraction.

Low-grade chondrosarcomas can be difficult to differentiate from benign but cellular cartilage lesions such as chondromas. Experience and long follow-up studies have shown that different rules apply in different locations. For example, cartilage tumors of the sternum are almost always malignant, regardless of the histologic appearance. On the other hand, chondromas of the hands and feet, periosteal chondromas, enchondromas of Ollier's

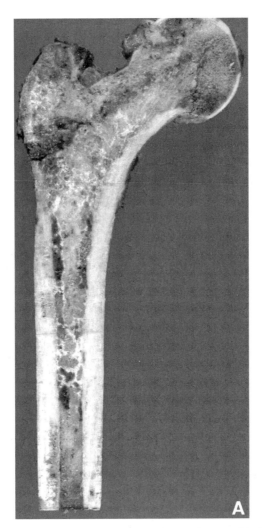

Figure 3. Low-grade chondrosarcoma (gross and photomicrograph). (A) One can identify a residual pin track (from a dynamic hip screw) where the lesion was internally fixed because of a mistaken belief that it was a metastases to the femur. *(Figure continues)*

disease and Maffuci's syndrome, synovial chondromatosis, and soft-tissue chondromas of the hands and feet are usually benign, despite the sometimes alarming cellularity. In making a distinction from benign chondromas, permeation, and the presence of myxoid change is helpful in raising the suspicion of malignancy.

2. Differential Diagnosis

As mentioned previously, the greatest difficulty involves the distinction of benign, atypical cartilage (for example, as seen in enchondromas, chondromyxoid fibromas, osteochondromas, and Nora's lesion) from low-grade chondrosarcomas. Radiological and growth characteristics are extremely important in making this distinction. The histologic clues regarding the aggressiveness of a cartilage lesion include an infiltrative

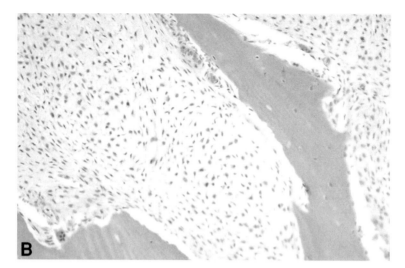

Figure 3. *(Continued)* A biopsy at the time (B) revealed a primary cartilaginous tumor. This led to a resection of the upper femur; limb salvage was possible despite the tumor spillage during the pinning. Sometimes, however, an improperly situated biopsy or the lack of an accurate pre-operative diagnosis may preclude proper planning and execution of a limb-salvage procedure.

margin and entrapment of (necrotic) bone. Infiltration of the Haversian system is particularly important. A periosteal chondroma should be distinguished from a chondrosarcoma. Clues that can help in this distinction include size (periosteal chondromas are most often less than 3 cm, and the reverse is true of chondrosarcomas, which are mostly over 5 cm) and sharp demarcation on X-ray in benign lesions, whereas chondrosarcomas are usually poorly marginated. An osteochondroma should also be distinguished from a secondary chondrosarcoma, and this is best done by paying attention to the thickness of the cartilage cap. A cap wider than 1 cm should raise suspicion, and those over 3 cm are almost always chondrosarcomas. Other features used for differentiation are listed here. A chondroblastic osteosarcoma may enter the differential with chondrosarcomas. Locating typical areas of malignant osteoid formation would be required for this distinction (however, it must be remembered that metaplastic osteoid can sometimes be seen in chondrosarcoma). Another entity that sometimes may be mistaken for chondrosarcoma is tophaceous pseudogout. This is generally distinguishable through the finding of crystals by polarized microscopy and the presence of a granulomatous response. It should be remembered that the tissue-processing for regular histology may dissolve the crystals, making the diagnosis difficult.

3. Management

Wide excision (amputation or resection) is the preferred therapy. Marginal or intra-lesional procedures have a high rate of recurrence, although an extremely thorough curettage with cryotherapy in selected cases have in some cases yielded acceptable results. Chemotherapy has not been effective in chondrosarcomas.

4. Clear-Cell Chondrosarcoma

Clear-cell chondrosarcomas are malignant, slow-growing tumors, composed of neo-plastic chondrocytes with abundant clear cytoplasm, with a sparse intercellular matrix.[14,93] Foci of conventional chondrosarcoma may also be present. These tumors are often mistaken clinically as well as histologically for chondroblastomas and osteoblastomas.

Most patients are in the third or fourth decades, with a slight male predominance. The presentation is usually with pain and joint symptoms. The joint symptoms reflect the preferred localization of these neoplasms to the epiphyseal regions of long tubular bones.

Radiologically, the epiphysis is the epicenter of these tumors, a location shared by the chondroblastoma and giant-cell tumor. They are usually geographic, lytic, expansile, and focally calcified neoplasms. The margins are well-defined, but sclerosis around the edge is rare.

Grossly, the appearance is tan, soft, and granular. Small foci of hyaline cartilage formation may be found, and cystic change is sometimes present.

Microscopically, unlike conventional chondrosarcomas, the clear-cell variant can be quite rich in multinucleated giant cells. This explains why, in the past, this tumor has been referred to as an atypical chondroblastoma. New bone formation may occur centrally within the tumor. The dominant cell is the "clear cell" chondrocyte, with a sharp cell border and a round, vesicular nucleus, with a prominent nucleolus. Powdery cytoplasm may be aggregated near the cell border or the nuclear membrane. There may be cells with a powdery eosinophilic cytoplasm scattered throughout the lesion. Mitotic figures are rare. Matrix is sparse, and may be focally calcified. Foci of conventional (Grade 1) chondrosarcoma may be present, and can be seen in up to one-half the cases (Fig. 4).

A. DIFFERENTIAL DIAGNOSIS

The characteristic location and radiological picture is helpful in making the diagnosis. Histologically, metastatic clear-cell carcinoma may enter the differential diagnosis; however, metastatic deposits are more frequently metaphyseal. Again, identifying areas of gland formation and the positivity of the carcinomas for epithelial markers would aid excluding them. In practice, the lobulated appearance of a clear-cell chondrosarcoma along with areas of bone formation are quite different from the appearance of a renal-cell carcinoma, and the use of immunohistochemistry is generally not required.

B. MANAGEMENT

These neoplasms are usually managed by wide resection. There appear to be no histologic markers for prognosis or predicting lesions that are likely to metastasize. Late metastases have been reported—and can occur up to 15 yr after initial surgery.

5. Dedifferentiated Chondrosarcoma

Dedifferentiated chondrosarcoma is a lesion with a high-grade, non-chondromatous sarcoma (such as osteosarcoma, malignant fibrous histiocytoma (MFH), and rhab-domyosarcoma) associated with, and presumably arising from, a low-grade cartilaginous neoplasm.[2,16,29] The term should not be used to designate high-grade *chondrosarcoma* arising in a benign cartilaginous neoplasm (such neoplasms are known as secondary chondrosarcomas).

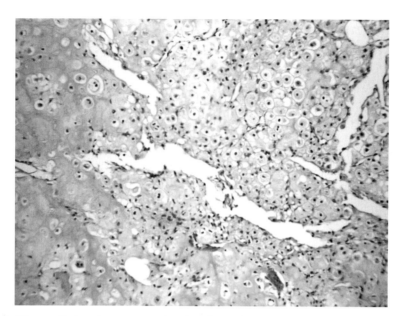

Figure 4. Clear-cell chondrosarcoma showing the typical proliferation of chondrocytes with a clear cytoplasm.

Most patients are over 50 yr of age. Pain and pathologic fractures are the most common presenting features. The skeletal distribution of these lesions parallels the distribution of conventional chondrosarcomas.

Radiographically, dedifferentiated chondrosarcomas are often large lesions with an associated soft-tissue mass. The typical radiographic appearance is that of a bi-morphic lesion, but this is not present in all cases. In the typical (bi-morphic) cases, a lytic mass or a soft-tissue mass is often seen in continuation with or adjacent to a lesion with features of a chondrosarcoma.

Grossly, the lesion reflects the radiological appearance. The two components (low-grade chondrosarcoma and high-grade sarcoma) are usually easily identified, the cartilage appearing translucent and lobular. The cartilage component is mostly centrally located, and may be extremely small and easily overlooked. The high-grade sarcoma is usually tan in color, hemorrhagic, and focally necrotic. The fleshy, anaplastic sarcomatous component often destroys the cartilaginous component. In a few cases, the reverse is true, with the anaplastic component being minor and the majority of the lesion being that of a well-differentiated chondrosarcoma.

Microscopically, the lesion has two components: a chondrosarcoma and a high-grade sarcoma. The chondrosarcoma component is most frequently low-grade (about three-fourths are Grade 1, the remainder Grade 2). The junction between the two components is most often quite sharp (Fig. 5). Fibrosarcoma and MFH are the most frequent supervening sarcomas, but osteosarcoma, rhabdomyosarcoma, and angiosarcoma have also been described. Some lesions may cluster, suggesting a metastatic carcinoma. In this regard, it is important to remember that some lesions can be positive for cytokeratins,

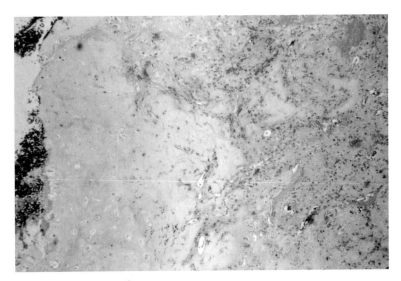

Figure 5. Dedifferentiated chondrosarcoma. The high-grade sarcomatous component on the left is seen immediately juxtaposed with the low-grade hyaline cartilage chondrosarcoma on the right.

thus reinforcing the potential misdiagnosis of metastatic carcinoma. Attention is given to the radiographic appearance, suggesting that chondrosarcoma is extremely helpful in making the correct diagnosis.

A. DIFFERENTIAL DIAGNOSIS

Dedifferentiated chondrosarcoma may be confused with mesenchymal chondrosarcoma and chondroblastic osteosarcoma. Mesenchymal chondrosarcoma is a small-cell neoplasm, with the admixture of low-grade cartilage and a spindle or round-cell neoplasm, the latter frequently arranged in a hemangiopericytomatous pattern. The small-cell component of a mesenchymal chondrosarcoma can easily be distinguished from the sarcomatous component of a dedifferentiated chondrosarcoma. In chondroblastic osteosarcoma, the cartilage component is most frequently of a high grade. Again, the irregular mixing of the various components should be sought in order to arrive at a correct diagnosis.

Fibrosarcoma and MFH may enter the differential, but the absence of a neoplastic cartilage component in these should help to delineate these two entities from a dedifferentiated chondrosarcoma.

B. MANAGEMENT

The management is that of high-grade sarcomas. The prognosis is dismal, and the rapid occurrence of widespread metastases is common. Chemotherapy has been used, and may be advantageous, however, the results of pre-operative chemotherapy have not been very encouraging.

6. Mesenchymal Chondrosarcoma

Mesenchymal chondrosarcomas are malignant cartilage-forming tumors that are primarily composed of small round to oval cells arranged in a hemangiopericytoma-like

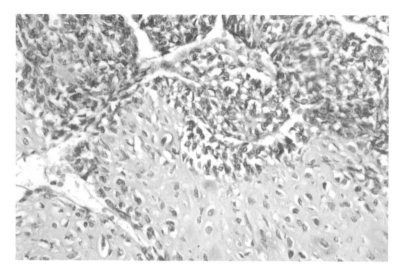

Figure 6. Mesenchymal chondrosarcoma. The two components of the tumor are the hyaline cartilage, and the small-cell proliferation; seen here, they are adjacent to each other.

pattern. Small areas of osteoid may be present. There is an abrupt transition to benign-appearing or low-grade cartilage from these small round-cell areas.[1,10,12,19,33,60,95] The tumors were first described by Lichtenstein and Bernstein in 1959.

The majority of the patients are below the age of 40 yr. The favored sites are maxilla, mandible, ribs, vertebrae, pelvis, and femur. Involvement of other long and short tubular bones, including multicentric lesions, has been reported. About one-third of the lesions occur in the soft tissues.

Radiologically, a lytic defect with small foci of mineralized cartilage is frequently seen. The margins are frequently sharp and very occasionally sclerotic.

Grossly, the sample may appear lobulated. Cartilage is usually not identified grossly. The appearance may be soft, gray or tan, and often is well-demarcated. Microscopically, the tumor is composed of a combination of anaplastic, small stromal cells and islands of benign-appearing chondroid (or sometimes that of a low-grade chondrosarcoma). The stromal cells may vary from "small, round, blue" cells to spindle-shaped cells. The stromal cells are often arranged in a hemangiopericytoma, or less commonly, an alveolar or even a herringbone fashion. Interspersed within these is low-grade cartilage, which may form only a small component of the neoplasm. The cartilage component may sometimes be calcified, or even ossified (Fig. 6).

A. DIFFERENTIAL DIAGNOSIS

Several tumors enter the differential diagnosis. Both mesenchymal chondrosarcoma and Ewing's tumor contain glycogen. In small biopsies, where the cartilage component is not present, this may prove a problem. Small-cell osteosarcoma and other "small blue-cell" tumors enter the differential in the same way. Small-cell osteosarcoma is distinguished by the presence of lacy osteoid and the absence of cartilage. Lymphomas and undifferentiated carcinomas may also enter the differential, but the presence of cartilage is helpful in differentiating these. In some selected cases, with very small biopsies, the use of immunohistochemistry may be helpful. If the roentgenograms demonstrate cartilage matrix within the lesion, then the diagnosis becomes more straightforward.

B. Management

Wide resection (sometimes followed by chemotherapy) has been the mainstay of treatment. The outcome of this tumor is extremely unpredictable, the number of cases studied have been small, and insufficient to give generalizations.

VII. BONE-FORMING TUMORS

A. *Osteoid Osteoma*

An osteoid osteoma is a benign neoplasm consisting of a nidus, which may be surrounded by reactive, sclerotic bone. The nidus is a highly vascular, sharply defined osteoblastic proliferation that is usually less than 1.5 cm.

The majority of osteoid osteomas are found within the first three decades of life. The classic presentation of the patient is with severe, unremitting pain, especially at night, often relieved by aspirin and completely cured by excision of the lesion. Undiagnosed osteoid osteomas may present with scoliosis or joint flexion contractures.

The most classic location is in the diaphyseal cortex of long bones, where it often has sclerotic borders on X-rays; but may it be found in short bones or in a peri-articular location. Osteoid osteomas of the joints can be difficult to detect through plain films.[45] The nidus is radiolucent on X-rays, and may have a small central spot of calcification. The nidus may require tomograms or computerized tomography (CT) scans to demonstrate it well. Since osteoid osteomas are "hot" on Technetium pyrophosphate bone scans, this modality becomes useful in locating osteoid osteomas in difficult cases (such as intra-articularly).

Finding the nidus is important, since this is diagnostic and also confirms that the lesion has been removed. Recurrence may follow (or the symptoms are unrelieved) if the nidus is not completely excised.

Grossly, the nidus is red, spherical, and gritty. It can often be shelled out from the surrounding bone. Microscopically, there is a sharp demarcation of the nidus from the surrounding sclerotic bone. The nidus may be poorly ossified and have a richly vascularized stroma, or, it may have variable amounts of osteoid rimmed with plump osteoblasts (Fig. 7). Cartilage is absent unless there has been a fracture, previous surgery, or if the lesion is intra-articular. Marrow hematopoietic elements and fat are also absent. Scattered lymphocytes and plasma cells may be found, but acute inflammation is absent. Surrounding the nidus is a 0.1–0.2-cm zone of less trabeculated fibrovascular tissue. Outside this, is sclerotic compact or spongy lamellar bone.

The differential diagnosis includes intracortical abscess or osteomyelitis and osteoblastoma and intracortical osteosarcomas. Osteoblastomas may be indistinguishable form osteoid osteomas (thus the size criteria—lesions below 1.5 cm are almost always osteoid osteomas, and those above are almost always osteoblastomas). Some osteoblastomas have a lobulated margin, and trabeculae tend to be more haphazard than in osteoid osteomas. Osteosarcomas are only rarely smaller than 1 cm and almost never completely intracortical. The prominent vascular stroma, the overall organization, circumscription, lack of

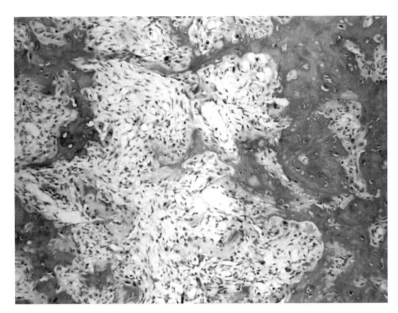

Figure 7. Osteoid osteoma. The nidus is seen here composed of a highly vascularized tissue with woven bone lined by osteoblasts.

atypia, and prominent osteoblastic rimming are all features that should lead away from the diagnosis of osteosarcoma.

Although some authors have suggested that osteoid osteomas may regress spontaneously (after many years), the majority of them are extremely painful, so most osteoid osteomas are managed operatively. Marginal excision is adequate in most cases. The entire nidus should be removed. CT-guided drilling, or microwave ablation are additional methods.[6,17,23,32,41,85]

B. Osteoblastoma

Osteoblastomas are benign or sometimes locally aggressive osseous lesions, with microscopic similarity to the osteoid osteomas, but larger than 1.5 cm.[8,27,42,56,69,91]

The majority of these tumors are seen in patients below the age of 30 yr, with a male predominance. The presentation is with pain, but often less intense than that of osteoid osteoma. There is a predilection for the axial skeleton, with a majority of cases affecting the posterior elements of the spine. Osteoblastomas can be metaphyseal or diaphyseal. Epiphyseal osteoblastomas are less common, except for the short, tubular bones of the hands and feet. Some cases have been associated with a paraneoplastic syndrome.

Radiologically, most lesions are geographic, expansile, lucent lesions and are cortical. About one-third may be intramedullary. There may be a stippled calcification in the matrix of the lesion. Grossly, the lesions show circumscription, and typically measure 2–10 cm (by definition they are over 1.5 cm). A secondary cystic change (ABC) may supervene in some of these tumors.

Microscopically, osteoblastomas are composed of anastamosing bony trabeculae in a fibrovascular stroma and are well-circumscribed, with the edges merging into the adjacent bone. There is no evidence of permeation. The bony trabeculae are variably calcified. Some lesions are heavily mineralized, whereas others may be made of osteoid seams. There is considerable intralesional variation in trabeculum size. Plump, mitotically active osteoblasts line these trabeculae. This rimming is considered an important feature in favor of benignity. Early lesions may be rich in giant cells. Chondroid differentiation may occur, but is unusual in the absence of fracture. Bizarre pleomorphic nuclei (degenerative change) may occur in some cases, but sheets of osteoblasts or sarcomatous stroma is absent. Secondary ABC-like change occurs in about 10% of cases.

A subgroup of "aggressive" osteoblastomas has also been hypothesized. These have been termed malignant osteoblastomas or low-grade osteosarcomas by other authors. These variants contain epithelioid osteoblasts and a tendency to wider and more irregular trabeculae. However, criteria for distinguishing this group are not well-defined and are somewhat subjective.

1. Differential Diagnosis

The differential diagnosis includes osteoid osteomas and osteosarcoma (of the low-grade variety). In limited material, the distinction between osteoblastoma and osteosarcoma can be extremely difficult to make.[4,9,18,74] Features that favor benignity include circumscription, loose arrangement of the tissue with trabeculae that seem embedded in it, and the osteoblastic rimming around the trabeculae. If sheets of osteoblasts are seen, then the diagnosis of osteosarcoma should be considered. The single most important feature, however, is permeation. Permeation, if present, helps make the diagnosis of osteosarcoma over osteoblastoma.

The mainstay of treatment is operative. Wide local resection is preferred. Adjunct treatment modalities such as cryosurgery or methyl methacrylate (MMA) packing may be considered. Lesions not amenable to surgery have occasionally been irradiated. However, this method of treatment is controversial, and the possibility of post-radiation sarcoma should be considered.

C. Osteosarcoma and Its Variants

Osteosarcomas are malignant neoplasms of bone that are composed of proliferating cells that produce osteoid, at least focally. Several subtypes exist, but in the conventional (high-grade, intramedullary) variant, the histologic pattern may be chondroblastic, osteoblastic, fibroblastic, or fibro-histiocytic. Such descriptors of the predominant patterns usually have no prognostic significance.

Other variants include: Small-cell, well-differentiated, intracortical, surface (parosteal and periosteal), multifocal, and pure telangiectatic varieties.

1. Conventional Osteosarcoma

Osteosarcomas may arise *de novo* or develop *secondarily* on other lesions such as irradiated bone, Paget's disease, osteogenesis imperfecta, bone infarct, chronic osteomyelitis, fibrous dysplasia, giant-cell tumor, or osteoblastoma. Traditionally, osteosarcomas that have arisen upon an underlying low-grade chondrosarcoma have been termed dedifferentiated chondrosarcoma. There is also an association with prior radiation therapy, and possibly with metallic or other orthopedic implants. There may be a relationship with trauma, but if so it is poorly documented and understood (it is more likely that the trauma brings to attention a mass in the area).

Some cases of osteosarcoma may be familial. Children with bilateral retinoblastomas have an incidence several hundredfold that of the normal control population. There may be a predisposition to osteosarcoma in genetic conditions such as the Li-Fraumeni, Rothmund-Thomson, and Bloom syndromes.

The majority of patients with conventional osteosarcoma, are below the age of 30 yr (over 85%). The long tubular bones, in the active growth phase (second decade) appear to be most at risk (about three-quarters of all tumors). The metaphyseal region is the site of more than 85% of these tumors, with the diaphysis being the primary site in about 10%. Epiphyseal location is rare.

The secondary osteosarcomas, the involvement of flat bones and diaphyses is much higher. The incidence of osteosarcoma (in fact, of all malignant bone tumors) in the distal appendicular skeleton, such as the hands and feet, is very low.

Pain is the most frequent presenting symptom, with or without swelling. The duration of the symptoms is usually less than 1 yr, most often a period ranging from a few weeks to months. Pathologic fractures may be the presentation in about 5% of cases.

The serum alkaline phosphatase (ALP) may be raised in the more heavily osteoblastic tumors, but is often normal in the lytic examples. A rise in ALP following excision may herald a recurrence.

Radiographic appearances are diagnostic in about two-thirds of osteosarcomas. The classic radiograph is that of an intramedullary, lytic, and sclerotic lesion, which demonstrates cortical breakthrough and is associated with matrix bone formation (Fig. 8A). Some lesions may be purely lytic or purely sclerotic. The margins vary from well-defined (but not sclerotic) to permeative. The periosteum is often lifted to form a Codman's triangle, or alternatively, may show other patterns associated with rapid growth such as a sunburst. Rare cases can be deceptively bland on X-rays. Telangiectatic osteosarcomas, may simulate ABCs on radiological studies. Skip lesions are rarely found, but are important potential causes of recurrent disease.

The gross appearance of the tumor depends on the predominant differentiation, and is frequently variegated—areas of lobular cartilaginous growth and gritty bone may be found within the same mass. Foci of hemorrhage and necrosis are common. Large, blood-filled areas may represent a telangiectatic component. The periosteal reaction is frequently visible as spicules or lamellae of bone. Epiphyseal penetration is rare, especially at the gross level, but occasionally joint extension may occur along the intra-articular ligaments (ligamentum teres in the femoral head, or the cruciate ligaments in the knee) (Fig. 8B). Because pre-operative chemotherapy is often utilized, it is rare to see osteosarcomas today in their native viable form.

Microscopically, osteosarcomas are usually high-grade, anaplastic tumors, and frequently show unequivocal osteoid production (Fig. 8C). Osteoblastic, chondroblastic, and fibroblastic differentiation is commonly admixed. Sometimes the amount of osteoid production can be minimal or absent in otherwise typical osteosarcomas (such lesions produce heavily ossified metastases, although the primary tumor has little or no bone production).

Osteosarcomas of the jawbones (gnathic osteosarcomas) are frequently chondroblastic, and are reputed to have a somewhat better outcome. The average age of such patients is usually higher than seen in conventional osteosarcomas. The tumors usually have less

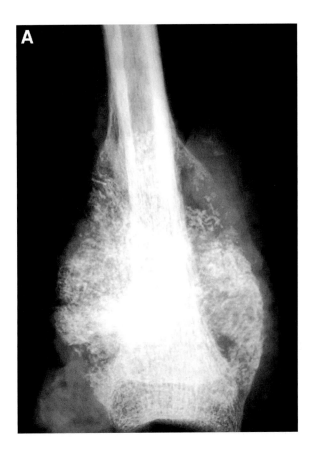

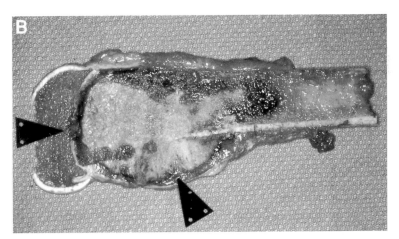

Figure 8. Osteosarcoma. (A) shows the roentgenographic appearance of a typical conventional osteosarcoma. The tumor has abundant mineralized osseous matrix, and breaks through the cortices to lift up the periosteum in the form of "Codman's triangles." (B) shows the resection specimen from a case showing extensive cortical breakthrough (lower arrow) and only minimal invasion of the physeal plate (arrow at left), which forms a relative barrier to epiphyseal extension of the tumor. *(Figure continues)*

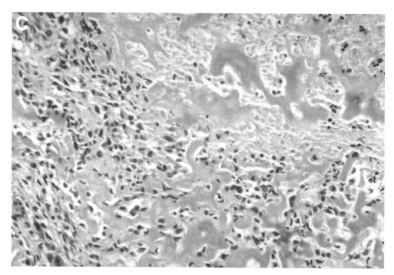

Figure 8. *(Continued)* (C) shows the microscopic appearance of a typical high-grade osteosarcoma.

anaplasia, and are often diagnosed as a lower grade. Cartilage differentiation in the jaw should always be viewed with suspicion, since many such lesions represent a chondroblastic osteosarcoma. The better outcome of jaw osteosarcomas does not extend to skull osteosarcomas, because the latter are highly malignant tumors.[7,21,63,82,89,90]

The neoplastic cells of the osteosarcoma are spindled or oval. They often have marked nuclear pleomorphism, a high mitotic rate, and atypical mitotic forms. These cells are easier to identify in the areas away from the bone trabeculae or osteoid formation. Occasional osteosarcomas, however, are cytologically bland. This makes small, fragmented biopsies treacherous to interpret, and the clinical context must be considered. A well-recognized phenomenon known as normalization is seen in most osteosarcomas. This refers to the tendency of the osteoblasts to become smaller and less pleomorphic as they are incorporated into the osteoid. Another feature that may be helpful is the presence of osteoid lacking an osteoblastic rimming. This can be helpful in differentiating neoplastic from reactive osteoid or woven bone.

Osteoid may have variable thickness and degrees of mineralization. A thin, highly mineralized pattern (the filigreed pattern) is highly suggestive of neoplastic osteoid if found. Other tumors can be very heavily ossified. Some osteosarcomas can resemble osteoblastomas. Although the chondroblastic, fibroblastic, and malignant fibrous histiocytoma-like (MFH-like) osteosarcomas are familiar to most pathologists, one histologic subtype is particularly troublesome. This is the giant-cell type, characterized by a proliferation of bland giant cells amidst a sarcomatous stroma. Osteoid production is usually sparse. If attention is not given to the stromal anaplasia, an incorrect interpretation of this lesion as a giant-cell tumor will result. Usually, but not always, these tumors are metaphyseal (like conventional osteosarcomas) rather than epiphyseal (like other giant-cell tumors), and this location gives a clue to their true nature. Unfortunately, there are examples where this is not the case, and some tumors have all the X-ray features of giant-cell tumors.

Osteosarcomas that resemble chondroblastomas are rarely seen. Such tumors can be correctly diagnosed if attention is given to the permeative nature. Sheets of osteosarcoma cells should provide a clue to malignancy, since chondroblastomas have a loose arrangement of cells. Frequently, however, the diagnosis is only made with the benefit of hindsight, when a tumor diagnosed as a chondroblastoma recurs or metastasizes and the metastasis has the more typical appearance of an osteosarcoma.

Some osteosarcomas are composed of epitheloid-looking cells. A rosette formation may give the appearance of gland formation, and immunohistochemical markers may be positive for epithelial differentiation. Such osteosarcomas can be also seen as part of the sarcomatous component of a dedifferentiated chondrosarcoma.

It is important to recognize and quantitate chemonecrosis of the tumor (following neoadjuvant therapy). The appearance of the tumor after chemotherapy depends upon its original morphology. Chondroblastic foci have the appearance of acellular chondroid, often with ghost cells in the lacunae. Telangiectatic foci appear as acellular blood-filled cysts. Osteoblastic foci appear as acellular osteoid matrix. Atypical stromal cells may be scattered in all these foci, and the biologic significance of these cells is unclear (Fig. 9).

A. DIFFERENTIAL DIAGNOSIS

Osteoblastomas:[4,5,9,18,20,24,89,90] About 10% of osteosarcomas may appear radiologically benign, and conversely about one-quarter of osteoblastomas may be worrisome on roentgenograms. The most important histological feature differentiating the two is permeation. Additionally, osteoblastomas are composed of trabeculae and intervening stroma, and the two components are frequently of equal width, yet osteosarcomas tend to be more haphazard and irregular in arrangement. Osteoblastic rimming is characteristic of osteoblastomas, whereas extensive pleomorphism and atypical mitotic figures are features that warrant the diagnosis of osteosarcoma. Another entity to differentiate is fracture callus—callus can be extremely hypercellular, from compact masses of osteoid, and contain a mitotically active stroma. The finding of zonation (a pattern of peripheral ossification with a fibrous or less ossified center) or osteoblastic rimming can be helpful in recognizing callus. Cartilage can be present in both entities, but atypical or frankly malignant cartilage is not seen in fractures.

Giant-Cell Tumor: Clues to the sarcomatous nature of tumors containing osteoclastic giant cells come from the radiograms. Evidence of destruction, infiltration, and the lack of an epicenter in the epiphysis should make the observer reconsider a diagnosis of giant-cell tumor. Histologically, the presence of a sarcomatous stroma and osteoid is diagnostic, and the reactive osteoclasts should be ignored. Another entity that should be kept in mind is an osteogenic melanoma (malignant melanoma-forming bone).[55] A search for junctional activity will be helpful in establishing this diagnosis.

B. MANAGEMENT

Wide resection along with neoadjuvant and adjuvant chemotherapy is utilized. The current survival of osteosarcoma is approaching 70–80% survival at 10 yr. Necrosis following neoadjuvant chemotherapy may be used both as a prognostic marker and to tailor the postoperative chemotherapy regime.

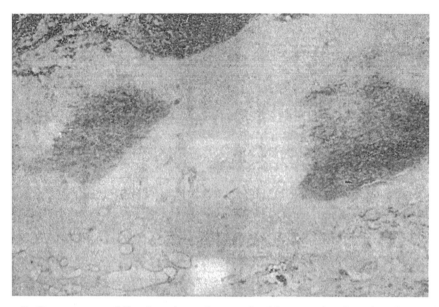

Figure 9. Osteosarcoma following chemotherapy. In this example, there is a hypocellular matrix with blood-filled spaces.

2. Multifocal Osteosarcoma

This is a small but distinct subgroup of osteosarcomas, which has traditionally been divided into the synchronous and the metachronous types. Synchronous lesions appear to arise (or are discovered) more or less simultaneously (or at least within 6 mo of each other). It is unclear whether multifocal osteosarcomas represent multiple primary sarcomas or whether they are metastatic deposits of single primary tumor. Morphologically, the individual lesions of multifocal osteosarcoma resemble the conventional osteosarcoma.

3. Telangiectatic Osteosarcoma

The terms refers to an osteosarcoma that is entirely (or very largely) composed of blood-filled spaces. The criteria for this entity have been very varied, and some authors have been extremely liberal with the diagnosis of this variant. The incidence is therefore difficult to estimate, but is probably less than 10%. Patients with the telangiectatic variant are more likely to present with a pathologic fracture than those with a conventional osteosarcoma (around 25%). The age and location of the tumors are similar to the conventional variant.

Radiologically, these tumors are purely lytic. They present features of rapid growth, such as permeative margins, cortical destruction, and soft-tissue extension. Any sclerosis on the X-ray should preclude the diagnosis of telangiectatic osteosarcoma.

Grossly, the tumor may appear as a blood clot, be a hemorrhagic-necrotic mass, or be multicystic with blood-filled spaces or ABC-like, resembling a blood-filled sponge.

Microscopically, the tumor may be hemorrhagic and necrotic, and the low-power view may be that of an ABC. The malignant cells are present in septae, in a background of blood and necrotic tissue. However, it may require careful observation at high power to appreciate the malignant cells within the cyst wall. Delicate osteoid is often appreciable, at least focally within the malignant cells. Benign giant cells are often present.

A. MANAGEMENT

The treatment is similar to that of conventional osteosarcoma. The biologic behavior and spread of this variant appear to be similar—according to presently available date—to a conventional osteosarcoma.

4. Small-Cell Osteosarcoma

A microscopically distinct variant of a high-grade intramedullary osteosarcoma consisting of small, round cells but showing at least focal osteoid production.[59,84]

The relationship with Ewing's sarcoma is unclear, although some studies have suggested that they share the t(11;22) chromosomal translocation.[62,81] Although approx 70% of the patients are in the first two decades of life, cases have been reported up to the age of 80. The presentation and sites of the lesions are similar to those of the conventional osteosarcoma.

Radiologically, the lesions show permeative margins with cortical destruction. Extraosseous extension is common. Most exhibit focal bone-forming matrix on X-ray and sometimes this can be extensive.

Grossly, the lesions cannot be differentiated from the conventional variant. Microscopically, the tumor resembles Ewing's sarcoma, but unequivocal osteoid must be found for the diagnosis.

5. Intra-osseous Well-Differentiated Osteosarcoma

Intra-osseous well-differentiated osteosarcoma is a term given to an intramedullary variant composed of low-grade, fibrous, and osseous tissue with only minimal cytological atypia.[49,65,67,68,76,89] Patients with this subtype usually do better than those with conventional osteosarcomas. Chemotherapy does not seem to materially alter the outcome.

There is a tendency to a slightly older age and slightly longer symptomology as compared to the conventional osteosarcoma. However, the sites of involvement and other clinical features are similar.

Radiographically, the lesions are intramedullary and some may be eccentrically situated. The margins may be well-defined, although they usually are not sclerotic. A mineralized matrix is present in the majority of cases.

Grossly, the tumors are often well-demarcated and gritty or whorled, resembling the gross appearance of desmoid tumor. Cortical breakthrough and soft-tissue extension may be seen.

Microscopically, fibrous tissue and osteoid form the bulk of the tumor. Cartilage differentiation is infrequent. A pattern of infiltration into the pre-existing lamellar bone or fatty marrow is diagnostic. There is only slight atypia, and the mitotic rate is low. The osteoid component is often mineralized and may appear mature (lamellar). About one-third have a fibroblastic stroma that resembles a desmoid or desmoplastic fibroma. Rarely, a fibrous dysplasia like pattern of "Chinese alphabet"-like bone may be seen embedded in a fibrous stroma. The most important histologic finding is that of a permeative growth pattern.

6. Periosteal Osteosarcoma

This subtype of surface osteosarcoma is characterized by a predilection for the diaphysis of long bones and for prominent chondroblastic differentiation. Some of these lesions have been mistakenly called juxtacortical chondrosarcoma. The age range and clinical presentation are similar to those of conventional osteosarcoma.

Radiographically, the tumors are located on the external surface of the cortex, and extend into the surrounding soft tissues. The lesions are predominantly lucent, and mineralization may be present at the base of the tumor with a characteristic radiating pattern, oriented perpendicular to the cortex. Intramedullary extension is absent or minimal.

Grossly, the tumors are sharply demarcated, lobulated, and cartilaginous. Microscopically, there is osteoid formation, at least focally. Typically cartilage lobules show central ossification and peripheral hypercellularity with some spindling.

7. High-Grade Surface Osteosarcoma

This is a rare variant of an osteosarcoma, that arises from the outer cortex of the bone and has a microscopic appearance similar to that of the conventional high-grade osteosarcoma. Intramedullary extension is absent or minimal. The lesions are often diaphyseal, and the presentation and location are otherwise similar to the high-grade. conventional intramedullary osteosarcoma.

8. Parosteal Osteosarcoma

A parosteal osteosarcoma is a well-differentiated low-grade (usually Grade 1), fibroosseous variant of surface osteosarcoma. This is considered to be a special variant of osteosarcoma, since the prognosis is much better than for conventional osteosarcoma.

The presentation is often a painless mass, usually situated in the posterior lower femur, the site of over two-thirds of these tumors. Other common sites include the tibia and humerus. The patients are usually symptomatic for longer periods than the conventional osteosarcoma. Most studies have shown a tendency to involve slightly older age groups as compared to the conventional osteosarcoma.

Radiographically, these lesions are characterized by a dense mass of bone attached to the outer metaphyseal cortex by a broad base. There is dense mineralization, which is often less prominent peripherally. On plain films, a lucent line between the mass and the bone can be seen, which indicates the tendency of the lesion to wrap around the bone. CT scanning can also demonstrate this feature. Intralesional lucencies are rare, and should raise the possibility of de-differentiation within the tumor.

Grossly, a large ossified exophytic mass with a broad base or, less often, demonstrating encirclement is identified. It may resemble an osteochondroma, including the presence of a cartilaginous cap. The lesions are heavily ossified, and may be lobulated. Less ossified areas may represent cartilage, fibrous tissue, fat, or dedifferentiation. Areas of intramedullary spread should be documented.

On microscopy, parosteal osteosarcomas show long, narrow trabeculae, or poorly defined areas of osteoid and woven bone separated by a fibrous stroma. The trabeculae may show maturation (normalization), which may result lamellar bone. The spaces between the trabeculae are often filled with spindled fibroblastic tissue that shows only minimal cytological atypia. Most lesions are Grade 1 osteosarcomas.

About one-half of the lesions in some series have shown the presence of cartilage. In about one-third, this was present peripherally, simulating the cap of an osteochondroma. In others, it was admixed with the tumor. The islands of cartilage, or the cartilage cap, are low-grade. High-grade areas resembling conventional osteosarcomas should be interpreted as evidence of dedifferentiation.

A. Differential Diagnosis

The lesions should be differentiated from high-grade surface osteosarcomas, osteo-chondromas, and reactive conditions such as myositis/Nora's lesion. Microscopically, osteochondromas lack an atypical fibrous stroma/osteoid and are composed of bone marrow and bone. Bone marrow is usually (but not always) absent in parosteal osteosarcomas. Myositis ossificans and reactive periostitis show zonation and lack a sarcomatous stroma.

B. Management

The tumor is generally managed with wide local excision without adjuvant chemotherapy.

VIII. FIBROGENIC AND FIBRO-HISTIOCYTIC TUMORS

A. Desmoplastic Fibroma

This type of lesion is intraosseous, non-metastasizing, but locally aggressive, and is composed of cytologically bland fibroblasts in an abundantly collagenized stroma resembling a soft-tissue desmoid.

Patients age from 1–70 yr, but most occur by the of 40 yr. Presentation includes swelling, pain, or fracture, and the patients have often been symptomatic for 2–3 yr.

The lesions are most frequent in the metaphysis of the long bones. The mandible, pelvis, ribs, vertebrae, or the small tubular bones of the hands and feet are less frequently involved. Radiographically, the lesions are lucent, and may expand the bone. The lesions frequently have coarse trabeculations that course the lytic areas (Fig. 10A). A periosteal reaction is usually absent. The margins are usually sharp, but may occasionally be more aggressive. CT scans usually demonstrate a soft-tissue shadow.

Grossly, the tumor is gray/fibrous and may be whorled, as in the soft-tissue desmoid.

Microscopically, the tumors are hypocellular. They demonstrate a proliferation of spindle cells separated by abundant collagen. Entrapped bone may be present. Soft-tissue extension is often seen. Nucleoli and mitotic figures are inconspicuous or absent. There are small thin-walled vessels, similar to the soft-tissue desmoid (Fig. 10B).

1. Management

Wide excision is the preferred treatment. Radiation and chemotherapy are not indicated.

B. Fibrosarcoma

This malignant spindle-cell lesion exclusively exhibits fibrous differentiation. Osteoid and chondroid matrices are absent.

The skeletal-site distribution is similar to osteosarcoma, but the age is more evenly distributed from the second to the seventh decades.

Presentation usually occurs with pain and swelling. About 25% of lesions in the Mayo Clinic files arose from pre-existing osseous lesions such as giant-cell tumors, Paget's disease, fibrous dysplasia, bone infarct, and radiation.

Radiologically, the lesions usually show aggressive, permeative margins.

Grossly, most tumors are gray, firm lesions, although some tumors may be more soft and fleshy. The tumors have infiltrative margins. Areas of hemorrhage or necrosis may be present in high-grade tumors. Microscopically, some tumors are paucicellular and collagenized, merging toward desmoplastic fibromas. Others are more cellular, with mitotically

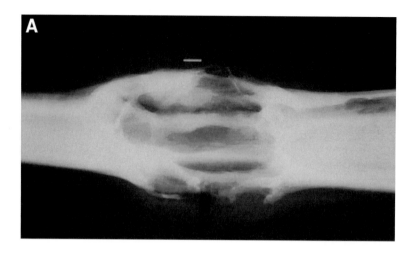

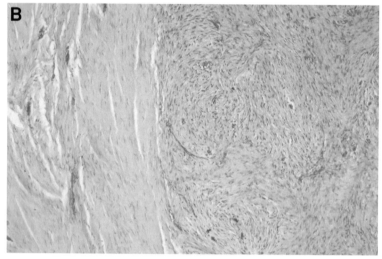

Figure 10. Desmoplastic fibroma. (A) shows the roentgenographic appearances with bony expansion and coarse trabeculations. (B) is the corresponding photomicrograph showing a lesion similar to the soft-tissue desmoid counterpart.

active spindle cells with considerable cytological atypia. The spindle cells are arranged in a "herringbone" fashion of interlacing fascicles. Some tumors may be myxoid. Most tumors show evidence of cortical breakthrough. Grading of the tumors is based upon the atypia and proliferative activity.

C. Benign Fibro-Histiocytic Tumors

These are very rare benign tumors with the microscopic appearance of a spindle-cell lesion in a storiform arrangement, giant cells, and foam cells (resembling a metaphyseal fibrous defect) that affect bones such as the pelvis and spine. They do not radiographically show features of a metaphyseal fibrous defect, and thus are separable.

D. Malignant Fibrous Histiocytoma

This entity (analogous to its soft-tissue counterpart) is a high-grade sarcoma with features merging between fibrosarcoma and fibroblastic osteosarcoma. Foam cells and benign giant cells may be found, and there may be a storiform arrangement. Chondroid and osteoid matrix is absent by definition. These tumors present in any age group as a lytic lesion, often in the appendicular skeleton, and may develop secondarily on other bone lesions (such as infarct) or in the setting of radiation. The most important differentials include malignant lymphoma and metastatic sarcomatoid carcinoma.

IX. MYELOMA AND LYMPHOMA

These are tumors of the hematopoietic system, and specialized texts on these topics cover these entities more thoroughly. This section discusses the surgical pathology of their presentation as bone lesions.

A. Myeloma

Although these are relatively common bone lesions (about 40% of all bone tumors were myeloma in the Mayo Clinic series), their presentation limited to bone (solitary plasmacytoma) is far less common. Patients are mostly older than 40 yr (however, the youngest patient in the Mayo Clinic series was 16 yr of age). There is clearly a male predisposition. Bone pain, pathologic fractures, vertebral compression, lytic bone lesions, anemia, and electrophoretic abnormalities of the serum and/or urine are among the usual clinical presentations. Bone lesions include punched-out lysis, diffuse osteopenia, and rarely, sclerotic lesions. In the so-called POEMS syndrome, there is *p*olyneuropathy, *o*rganomegaly, *e*ndocrinopathy, *M*-protein, and *s*kin changes, and the bone lesions are typically sclerotic. Solitary plasmacytomas are usually, seen in somewhat younger patients, and more often in the spine.

Grossly, the material often resembles "red currant jelly," but may resemble the fish-flesh more typically associated with lymphomas. Microscopically, the lesions vary from those resembling normal plasma cells to more anaplastic variants. They often have an eccentric nucleus with clumped chromatin, and may exhibit multinucleation. Often, there is a prominent sinusoidal vascular pattern similar to neuroendocrine neoplasms. About 10–15% of cases have some amyloid deposition, which could be associated with a giant-cell reaction and they are occasionally massive.

B. Lymphoma

Malignant lymphoma accounted for 7% of all malignant bone neoplasms in the Mayo Clinic series. The disease has a wide age range, with a slight male predominance. Roentgenograms show extensive bone involvement with a destructive permeative process, (or a combination of lysis and sclerosis). However, in some cases the findings on plain films may be subtle or even absent. In cases in which the plain X-rays show minimal or no changes, the other scanning studies (especially MRI or bone scan) may be obvious.

The gross appearances are usually described as "fish-flesh," but may show extensive bony sclerosis. Microscopically, the tumor is composed of small or slightly larger round cells (often a mixture), and shows permeation with or without some amount of trabecular bone thickening. Some extensively fibrotic lymphomas may show some spindling of the cells. The differential diagnosis includes chronic osteomyelitis, granulocytic sarcoma, and carcinoma. Lymphoma lacks the granulation-tissue appearance of osteomyelitis. Granulocytic sarcoma can sometimes be a difficult problem, but in most cases some differentiation along the myeloid lines can be identified. A judicious use of immunohistochemical stains can be helpful in distinguishing these entities in selected cases. Outcome is dependent upon stage and whether the lesion develops secondary to an underlying lymphoma of the solid organs or lymph nodes. Primary bone lymphomas usually do better than those that develop secondarily.

X. EWING'S SARCOMA

Ewing's sarcoma accounted for about 6% of all bone tumors in the Mayo Clinic series. It is a primary osseous neoplasm composed of small round cells with no matrix production. It bears a close relationship and may be identical to the peripheral neuro-ectodermal tumor (PNET).

Chromosomal translocations characteristic of Ewing's sarcoma have been recently identified. One of these is the t(11;22) chromosomal translocation, which is seen in the majority of cases. This abnormality has been seen in PNETs, thus strengthening the belief that all these tumors are either identical or at the very least related. The sensitivity/specificity of the translocation and whether this translocation also occurs in entities such as small-cell osteosarcomas, or mesenchymal chondrosarcomas is not yet known.[26,48,51,58,59,64,70,88,94]

By molecular methods, this chromosomal abnormality corresponds to the EWS/FL1 gene fusion. The EWS gene (located on chromosome 22 at q12) is translocated to the FL1 (a gene of the ETS family located on chromosome 11). This results in the formation of a chimerical protein product, and is seen in about 85% of patients. A second translocation that has been identified in about 15% of patients, is the t(21;22) translocation, which fuses the EWS gene with a different member of the ETS family, the ERG gene located on chromosome 21 at q22. This yields a hybrid EWS/ERG product. Whether these two types of Ewing's sarcoma (at the molecular level) behave differently clinically is unknown. These two types cannot be distinguished at the light microscopic level. Diagnostically, this is a convenient method to confirm or establish the diagnosis of Ewing's tumor in selected cases.

Ewing's sarcoma usually afflict patients at young ages. The majority of patients are in the first two decades of life. In children below 5 yr of age, metastatic neuroblastoma should be excluded. Localized pain and a mass are the most common presenting symptoms. There may be fever, leukocytosis, and a raised sedimentation rate. These bring up the clinical differential of acute osteomyelitis, an entity that can mimic Ewing's tumor both clinically and radiologically. Up to 10% of patients may have skeletal metastases at the time of presentation.

The tumor involves the long tubular bones such as the femur, as well as some flat bones such as the pelvis and ribs, in greater frequencies than the short tubular bones of the hands and feet or sites such as the skull, vertebrae, or sternum—yet any bone may be affected. Although diaphyseal location is more common, tumors may also occur in the metaphysis. Epiphyseal location is rare.

Radiologically, the lesions are poorly defined and are lytic, with permeative margins. A periosteal reaction, if present, may affect the onionskin, sunburst, or other rapidly growing type. A soft-tissue component is often present, and is easily detected by CT or MR

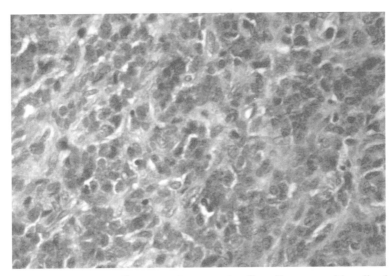

Figure 11. Ewing's sarcoma. The tumor is a round-cell malignancy with cells showing no matrix formation.

scans. The extent of involvement by MR is frequently far greater than that demonstrated by plain X-rays.

Grossly, the tumor may be firm or glistening, or more friable, mimicking pus. Hemorrhage and cystic change may be evident.

Microscopically, the classic form is very cellular, and consists of sheets and large nests of uniform, small, round to polygonal cells with scanty cytoplasm (Fig. 11). The chromatin is finely dispersed, usually with no nucleoli and a variable number of mitotic figures. Perivascular cuffing may be evident in areas of necrosis. Rosettes are seen in a small minority of cases, and should not be taken to diagnose the lesion as a metastatic neuroblastoma.

Cytoplasmic glycogen demonstrated by the periodic acid-Schiff (PAS) stain is evident in many but not all cases, especially in alcohol-fixed material. Variants from this classic pattern include a atypical Ewing's (large-cell Ewing's) and a filigree pattern. The filigree pattern refers to a bicellular architecture, separated by stroma. These tumors are generally positive for glycogen by PAS stain, but may require electron microscopy to demonstrate this on occasion. Atypical Ewing's sarcoma is characterized by one or more of the features—lack of glycogen, brisk (over two per high-power field) mitoses, neoplastic vascular formation, spindling at the periphery of the tumor, some amount of extracellular matrix (ECM), lobular architecture, or alveolar pattern.[61] Spindle-cell cytology, differentiation into muscle or ganglion cells or ECM are always absent by definition in all forms.

An immunohistochemical stain, Mic 2 (CD 99), has become available for use in formalin-fixed paraffin-embedded tissue. This stains the protein expression of a pseudoautosomal gene located on the X- and the Y-chromosomes. Limited experience with this stain shows it to be positive in the large majority of Ewing's sarcoma and PNETs. This immunomarker also stains the cells from some other sarcomas such as rhabdomyosarcomas, epithelioid osteosarcoma, thymic lymphocytes, and cells from acute lymphoblastic leukemia. Rare cases may express weak-focal staining for cytokeratin (up to 25% in some series,[35] but closer to 2% in our experience). Neuron-specific enolase and other neural-specific markers may be positive. Leukocyte Common Antigen, and markers of muscle and blood-vessel differentiation should be absent.

A. Differential Diagnosis

Small-cell osteosarcoma and mesenchymal chondrosarcoma are distinguished by their production of osteoid or cartilage matrices. Lymphoma is differentiated on the basis of the standard immunohistochemical markers for the various lymphoma entities, and on the basis of Mic 2 negativity in lymphoma. Ewing's sarcoma is negative for the leukocyte common antigen (CD 45). It is important to remember that CD 99 stains thymic lymphocytes and acute lymphoblastic leukemia.

Metastatic neuroblastoma has Homer-Wright pseudo-rosettes and a pink fibrillary background, and may have ganglion cells. Immunohistochemically, neural markers such as neuron-specific enolase may be present in both neuroblastoma and Ewing's sarcoma, and thus are not helpful. Ultrastructurally, the neuroblastoma may show neuritic-cell processes containing neurofilaments, neural tubules, and dense-core granules. However, these are found in PNETs. Biochemical demonstration of raised catecholamine metabolite levels or CT scan demonstration of an adrenal mass may be helpful in this differentiation.

The primary modality of treatment of Ewing's sarcoma has shifted from radiation to surgery over the past two decades. Chemotherapy (with or without radiation) is used in a neoadjuvant and adjuvant setting. As life expectancy increases, the problem of second malignancies is also increasing.

XI. GIANT-CELL TUMOR (OSTEOCLASTOMA)

Giant-cell tumor is a locally aggressive neoplasm characterized by large numbers of uniformly distributed osteoclast type giant cells in a population of plump epitheloid or spindle-stromal cells. Giant-cell tumors are more common in the skeletally mature adult population (peak 3rd decade). In this age group they occur in the region of the epiphysis. Only about 15% of the patients are less than 20 yr, and less than 5% have open epiphyses at diagnosis. They usually involve the long tubular bones, but occasionally involve flat bones, especially the sacrum. Cranio-facial involvement is unusual except in the context of Paget's disease. Most giant-cell lesions of the gnathic skeleton are believed to be giant-cell reparative granulomas rather than true giant-cell tumors. The same may be true of giant-cell tumors of the hands and feet. True giant-cell tumors of the hands and feet may behave more aggressively.[96]

Patients may present with pain or a mass. About 10% of patients present with a pathologic fracture. Serum chemistries are generally normal. An elevated serum Ca^{2+} should raise the possibility of hyperparathyroidism, and an elevated serum ALP in an older patient should raise the possibility of Paget's disease. Although as a group, multicentric tumors are uncommon (once hyperparathyroidism is excluded), these tumors may occur in the peripheral appendicular skeleton, and often pursue an aggressive course.

Giant-cell tumors may rarely arise in the context of Paget's disease of bone. Rarely, even histologically typical giant-cell tumors can metastasize, and in this situation they often behave indolently ("benign" metastasizing tumors).

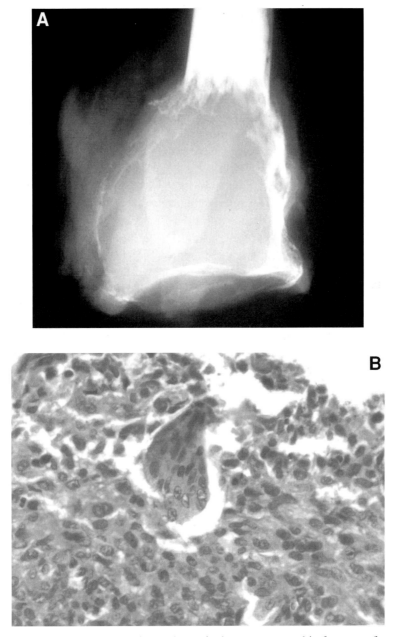

Figure 12. Giant-cell tumor. (A) shows the typical roentgenographic features of an example that involved the epiphysis of the distal radius. (B) shows the microscopic appearance of the tumor. There are numerous stromal cells in this field.

Radiographically, most lesions are lytic epiphyseal lesions, often extending into the metaphysis (Fig. 12A). They may show trabeculations or some fluid levels with a secondary ABC formation. Aggressive periosteal reactions and calcifications (sunburst, onion-skinning, or Codman's angles) are unusual, and should make the diagnosis suspect.

Lesions extending into the soft tissue often have a thin rim of bone (the "egg-shell"). There have been several attempts at predicting the aggressiveness of these tumors pre-operatively.[40,73] Ennekings system conceives of three kinds (or stages) of lesions. These are known as benign latent, benign active, and aggressive giant-cell tumors.

Grossly, the giant-cell tumors may be dark brown or have areas of hemorrhage, and ABC formation. Some may be tan or fleshy. The tumor may abut the cartilage—extension through the cartilage into the joint occurs, but only rarely. The tumor may extend along the cruciates or other intra-articular ligaments, or alternatively extend into the joint from the lateral side. Expansion of the bone is common, but extension through the periosteum into the soft-tissues is unusual, even with large lesions.

Microscopically, the diagnosis is made on the background population of stromal cells. These are round to oval, with nuclei resembling those of the giant cells (Fig. 12B). Occasionally, the stromal cells appear more spindled. Mitotic figures may be abundant, with two to three per high-power field. A high mitotic rate does not correlate with outcome. Giant cells are numerous, diffusely distributed, and contain a few to hundreds of nuclei (which resemble the nuclei of the stromal cells). Occasional cases may have broad bands collagen coursing through, especially in recurrent tumors. About one-half the giant-cell tumors contain reactive osteoid and woven bone, especially at the advancing edge of the lesion and in areas of soft-tissue extension. Reactive woven bone and osteoid may also be seen in the "benign" metastases in the lung, but do not warrant a revision of the diagnosis to osteosarcoma, provided the stromal cells show no cytological atypia. Cartilage is absent, except with fracture. Areas of infarct-like necrosis and foam cells are common.

The stroma of giant-cell tumors is usually vascular, and contains numerous thin-walled capillaries, areas of hemorrhage, and foamy or hemosiderin-laden macrophages. There may be focal vascular invasion (which might explain the "benign" metastases of a giant-cell tumor). This phenomenon, however, has not been associated with more aggressive behavior. Giant-cell tumors may be associated with a secondary ABC-like change. Histologic grading of giant-cell tumors has not been found to correlate with metastasis, recurrence, or local aggressiveness.

The term "malignant" giant-cell tumor (or malignancy in giant-cell tumor) refers to focal spindle-cell sarcoma arising at the site of a previously documented giant-cell tumor (secondarily) or present focally in an otherwise typical giant-cell tumor.

About 1–2% of otherwise typical giant-cell tumors may metastasize. Most are detected within 1 yr of resection, but some occur up to a decade later. There are no microscopic features to predict this phenomenon. Such metastases are indolent and amenable to resection. A sarcomatous transformation should be excluded in these cases.

A. Differential Diagnosis

Giant-cell tumors have to be differentiated from a variety of tumors containing giant cells. On the benign end, there are the giant-cell reparative granulomas and the brown tumors of hyperparthyroidism. True giant-cell tumors usually have a more uniform distribution of giant cells, often with more nuclei. In the reparative granulomas, they tend to be aggregated, mostly around areas of hemorrhage. The stroma of giant-cell tumors contains less fibrosis and is composed of characteristic mononuclear cells. In contrast, in the reparative granulomas, there is a fibrotic stroma, hemorrhage, and hemosiderin deposition. Foci of reactive bone are more common in reparative granulomas.

Metastatic carcinoma with osteoclast-type giant cells has been seen in some locations (especially the breast, thyroid, and pancreas). Metastatic carcinoma rarely affects the epiphysis. This entity may be excluded by a good history and if needed by appropriate immunostains.

ABC formation in a giant-cell tumor is not unusual. Differentiation from a true ABC may be difficult. Epiphyseal tumors with such changes are usually easily interpreted. The problem occurs in locations such as the spine. True giant-cell tumors have characteristic stromal cells, whereas ABCs have a more fibrotic reactive type of stroma.

The giant-cell tumors must also be differentiated from osteosarcomas with prominent giant cells. This is a serious diagnostic pitfall. In such osteosarcomas, there may be sheets of giant cells, and most of them are histologically bland. Osteoid production may be minimal. It may be limited to thin strands encircling mononuclear pleomorphic stromal cells. The latter usually have hyperchromatic nuclei, often with numerous atypical mitoses. The radiographic pattern suggests a permeative growth, not extending into the epiphyses.

1. Management

The lesions are treated by complete removal by currettage (followed by burring, thermal, or chemical ablation) or en-bloc resection. Recurrence has been linked to the types of surgical procedures done (intralesional, marginal, or wide). Adequacy of excision and absence of residual tumor are clearly important. Tumor spillage during surgery may lead to recurrences. Radiotherapy has had a low cure rate, with an approximate 5% rate of sarcomatous transformation.

XII. CHORDOMA

This is a low-grade malignant tumor that occurs predominantly in the axial skeleton, in the region of the embryonic notochord. There is a particular predilection to the caudal and cranial extremes, and the clivus and the sacrum are the most common sites. These have a differentiation toward (but not identical to) the fetal notochord. Vestigial rests of notochord-like tissue, located in the spheno-occipital region, are sometimes found and termed "ecchordosis physaliphora." There is a chondroid variant of chordoma that has foci of cartilaginous differentiation. This chondroid chordoma has a predilection for the spheno-occipital region.

Symptoms are a reflection of the anatomic location of the tumor. Thus, those that are located at the spheno-occipital region result in headache, cranial-nerve palsies, visual-field disturbances, and endocrinopathies. Cervical tumors may result in spinal-cord compression. Sacrococcygeal tumors may produce lower back pain, urinary bladder or bowel dysfunction, paresthesias, or a pelvic or sacral mass.

Radiologically, chordomas are midline tumors that expand and destroy bone. About one-half of the lesions in most series occur in the sacrum, and the other half are localized to the clivus. Locations other than these are exceedingly rare. Matrix calcifications are sometimes present in the clivus region.

Grossly, they are lobulated, soft, myxoid masses, and may mimic a chondrosarcoma. Microscopically, the lesions are lobulated, and have a myxoid background. The lobules are separated by fibrous septa. The tumor frequently extends beyond the grossly identified margins. Within these lobules are cells arranged in cords or sheets, or occasionally, haphazardly. At least some of these cells contain vacuolated cytoplasm (physaliphorous cells). Some cells may have abundant eosinophilic cytoplasm, or may mimic signet-ring cells. Nuclear pleomorphism is mild, and mitotic activity is low to absent. Some cases are seen with considerable "degenerative" atypia present in the tumor cells. Such lesion should not be considered as dedifferentiated.

A. Differential Diagnosis

Metastatic adenocarcinomas have a greater degree of cytological atypia than chordomas, and lack the lobulated growth pattern. The vacuolated cells of chordoma may be mistaken for a liposarcoma; however, a lobular growth pattern favors a chordoma. Myxoid chondrosarcoma is not common in the axial skeleton; however, the lobular pattern, the cord-like arrangement of cells, and S-100 positivity are common to both. Physaliphorous cells are seen in chordomas, but not in chondrosarcoma. Positive cytokeratin staining is not characteristic of chondrosarcoma. Myxo-papillary ependymoma enters the differential in the sacrum; however, it lacks the physalipherous cells and stains positively with glial fibrillary acid protein (GFAP). Chordoid meningioma is a rare type of meningioma that mimics chordoma. The location (a well-circumscribed mass attached to dura) helps to distinguish this lesion. Additionally, chordoid meningiomas often have more typical areas, are rich in a lympho-plasmacytic infiltrate, and are generally negative for cytokeratin.

B. Management

Wide excision is the optimal treatment. Because of the anatomic site however, this is not always possible in many cases. In these cases, debulking followed by radiation has been attempted. Some cases can undergo dedifferentiation to a MFH. This change is seen in a proportion of patients who have received radiation therapy, or have had multiple recurrences. However, some chordomas have dedifferentiated without either of these factors being applicable. The outcome for these patients is predictably poor.

XIII. VASO-FORMATIVE TUMORS

A. Benign Vascular Tumors

1. Lymphangioma and Hemangiomas

Lymphangioma and hemangiomas are a benign proliferation of lymphatic or vascular channels that occur in and replace bone. Some lesions occur in the form of polyostotic angiomatosis, and are associated with soft-tissue lesions. Gorham's disease (disappearing bone disease) may be related to angiomatosis.

Hemangiomas may be incidental findings on roentgenograms, or may present with pain. The spine, pelvis, and the long bones of the appendicular skeleton are the most frequent sites.

Radiologically, these lesions are lytic and may occupy most of the medullary cavity, or they may be seen as small intracortical lytic defects. There may be characteristically thickened vertical striations (corduroy cloth pattern). On CT scan, this translates into a polka-dot appearance. In the vertebrae, they are mostly confined to the body, with possible spread into the laminae. In the calvaria, the lesions are centered in the diploe, but there may be "bulges" of the outer and the inner tables. A periosteal reaction, if present, may be of the "sunburst" type. Frequent sites of hemangiomas include the calvaria, temporal bone (may present with facial palsy) and vertebra. Other sites include the ribs, femur, humerus, and pelvis.

Grossly and microscopically, these lesions correspond to the soft-tissue counterparts. They are hemorrhagic lesions, with either a capillary or cavernous growth pattern.

B. Hemangioendothelioma

This term has been used in several different ways by other authors, but we have considered it synonomous with angiosarcoma and hemangio-endotheliosarcoma.

This is a high-grade (sometimes surface) sarcoma of bone composed of atypical endothelial cells. Any bone can be affected, and often there is multicentric disease. Premalignant conditions are believed to include radiation, long-standing chronic osteomyelitis, and possibly benign vascular lesions. Such secondary angiosarcomas are extremely rare.

There is a wide age range, but most patients are over the age of 30 yr. Pain is the typical presenting complaint.

Radiographically, these are lytic, destructive, and permeative lesions, and soft-tissue extension often occurs.

Grossly, the lesions are soft, red/gray, spongy and focally firm, and solid. Microscopically, the diagnosis is usually not difficult. There are areas of well-formed anastomosing vascular channels lined by atypical endothelial cells, with large vesicular or hyperchromatic nuclei. Inflammatory cells, including eosinophils, are often seen. Sometimes the lesions are solid, poorly differentiated areas where the vasoformative nature may be more difficult to diagnose. Immunostains for endothelial markers (such as CD 31, CD 34 and Factor VIII-related antigen) may be helpful in establishing the diagnosis in selected cases. In other examples, the lesions have epithelioid cells and a myxoid background.

Treatment is usually surgical, although radiation has occasionally been successful. The outcome depends upon the involvement of multiple sites (especially deep organs), in which case the outcome is poor. It also depends upon the grade of the tumor. High-grade hemangioendotheliomas have a dismal prognosis.

XIV. ADAMANTINOMA

Adamantinoma is considered to be a low-grade malignant neoplasm with epithelial differentiation. It has an uncertain and controversial relationship with Campanacci's disease or osteofibrous dysplasia.[37,44,71,92] It arises in patients somewhat older than those with osteofibrous dysplasia, but shares the same predilection for the tibia.

The tumor is probably an entirely different entity from the adamantinoma (ameloblastoma) seen in the jaw.

The uncertain relationship with osteofibrous dysplasia is mostly based upon clinical studies. A possibility suggested is that osteofibrous dysplasia is a regressed form of adamantinoma.

Patients display a wide age range, but most cases occur in the second and third decades of life. Presentation can be with pain, fracture or be discovered incidentally.

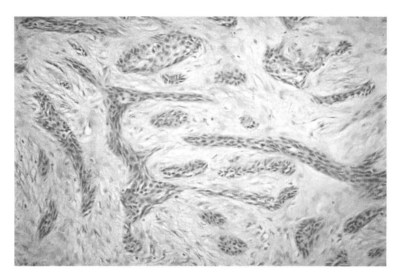

Figure 13. Adamantinoma of the tibia. The lesion shows epithelial islands in a fibrous stroma.

Radiologically, most lesions affect the tibial diaphysis. A very small number of cases have involved bones other than the tibia, these bones include the fibula, femur, other long bones, pelvis, and the short tubular bones. The lesions are often diaphyseal, eccentric, and epicentered in the cortex, with a "soap-bubble" appearance. Primary intramedullary origin or cortical breakthrough is seen in a small number of cases. The lesions usually show a geographic margin, usually without sclerosis.

Grossly, the tumor is well-demarcated in resection specimens. A lobular growth pattern may be evident. Cystic spaces and hemorrhage are common. Microscopically, the tumor consists of epithelial islands in a fibrous stroma (Fig. 13). The nuclei of adamantinoma are usually bland, and the mitotic rate is usually low in most cases. A variety of growth patterns may be evident in the epithelial component. These include spindled, basaloid, tubular, and squamoid or spindled patterns. Anastamosing spaces with the appearance of vascular channels are seen in some cases.

The differential diagnosis includes osteofibrous dysplasia and metastatic carcinoma. Osteofibrous dysplasia has no epithelial islands or differentiation. Stains for cytokeratin may be helpful in this distinction. Metastatic carcinoma is rare in the distal appendicular skeleton (such as the tibia). The co-existance of osteofibrous-like areas would argue against metastatic carcinoma. The epithelial component of the synovial sarcoma may be indistinguishable from that of adamantinoma. The mesenchymal component of a synovial sarcoma, however, tends to be far more cytologically atypical than the osteofibrous dysplasia-like bland stroma of an adamantinoma. Synovial sarcomas are epicentered in the soft tissues, and do not usually invade the bone to a great extent.

The treatment of adamantinoma is essentially surgical. Adamantinoma is a lesion prone to recurrences. Occasional cases metastasize to the lungs, lymph nodes, or other bones. At present, there seem to be no consistent histologic or clinical markers to predict the lesions that would be more likely to show an aggressive biologic behavior.

XV. NEUROGENIC TUMORS

Intraosseous schwannomas are very unusual lesions, but have been described especially in the mandible and sacrum. Neurofibromas are extremely rare, even in neurofibromatosis. However, neurofibromas have occasionally been described in the tissue present in congenital pseudarthrosis of the tibia in infancy. Generally, this tissue is fibrous, and we have not seen a *bonafide* neurofibroma even in this situation.

XVI. LIPOGENIC TUMORS

Benign lipomas are rare lesions that seem to have a predilection for the calcaneus. Radiologically, the lesions resemble infarcts, with a geographic margin and a central area of calcification. Microscopically, cancellous bone is replaced by fat. There may be fat necrosis and dystrophic calcification.

XVII. CONDITIONS THAT SIMULATE PRIMARY BONE TUMORS

A. Metastases

Osseous metastases may occur with a variety of primary tumors, and the frequency of each depends upon the age of the patient. For example, in young children, neuroblastoma is common, whereas in older adults, metastatic carcinoma predominates. The majority of metastases present as multiple lesions and can be identified on X-rays, bone scans, or more sensitively by MR scans.

1. Tumors Metastasizing to Bone

The incidence of osseous metastatic disease at autopsy is far higher than the clinical incidence (it may be up to 70% in some series). In adults, the primary lesions that are most frequently present with metastatic bone disease include breast, lung, prostate, kidney, and thyroid.

The hypothesized mechanism of spread in most malignancies occurs via the hematogenous route. This includes the arterial as well as the venous system, especially the vertebral venous plexus of Batson. In addition, the location and spread pattern of tumors is probably dependent upon a variety of local factors, such as adhesion molecules and certain members of the cadherin, immunoglobulin, integrin, selectin, hyluronate receptor, and sialomucin families. Once the carcinoma has adhered to bone, a variety of bone-derived growth factors may help in carcinoma cell growth. Factors such as transforming growth factor β (TGF-β), insulin-like growth factors (IGF)-I and -II and platelet-derived growth factors have been mitogenic or supportive of tumors in vitro.

2. Blastic and Lytic Metastases

Carcinomas and other metastatic tumors stimulate or secrete a variety of cytokines when in contact with bone. These in turn influence the bone that produces and resorbs cells locally. Thus, they are responsible for the various osteoblastic and osteoclastic effects seen histologically. Such effects are also reflected on the blastic and lytic lesions seen radiologically, as well as the cold and hot scans seen by radioisotope scans.

A. SYSTEMIC EFFECTS

Certain tumors can cause large amounts of osteolysis, and may result in generalized osteoporosis or hypercalcemia. This is probably done by the secretion of humoral factors such as parathyroid hormone, TGF-α, vitamin D, cathepsin D, colony-stimulating factors, E-series prostaglandins, IL-1, IL-6, and tumor necrosis factors (TNFs) α and β.

Adult patients commonly present with pain, swelling, tenderness, or pathologic fracture. The same can occur in children, but many cases are detected in this age group as part of a work-up for a known malignancy. Although any site can be involved, the bones of the axial skeleton and proximal appendicular skeleton are more frequently affected.

Radiologic findings vary. Blastic, lytic, or mixed lesions are possible. The majority of lesions are lytic, especially those from kidney, thyroid, and the gastrointestinal tract. Carcinomas of the breast and prostate as well as carcinoid tumors and medulloblastomas sometimes produce blastic metastases. Some carcinomas, such as breast, may produce either blastic or lytic lesions. Periosteal reactions are rare; the lesions are often geographic and occasionally expansile.

Grossly, it is often impossible to differentiate secondary tumors from primary ones. Some primary tumors are more sharply demarcated (for example, many lytic tumors), and some tend to be extremely vascular (kidney and thyroid tumors) but in many cases no general rules can be made. Carcinomas that are metastatic to bone can vary from hard, bony tumors to soft, fleshy, or friable.

Microscopically, well-differentiated metastatic tumors do not pose a problem. For example, renal-cell or thyroid carcinomas can often be diagnosed, and the primary sites can be identified even without resorting to immunohistochemistry. Spindle-cell carcinomas and undifferentiated neoplasms pose a special problem because they mimic sarcomas. Reactive bone formation may mimic osteosarcoma. It is important to also, remember that some sarcomas can be positive for epithelial markers, such as cytokeratin-leiomyosarcomas, MFH, epitheloid osteosarcomas, and epitheloid hemangioendotheliomas.

Management of metastatic tumors includes attempts to identify the primary site and give appropriate chemotherapy, and in certain cases, endocrine therapy. This process involves imaging methods and biopsies of the primary and metastatic sites. Pain management is important, and can be done via surgical (resection, stabilization, or other) means. Radiation therapy may occasionally be required. Impending pathologic fractures, especially in weight-bearing bones, may require prophylactic stabilization. However, predicting the fracture risk is difficult. Existing guidelines suggest stabilization for diaphyseal lesions greater than 2.5 cm or those with over 50% cortical destruction. Some cases require the use of bisphosphonates to limit the amount of bone pain or hypercalcemia.

B. Cysts

1. Simple (Unicameral) Bone Cyst (UBC)

A unicameral bone cyst (UBC) is an intramedullary cystic cavity that is often unilocular, filled with clear or straw-colored fluid. A thin fibrovascular membrane lines the cavity. The possibility that these are related to a developmental or traumatic defect has been considered. The presentation includes pain, stiffness, and pathological fracture, and sometimes occurs as an incidental finding on X-rays. Most patients are within the first two decades of life. About 80% of cases are seen in either the humerus or femur. In older age groups, lesions of the ilium and calcaneus are sometimes also seen. The involvement of other bones is rare.

Radiologically, UBCs are often metaphyseal, and may encroach the epiphysis in skeletally immature individuals. As the bone lengthens at the physeal end, the cyst may appear to "move" into a diaphyseal location. The cysts size varies from a few to several centimeters. Fragments of bone may be present within the cyst, and can be visualized as "fallen fragments" by X-ray.

It is most unusual to receive intact gross specimens, since these lesions are rarely resected. Curetted material, if received, often consists of irregular fragments of membranous fibrovascular tissue. Hemosiderin, granulation tissue, or mild focal chronic inflammatory cells may be present. Some cases have pink cementum-like rounded material.

A. MANAGEMENT

Aspiration of the cyst followed by steroid injections is currently the most popular method of treatment.

2. Subchondral (Synovial) Cyst

These are small cysts, usually adjacent to the articular cartilage and associated with degenerative joint disease. Microscopically, they appear as defects in the bone, often with no discernible lining.

3. Intraosseous Ganglion

These are intramedullary, mucin-filled, fibrous-lined lesions. There is a wide age range, and the presentation often occurs with pain or as an incidental finding. The distal and proximal tibia, femur, ulna, and the hands and feet are commonly involved. Microscopically, the tissue is mainly myxoid, mixed with fibroblasts. Fibrous tissue may be haphazardly interspersed, or may be arranged in the form of septa. The outer layer is often heavily collagenized.

4. Aneurysmal Bone Cyst (ABC)

An ABC is a benign (and probably non-neoplastic) lesion, which is often multicystic, rapidly expansile, and locally destructive. The walls of the cyst are composed of spindle cells, as well as osteoid, and multinucleate giant cells.

The histogenesis of this lesion has been controversial. Some advocate the possibility of this representing a change secondary to an arteriovenous malformation. Some lesions arise in association with a variety of bone neoplasms. These lesions include giant-cell tumor, non-ossifying fibroma, giant-cell reparative granuloma, fibrous dysplasia, chondromyxoid fibroma, chondroblastoma, osteoblastoma, UBC, hemangioma, and osteosarcoma. It is essential to search for and exclude these underlying lesions.

These cysts are found to exist through a broad age range, but mostly occur between the ages of 5 and 25 yr. Pain of a few weeks duration is the most common presenting complaint. Visible swelling, and throbbing are not infrequent. Almost any bone can be involved. In the vertebrae, multiple bones may be involved. Lesions in this location are more likely to involve the posterior arch and spinous processes. Most primary ABCs of long bones are metaphyseal. Secondary ABCs follow the site of predilection of their primary lesions.

Radiologically, the lesions may be eccentric (often seen in long bones), central, or parosteal (a rare location). In the initial (or incipient) phase, there is a small lytic lesion, which does not expand the bone. In the growth phase, there is rapid growth and lysis of bone, and there may be cortical "blowout." The intramedullary component is usually well-circumscribed, and this may help establish the diagnosis. In the stable phase, the X-rays have a characteristic picture with expanded bone and a "shell" around the lesion, along with trabeculations coursing within it. Finally, there is a healing phase, in which there is progressive ossification, resulting in a coarsely trabeculated bony mass.

Grossly (if intact), the lesions can be seen to have thin osseous bony shell surrounding a honeycombed mass with cavernous vascular spaces that "ooze" blood like a veritable sponge. Older cysts may have sero-sanguinous fluid instead of blood. Microscopically, the main feature is the presence of carvernous spaces that are filled with blood but lack the smooth-muscle wall and endothelial cells of blood vessels. Fibrous walls that contain osteoid, chondroid, and giant cells in varying proportions and combinations surround these spaces. Sometimes, the mineralizing component has a chondroid aura, rarely found in any other lesion. The cyst may extend into the soft tissue. Osteoid may be present, and a calcification frequently occurs in long, linear depositions. Mitotic figures may be numerous; however, the stromal cells lack atypia, atypical mitoses, and anaplasia. These are important features to search for, because the possibility of telangiactatic osteosarcoma must be considered if they are found. A solid variant of an ABC has been described that is probably identical to a reparative giant-cell granuloma.

A. MANAGEMENT

Intralesional procedures such as curettage or sclerotherapy, via feeding vessels, have been advocated. Radiation carries a risk of postradiation sarcoma transformation.

C. Metaphyseal Fibrous Defect

A metaphyseal fibrous defect is an intracortical proliferation of fibrous tissue and histiocytes. Larger lesions may involve the medullary cavity. There have been suggestions that metaphyseal defects can move from the metaphysis to the diaphysis (as the bone grows) with time. Lesions arising in the context of cafe-au-lait spots have been called the Jaffe-Campanacci syndrome.

The incidence of these lesions may be age-related. Up to 35% of all children (if screened) are said to have these lesions. They are most common between the ages of 4 and 8 yr. The majority of the lesions in this group are less than 0.5 cm. The incidence falls below 2 and above 14 yr of age. Most lesions last about 2 yr before disappearing by healing by sclerosis (the healing phase or the so-called ossifying non-ossifying fibromas). Symptomatic cases usually have larger lesions, and may present with pain or pathologic fracture. The distal femur, distal tibia, proximal tibia, and fibula account for the vast majority of lesions.

Radiographically, most lesions are geographic, lytic lesions with well-demarcated sclerotic margins. In the healing phase, there may be varying amounts of sclerosis within the lesion.

Microscopically, the lesions are predominantly fibrous, often with a storiform arrangement. Foamy histiocytes (xanthoma cells), hemosiderin-laden macrophages, and multinucleated giant cells are present in varying proportions. In the presence of fracture or in the healing phase, reactive woven bone may be present.

D. Fibrous Dysplasia

Fibrous dysplasia (FD) is a benign, mono-ostotic (80% of cases) or poly-ostotic (20% of cases) proliferation of fibrous tissue and bone. The osseous component is irregularly distributed, and consists of woven bone with inconspicuous osteoblastic rimming. Cartilage formation (fibro-cartilaginous dysplasia) is seen in less than 10% of cases.

Mono-ostotic FD may be seen at any age, although most cases occur below 30 yr of age. Poly-ostotic FD generally presents before the age of puberty. Presentation may be with pain, pathologic fracture, or deformity (especially gnathic or upper femoral FD), or be asymptomatic. A reduction in activity with age is seen in many lesions, with a possible re-activation at the time of pregnancy. Poly-ostotic FD with macular skin lesions, precocious puberty, and with or without fibromyxomatous soft-tissue tumors and endocrinopathies, is known eponymically as McCune-Albright syndrome. The association of FD with a soft-tissue or intramuscular (im) myxoma is known as the Mazabraud syndrome. Very rarely, secondary sarcomas may develop on FD.

About one-third of mono-ostotic FD involves the craniofacial bones, another third the tibia/femur, and about 20% involves the ribs. In patients with poly-ostotic FD, the femur, tibia, and pelvis are commonly involved. In many of these cases, small bones of the hands and feet, the ribs, and the skull may also exhibit lesions.

The pathogenesis and molecular basis of FD is poorly understood, and may be related to mutation in G-proteins (guanine nucleotide-binding proteins) and certain growth factors.[3,11,46,50,78,79,86]

The radiologic appearances can be variable. The majority of cases are intramedullary, geographic lesions with sclerotic or well-defined margins and a "ground-glass" matrix. These are intensely hot on bone scans. A few lesions may be more sclerotic or show calcified cartilage. Bony expansion is marked in some examples, especially lesions involving the ribs. FD of the femoral neck (and sometimes other bones) is often accompanied by a pathologic fracture.

Grossly FD is firm, fibrous white or red, with a variable amount of "grittiness." Secondary cyst formation is occasionally seen. Some lesions contain grossly visible cartilage. Microscopically, there are trabeculae of woven bone in a background of moderately cellular fibrous tissue. The trabeculae often take a variety of shapes (C's or circles) and are sometimes referred to as "Chinese-letters." Osteoblasts are interspersed in the woven bone, but are not conspicuous around the trabeculae. The latter feature, called rimming, is more commonly seen in other examples of woven bone formation such as fracture-callus or myositis ossificans. In some cases of FD, small foci of lamellar bone may also be seen. The fibrous stroma may be highly or sparsely cellular or myxomatous, or may show considerable collagenization. The fibroblasts usually have plump ovoid nuclei, but may show elongated narrow ones in some cases or in some areas. Multinucleate osteoclast-type giant cells may be present. Cartilage with peripheral enchondral ossification is sometimes present. The cartilage may be present in long islands, rounded nodules or simulate a growth plate, and collections of foam cells are common. They may be mistaken for metastatic clear-cell carcinoma in small biopsy samples.

The lesion is benign, and if indicated (such as in impending fracture or doubtful diagnosis), can be curetted.

REFERENCES

1. Aigner T, Loos S, Muller S, et al: Cell differentiation and matrix gene expression in mesenchymal chondrosarcomas. *Am J Pathol* 156:1327–1335, 2000.
2. Aigner T, Unni KK: Is dedifferentiated chondrosarcoma a 'de-differentiated' chondrosarcoma? *J Pathol* 189:445–447, 1999.
3. Alman BA, Greel DA, Wolfe HJ: Activating mutations of Gs protein in monostotic fibrous lesions of bone. *J Orthop Res* 14:311–315, 1996.
4. Angervall L, Persson S, Stenman G, et al: Large cell, epithelioid, telangiectatic osteoblastoma: a unique pseudosarcomatous variant of osteoblastoma. *Hum Pathol* 30:1254–1259, 1999.
5. Bacchini P, Inwards C, Biscaglia R, et al: Chondroblastoma-like osteosarcoma *Orthopedics (Thorofare, NJ)* 22:337–339, 1999.
6. Barei DP, Moreau G, Scarborough MT, et al: Percutaneous radiofrequency ablation of osteoid osteoma. *Clin Orthop* 373:115–124, 2000.
7. Bennett JH, Thomas G, Evans AW, et al: Osteosarcoma of the jaws: a 30-year retrospective review. *Oral Surg Oral Med Oral Pathol Oral Radiol Endod* 90:323–332, 2000.
8. Bertoni F, Unni KK, Lucas DR, et al: Osteoblastoma with cartilaginous matrix. An unsual morphologic presentation in 18 cases. *Am J Surg Pathol* 17:69–74, 1993.
9. Bertoni F, Unni KK, McLeod RA, et al: Osteosarcoma resembling osteoblastoma. *Cancer* 55:416–426, 1985.
10. Biagini R, Orsini U, Demitri S, et al: Mesenchymal chondrosarcoma of the sacrum: a case report and review of the literature. *Tumori* 86:75–78, 2000.
11. Bianco P, Riminucci M, Majolagbe A, et al: Mutations of the GNAS1 gene, stromal cell dysfunction, and osteomalacic changes in non-McCune-Albright fibrous dysplasia of bone. *J Bone Miner Res* 15:120–128, 2000.
12. Bingaman KD, Alleyne Jr., CH, Olson JJ: Intracranial extraskeletal mesenchymal chondrosarcoma: case report. *Neurosurgery* 46:207–211; discussion 11–2, 2000.
13. Bjornsson J, McLeod RA, Unni KK, et al: Primary chondrosarcoma of long bones and limb girdles. *Cancer* 83:2105–2119, 1998.
14. Bjornsson J, Unni KK, Dahlin DC, et al: Clear cell chondrosarcoma of bone. Observations in 47 cases. *Am J Surg Pathol* 8:223–230, 1984.
15. Boriani S, De Iure F, Bandiera S, et al: Chondrosarcoma of the mobile spine: report on 22 cases. *Spine* 25:804–812, 2000.
16. Bovee JV, Cleton-Jansen AM, Rosenberg C, et al: Molecular genetic characterization of both components of a dedifferentiated chondrosarcoma, with implications for its histogenesis *J Pathol* 189:454–462, 1999.
17. Campanacci M, Ruggieri P, Gasbarrini A, et al: Osteoid osteoma. Direct visual identification and intralesional excision of the nidus with minimal removal of bone. *J Bone Joint Surg [Br]* 81:814–820, 1999.
18. Cheung FM, Wu WC, Lam CK, et al: Diagnostic criteria for pseudomalignant osteoblastoma. *Histopathology* 31:196–200, 1997.
19. Chidambaram A, Sanville P: Mesenchymal chondrosarcoma of the maxilla. *J Laryngol Otol* 114:536–539, 2000.
20. Chow LT, Lin J, Yip KM, et al: Chondromyxoid fibroma-like osteosarcoma: a distinct variant of low-grade osteosarcoma. *Histopathology* 29:429–436, 1996.
21. Clark JL, Unni KK, Dahlin DC, et al: Osteosarcoma of the jaw. *Cancer* 51:2311–2316, 1983.
22. Coates HL, Pearson BW, Devine KD, et al: Chondrosarcoma of the nasal cavity, paranasal sinuses, and nasopharynx. *Trans Am Acad Opthalmol* 84:ORL919–926, 1977.
23. Cove JA, Taminiau AH, Obermann WR, et al: Osteoid osteoma of the spine treated with percutaneous computed tomography-guided thermocoagulation. *Spine* 25:1283–1286, 2000.
24. Dahlin DC, Unni KK: Osteosarcoma of bone and its important recognizable varieties. *Am J Surg Pathol* 1:61–72, 1977.

25. Damron TA, Sim FH, Unni KK: Multicentric chondrosarcomas. *Clin Orthop* 328:211–219, 1996

26. De Alava E, Gerald WL: Molecular biology of the Ewing's sarcoma/primitive neuroectodermal tumor family. *J Clin Oncol* 18:204–213, 2000.

27. El-Mofty SK: Cemento-ossifying fibroma and benign cementoblastoma. *Semin Diagn Pathol* 16:302–307, 1999.

28. Enneking WF: A system of staging musculoskeletal neoplasms. *Clin Orthop* 204:9–24, 1986.

29. Frassica FJ, Unni KK, Beabout JW, et al: Dedifferentiated chondrosarcoma. A report of the clinicopathological features and treatment of seventy-eight cases. *J Bone Joint Surg [Am]* 68:1197–1205, 1986.

30. Gadwal SR, Fanburg-Smith JC, Gannon FH, et al: Primary chondrosarcoma of the head and neck in pediatric patients: a clinicopathologic study of 14 cases with a review of the literature. *Cancer* 88:2181–2188, 2000.

31. Garrison RC, Unni KK, McLeod RA, et al: Chondrosarcoma arising in osteochondroma. *Cancer* 49:1890–1897, 1982.

32. Gil S, Marco SF, Arenas J, et al: Doppler duplex color localization of osteoid osteomas. *Skeletal Radiol* 28:107–110, 1999.

33. Granter SR, Renshaw AA, Fletcher CD, et al: CD99 reactivity in mesenchymal chondrosarcoma. *Hum Pathol* 27:1273–1276, 1996.

34. Green P, Whittaker RP: Benign chondroblastoma. Case report with pulmonary metastasis. *J Bone Joint Surg [Am]* 57:418–420, 1975.

35. Gu M, Antonescu CR, Guiter G, et al: Cytokeratin immunoreactivity in Ewing's sarcoma: prevalence in 50 cases confirmed by molecular diagnostic studies. *Am J Surg Pathol* 24:410–416, 2000.

36. Hammad HM, Hammond HL, Kurago ZB, et al: Chondromyxoid fibroma of the jaws. Case report and review of the literature. *Oral Surg Oral Med Oral Pathol Oral Radiol Endod* 85:293–300, 1998.

37. Hazelbag HM, Wessels JW, Mollevangers P, et al: Cytogenetic analysis of adamantinoma of long bones: further indications for a common histogenesis with osteofibrous dysplasia. *Cancer Genet Cytogenet* 97:5–11, 1997.

38. Hecht JT, Hogue D, Strong LC, et al: Hereditary multiple exostosis and chondrosarcoma: linkage to chromosome 11 and loss of heterozygosity for EXT-linked markers on chromosomes 11 and 8. *Am J Hum Genet* 56:1125–1131, 1995.

39. Hecht JT, Hogue D, Wang Y, et al: Hereditary multiple exostoses (EXT): mutational studies of familial EXT1 cases and EXT-associated malignancies. *Am J Hum Genet* 60:80–86, 1997.

40. Hudson TM, Schiebler M, Springfield DS, et al: Radiology of giant cell tumors of bone: computed tomography, arthro-tomography, and scintigraphy. *Skeletal Radiol* 11:85–95, 1984.

41. Katz K, Kornreich L, David R, et al: Osteoid osteoma: resection with CT guidance. *Isr Med Assoc J* 2:151–153, 2000.

42. Kawaguchi K, Oda Y, Miura H, et al: Periosteal osteoblastoma of the distal humerus. *J Orthop Sci* 3:341–345, 1998.

43. Keel SB, Bhan AK, Liebsch NJ, et al: Chondromyxoid fibroma of the skull base: a tumor which may be confused with chondroma and chondrosarcoma. A report of three cases and review of the literature. *Am J Surg Pathol* 21:577–582, 1997.

44. Keeney GL, Unni KK, Beabout JW, et al: Adamantinoma of long bones. A clinicopathologic study of 85 cases. *Cancer* 64:730–737, 1989.

45. Khurana JS, Mayo-Smith W, Kattapuram SV: Subtalar arthralgia caused by juxtaarticular osteoid osteoma. *Clin Orthop* 252:205–208, 1990.

46. Kim IS, Kim ER, Nam HJ, et al: Activating mutation of GS alpha in McCune-Albright syndrome causes skin pigmentation by tyrosinase gene activation on affected melanocytes. *Hormone Res* 52:235–240, 1999.

47. Koh JS, Chung JH, Lee SY, et al: Parachordoma of the tibia: report of a rare case. *Pathol Res Pract* 196:269–273, 2000.
48. Kovar H: Ewing's sarcoma and peripheral primitive neuroectodermal tumors after their genetic union. *Curr Opin Oncol* 10:334–342, 1998.
49. Kurt AM, Unni KK, McLeod RA, et al: Low-grade intraosseous osteosarcoma. *Cancer* 65:1418–1428, 1990.
50. Levine MA: Clinical implications of genetic defects in G proteins: oncogenic mutations in G alpha s as the molecular basis for the McCune-Albright syndrome. *Arch Med Res* 30:522–531, 1999.
51. Lin PP, Brody RI, Hamelin AC, et al: Differential transactivation by alternative EWS-FLI1 fusion proteins correlates with clinical heterogeneity in Ewing's sarcoma. *Cancer Res* 59:1428–1432, 1999.
52. Liu J, Hudkins PG, Swee RG, et al: Bone sarcomas associated with Ollier's disease. *Cancer* 59:1376–1385, 1987.
53. Lodwick GS: Radiographic diagnosis and grading of bone tumors, with comments on computer evaluation. *Proc Natl Cancer Conf* 5:369–380, 1964.
54. Lodwick GS: A probabilistic approach to the diagnosis of bone tumors. *Radiol Clin North Am* 3:487–497, 1965.
55. Lucas DR, Tazelaar HD, Unni KK, et al: Osteogenic melanoma. A rare variant of malignant melanoma. *Am J Surg Pathol* 17:400–409, 1993.
56. Lucas DR, Unni KK, McLeod RA, et al: Osteoblastoma: clinicopathologic study of 306 cases. *Hum Pathol* 25:117–134, 1994.
57. McAfee MK, Pairolero PC, Bergstralh EJ, et al: Chondrosarcoma of the chest wall: factors affecting survival. *Ann Thorac Surg* 40:535–541, 1985.
58. Montanaro L, Pession A, Trere D, et al: Detection of EWS chimeric transcripts by nested RT-PCR to allow reinfusion of uncontaminated peripheral blood stem cells in high-risk Ewing's tumor in childhood. *Haematologica* 84:1012–1015, 1999.
59. Nakajima H, Sim FH, Bond JR, et al: Small cell osteosarcoma of bone. Review of 72 cases. *Cancer* 79:2095–2106, 1997.
60. Nakashima Y, Unni KK, Shives TC, et al: Mesenchymal chondrosarcoma of bone and soft tissue. A review of 111 cases. *Cancer* 57:2444–2453, 1986.
61. Nascimento AG, Unii KK, Pritchard DJ, et al: A clinicopathologic study of 20 cases of large-cell (atypical) Ewing's sarcoma of bone. *Am J Surg Pathol* 4:29–36, 1980.
62. Noguera R, Navarro S, Triche TJ: Translocation (11;22) in small cell osteosarcoma. *Cancer Genet Cytogenet* 45:121–124, 1990.
63. Nora FE, Unni KK, Pritchard DJ, et al: Osteosarcoma of extragnathic craniofacial bones. *Mayo Clin Proc* 58:268–272, 1983.
64. Obata K, Hiraga H, Nojima T, et al: Molecular characterization of the genomic breakpoint junction in a t(11;22) translocation in Ewing sarcoma. *Genes Chromosomes Cancer* 25:6–15, 1999.
65. Ogose A, Hotta T, Emura I, et al: Repeated dedifferentiation of low-grade intraosseous osteosarcoma. *Hum Pathol* 31:615–618, 2000.
66. Ogose A, Unni KK, Swee RG, et al: Chondrosarcoma of small bones of the hands and feet. *Cancer* 80:50–59, 1997.
67. Okada K, Nishida J, Morita T, et al: Low-grade intraosseous osteosarcoma in northern Japan: advantage of AgNOR and MIB-1 staining in differential diagnosis. *Hum Pathol* 31:633–639, 2000.
68. Ostrowski ML, Johnson ME, Smith PD, et al: Low-grade intraosseous osteosarcoma with prominent lymphoid infiltrate. *Arch Pathol Lab Med* 124:868–871, 2000.
69. Papagelopoulos PJ, Galanis EC, Sim FH, et al: Clinicopathologic features, diagnosis, and treatment of osteoblastoma. *Orthopedics (Thorofare, NJ)* 22:244–247; quiz 8–9, 1999.

70. Park YK, Chi SG, Park HR, et al: Detection of t(11;22)(q24;q12) translocation of Ewing's sarcoma in paraffin embedded tissue by nested reverse transcription-polymerase chain reaction. *J Korean Med Sci* 13:395–399, 1998.

71. Park YK, Unni KK, McLeod RA, et al: Osteofibrous dysplasia: clinicopathologic study of 80 cases. *Hum Pathol* 24:1339–1347, 1993.

72. Patino-Cordoba JI, Turner J, McCarthy SW, et al: Chondromyxoid fibroma of the skull base. *Otolaryngol—Head Neck Surg* 118:415–418, 1998.

73. Present D, Bertoni F, Hudson T, et al: The correlation between the radiologic staging studies and histopathologic findings in aggressive stage 3 giant cell tumor of bone. *Cancer* 57:237–244, 1986.

74. Ramirez JA, Sandoz JC, Kaakaji Y, et al: Case 3: Aggressive osteoblastoma. *Am J Roentgenol* 171:863, 7–8, 1998.

75. Raskind WH, Conrad EU, Chansky H, et al: Loss of heterozygosity in chondrosarcomas for markers linked to hereditary multiple exostoses loci on chromosomes 8 and 11. *Am J Hum Genet* 56:1132–1139, 1995.

76. Raubenheimer EJ, Noffke CE: Low-grade intraosseous osteosarcoma of the jaws. *Oral Surg Oral Med Oral Pathol Oral Radiol Endod* 86:82–85, 1998.

77. Riddell RJ, Louis CJ, Bromberger NA: Pulmonary metastases from chondroblastoma of the tibia. Report of a case. *J Bone Joint Surg [Br]* 55:848–853, 1973.

78. Riminucci M, Fisher LW, Shenker A, et al: Fibrous dysplasia of bone in the McCune-Albright syndrome: abnormalities in bone formation. *Am J Pathol* 151:1587–1600, 1997.

79. Riminucci M, Liu B, Corsi A, et al: The histopathology of fibrous dysplasia of bone in patients with activating mutations of the Gs alpha gene: site-specific patterns and recurrent histological hallmarks. *J Pathol* 187:249–258, 1999.

80. Robinson LH UKK, O'Laughlin S, Beabout JW, et al: Surface chondromyxoid fibroma of bone. *Mod Pathol* 7:1994.

81. Roessner A, Jurgens H: Round cell tumours of bone. *Pathol Res Pract* 189:111–136, 1993.

82. Saito K, Unni KK, Wollan PC, et al: Chondrosarcoma of the jaw and facial bones. *Cancer* 76:1550–1558, 1995.

83. Shek TW, Peh WC, Leung G: Chondromyxoid fibroma of skull base: a tumour prone to local recurrence. *J Laryngol Otol* 113:380–385, 1999.

84. Sim FH, Unni KK, Beabout JW, et al: Osteosarcoma with small cells simulating Ewing's tumor. *J Bone Joint Surg [Am]* 61:207–215, 1979.

85. Simon MA: Percutaneous radiofrequency coagulation of osteoid osteoma compared with operative treatment *J Bone Joint Surg [Am]* 81:437–438, 1999.

86. Spiegel AM: G protein defects in signal transduction. *Horm Res* 53:17–22, 2000.

87. Sun TC, Swee RG, Shives TC, et al: Chondrosarcoma in Maffucci's syndrome. *J Bone Joint Surg [Am]* 67:1214–1219, 1985.

88. Thompson AD, Teitell MA, Arvand A, et al: Divergent Ewing's sarcoma EWS/ETS fusions confer a common tumorigenic phenotype on NIH3T3 cells. *Oncogene* 18:5506–5513, 1999.

89. Unni KK: Osteosarcoma of bone. *J Orthp Sci* 3:287–294, 1998.

90. Unni KK, Dahlin DC: Premalignant tumors and conditions of bone. *Am J Surg Pathol* 3:47–60, 1979.

91. Unni KK, Dahlin DC: Osteosarcoma: pathology and classification. *Semin Roentgenol* 24:143–152, 1989.

92. Unni KK, Dahlin DC, Beabout JW, et al: Adamantinomas of long bones. *Cancer* 34:1796–1805, 1974.

93. Unni KK, Dahlin DC, Beabout JW, et al: Chondrosarcoma: clear-cell variant. A report of sixteen cases. *J Bone Joint Surg [Am]* 58:676–683, 1976.

94. Urano F, Umezawa A, Yabe H, et al: Molecular analysis of Ewing's sarcoma: another fusion gene, EWS-E1AF, available for diagnosis. *Jpn J Cancer Res* 89:703–711, 1998.

95. Vencio EF, Reeve CM, Unni KK, et al: Mesenchymal chondrosarcoma of the jaw bones: clinicopathologic study of 19 cases. *Cancer* 82:2350–2355, 1998.
96. Wold LE, Swee RG: Giant cell tumors of the hands and feet. *Semin Diagn Pathol* 1:173–184, 1984.
97. Wu CT, Inwards CY, O'Laughlin S, et al: Chondromyxoid fibroma of bone: a clinicopathologic review of 278 cases. *Hum Pathol* 29:438–446, 1998.
98. Young CL, Sim FH, Unni KK, et al: Chondrosarcoma of bone in children. *Cancer* 66:1641–1648, 1990.

VII Electron Microscopy and Radiography

34

Methods for Transmission and Scanning Electron Microscopy of Bone and Cartilage

Helen E. Gruber[1] and Winston W. Wiggins[2]

[1]*Orthopaedic Research Biology, Carolinas Medical Center, Charlotte, NC, USA*
[2]*Electron Microscopy Laboratory, Carolinas Medical Center, Charlotte, NC, USA*

I. INTRODUCTION

Ultrastructural studies of bone and cartilage using transmission electron microscopy (TEM) and scanning electron microscopy (SEM) present unique challenges for technical preparation and scientific interpretation. Preparative methods have been described elsewhere; space limitations do not allow us to cite all authors who have contributed to this field. Chemical fixation and specimen preparation for TEM for bone studies have been reviewed by several authors.[3,14,15,23] Reviews of preparation methods for SEM have been published by Boyde et al.[7,9,10] Specialized techniques directed toward preserving the bone-cell-implant interface are discussed elsewhere in this volume.

II. METHODS FOR TEM STUDIES OF BONE AND CARTILAGE

Most studies rely upon traditional tissue-processing methods for bone and cartilage. Fetal bone, because of its lower mineral content, can be successfully sectioned with diamond knives, but pediatric specimens and specimens from older age groups require decalcification. In undecalcified preparations processed with traditional heavy-metal stains, electron-dense, needle-like mineralization crystals are retained. Decalcified specimens, however, usually fail to preserve this feature.

A. Formalin-Fixed Tissue

If only formalin-fixed or paraffin-embedded tissue is available on a critical clinical specimen, tissue can be retrieved and prepared for TEM using the methods listed in the Appendix (*see* p. 502). Although preservation will certainly not be optimal, retrieval can offer insight into the presence of inclusion bodies in chondrocytes from biopsies or pathology specimens in cases in which skeletal dysplasias are suspected.

B. Fixation Methods, Decalcification and Embedding

Although mechanical saw or blade cutting of bone is necessary in order to allow fixative penetration into dense bone, these preparative techniques usually cause artifacts.

From: *Handbook of Histology Methods for Bone and Cartilage*
Edited by: Y. H. An and K. L. Martin © Humana Press Inc., Totowa, NJ

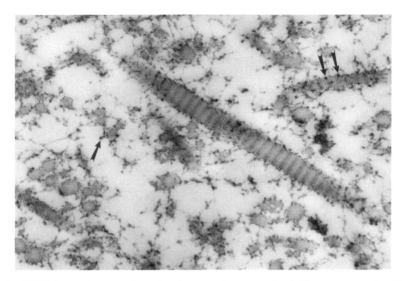

Figure 1. TEM from the annulus of a human intervertebral disc processed with ruthenium red to enhance proteoglycans. Proteoglycans appear as dark dots (arrows). Magnification ×43,660.

Perfusion techniques for animal specimens can achieve good fixation, but require additional harvest time and equipment. Traditional primary fixation with glutaraldehyde/paraformaldehyde fixatives and secondary (post-) fixation with osmium tetroxide work well with bone and cartilage if the specimen has been trimmed into small cubes to allow adequate fixative penetration. Embryonic chick bone has successfully been fixed with acrolein vapors for TEM examination.[26]

The organic matrix of bone was tested by Bonucci and Silvestrini[6] following *en bloc* treatment with acetone solutions of $KMnO_4$, and aqueous or alcoholic solutions of phosphotungstic acid or uranyl acetate, with special attention to woven bone. Extraction of proteoglycans, especially in cartilage and intervertebral disc tissue, can be overcome by specialized application of cationic stains, which can be combined with osmium tetroxide.[27,36] Ruthenium hexamine trichloride, evaluated for the preservation of avian physeal cartilage,[30] was found to be consistent and to provide good overall fixation. We routinely use ruthenium red in our processing of human intervertebral disc tissue to gain a better appreciation of proteoglycan content (Fig. 1). Shepard and Mitchell[38] found that osmium-potassium ferrocyanide fixation afforded improved chondrocyte preservation and stabilization of cartilage proteoglycans. As noted by Hunziker et al.,[21] it is important to test whether dye-proteoglycan complexes continue to be stable during post-fixation processing steps.

The pre-embedding decalcification most often used today traditionally employs ethylenediaminetetraacetic acid (EDTA). As with any decalcification of bone or calcified cartilage specimens, it is important that complete decalcification be achieved prior to embedding. A variety of embedding resins popular with specific laboratories have successfully been used for bone and cartilage studies. In our laboratory, Spurr's resin, with its ability to achieve various hardness formulations, is the resin routinely used. Other methods have been reviewed by Dickson.[14] Fig. 2 illustrates a human chondrocyte with

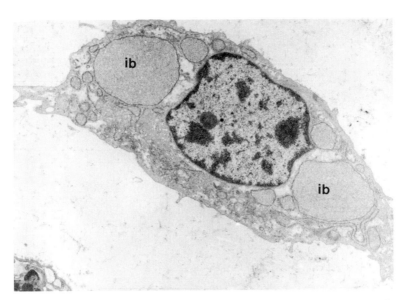

Figure 2. TEM of a human chondrocyte in resting cartilage. Large inclusion bodies (ib) are indicative of the achondrogenesis II-hypochondrogenesis spectrum of chondrodysplasias. Magnificaiton ×7,600.

large inclusion bodies characteristic of the achondrogenesis II-hypochondrogenesis type of chondrodysplasia.

Important specialized techniques are also available for the examination of bone and cartilage. Cryoultramicrotomy of bone and cartilage, as well as high-pressure freezing, freeze substitution, and low-temperature-embedding methods,[20] require specialized specimen preparative techniques and microtomy systems.[5,19,23] Ultrathin cryosections can also be used in conjunction with quantitative electron-probe analysis to provide analysis of cytoplasmic and matrix levels of Ca, K, Cl, S, P, Mg, and Na.[17] Hunziker et al. have used cryotechniques to examine adult human articular cartilage,[22] which offered an improved visualization of the collagen fibrillar network.

III. METHODS FOR SEM STUDIES OF BONE AND CARTILAGE

A. General Applications

Boyde has summarized many of the methodologies for the examination of bone and cartilage with SEM.[7,9,10] SEM examination of bone can be carried out either with marrow and bone cells intact or following removal of marrow and cellular elements to expose the bone surface. The latter can be easily achieved by taking a fixed specimen, rinsing it three times in distilled water (15 min/rinse), placing the specimen in 5% sodium hypochlorite, and shaking it for 1 h. After the bleach step, examination with a dissecting scope helps to determine whether further incubation is required. The specimen is then ready for further processing, either by critical-point drying or other chemical methods. Regions of resorption appear as scalloped depressions (Fig. 3), and endosteal surfaces with no bone turnover appear smooth (Fig. 4).

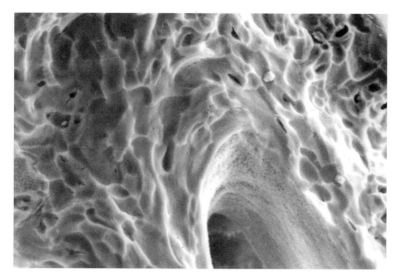

Figure 3. SEM of a bone specimen following removal of marrow and bone cells. Numerous scalloped pits mark sites of bone resorption. Magnification ×560.

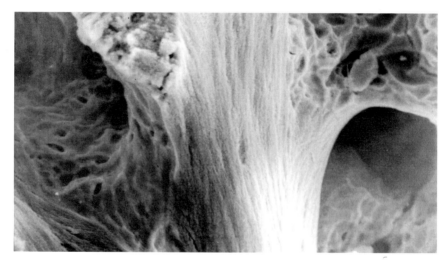

Figure 4. SEM of a bone specimen following removal of marrow and bone cells. The central portion of the micrograph shows a large, smooth expanse of neutral bone surface. Magnification ×350.

Scanning studies require that specimens be trimmed to a size that can be examined in the SEM chamber. Our routine processing uses specimens fixed in 2.5% glutaraldehyde in 0.1 M phosphate buffer, rinsed three times in phosphate buffer, 15 min each change, bleached to remove cellular components as described previously, if desired, and dehydrated through graded acetones (30%, 50%, 70%, 90%, and three 100% changes, 15 min each). The specimen is then ready for critical-point drying, mounting, and sputter-coat application.

B. Application of SEM to the Study of the Bone Surface and Bone Cells

The surface topography of bone made visible with SEM provides an exciting way to visualize the past metabolic activity of the bone cells over relatively large bone surfaces (Fig. 3). Bone surfaces undergoing resorption show scalloped pits; sites of bone formation exhibit "knobby projections" in sites of mineralization. The surface of quiescent bone appears smooth. Marks et al.[28] made use of these attributes in their SEM study of alveolar bone involved in tooth eruption. Reid has used bone-surface characterization in an aging study of the endosteal features of the human rib.[33,34] SEM has also been used to detect fatigue fractures.[39] The often-aggressive surface cleaning of anthropologic bone specimens can often introduce artifacts,[12] and the value of a more gentle cleaning procedure for such specimens is suggested.

Experimental application of SEM in the study of bone resorption has made use of examination and/or quantification of the resorption pits formed by osteoclasts in vitro. As noted by Jones et al., this is an important tool for osteoclast studies because the technique enables the investigator to control the type of substrate on which the osteoclasts are plated, and to vary experimental culture conditions and times.[24] An extension of this type of study has been performed using automated three-dimensional (3D) characterization of osteoclast resorption pits using stereoscopic SEM.[16]

The backscattered electron (BSE) detector in SEM is a new tool that allows evaluation of mineral-density distribution patterns within bone. In this methodology, bone is cut and polished (micromilled). The resulting images have a higher spatial resolution than older microradiographs because BSE signals are collected from a thin surface layer.[8,18,34] Reid and Boyde have applied this technique to a study of the rib from humans age 8 wk to 59 yr, and found that the greatest low-density mineral fraction in adult bone was detected in specimens from the oldest subjects.[34] This method thus discriminates between the bone of various age groups.

Preparative methods to examine bone cells with SEM have been published by Abe et al.[1] With their method, bone collagen was removed with EDTA, and the specimen was split to reveal only the cell-surface area.

C. SEM Studies of Cartilage

The SEM of cartilage has been reviewed by Boyde and Jones.[9] Because of its high water content, cartilage presents a challenge for SEM examination. Microwave fixation of articular cartilage has been found to produce good structural preservation with reliable and rapid processing.[35] Specialized methods for high-resolution studies of organic cartilage components have been developed using ruthenium red combined with glutaraldehyde.[37] Freeze fracture and freeze-substitution SEM techniques have been used to evaluate deformation of articular cartilage during loading.[29] Backscatter SEM (BSEM) has been used to examine cell patterns on the articular surface of the rabbit hip and knee. This method improved the ability to study the relationship between surface contour and underlying chondrocytes.[13]

IV. QUANTITATIVE ELEMENTAL ANALYSIS

The application of electron probe X-ray microanalysis in bone and cartilage research has been reviewed.[25,32] For such studies, careful attention is needed for specimen preparation and microprobe calibrations. Boyde and Shapiro analyzed Ca, S, and K in fragments of growth plate.[11] Obrant and Odselium have used energy-dispersive X-ray microanalysis to evaluate the chemical staining features of Goldner's trichrome and von Kossa stains, with special reference to calcium distribution features in human bone biopsies from osteoporotic patients.[31] In other studies of osteoporotic bone, Ca and P contents were found to be similar to levels in control specimens.[4] More recently, energy-dispersive X-ray microanalysis (EDX) of human trabecular bone was compared to neutron activation analysis. EDX was found to be excellent for major bone constituents (Ca and P), but neutron activation was more sensitive for trace element determinations.[2]

APPENDIX I

Retrieval of Specimens from Formalin and Paraffin for TEM Examination

Specimens can be retrieved from a 5-μm *paraffin section* on a slide by removing the paraffin with three 30-min changes of xylene and rehydrating the specimen with graded alcohol changes. Fix the specimen with 2.5% glutaraldehyde overnight, rinse three times with phosphate buffer (15 min each), and post-fix with a 1:1:1 mixture of 3% OsO_4, distilled water, and phosphate buffer for 30 min. Rinse three times, 15 min each, with distilled water, and dehydrate with 15-min changes of acetone in the following concentrations: 50%, 70%, 90%, 100%, 100%, and 100%. Infiltrate in Spurr's and acetone (1:1) for 1 h, 100% Spurr's for 10 min, and 100% Spurr's for 1 h. Embed and polymerize in an oven at 60°C under vacuum for 24 h.

For specimens that have been *stored in formalin,* trim the tissue into 2–3 mm × 0.5–1.0 mm blocks and place in a specimen bottle covered with gauze. Wash in running water overnight, and rinse three times with phosphate buffer, 15 min each change. Post-fix with a 1:1:1 mixture of 3% OsO_4, water, and phosphate buffer for 2 h, rinse three times with distilled water, 15 min each rinse. Dehydrate with 15-min changes of acetone in the following concentrations: 50%, 70%, 90%, 100%, 100%, and 100%. Infiltrate in Spurr's and acetone (1:1) for 1 h, 100% Spurr's for 10 min, and 100% Spurr's for 1 h. Embed and polymerize in an oven at 60°C under vacuum for 24 h.

REFERENCES

1. Abe K, Hashizume H, Ushiki T: An EDTA-KOH method to expose bone cells for scanning electron microscopy. *J Electron Microsc* 41:113–115, 1992.
2. Akesson K, Grynpas MD, Hancock RGV, et al: Energy-dispersive X-ray microanalysis of the bone mineral content in human trabecular bone: a comparison with ICPES and neutron activation analysis. *Calcif Tissue Int* 55:236–239, 1994.
3. Anderson C: *Manual for the Examination of Bone.* CRC Press, Inc., Boca Raton, FL, 1982:81–92.
4. Baslé MF, Mauras Y, Audran M, et al: Concentration of bone elements in osteoporosis. *J Bone Miner Res* 5:41–47, 1990.
5. Boivin G, Morel G, Meunier PJ, et al: Ultrastructural aspects after cryoultramicrotomy of bone tissue and sutural cartilage in neonatal mice calvaria. *Biol Cell* 49:227–230, 1983.
6. Bonucci E, Silvestrini G: Ultrastructure of the organic matrix of embryonic avian bone after en bloc reaction with various electron-dense "stains." *Acta Anat (Basel)* 156:22–33, 1996.
7. Boyde A: Methodology of calcified tissue specimen preparation for scanning electron microscopy. In: Dickson GR, ed: *Methods of Calcified Tissue Preparation.* Elsevier, Amsterdam, The Netherlands, 1984:251–307.

8. Boyde A, Jones SJ: Back-scattered electron imaging of skeletal tissues. *Metabol Bone Dis Rel Res* 5:145–150, 1983.
9. Boyde A, Jones SJ: Scanning electron microscopy of cartilage. In: Hall BK: *Cartilage, Vol. I. Structure, Function, and Biochemistry.* Academic Press, New York, NY, 1983:105–148.
10. Boyde A, Maconnachie E, Reid SA, et al: Scanning electron microscopy in bone pathology: review of methods, potential and applications. *Scanning Electron Microsc* 4:1537–1554, 1986.
11. Boyde A, Shapiro IM: Energy dispersive X-ray elemental analysis of isolated epiphyseal growth plate chondrocyte fragments. *Histochemistry* 69:85–94, 1980.
12. Bromage TG: Interpretation of scanning electron microscopic images of abraded forming bone surfaces. *Am J Phys Anthropol* 64:161–178, 1984.
13. Clark JM, Rudd E: Cell patterns in the surface of rabbit articular cartilage revealed by the backscatter mode of scanning electron microscopy. *J Orthop Res* 9:275–283, 1991.
14. Dickson GR: Chemical fixation and the preparation of calcified tissues for transmission electron microscopy. In: Dickson GR, ed: *Methods of Calcified Tissue Preparation.* Elsevier, Amsterdam, The Netherlands, 1984:79–148.
15. Doty SB, Schofield BH: Ultrahistochemistry of calcified tissues. In: Dickson GR, ed: *Methods of Calcified Tissue Preparation.* Elsevier, Amsterdam, the Netherlands, 1984:149–198.
16. Fuller K, Thong JTL, Breton BC, et al: Automated three-dimensional characterization of osteoclastic resorption lacunae by stereoscopic scanning electron microscopy. *J Bone Miner Res* 9:17–23, 1994.
17. Hargest TE, Gay CV, Schraer H, et al: Vertical distribution of elements in cells and matrix of epiphyseal growth plate cartilage determined by quantitative electron probe analysis. *J Histochem Cytochem* 33:275–286, 1985.
18. Hashizume H, Abe K, Ushiki T: Detection of mineral density on the surface of mouse parietal bones: Backscattered electron imaging of low accelerating voltage scanning electron microscopy. *Arch Histol Cytol* 60:195–204, 1997.
19. Höhling HJ, Krefting ER: Cryopreparation for microprobe analysis of calcified tissue. In: Dickson GR, ed: *Methods of Calcified Tissue Preparation.* Elsevier, Amsterdam, The Netherlands, 1984:219–249.
20. Hunziker EB, Herrmann W, Schnek RK, et al: Cartilage ultrastructure after high pressure freezing, freeze substitution, and low temperature embedding. I. Chondrocyte ultrastructure— Implications for the theories of mineralization and vascular invasion. *J Cell Biol* 98:267–276, 1984.
21. Hunziker EB, Ludi A, Herrmann W: Preservation of cartilage matrix proteoglycans using cationic dyes chemically related to ruthenium hexaammine trichloride. *J Histochem Cytochem* 40:909–917, 1992.
22. Hunziker EB, Michel M, Studer D: Ultrastructure of adult human articular cartilage matrix after cryotechnical processing. *Microsc Res Technol* 37:271–284, 1997.
23. Hunziker EB, Schenk RK: Cryomethods for transmission electron microscopy of calcifying cartilage. In: Dickson GR, ed: *Methods of Calcified Tissue Preparation.* Elsevier, Amsterdam, The Netherlands, 1984:199–218.
24. Jones SJ, Boyde A, Ali NN, et al: Variation in the sizes of resorption lacunae made in vitro. *Scanning Electron Microsc* 4:1571–1580, 1986.
25. Landis WJ: Application of electron probe X-ray microanalysis to calcification studies of bone and cartilage. *Scanning Electron Microsc* 2:555–570, 1979.
26. Landis WJ, Paine MC, Glimcher MJ: Use of acrolein vapors for the anhydrous preparation of bone tissue for electron microscopy. *J Ultrastruct Res* 70:171–180, 1980.
27. Leng CG, Yu Y, Ueda H, et al: The ultrastructure of anionic sites in rat articular cartilage as revealed by different preparation methods and polyethyleneimine staining. *Histochem J* 30:253–261, 1998.

28. Marks SC Jr, Cielinski MJ, Sundquist KT: Bone surface morphology reflects local skeletal metabolism. *Microsc Res Technol* 33:121–127, 1996.
29. Notzli H, Clark J: Deformation of loaded articular cartilage prepared for scanning electron microscopy with rapid freezing and freeze-substitution fixation. *J Orthop Res* 15:76–86, 1997.
30. Nuehring LP, Steffens WL, Rowland GN: Comparison of the ruthenium hexammine trichloride method to other methods of chemical fixation for preservation of avian physeal cartilage. *Histochem J* 23:201–214, 1991.
31. Obrant KJ, Odselius R: Electron microprobe analysis and histochemical examination of the calcium distribution in human bone trabeculae: a methodological study using biopsy specimens from post-traumatic osteopenia. *Ultrastruct Pathol* 7:123–131, 1984.
32. Ozawa HYT: An application of energy-dispersive X-ray microanalysis for the study of biological calcification. *J Histochem Cytochem* 31:210–213, 1983.
33. Reid SA: Micromorphological characterization of normal human bone surfaces as a function of age. *Scanning Microsc* 1:579–597, 1987.
34. Reid SA, Boyde A: Changes in the mineral density distribution in human bone with age: Image analysis using backscattered electrons in the SEM. *J Bone Miner Res* 2:13–22, 1987.
35. Richards RG, Kääb MJ: Microwave-enhanced fixation of rabbit articular cartilage. *J Microsc* 181:269–276, 1995.
36. Sauren YMHF, Mieremet RHP, Groot CG, et al: An electron microscopical study on the presence of proteoglycans in the calcified bone matrix by use of cuprolinic blue. *Bone* 10:287–294, 1989.
37. Segawa K, Takiguchi R: A method for high-resolution scanning electron microscopy of organic cartilaginous components. *J Electron Microsc Techn* 18:203–204, 1991.
38. Shepard N, Mitchell N: Improved chondrocyte morphology and glycogen retention in the secondary center of ossification following osmium-potassium ferrocyanide fixation. *J Electron Microsc Techn* 11:83–89, 1989.
39. Tomlin JL, Lawes TJ, Blunn GW, et al: Fractographic examination of racing greyhound central (navicular) tarsal bone failure surfaces using scanning electron microscopy. *Calcif Tissue Res* 67:260–266, 2000.

35

SEM Methods for Observation
of the Bone-Implant Interface

Masashi Neo and Takashi Nakamura

Department of Orthopaedic Surgery, Kyoto University, Kyoto, Japan

I. INTRODUCTION

There is currently considerable debate concerning implant-bone interfaces, especially on bioactive material-bone interfaces. Bioactive materials are known to bond to bone directly, as proven by conventional histology and mechanical testing, but the precise bonding mechanism is unclear. In order to study the precise mechanism, the ultrastructure of the bioactive material-bone interface has been examined using scanning and transmission electron microscopy (SEM and TEM). These methods provide the proof of direct bonding at the ultrastructural level, as well as additional information that helped in the study of the mechanism of bone bonding.

Two methods have been used for the observation of the implant-bone interface using SEM. One is to observe the fractured surface (Fig. 1A).[3,4,6,7] In this method, the implanted bone is first excised, fixed, and freeze-fractured in liquid nitrogen. If the focus is on the mineral component, treatment with a 5–10% solution of sodium hypochlorite (NaOCl) dissolves both the cells and the organic component, exposing the surface of the mineral component.[1] The specimen is then dehydrated, dried at the critical point, and coated with carbon and/or gold. Then the exposed surface across the material-bone interface is examined using SEM. In this method, the changes of the material surface in vivo can be observed. For example, material surface degradation, deposition of some proteins or calcium phosphate (CaP) crystals, or a new layer formed by chemical changes to the material surface in vivo can be studied. The adsorption of cells and their structural characteristics, or the pattern of bone formation on the material surface, can also be observed. Similarly, a surface detached by a mechanical test can be analyzed.[2,5,10] After bone is detached from the material, the exposed surface of the material is fixed, dehydrated, dried at the critical point, coated, and observed using SEM. In the case of bioactive materials, a bone portion sometimes bonds to the material even after detachment, and the material-bone interface can be studied.

Another method is to observe the surface cut perpendicular to the interface (Fig. 1B).[8,9,11–16] Embedding the material-bone complex into a resin makes the cutting possible without destroying the interface. Although this method provides only a two-dimensional

From: *Handbook of Histology Methods for Bone and Cartilage*
Edited by: Y. H. An and K. L. Martin © Humana Press Inc., Totowa, NJ

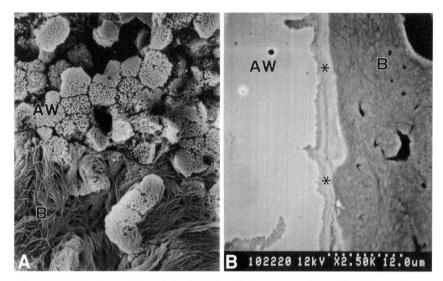

Figure 1. (A) SEM observation of the interface between apatite- and wollastonite-containing glass-ceramic (A-W GC "AW") and mouse bone "B" 4 wk after implantation. (Original magnification ×3000). The specimen was prepared by a fracture method with hypochlorite (NaOC1) treatment. This figure demonstrates surface structural change of A-W GC, and the collage fiber pattern of new bone formed on the material. (This photo was contributed by Masahiro Kokaji, M.D., Department of Orthopaedic Surgery, Bibai Rosai Hospital, Japan). (B) SEM observation of the interface between A-W GC "AW" and rat bone "B" 8 wk after implantation. (Original magnification ×2500). Direct material—bone bonding through a CaP-rich layer (asterisks) is demonstrated.

(2D) image, it enables us to observe the change from the depths of the material to the surface and then to bone, continuously. This is particularly important in studying the surface-active materials because they bond to bone through a CaP rich layer (apatite layer) formed on the surface in vivo. If an energy-dispersive electron probe X-ray microanalyzer (EDX) is utilized, the elemental analysis across the interface gives more precise information. The sample preparation is also quite easy and reproducible, and is different from the first method, in which the obtained images depend on the accidentally formed interfaces by fracture or detachment. Therefore, the second method is preferred, and is the focus of this chapter. Many types of bioactive and resorbable materials have been studied using this method.

II. SAMPLE PREPARATION

The bone-implant complex is excised and trimmed. It is then fixed, dehydrated, defatted, and embedded in polyester resin according to the manufacturer's instructions. The following is the procedure used in our laboratory. The duration of each step depends on the size of the specimens. For example, for rat tibia it takes 1 d, and for dog femur it takes several days for each step.

A. Fixation, Dehydration, Defatting

1. Fix in 10% phosphate-buffered formalin solution (3–10 d).
2. Wash in running water (12–24 h).
3. Trim the specimen if necessary.

  4. 70% ethanol.
  5. 80% ethanol.
  6. 90% ethanol.
  7. 99% ethanol.
  8. 100% ethanol (with copper sulfate (II) anhydrate) (first change).
  9. 100% ethanol (with copper sulfate (II) anhydrate) (second change).
 10. Styrene 50% + ethanol 50%.
 11. Styrene 80% + ethanol 20%.
 12. Styrene 100% (1).
 13. Styrene 100% (2).

The following steps (14–17) are carried out at 4°C.

 14. Polyester resin 50% + styrene 50%.
 15. Polyester resin 80% + styrene 20%.
 16. Polyester resin 100% (first change).
 17. Polyester resin 100% (second change).

B. Embedding

  1. In a tissue-embedding mold (Peel-A-Way®, Polysciences, Inc.), pour polyester resin (with polymerization initiator) to the height of about 5 mm and polymerize it at 60°C (1–2 d) in advance.
  2. Put the specimen into the prepared mold and pour polyester resin (with polymerization initiator) over the specimen until it is covered completely. Polymerize the resin at 37°C for 1 d, then 60°C for 2 d.
  3. Remove the hardened specimen from the mold.

C. Cutting and Polishing

  1. Cross-sections (0.5–3 mm in thickness) are made using a band saw (BS-3000, Exakt, Norderstedt, Germany) so that the material-bone interface is exposed to the cutting surface.
  2. The surface of the sections are polished to a mirror surface using #400, #1000, and #2000 abrasive paper, 3-µm diamond paste, and 1-µm diamond paste in that order. This step is important in order to get a clear SEM image.

D. Observation Using SEM

  1. The specimen is attached to an aluminum holder with double-sided adhesive tape.
  2. Sufficient silver paste is applied to the side of the specimen to earth the electric charge.
  3. The specimen is coated with a thin layer of carbon in an evaporator. If EDX is to be used to perform the analysis, avoid coating with gold because a peak of phosphate is indistinguishable from a peak of gold. If not, coating with gold is easier and also works well.
  4. Observe the specimen with conventional SEM according to the manufacturer's instructions. A backscattered image may provide a clearer image without electron charge.
  5. Elemental analysis is also performed with EDX according to the manufacturer's instructions. An electron beam is maintained at 2×10^{-10} amp, and the accelerating voltage is 12 kV.

III. EXAMPLES OF THE SEM OBSERVATION OF THE MATERIAL—BONE INTERFACE

Fig. 2A demonstrates the interface between Bioglass®-type glass and rat bone at 8 wk after the material particles were implanted. Bioglass® is a surface-active material that bonds to bone directly through a CaP-rich layer. This layer is formed on the material surface after implantation by chemical change of the surface. The figure shows that

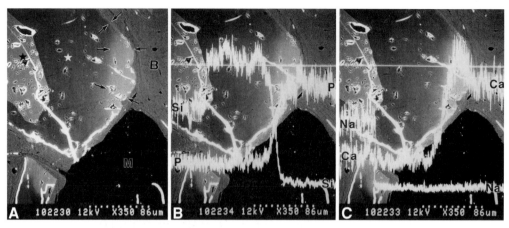

Figure 2. SEM (A) and SEM-EDX (B, C) of the interface between Bioglass®-type glass and rat bone "B" 8 wk after implantation. (B) elemental analysis of Si and P, and (C) that of Ca and Na. Three layers, namely a CaP-rich layer (between arrows), a Si-rich layer (white asterisk), and the original glass (black asterisk) are demonstrated. M: bone marrow.

Bioglass®-type glass bonds to bone without intervention of soft tissue. Bone is demonstrated as a feathery matrix containing osteocyte lacunae and bone canaliculi. Three distinct layers are also clearly demonstrated in the material—from the surface to the center of the material: a gray layer, a dark layer, and the original core material. A line elemental analysis by EDX (Fig. 2B,C) demonstrates that the gray layer is Ca- and P-rich with a low content of silicon (Si), corresponding to a CaP-rich layer, whereas the dark layer is Si-rich with low Ca and P content—a Si-rich layer.

Fig. 3 demonstrates a β-tricalcium phosphate (TCP)-rat bone interface 8 wk after implantation. TCP is an absorbable material, and it is gradually absorbed and replaced by bone when it is implanted into bone. The figure demonstrates that TCP makes direct contact to bone without a CaP-rich layer different from surface-active materials. It also shows how the material is absorbed in bone, retaining its direct contact with bone. The surface of the material is fragmented into small pieces, but bone grows into the very fine surface irregularities thus formed without soft-tissue interposition.

Fig. 4 demonstrates the interface between apatite- and wollastonite-containing glass-ceramic (A-W GC) and rat bone 96 wk after implantation. The A-W GC is also a surface-active material and bonds to bone through a CaP-rich layer (Fig. 1B). The figure demonstrates a mixture of the CaP-rich layer and bone at the interface, suggesting that the CaP-rich layer has been gradually replaced by bone. However, EDX showed that this intermingled zone had the same elemental level as the bone.

IV. DISCUSSION AND CONCLUSION

Generally speaking, SEM features the ability to demonstrate the three-dimensional (3D) image of the surface of specimens, and ground or polished sections have little place in the procedure. Further, cutting and polishing procedures damage the details of the surface. However, as demonstrated here, the SEM method becomes a strong weapon when

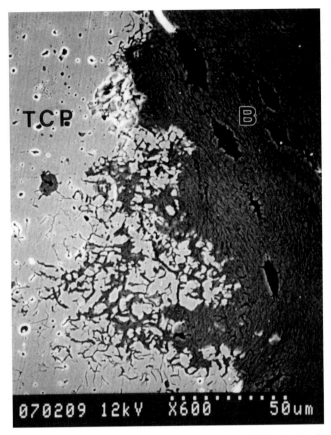

Figure 3. SEM of the interface between TCP and rat bone "B" 8 wk after implantation. The surface is fragmented into small pieces, demonstrating material degradation. Bone has grown into fine surface irregularities, suggesting bone remodeling.

analyzing the material-bone interface, especially when it is used with EDX apparatus. It clearly shows not only direct bonding between material and bone at the ultrastructural level, but also chronological changes occurring at the interface in vivo. For example, the formation of a Si-rich layer or CaP-rich layer, surface degradation of the material, replacement of the material with bone (remodeling), and so on. These findings are important in studying the behavior of many types of materials in vivo, clarifying the bonding mechanism and bioactivity of the materials.

Another advantage of this method is its reproducibility. Specimen preparation is quite easy, and many interfaces can be observed from one specimen. On the contrary, the observation of a fractured or detached surface depends on the accidentally exposed interface, which makes the results less convincing.

However, a major disadvantage of this method is the impossibility to observe cells and soft tissue. Therefore, observation of early biological reaction around material, such as cell (macrophages, mesenchymal cells, osteoblasts, and so on) adsorption or osteoid formation, is not possible. Nonbioactive material-bone interfaces, in which some kinds of cells or fibrous tissue intervene, are also poor candidates for this method.

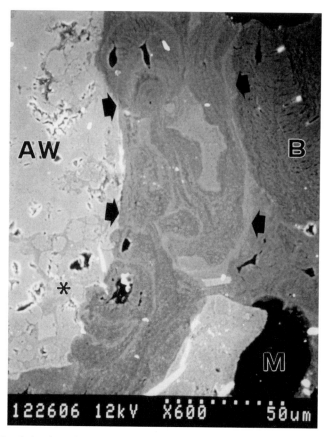

Figure 4. SEM of the interface between A-W GC "AW" and rat bone "B" 96 wk after implantation. An intermingled layer of the material and bone (between arrows) is evident between them, suggesting that the CaP-rich layer (asterisk) is absorbed and replaced by bone in the same way as for bone remodeling. M: bone marrow.

As shown in Fig. 1, the images obtained are strikingly different between the two methods, which results in confusion in the interpretation and causes some debate concerning the material-bone interface. Therefore, deliberate further analysis is necessary, hopefully using both SEM methods and other methods such as TEM.

In conclusion, SEM observation of a cut and polished surface across the material-bone interface is a useful method especially for analyzing the bioactive material-bone interface.

REFERENCES

1. Boyde A: Scanning electron microscope studies of bone. In: Bourne GH, ed: *The Biochemistry and Physiology of Bone, Vol. I.* Academic Press, New York, NY, 1972:259.
2. Davies JE, Nagai N, Takeshita N, et al: Deposition of cement-like matrix on implant materials. In: Davies JE, ed: *The Bone-Biomaterial Interface.* University of Toronto Press, Toronto, Canada, 1991:285.
3. Davies JE, Baldan N: Scanning electron microscopy of the bone-bioactive implant interface. *J Biomed Mater Res* 36:429–440, 1997.

4. de Bruijn JD, Davies JE, Klein CPAT, et al: Biological responses to calcium phosphate ceramics. In: Ducheyne P, Kokubo T, van Blitterswijk CA, eds: *Bone-Bonding Biomaterials.* Reed Healthcare Communications, Leiderdorp, The Netherlands, 1992:57.
5. Edwards JT, Brunski JB, Higuchi HW: Mechanical and morphological investigation of the tensile strength of a bone-hydroxyapatite interface. *J Biomed Mater Res* 36:454–468, 1997.
6. Gross UM, Muller-Mai C, Voigt C: Comparative morphology of the bone interface with glass ceramics, hydroxyapatite, and natural coral. In: Davies JE, ed: *The Bone-Biomaterial Interface.* University of Toronto Press, Toronto, Canada, 1991:308.
7. Hench LL, Clark AE: Adhesion to bone. In: Williams DF, ed: *Biocompatibility of Orthopedic Implants, Vol. 2.* Franklin Book Co., Elkins, PA, 1981:129.
8. Kitsugi T, Nakamura T, Yamamuro T, et al: SEM-EPMA observation of three types of apatite-containing glass-ceramics implanted in bone: the variance of a Ca-P-rich layer. *J Biomed Mater Res* 21:1255–1277, 1987.
9. Kobayashi M, Shinzato S, Kawanabe K, et al: Alumina powder/Bis-GMA composite: effect of filler content on mechanical properties and osteoconductivity. *J Biomed Mater Res* 49:319–327, 2000.
10. Nakamura T, Yamamuro T, Higashi S, et al: A new glass-ceramic for bone replacement: evaluation of its bonding to bone tissue. *J Biomed Mater Res* 19:685–698, 1985.
11. Neo M, Kotani S, Fujita Y, et al: Differences in ceramic-bone interface between surface-active ceramics and resorbable ceramics: a study by scanning and transmission electron microscopy. *J Biomed Mater Res* 26:255–267, 1992.
12. Neo M, Kotani S, Nakamura T, et al: A comparative study of ultrastructures of the interfaces between four kinds of surface-active ceramic and bone. *J Biomed Mater Res* 26:1419–1432, 1992.
13. Neo M, Nakamura T, Ohtsuki C, et al: Ultrastructural study of the A-W GC-bone interface after long-term implantation in rat and human bone. *J Biomed Mater Res* 28:365–372, 1994.
14. Ohura K, Nakamura T, Yamamuro T, et al; Bone-bonding ability of P_2O_5-free $CaO \bullet SiO_2$ glasses. *J Biomed Mater Res* 25:357–365, 1991.
15. Ohura K, Nakamura T, Yamamuro T, et al: Bioactivity of $CaO \bullet SiO_2$ glasses added with various ions. *J Mater Sci Med Mater* 3:95, 1992.
16. Shinzato S, Kobayashi M, Mousa WF, et al: Bioactive polymethyl methacrylate-based bone cement: comparison of glass beads, apatite- and wollastonite-containing glass-ceramic, and hydroxyapatite fillers on mechanical and biological properties. *J Biomed Mater Res* 51:258–272, 2000.

36

TEM Methods for Observation
of the Bone-Implant Interface

Joseph Hemmerlé

Institut National de la Santé et de la Recherche Médicale U424, Strasbourg, France

I. INTRODUCTION

Numerous alloplastic biomaterials, ranging from bone-grafting materials to joint replacement prostheses, have been developed for the treatment of skeletal deficiencies. A literature survey shows that sustained efforts have been made to evaluate the biological and biophysical processes occurring at the bone-implant interface. One can also note the growing demand of clinicians to visualize the host response and to analyze the long-term behavior of the implanted biomaterials. Thus, the microstructural features of the bone-implant interface receive the eager attention of electron microscopists. Indeed, transmission electron microscopy (TEM) allows the histological, crystallographic, and chemical characterization of the interfaces, thus enabling a better understanding of the bone-bonding mechanism. However, electron microscopy methods used in the field of implantology cannot merely be drawn in the form of a sole and permanent protocol, mainly for two reasons: first, there are almost as many types of interface as there are variations of prosthetic devices; second, technical improvements and up-to-date preparation methods are regularly published. Moreover, the study of the bone-implant interface is an interdisciplinary subject involving the physicians, biologists, and physicists. This chapter will focus on the major microscopy-related aspects of the bone-implant interface. First, several biomaterials as well as the osseointegration process are considered briefly. Second, the available TEM methods, including fixation, embedding and sectioning are fully discussed. Third, rational and proven preparation methods, supplemented by technical hints and tips, are suggested and illustrated.

II. THE BONE-IMPLANT INTERFACE

A. Various Implant Materials

Among the numerous available biomaterials used for bone repair, only the following classes, of paramount interest, will be taken into account for the discussion of TEM preparation methods.

1. Synthetic and Natural Ceramics

Synthetic calcium phosphates (CaPs) present a compositional resemblance to the mineral phase of the bone tissue. Particular attention has been given to hydroxyapatite corresponding

From: *Handbook of Histology Methods for Bone and Cartilage*
Edited by: Y. H. An and K. L. Martin © Humana Press Inc., Totowa, NJ

to the chemical formula $Ca_{10}(PO_4)_6(OH)_2$ with a molar ratio of 10/6. CaPs have been successfully used as bone-defect fillers.[36] Hydroxyapatite has even been used in association with collagen and glycosaminoglycans (GAGs) to form a composite bone-filling biomaterial.[21,45] Ogiso et al.[37] report a chemical bonding between newly formed bone and a dense hydroxyapatite dental implant. Although CaPs are mostly used to fill bone cavities, a machinable and uniformly microporous hydroxyapatite usable in dental surgery has been reported.[47] However, hydroxyapatite can be employed for the coating, by plasma spraying, of metal implants to produce a physical barrier against metal ion release.[48] Augat et al.[4] investigated the effectiveness of hydroxyapatite-coated bone screws used for external fixation of fractures. CaP coatings, which are believed to enhance biocompatibility and to produce a fast bony adaptation, can also be obtained successfully by other deposition means such as the pulsed laser deposition process[54] or the ion-beam-assisted deposition method.[12]

Natural aragonite has been tested as a bone-graft substitute, and found to be a biocompatible, biodegradable, and osteoconductive material.[30] These conclusions are supported by clinical evaluations of coralline calcium carbonate used as a bone replacement material in periodontal defects.[53] The combination of natural coral with GAGs also shows promise for regeneration therapy in orthopedics and dentistry.[51] Camprasse et al.[9] even claim that artificial dental roots machined from non-biodegradable natural calcium carbonate are exceptional substitutes that match the biological properties of natural bone.

2. Titanium and Titanium Alloy

Commercially pure titanium, a corrosive-resistant metal, and Ti-6Al-4V, a titanium alloy having superior mechanical properties, are commonly used metal implants. An extremely adherent passivation oxide film, about 5 nm in thickness, forms spontaneously at a titanium-air or titanium-water interface.[42] The biocompatibility of titanium in clinical use is a result of the surface oxide layer, which is very resistant against chemical attack. According to Hanawa,[20] CaP forms naturally at the passive oxide surface layers of titanium and its alloys immersed in a neutral electrolyte solution. Moreover, Ellingsen[17] suggests that the calcium from the body fluids which reacts with a titanium oxide film may be a possible mechanism for the initial adsorption of macromolecules onto titanium implants The surfaces of titanium implants are usually polished, textured, or covered with a porous coating.[10] The latter coating can be achieved by plasma-spraying, either with CaPs[25] or with titanium hydride.[13]

B. Bone Bonding to Biomaterials

It is expected that any bone implant, regardless of its nature, type, or design, will be well-integrated in the surrounding bone tissue. That condition could be summarized by the statement of Brånemark,[8] considering that osseointegration involves a direct structural connection between bone and the surface of endosteal devices. Nevertheless, it is important to remember that the bony mineralized matrix is an ordered mineral-organic composite material with a complex hierarchical structure and that an adaptive bone remodeling does occur with time. Thus, the description of bone anchorage strongly depends on implantation period as well as on the investigation level—i.e., clinical, radiographic, histologic, or crystallographic.

The fact remains that the bone-bonding process has been documented in TEM since it became possible to achieve ultrathin sections of intact bone-implant interfaces. For example, in the case of calcium phosphate ceramics, Piattelli et al.[40] state that an organic bonding between hydroxyapatite and bone may be hypothesized, whereas Oguchi et al.[39] mention either bone directly bound to hydroxyapatite ceramics or the presence of an intervening electron-dense material at the interface. Ogiso et al.[38] show a chemical bonding between a dense hydroxyapatite dental implant and human bone after long-term use, and Kotani et al.[28] suggest a micro-anchoring mechanism between β-tricalcium phosphate and bone. Concerning titanium-based implants, TEM reports dealing with intact metal-implant interfaces are scarce. In a study of the titanium-bone interface in rat tibiae, Murai et al.[35] observed a thin amorphous zone, a slender cell layer, and/or a poorly mineralized zone interposed between the titanium surface and lamellar bone, whereas Leize et al.[29] observed CaP crystallites within a porous surface layer made of titanium grains, which they interpreted as a bone ingrowth process.

C. A Wide Range of Approaches

TEM assessments of implanted ceramics do not present insurmountable difficulties, because laboratories where ultrathin preparation techniques and skills for mineralized tissues are available are also in a position to treat ceramic-bone interfaces. More rarely, some preparation methods recommend a demineralization stage for the removal of the ceramic material prior to ultrathin sectioning, when artifacts caused by the presence of a dense implant are suspected.[15] On the contrary, overwhelming difficulties are encountered when ultrathin investigations are to be carried out on metal-bone interfaces. For that reason, several technical strategies that are sometimes unorthodox have been employed to overcome the thinning of implant materials. In 1983, Linder et al.[31] used machined polycarbonate covered by evaporation with a 120–250-nm-thick layer of pure titanium as implants. Some years later, Albrektsson and Hansson[1] employed a similar method, but covered plastic plugs with a 100-nm-thick layer of titanium by using the sputtering technique. Listgarten et al.[32] fabricated epoxy resin replicas from cylindrical titanium implants with a plasma-sprayed apical portion. These replicas were then coated with a 90–120-nm-thick layer of titanium using an electron-beam evaporator. Sennerby et al.[44] employed an electropolishing procedure to electrochemically dissolve the bulk metal of retrieved titanium implants, leaving the surface oxide layer in the surrounding biological tissues and thus allowing further sectioning for TEM. In 1993, Steflik et al.[49] used a cryofracture method to separate endosteal dental implant material from the adjacent tissues. Sections 500 nm thick obtained from the interfacial tissues previously lining the implant surface were then examined in a high-voltage electron microscope operating with an accelerating voltage of 1 MV. Another attempt consisted of first separating the bone tissue from the titanium implant material, which is subsequently replaced by epoxy-embedding resin to protect the interfacial zone before ultrathin sectioning.[46]

III. ACHIEVEMENT OF ULTRATHIN INTACT INTERFACES

This section has two goals: to provide a step-by-step presentation of straightforward electron microscopy preparation methods, and to get acquainted with methods specifically related to ultrathin sectioning of intact bone-implant interfaces.

A. Recommended Fixation

Optimal fixation is the prerequisite for the preservation of ultrastructural details. A biopsy composed of an implanted material with the surrounding bone tissue should be as small as possible, and must undergo immediate primary fixation. A solution of 2% paraformaldehyde and 2% glutaraldehyde buffered at pH 7.4 with 0.1 *M* sodium cacodylate constitutes a well-tried primary fixative. Formaldehyde, obtained by depolymerizing powdered paraformaldehyde, is advisable for its fast penetration rate and glutaraldehyde, a dialdehyde, because it is an effective crosslinking agent for proteins, thus stabilizing tissue structures. Cacodylate buffer inhibits microbial growth. Duration of fixation depends on the volume to be infiltrated. When fixation is carried out at room temperature, it is generally accepted that the penetration rate is in the order of 1 mm/h. In other words, aldehyde fixation time, in hours, corresponds roughly to the radius, expressed in millimeters, of the biopsy. This indication can be lengthened somewhat without deleterious effects at the morphologic point of view. Nevertheless, according to Massa and Arana-Chavez,[33] processing time can be significantly reduced (two periods of 20 s each) and preservation of mineralizing tissues remains excellent when microwave irradiation is employed. The fixative solution should be freshly prepared. After primary fixation, the specimens are rinsed three times (20 min each change) in 0.1 *M* cacodylate buffer solution. Secondary fixation is performed in 1% osmium tetroxide in 0.1 *M* cacodylate buffer for periods ranging from 30 min to 2 h, depending on the size of the specimen. An exaggerated post-fixation time tends to make samples brittle. Osmium tetroxide particularly reacts with lipids, thus having the advantage of revealing cellular membranes under the electron microscope. However, it has the drawback of turning tissues black, which may complicate specimen orientation for further sectioning

B. Embedding Procedure

The goal of this stage is to bring the biopsy to a non-aqueous state, to infiltrate it with a fluid resin, and finally to harden the resin-penetrated specimen to produce a solid and sectionable block. Dehydration is performed in a series of graded ethanol solutions. The dehydration agent is then replaced by propylene oxide (1,2-epoxypropane) to gradually infiltrate the specimen with epoxy-embedding resin. However, as the transitional solvent (propylene oxide) may dissolve polymer biomaterials or substrates, some authors suggest replacing it with butyl-2,3-epoxypropylether[6] or with ethanol.[52] Epoxy resins are often used since they cause little shrinkage and offer adequate stability under the electron beam. Toughness of the embedding medium must be adapted to the hardness of the specimen to be sectioned. For ceramic and metallic biomaterials as well as for hard tissues, the "B" mixture (refer to supplied instructions) of Epon 812 resin is indicated. Several precautions must be taken when preparing and curing Epon 812 embedding resin:

- Thoroughly mix the different ingredients without introducing air bubbles.
- Cure the embedded specimen very slowly (four temperature stages).
- Although batches of embedding medium may be stored frozen for several weeks at –20°C in tightly capped disposable syringes, freshly prepared epoxy blends should be used whenever possible.

Fig. 1 shows the presence of holes in a trimmed epoxy block, resulting from inappropriate stirring and too quickly curing the resin. An embedded specimen like this would be very difficult to section. The following dehydration, infiltration, and polymerization schedule has proven satisfactory for bone-implant interfaces:

1. Dehydrate in a graded series of ethanol (50%, 70%, 90%, 100%, and 100%, for 15 min each).
2. Replace absolute ethanol by propylene oxide (two rinses of 15 min each).

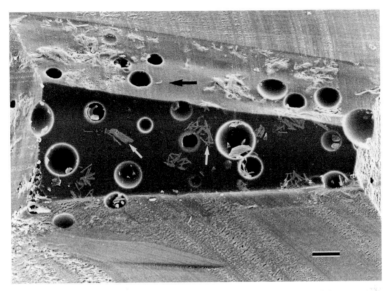

Figure 1. Scanning electron micrograph of hydroxyapatite powder (white arrows) embedded in Epon 812 resin. Note the presence of numerous spherical holes resulting from air bubbles introduced by too energetic mixing of the ingredients. The darker trapezoidal area corresponds to the sectioning plane of the trimmed block. Black arrow indicates cutting direction. Bar = 100 μm.

3. Place specimen in 1:1 (by volume) mixture of propylene oxide and embedding resin in covered vials for several hours. Epon 812 resin is blended as follows:
   a. 20 mL of Epon resin (glycerol-based aliphatic epoxy resin).
   b. 18 mL of hardener (nadic methyl anhydride).
   c. 1.7% (v/v) of DMP-30 accelerator (2,4,6-tri(dimethylaminomethyl) phenol).
   d. Accelerator is added just before use. Resin is mixed thoroughly but carefully!
4. Mount vials on a slow speed rotator for 24 h, leaving them uncovered to allow propylene oxide to evaporate.
5. Transfer the specimens to gelatin capsules or pyramid-shaped polyethylene molds filled with freshly prepared embedding resin and leave at room temperature for 24 h.
6. Place embedding medium-infiltrated specimens in an oven for three-step curing (24 h at 35°C, 24 h at 45°C, and 24 h at 60°C).

C. Ultramicrotomy Guidelines

   In TEM, object thickness can be a limiting factor for resolution because the energy losses of electrons passing through the specimen induce chromatic spreading. A sample is usable if its thickness is below 100 nm for conventional TEM and measures only a few tens of nanometers for high-resolution TEM. However, it is important to note that for specimens of the same thickness, the transmitted intensity decreases with the atomic number of the irradiated area. This is of paramount interest when considering microscopic evaluations of interfaces. Ultramicrotomy is a technique that produces very thin slices by a direct cutting procedure using a diamond knife. It is routinely and successfully employed for the sectioning of all types of biological tissues. Nevertheless, several research groups introduced that slicing tool for specimen preparation of many diverse

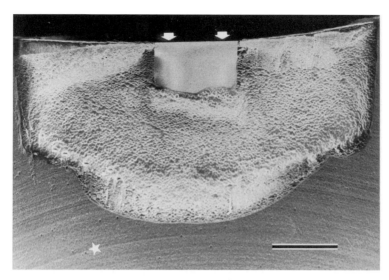

Figure 2. Scanning electron micrograph of a diamond knife with a size of 1.2 mm. Arrows show the cutting edge, and the star represents the bottom of the reservoir. Bar = 1 mm.

materials. In that way, Frank et al.[18] investigated the gingival reaction to gold foil restorations, and Ehret et al.[16] evaluated leached glasses. Diamond knives with different edge angles are commercially available. For routine work, knives are manufactured with an angle of 45°, for sectioning hard materials such as ceramics cutting edges of 55° are used, and for ductile metals a 35° angle is usually suggested. For instance, Jésior[26] states that a low-angle (28.6°) diamond knife strongly diminishes curling of copper sections. On the other hand, personal experience revealed that a 45° knife edge is usable for hard tissues, for CaP ceramics[23,24] and for titanium implants.[22,29] Fig. 2 shows the sectioning facet of a typical diamond knife. When using a diamond knife, it is highly recommended that the trimmed block face have a width less than one-half the length of the cutting edge. This allows three-step wearing of the diamond edge. During the first period, only the left part of the knife will be used, then the right half will be employed and finally the middle area of the knife edge will be put into service. The knife trough is generally filled with distilled water, which has a surface tension that is adequate for floating ultrathin sections prior to collecting them on TEM grids. The trough liquid must be precisely level with the knife edge. If the tip of the sectioning facet (Fig. 2) of the diamond remains dry the resulting sections will be creased. On the other hand, a water level that is too high risks wetting the specimen's surface, which would seriously impair cutting. To prevent demineralization of calcified tissue sections, some authors use a saturated CaP solution as the trough liquid.[7]

Below are listed the major rules to apply for achieving ultrathin preparations of hard biological tissues, ceramics, and metals by using an ultramicrotome:

1. The surface to be sectioned must be as small as possible. When sectioning oxidic thin films on glass, Becker and Bange[5] prepared surfaces as small as 200 μm in width and 300 μm in length.
2. The tip of the trimmed block should end with a plane having a trapezoidal shape (Fig. 1). The knife should first cut the shortest of the parallel sides of the trapeze to begin sectioning with minimal shearing strain. The axis of the interface should be oriented perpendicular to the cutting edge to apply a constant, even stress on the knife.

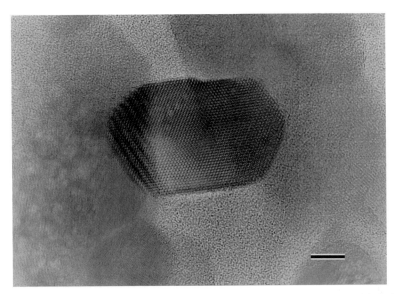

Figure 3. High-resolution TEM micrograph of a hydroxyapatite crystallite with well-faceted hexagonal habit. Bar = 10 nm.

3. To avoid vibration of the block during sectioning, the embedded specimen must be pushed firmly in its holder and locked in place. The block must also be trimmed in the form of a short pyramid with gentle slopes instead of a long rod.
4. Cutting speed must be determined experimentally. An initial speed could be approx 2 mm/s. It is then progressively varied, according to the sectioning behavior, until the most consistent sections are produced.
5. Section quality may be improved by slightly reducing (such as 1° or 2°) the clearance angle value recommended by the manufacturer.

As porous ceramics can be impregnated by the embedding medium, the individual crystals are locked in the polymerized resin and can undergo ultramicrotomy. In this case, the thinning process is more like a cleavage mechanism than real slicing. Ultramicrotomy works well for small-sized crystals (Fig. 3), but it is likely to induce multiple breaks when larger ceramic particles are sectioned, as shown in Fig. 4. It must also be noted that the cutting process may be responsible for the introduction of artificial dislocations in broken particles of the embedded material.[19] A dislocation multiplication process, known as the "Frank-Read" mechanism, may generate numerous concentric dislocations during plastic deformation. These begin from the cutting impact side of the embedded particle and remain mainly located in the outer part of the crystal.[19] The characteristic configuration of these artificial dislocations makes them easily identifiable. Small crystallites are usually free of this highly specific artifact. Despite these artifacts, specimens prepared by ultramicrotomy disclose invaluable information about the bone-ceramic interfaces (Fig. 4). It has been successfully employed for the study of CaP bone-filling materials (Fig. 3) and for the investigation of the interfacial host response after their implantation.[21,24]

For the evaluation of the interface between bone tissue and a plasma-sprayed coating covering a metal implant (Fig. 5), the implementation of a two-stage embedding procedure is necessary.[23]

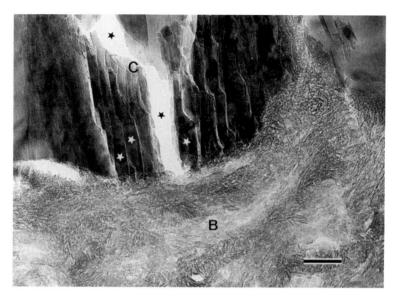

Figure 4. TEM micrograph of a calcium phosphate-bone interface. Note the presence of broken pieces (white stars) and even empty areas (black stars) within the implanted material. C = CaP ceramic. B = bone tissue. Bar = 100 nm.

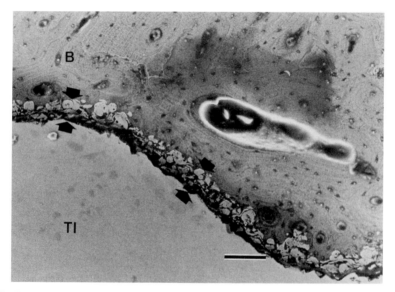

Figure 5. Scanning electron micrograph from a longitudinal section of a hydroxyapatite (between arrows) coated titanium alloy implant (TI) with surrounding bone tissue (B). Bar = 100 μm.

1. The retrieved implant with surrounding calcified bone matrix is fixed and embedded, and then sliced with a wire saw. A metal wire measuring 10 m in length and 0.17 mm in diameter encrusted with 30-μm diamond particles makes successive unwind-rewind cycles (automatic reversal of direction) and applies a very gentle strain to the specimen. The wire is water-cooled, so there are no heating effects on the sliced sample. The slices (about 300 μm thick)

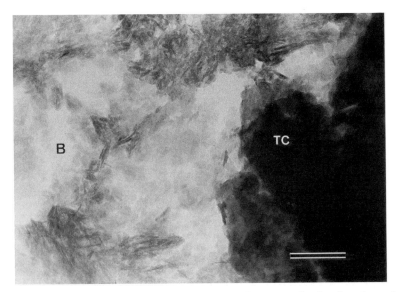

Figure 6. TEM micrograph revealing the interfacial features of a titanium-bone interface. TC = plasma-sprayed titanium coating. B = calcified bone matrix. Bar = 100 nm.

are subsequently cut in half, and are carefully plunged into liquid nitrogen until it stops boiling. The differential thermal expansion of the implant core and the coating shell generally produces a separation at the metal-ceramic interface.[14]
2. The recovered mineralized tissue with the attached CaP coating layer is then re-embedded and processed for further ultrathin sectioning. The specimen to be sectioned corresponds to a classic and intact bone-ceramic interface, as previously discussed.

The previous double-embedding preparation technique can be adapted for the observation of the bone tissue close to plasma-sprayed titanium.[22,29] Fig. 6 discloses the ultrastructural aspects of a titanium coating-bone interface. The re-embedded thin implant-bone slice, obtained by wire-sawing, undergoes very progressive grinding and polishing steps. After removal of the implant bulk metal, the remaining thin layer of titanium coating with the surrounding bone tissue can be prepared for the usual ultramicrotomy. The area to be sectioned should be preferably smaller than 200 μm^2.

D. Specimen Grids and Support Films

1. Specimen Grids

Copper grids consisting of a square array of bars are suitable for the majority of applications. Grids are quoted in bars per inch. A "100-mesh" grid is composed of 100 bars per inch. Its mesh size is thus 250 μm. The higher the mesh value (bars per inch), the better the specimen support, but the smaller the open area left free for viewing in TEM. The latter loss of opening can be compensated by the use of thinner bars. Bar widths usually range from 10 to 50 μm. Generally, one side of the grid has a shiny appearance because of a smooth surface finish, whereas the opposite side appears dull because of a rougher surface. It is good practice to apply the support films onto the matte face of a grid, which offers a larger contact surface compared to the glossy face. In the case of bone-implant sections, 300-mesh grids constitute a reasonable compromise between sufficient mechanical support and adequate transmission area.

2. Plastic Support Films

Although TEM observations can be carried out on ultrathin sections from specimens embedded in epoxy resin, which are mounted directly on grids of small mesh sizes (300 or greater mesh grids), the use of support films is highly recommended for electron microscopy assessments of bone-implant interfaces. These films are believed to enhance the mechanical stability of ultrathin sections, but must remain transparent enough to the electron beam to not hamper the imaging process. Based on personal experience, Formvar® (polyvinyl formal) best matches these criteria. Commercially ready-to-use microfiltered Formvar® solutions in ethylene dichloride are available in different concentrations. The more diluted the solution, the thinner and more transparent the plastic film, but the lower the mechanical strength. Dilutions of approx 0.25% can be considered as all-purpose solutions. The typical procedure is enumerated as follows.

1. Dip a clean, dry microscope slide half its length in the Formvar® solution.
2. Withdraw with a smooth motion and allow to dry for several minutes.
3. Using a razor blade, scrape the edges of the Formvar®-covered half of the glass slide.
4. Float off the polymer film by dipping slowly into a very clean water surface at a sharp angle (between 30° and 40°).
5. Align grids (matte side down) onto the floating film.
6. Place a piece of highly absorbent filter paper on the grid-covered film. When filter paper is saturated with water, catch the sandwiched grid with a pair of tweezers and place in a Petri dish.
7. After air-drying, store the filter paper holding coated grids in a dessiccator.

3. Holey Support Films

Unfortunately, support films superimpose background noise to the visualized structures of a specimen and reduce image contrast. That disadvantage can be overcome by employing holey support films. Fig. 7 clearly shows, at high magnification, the granular aspect of a support film. Holey Formvar® films are obtained by adding some glycerol (glycerol content of 2% for hole diameters expected in the μm range) to the previous Formvar® solution. The mixture is sonicated prior to use. The polymer film, covering the upper side of the glass side, is then exposed to a steam-jet for a minute or so before stripping on water surface. Such perforated support films are employed for high-resolution investigations of the bone-implant interface.[24]

Finally, an amorphous carbon layer is vacuum evaporated onto the continuous or Holey plastic films to reduce electron charge effects. Planarity of support films may be easily checked by using reflected light microscopy.[43]

E. Staining Methods

If only the crystallographic features of the calcified bone matrix at the interface are to be considered, then no further staining of the ultrathin sections is needed.[41] However, when histological aspects of the host response to the implanted material are of interest, then a staining step is needed. The very classic and widely used uranyl acetate followed by lead citrate double-staining is convenient for routine work. In the case of epoxy resin embedding, at room temperature, 20 min in saturated uranyl acetate in 50% ethanol followed by 10 min in lead citrate generally produces appropriate contrast. The staining

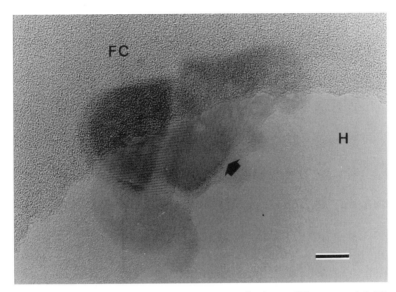

Figure 7. TEM micrograph of a synthetic hydroxyapatite bone-filling material. Note that the lattice fringes (arrow) are conspicuously more distinct in the hole region (H) of the carbon-coated Formvar® film (FC). Bar = 10 nm.

duration must be optimized for particular materials. Both staining solutions must be protected from bright light during storage and staining procedure. They should be filtered just before use. Moreover, lead staining must be performed in a carbon dioxide-free atmosphere to avoid precipitation of insoluble lead carbonate onto the sections being stained. To achieve this, staining is performed within a Petri dish containing several sodium hydroxide pellets. The grids to be stained are placed on drops of lead citrate distributed onto a sheet of Parafilm®.

If the organization and orientation of collagen fibrils along an interface or the penetration of collagen fibrils within a CaP repair material are to be studied, then phosphotungstic acid (0.5 g in 100 mL of 70% ethanol, for 2 min) can be used to stain decalcified sections (Fig. 8).

IV. TEM EVALUATION

A. Optimal TEM Operation

The following instrument recommendations provide a clue to optimal operating conditions for an electron microscope. This particular list of factors, avoiding theoretical intricacies, is mainly focused on biomaterials and hard-tissue specimens.

1. Choice of Accelerating Voltage

Increasing the accelerating voltage offers the advantage of increasing the illumination brightness, but has the drawback of lowering the amplitude contrast in the image. In fact, the higher the electron energy (i.e., the accelerating voltage), the smaller the scattering angle of incident electrons by a given object in the section, the smaller the quantity of

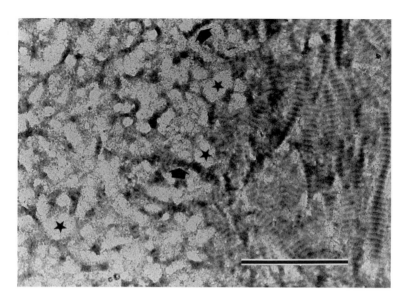

Figure 8. TEM micrograph of a phosphotungstic acid-stained decalcified section of a synthetic hydroxyapatite-bone interface. Empty spaces (stars) correspond to locations of demineralized repair material. Note that some collagen fibrils (arrow) encased between implanted crystals. Bar = 1 μm.

electrons being stopped by the objective lens aperture, and thus the lower the image contrast. Moreover, metallic, ceramic, and hard-tissue samples, even when very thin, require sufficient voltage to permit electrons to penetrate the specimen, especially when electron diffraction techniques are employed. For these reasons, it is advisable to work with the highest possible accelerating voltage and to secure enough contrast by using an adequate objective lens aperture and possibly staining the specimen.

2. Selecting Condenser Lens Aperture

The choice of the condenser lens aperture size must be consistent with specimen nature and thickness, radiation damage of sensitive materials, and illumination intensity at the highest required magnification. The smaller the aperture size, the smaller the beam divergence and the weaker the electron flux to be used on the sample, thus reducing image brightness. However, a smaller aperture angle will enhance image sharpness. It is common practice to choose a middle-sized aperture (for example, 200 μm in diameter) and to adjust the effective aperture angle by operating the condenser lens to yield minimum spot size.

3. Selecting Objective Lens Aperture

Usually, selecting the objective lens aperture is empirically defined by image contrast needs. For this reason, it is also called "contrast aperture." The smaller the aperture, the higher the contrast because of the stopping of scattered electrons. The choice of aperture is governed by precise rules whenever optimal performance is required for high-resolution electron microscopy. Actually, this small aperture reduces the beam divergence angle of the objective lens and in turn lowers spherical aberration. Moreover, there is an optimum aperture size consistent with spherical aberration and diffraction limitation. For conventional microscopy, nevertheless, the image contrast criterion is relatively efficient.

4. Magnification Calibration

The actual value of magnification must be calibrated for the employed accelerating voltage and objective lens settings by reference to a standard specimen with well-defined dimensional parameters. For low magnifications, one can use fine mesh grids. For example, a so-called "1000-mesh" grid presents a mesh-size of 25 μm, which is in the order of cellular dimensions. For high-magnification assessments, one can use lattice plane specimens such as asbestos crocidolite or potassium chloroplatinate. Lattice plane spacings are accurately known from X-ray measurements. A test specimen can even be placed directly on the grid supporting the studied sample. In this connection, Arends et al.[2] obtained a reproducibility of 0.8% in lattice parameter determination when synthetic hydroxyapatite was used as an internal reference for the measurement of the lattice space distances in human dental enamel.

5. Filling Refrigerant Tanks

Contamination is caused by poor vacuum in the microscope column. It corresponds to a carbon deposition at any exposed surface inside the microscope. Contamination becomes very problematic when it affects the objective lens aperture, and above all, the specimen itself. Column vacuum is improved when a cooling trap is mounted on the oil diffusion pump to prevent oil vapors from entering the microscope. Contamination is also appreciably reduced by placing a cooled metal blade between specimen holder and objective lens aperture. Both devices are cooled by liquid nitrogen. An obviously mundane but relevant recommendation is to regularly top up refrigerant tanks.

B. Analytical Facilities

Whenever an image is formed in a TEM, a concomitant diffraction pattern is located in the back focal planes of the different imaging lenses. Although this phenomenon, known as "electron diffraction," is available in all electron microscopes, biologists are often daunted by the mathematical aspects of the subject and hesitate to use this data source. Yet the type of diffraction pattern provides essential information about the three-dimensional (3D) arrangement of the atoms in the examined area. Structural data are of utmost interest when biomaterials and calcified tissues are investigated. The supplementary information they provide may be correlated with morphological findings for the characterization of given interfacial domains.[50] The selected area diffraction technique is particularly suitable for bone-implant interfaces, because it allows one to obtain electron diffraction patterns from very specific and minute areas.[34] At first glance, one can determine if an assessed zone contains ordered regions—i.e. whether it is amorphous, a single crystal, or polycrystalline. Closer analysis reveals crystallographic data, because there is a reciprocal relationship between the spacing of the diffraction spots or the radii of the diffraction circles and the various lattice parameters in the examined specimen area.

C. Interpreting Bone-Section Micrographs

Bone mineral crystals are of irregular plate-shaped morphology.[27] Depending on their orientation with respect to the incident electron beam, bone crystals will exhibit various habits and sizes. Crystallites observed edge-on show rod-like electron-opaque struc-

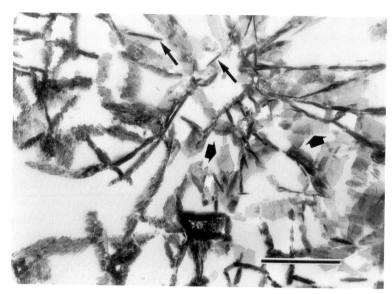

Figure 9. TEM micrograph from an ultrathin section of epoxy-embedded minute hydroxya-patite crystals. Thin arrows = edge-on view. Bold arrows = side-on view. Bar = 1 μm.

tures, whereas crystallites viewed side-on appear broad, flat, and pale. Moreover, oblique-sectioned crystallites may show peculiar aspects. As a result, the non-initiated observer may focus on the contrasted rods and draw misleading conclusions about crystal shapes and spatial distribution. Fig. 9 illustrates the different morphological features of plate-shaped crystallites according to their spatial orientation with regard to the sectioning plan.

In a conventional TEM, an ultrathin section of appropriate thickness will be sharply in focus throughout its thickness because of the very large depth of field of the electron microscope. Thus, the whole irradiated volume will be pictured in the form of a 2D projection. Because of their tiny size, bone crystals may thus overlap and consequently lead to distorted crystal habit images.[3] On the other hand, side-viewed bone crystals, which are of low density, may provide to weak contrast and remain unnoticed within the surrounding organic matrix. These two latter aspects correspond to the "Holmes effect," named after the geologist who first described it in the year 1930.[11] Therefore, preparation techniques, including cutting orientation, should be varied to produce corroborative and reliable findings.

REFERENCES

1. Albrektsson T, Hansson HA: An ultrastructural characterization of the interface between bone and sputtered titanium or stainless steel surfaces. *Biomaterials* 7:201–205, 1986.
2. Arends J, Voegel JC, Jongebloed W, et al: Determination and calibration of crystal lattice images of biological apatites. *J Biol Buccale* 10:125–133, 1982.
3. Arsenault AL: A comparative electron microscopic study of apatite crystals in collagen fibrils of rat bone, dentin and calcified turkey leg tendons. *Bone Miner* 6:165–177, 1989.
4. Augat P, Claes L, Hanselmann KF, et al: Increase of stability in external fracture fixation by hydroxyapatite-coated bone screws. *J Appl Biomater* 6:99–104, 1995.

5. Becker O, Bange K: Ultramicrotomy: an alternative cross section preparation for oxidic thin films on glass. *Ultramicroscopy* 52:73–84, 1993.

6. Blaauw EH, Oosterbaan JA, Schakenraad JM: Improved Epon embedding for biomaterials. *Biomaterials* 10:356–358, 1989.

7. Bodier-Houllé P, Steuer P, Voegel JC, et al: First experimental evidence for human dentine crystal formation involving conversion of octacalcium phosphate to hydroxyapatite. *Acta Cryst* D54:1377–1381, 1998.

8. Brånemark PI: Introduction to osseointegration. In: Brånemark PI, Zarb G, Albrektsson T, eds: *Tissue Integrated Prostheses.* Quintessence Publishing, Chicago, IL, 1985:11–76.

9. Camprasse S, Camprasse G, Pouzol M, et al: Artificial dental root made of natural calcium carbonate (Bioracine). In: Muster D, Hastings G, eds: *Interfaces in Biomaterials Sciences.* European Materials Research Society Symposia Proceedings. North-Holland, Amsterdam, The Netherlands, 1990:139–154.

10. Carlsson L, Regnér L, Johansson C, et al: Bone response to hydroxyapatite-coated and commercially pure titanium implants in the human arthritic knee. *J Orthop Res* 12:274–285, 1994.

11. Cau P: *Techniques En Microscopie Quantitative.* Les Editions INSERM, Paris, France, 1990.

12. Choi JM, Kim HE, Lee IS: Ion-beam-assisted deposition (IBAD) of hydroxyapatite coating layer on Ti-based metal substrate. *Biomaterials* 21:469–473, 2000.

13. Cochran DL, Hermann JS, Schenk RK, et al: Biologic width around titanium implants. A histometric analysis of the implanto-gingival junction around unloaded and loaded non-submerged implants in the canine mandible. *J Periodontol* 68:186–198, 1997.

14. Davies JE, Lowenberg B, Shiga A: The bone-titanium interface in vitro. *J Biomed Mater Res* 24:1289–1306, 1990.

15. De Lange GL, De Putter C, De Wijs FLJA: Histological and ultrastructural appearance of the hydroxyapatite-bone interface. *J Biomed Mater Res* 24:829–845, 1990.

16. Ehret G, Crovisier JL, Eberhart JP: A new method for studying leached glasses: analytical electron microscopy on ultramicrotomic thin sections. *J Non-Crystalline Solids* 86:72–79, 1986.

17. Ellingsen JE: A study on the mechanism of protein adsorption to TiO_2. *Biomaterials* 12:593–596, 1991.

18. Frank RM, Brion M, De Rouffignac M: Ultrastructural gingival reactions to gold foil restorations. *J Periodontol* 46:614–624, 1975.

19. Gu H, Ruault MO, Beriot E: Comparison of different TEM sample preparation methods for $YBa_2Cu_3O_{7-\delta}$ type materials. *Microsc Microanal Microstruct* 4:51–61, 1993.

20. Hanawa T: Titanium and its oxide film: A substrate for formation of apatite. In: Davies JE, ed. *The Bone-Biomaterial Interface.* University of Toronto Press, Toronto, Canada, 1991:49–61.

21. Hemmerlé J, Leize M, Voegel JC: Long-term behaviour of a hydroxyapatite/collagen-glycosaminoglycan biomaterial used for oral surgery: a case report. *J Mater Science Mater Med* 6:360–366, 1995.

22. Hemmerlé J, Voegel JC: Ultrastructural aspects of the intact titanium implant-bone interface from undecalcified ultrathin sections. *Biomaterials* 17:1913–1920, 1996.

23. Hemmerlé J, Önçag A, Ertürk S: Ultrastructural features of the bone response to a plasma-sprayed hydroxyapatite coating in sheep. *J Biomed Mater Res* 36:418–425, 1997.

24. Hemmerlé J, Cuisinier FJG, Schultz P, et al: HRTEM study of biological crystal growth mechanisms in the vicinity of implanted synthetic hydroxyapatite crystals. *J Dent Res* 76:682–687, 1997.

25. Jansen JA, Van der Waerden JPCM, Wolke JGC: Histologic investigation of the biologic behavior of different hydroxyapatite plasma-sprayed coatings in rabbits. *J Biomed Mater Res* 27:603–610, 1993.

26. Jésior JC: Use of low-angle diamond knives leads to improved ultrastructural preservation of ultrathin sections. *Scanning Microsc Suppl* 3:147–153, 1989.

27. Kim HM, Rey C, Glimcher MJ: Isolation of calcium-phosphate crystals of bone by non-aqueous methods at low temperature. *J Bone Miner Res* 10:1589–1601, 1995.

28. Kotani S, Fujita Y, Kitsugi T, et al: Bone bonding mechanism of β-tricalcium phosphate. *J Biomed Mater Res* 25:1303–1315, 1991.

29. Leize EM, Hemmerlé J, Leize M: Characterization, at the bone crystal level, of the titanium-coating/bone interfacial zone. *Clin Oral Impl Res* 11:279–288, 2000.

30. Liao H, Mutvei H, Sjöström M, et al: Tissue response to natural aragonite (Margaritifera shell) implants in vivo. *Biomaterials* 21:457–468, 2000.

31. Linder L, Albrektsson T, Brånemark PI, et al. Electron microscopic analysis of the bone-titanium interface. *Acta Orthop Scand* 54:45–52, 1983.

32. Listgarten MA, Buser D, Steinemann SG, et al: Light and transmission electron microscopy of the intact interfaces between non-submerged titanium-coated epoxy resin implants and bone or gingiva. *J Dent Res* 71:364–371, 1992.

33. Massa LF, Arana-Chavez VE: Ultrastructural preservation of rat embryonic dental tissues after rapid fixation and dehydration under microwave irradiation. *Eur J Oral Sci* 108:74–77, 2000.

34. Miake Y, Yanagisawa T, Yajima Y, et al: High-resolution and analytical electron microscopic studies of new crystals induced by a bioactive ceramic (diopside). *J Dent Res* 74:1756–1763, 1995.

35. Murai K, Takeshita F, Ayukawa Y, et al: Light and electron microscopic studies of bone-titanium interface in the tibiae of young and mature rats. *J Biomed Mater Res* 30:523–533, 1996.

36. Ogilvie A, Frank RM, Benqué EP, et al: The biocompatibility of hydroxyapatite implanted in the human periodontium. *J Periodontol Res* 22:270–283, 1987.

37. Ogiso M, Tabata T, Ichijo T, et al: Bone calcification on the hydroxyapatite dental implant and the bone-hydroxyapatite interface. *J Long Term Eff Med Implants* 2:137–148, 1992.

38. Ogiso M, Tabata T, Ichijo T, et al: Examination of human bone surrounded by a dense hydroxyapatite dental implant after long-term use. *J Long Term Eff Med Implants* 2:235–247, 1992.

39. Oguchi H, Ishikawa K, Mizoue K, et al: Long-term histological evaluation of hydroxyapatite ceramics in humans. *Biomaterials* 16:33–38, 1995.

40. Piattelli A, Piattelli M, Romasco N, et al: Histochemical and laser scanning microscopy characterization of the hydroxyapatite-bone interface: an experimental study in rabbits. *Int J Oral Maxillofac Implants* 9:163–168, 1994.

41. Prostak KS, Lees S: Visualization of crystal-matrix structure. In situ demineralization of mineralized turkey leg tendon and bone. *Calcif Tissue Int* 59:474–479, 1996.

42. Rupp BF, Geis-Gerstorfer J, Geckeler KE: Dental implant materials: surface modification and interface phenomena. *Adv Mater* 8:254–257, 1996.

43. Schmutz M, Lang J, Graff S, Brisson A: Defects of planarity of carbon films supported on electron microscope grids revealed by reflected light microscopy. *J Struct Biol* 112:252–258, 1994.

44. Sennerby L, Thomsen P, Ericson LE: Ultrastructure of the bone-titanium interface in rabbits. *J Mater Sci Mater Med* 3:262–271, 1992.

45. Serre CM, Papillard M, Chavassieux P, et al: In vitro induction of a calcifying matrix by biomaterials constituted of collagen and/or hydroxyapatite: an ultrastructural comparison of three types of biomaterials. *Biomaterials* 14:97–106, 1993.

46. Serre CM, Boivin G, Obrant KJ, et al: Osseointegration of titanium implants in the tibia. Electron microscopy of biopsies from 4 patients. *Acta Orthop Scand* 65:323–327, 1994.

47. Shareef MY, Messer PF, Van Noort R: Fabrication, characterization and fracture study of a machinable hydroxyapatite ceramic. *Biomaterials* 14:69–75, 1993.

48. Sousa SR, Barbosa MA: Effect of hydroxyapatite thickness on metal ion release from Ti6Al4V substrates. *Biomaterials* 17:397–404, 1996.

49. Steflik DE, Sisk AL, Parr GR, et al: Osteogenesis at the dental implant interface: high-voltage electron microscopic and conventional transmission electron microscopic observations. *J Biomed Mater Res* 27:791–800, 1993.

50. Suvorova EI, Buffat PA: Electron diffraction from micro- and nanoparticles of hydroxyapatite. *J Microscopy* 196:46–58, 1999.

51. Volpi N: Adsorption of glycosaminoglycans onto coral: a new possible implant biomaterials for regeneration therapy. *Biomaterials* 20:1359–1363, 1999.
52. Walboomers XF, Croes HJE, Ginsel LA, et al: Contact guidance of rat fibroblasts on various implant materials. *J Biomed Mater Res* 47:204–212, 1999.
53. Yukna RA: Clinical evaluation of coralline calcium carbonate as a bone replacement graft material in human periodontal osseous defects. *J Periodontol* 65:177–185, 1994.
54. Zeng H, Lacefield WR, Mirov S: Structural and morphological study of pulsed laser deposited calcium phosphate bioceramic coatings: influence of deposition conditions, laser parameters, and target properties. *J Biomed Mater Res* 50:248–258, 2000.

37

Radiological Examination of Calcified Tissues with Emphasis on Bone

Victor Fornasier and Charles L. Ho

*Department of Laboratory Medicine and Pathology, St. Michael's Hospital,
University of Toronto, Toronto, Ontario, Canada*

I. INTRODUCTION

The examination of hard/mineralized tissue has always been regarded as a challenge in the preparation of sections for histomorphopathological study in both clinical and research applications. The time required to decalcify tissue is a recognized extension of the turn-around time in processing, and as a result, a delay in analysis and report generation. Technically, the need for modified embedding (e.g., double embedding such as celloidin or methylsalicylate and paraffin wax) and the use of heavy-duty microtomes such as sledge) adds to the challenge of processing. The need for decalcification complicates the application of phenotypic methods of cell characterization. It is believed that decalcification methods such as acids or kelating agents damage antigenic components of cells and tissue. This would therefore preclude the use of immunohistochemistry or *in situ* hybridization in the assessment of disease processes in bone.

If one were able to examine mineralized tissue before any processing and be more selective in tissue blocks submitted for histological preparation, then one may well influence quality, specificity, and ease of preparation of specimen for histomorphopathological and microscopic study. If the method leading up to the selection of tissue blocks provided additional diagnostic benefit, then one would indeed have added a significant advantage. If one could add a factor of cost-effectiveness through such methodology, then one would certainly provide a very real benefit in the processing of mineralized/hard tissue for histomorphological examination. More detailed and more informative assessment would be the final outcome.

"Low energy" or "fine detail" radiology is a method of examining a large or small sample of tissue, of visualizing the internal structure of such tissue, and of enabling differentiation between normal and abnormal patterns. With such imaging, one could examine the internal structure of an entire femoral head, and not just see what is shown in the selected tissue block microscopically. A bone tumor can be "mapped" with an opportunity to record exactly where tissue blocks are taken, with knowledge of the features in each tissue block. This provides an opportunity for a correlation between gross, radiolog-

From: *Handbook of Histology Methods for Bone and Cartilage*
Edited by: Y. H. An and K. L. Martin © Humana Press Inc., Totowa, NJ

ical, and microscopic characteristics. The evaluation of bone density becomes more than the two-dimensional (2D) image seen in a histological section; it is a true measure of bone "quality" and density in the sample examined. The quantitation of porosity of bone and density of mineralization is the only objective measure of metabolic bone health or severity of disease. In the evaluation of implant anchorage or graft incorporation, one can specifically determine the appearance of the actual interface between the implant or the bone graft and the host bone. Such features are recorded, and can also be evaluated in a reproducible, quantitative manner. In the evaluation of metabolic diseases of bone, the fine-detail image provides a semi-quantitative measure of bone turnover. For example, in hyperparathyroidism the erosive changes can be visualized along the endosteal aspect of cortical and trabecular bone.

II. METHODS

The examination of tissues by radiological means requires an understanding of basic concepts of radiological imaging, with particular reference to individual disease processes and how they affect tissue. X-rays provide "shadows" that differentiate between varying densities in both bony and soft tissue. For this reason, it is possible to obtain images of soft or non-calcified tissues such as the kidney, lungs, or soft-tissue sarcomas. In the lungs, one can evaluate aeration or its absence in consolidating pneumopathies. In the kidney or lung, one can visualize and quantitate calcification. In tumors, one can separate hyalinized areas from cellular or fatty areas and cystic areas.

The use of appropriately adjusted, very low energy provides useful images that separate various tissue densities to reflect structure and architecture. In dealing with osseous tissues, one can identify changes in cortical and trabecular bone. Fibrosis and erosions point to hyperparathyroidism. Poor trabecular definition indicates a defect in mineralization (e.g., osteomalacia). Structured or unstructured mineralization in primary bone neoplasms distinguishes bone from cartilage content.

To achieve this, one must have an X-ray unit capable of delivering a low kilovoltage from the smallest possible point source. Mammography units approach this requirement. However, because of the time element involved in exposure with such a unit, one is limited to standard mammography-type film, which would not provide the resolution required to make the analysis useful. Equipment available on the market today can provide variable kilovoltage from a fixed-pinpoint source while operating on a standard 110/120-volt alternating current source. The variable voltage is needed to adjust for the size of the specimen and to specifically examine non-mineralized vs bone or mineralized tissue samples. It is preferable to use self-contained equipment that is safe in populated areas for laboratory applications. Standard radiological equipment is large, requires dedicated space, and does not provide a sufficiently small point source or the low levels of kilovoltage required for the examination of a sample of tissue. After all, they are intended for the examination of the entire patient. Radiation risk would be involved with standard radiological equipment. Currently available equipment suitable for tissue examination is "self-contained" in a format that provides an entirely safe environment at all its surfaces and with added safety "shut downs" if interfered with or if the door to the internal compartment is opened. The selection of equipment depends on the application and on the user's preference. Nevertheless, today's units are compact, and provide both manual and automatic exposure controls. Available units have a key-operated master switch, precluding the use of equipment by unauthorized personnel or anyone who is not familiar with its operation. The point source of our laboratory unit is approx 0.5 mm. It is entirely shielded to preclude any risk of radiation hazard, and has two independent cut-off switches, which would turn off the equipment before the door is opened enough to permit radiation to exit the compartment.

The range of kilovoltage is from 10–110 kV at a continuous current of 3 mA. This provides flexibility so that at the lower kilovoltages one can examine non-calcified soft tissues, and in the mid range one can examine small sections or slabs of tissue. At the upper end, one can examine large, bulky resection specimens such as neoplasms in amputated limbs.

The film used depends on the application. For large, bulky specimens, for which detail is not essential but a record of the architecture and structure is desired, film is not required to be of the highest sensitivity. Thus, the double-emulsion standard mammography-type film can be used in such applications. This can be developed in a standard developer, precluding the need for the time-consuming processing by hand in a dark room. Examples include Hewlett-Packard Cabinet X-ray System Faxitron Series and Kodak Professional Industry SR Film.

For greater detail, single-emulsion industrial-type film (very much like a black-and-white negative for photography) is best. Such high resolution is required in the examination of small samples, particularly in the evaluation of biopsies for metabolic bone disease, in order to identify adequacy of mineralization and trabecular structure. This is particularly useful in the primary assessment of bone architecture and quality, even before undecalcified plastic-embedded microtome or milled sections are prepared. Development of such film can also be undertaken in an automatic processor that has been adjusted to handle such films.

Voltages below 15 kV are only practical in "micro-radiography." In such cases, a very high-resolution emulsion is placed on a microscopic glass slide, and a section of tissue between 20 and 50 μm in thickness is placed directly onto the surface of the emulsion in a darkroom. The slide and tissue are placed in a light-sealed but radiolucent vacuum container, and the slide is subjected to radiographic exposure at very low kilovoltages (usually between 5 kV and 10 kV) to produce an "image" of the section. The slide with the exposed and developed emulsion can then be examined under the microscope in the quantitation of the adequacy of mineralization with densitometric techniques.

In preparing the tissue for radiological examination, great care must be taken to ensure uniformity of thickness of the specimen. Orientation of the specimen is important to show the area or structure of interest. It is possible to use both fixed and unfixed tissue. However, it is important to remember that one is often dealing with diseased tissue, and therefore, appropriate universal precautions must be undertaken, particularly in the case of unfixed tissue. In my experience, examination of unfixed tissue is useful in intra-operative consultations, when the goal is to identify an area that can be used for frozen-section examination or areas that can be used for special fixations (e.g., electron microscopy) or special procedures (e.g., molecular studies). However, it is preferable, if possible, to examine tissues that had been properly fixed and specifically prepared for radiological examination. The one exception is the identification of calcified foci in breast lumpectomy to direct tissue-block selection.

In the evaluation of bone biopsies for metabolic diseases, overnight fixation in formalin is adequate preparation. Even when one suspects the presence of crystals, fixation in formalin does not remove enough crystals to eliminate the possibility of identification of such crystals. The loss of crystals occurs primarily during the staining process, when a thin section only a few microns across is exposed to a number of water-based solutions. In practice, it is best to prepare and examine an unstained, mounted section under polarized light. With such preparation, the crystals are preserved. In larger samples, there is a balance to be drawn between sectioning fresh tissue or waiting long enough for penetration of formalin into the tissue to fix it. Handsaws are usually preferable to electrically operated oscillating circular or band saws in cutting fresh specimens, as the speed of the electrical equipment will create aerosol particles. Universal precautions would therefore be essential. In fixed tissue, there is less of a risk of aerosols if an appropriate saw with an appropriate band teeth distribution is selected. For both mineralized and unmineralized tissues, I have found that a bandsaw with no more than twelve teeth per inch and with a minimum of external curvature of the teeth is most effective. A larger number of teeth per inch is usually less efficient in tissue cutting, and generates heat as well as greater tissue fluid extraction. Too few teeth tend to rip tissue, thus widening the path of the blade and leading to a greater amount of tissue loss from the passage of the blade. Compact table-top bandsaws are now available. They are constructed of stainless steel or brushed aluminum with a well-sealed electrical compartment so that the machine can be quickly washed and sterilized following use. Cleanliness of the blade itself may be achieved with a brush, or by having blocks of soft wood available to cut between cases. This will ensure that tissue fragments are not transferred from one case to the next. The operator should be well-shielded and dressed, and the room should be well-ventilated.

In the examination of femoral heads removed at surgery and resected large osseous tumors, it is useful to radiograph the specimen as received for purposes of orientation and internal structure definition. This information can then be used in the selection of the plane of section to produce slabs and to match clinical imaging projection. The slabs should be approx 4–5 mm in thickness. Thicker specimens will produce overlap of trabeculae and detail of individual trabeculae will be lost. Sections that are too thin distort the appearance by providing a decrease in the overall amount of tissue to be examined. In bone, this may lead to mistaken interpretation of osteopenia, when in fact the lack of trabeculae is a technically produced artifact. The development of specific protocols of exposure are essential in order to address differences of methodology and application of techniques by different operators and for various types of specimens.

Once the films are developed, they are available for assessment and selection of histological sections (if required), and the provision of a preliminary assessment of the disease process.

The interpretation of radiological imaging can be an uncomfortable task for the pathologist. Most laboratory physicians are not accustomed to seeing black-and-white shadows without the esthetic characteristics of multicolored histologic sections. One must remember that one is seeing the shadow cast by tissues of different densities, and that one is evaluating the level of mineralization in the case of bone and cartilage (normal, reactive, or neoplastic). One cannot attempt to make a microscopic diagnosis based on the radiological examination.

The author's laboratory has 25 years of experience with this methodology, and in selected circumstances, the radiograph is sufficient to give the reporting pathologist confidence in not proceeding to histologic examination in many tissues. For example, the combination of the gross appearance and the radiological image provide sufficient data for the definitive reporting of many cases of degenerative joint diseases, particularly in tissue resected for knee or hip arthroplasties. Often one receives a large sample of fragmented tissue from a surgical procedure (e.g., tissue reamings or multiple curetted fragments). The X-ray is helpful in identifying the location of tissue that will be useful for histomorphologic assessment and the orientation for embedding.

The final benefit is economic. The X-ray provides an opportunity to examine a large sample of tissue in a very intimate way. One can often examine a complete specimen and identify areas of interest for blocking for histology. This process diminishes the number of sections that need to be taken. The fact that one has selected tissue blocks with knowledge of the internal structure of the tissue will ensure that the blocks selected are representative of the sample. This will obviate repeated return to the specimen for additional sections if the previous sections are inconclusive, since tissue blocks taken with radiological guide are invariably adequate to identify the expected diagnostic features. In the author's experience, the cost of the X-ray is roughly one-fifth the cost of a decalcified paraffin-embedded hematoxylin & eosin (H&E)-stained section.

In the case of metabolic bone diseases, it is possible to identify defects in mineralization and in bone resorption on the radiograph, and therefore in patients with defects in mineralization, bone resorption or even in patients with Paget's disease of bone, one can confidently provide a preliminary assessment of the tissue sample, literally within minutes of the arrival of the sample in the laboratory. The high-resolution film can be examined with up to 25× magnification without loss of detail. This can be achieved with a hand lens, dissecting microscope, or a very low-power objective lens in a standard lab microscope.

The following case reports illustrate the usefulness of fine detail radiography in the assessment of bone charges in disease. The illustrations will be limited to one specific area to show the various imaging characteristics that can be identified in one anatomic site as a result of disease.

III. CASE REPORTS

A. Case Report 1

A 71-yr-old male underwent total hip arthroplasty with pre-operative diagnosis of degenerative arthritis (osteoarthritis). The sections in the upper portion of the photograph are from the anterior half of the femoral head cut in the sagittal plane (Fig. 1A). The bottom sections are from the posterior part of the femoral head cut in the sagittal plane. The two central sections are coronal sections of the femoral head. This overview provides a clear representation of subchondral cysts, the extent of denudation of the articular surface, the severity of loss of substance in the weight-bearing zone, the pattern of osteophyte formation—including intra-cartilaginous ossification within the inferomedial portion of the articular surface as seen toward the right of the two coronal sections in the illustration—and the presence of a focus of increased mineralization at the margin of the calcarine trabecular radiation deep in the substance of the femoral head. This type of overview allows for sepcifically selected blocks for histologic examination. In this case, the interest would be in the floating fragment seen in the central section of the posterior part of the femoral head (lower part of the photograph) to determine if this is residual femoral head overhanging the subchondral cyst or whether it is a focus of avascular necrosis. A similar

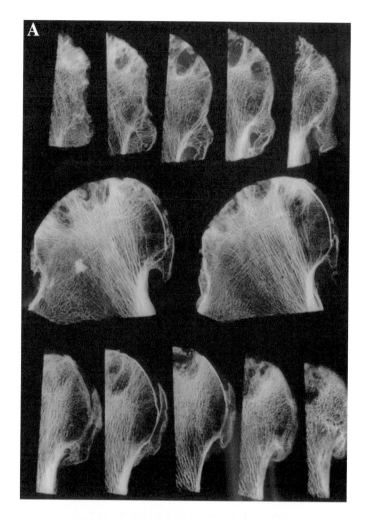

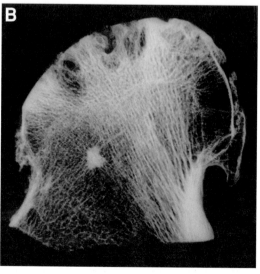

Figure 1. *See* case report 1.

floating fragment is seen in the central weight-bearing zone of the coronal section in the right center of the photograph, where an elongated ovoid nodule of osseous tissue appears to have collapsed into a lucent zone. The third area of interest would be the focus of enhanced mineralization within the spongiosa of the femoral head, as seen in the coronal section on the left of the photograph. This is the pattern of a solitary osteoma, which can be confirmed by histology. The changes resulting from osteoarthritis are well-illustrated, and may not require histologic sections for further evaluation or confirmation.

Fig. 1B shows one of the coronal sections of the femoral head in Fig. 1A. The fine-detail radiograph permits visualization of the combined lytic and sclerotic pattern in the weight-bearing zone. The lucent zones are caused by subchondral "cysts." Some of these so-called "cysts" are solid and composed of gelatinous fibrous tissue, and a minority actually are cystic. The thicker cortex of the calcar gives origin to the calcarine trabecular radiation, which extends to the weight-bearing zone that shows such advanced degenerative changes. Inferomedially in the femoral head (to the right in the illustration), there is a localized zone of osteopenia with few thin trabeculae. Nevertheless, in this area, the original subchondral bone plate is present as a white linear band. External to this, there is new bone coursing along the articular surface. This is in continuity with the osteophyte that overhangs inferomedially beyond the end of the joint. It is important to note that the presence of the localized area of density just adjacent to the superior margin of the calcarine trabecular radiation. The zone appears to extend along pre-existing trabeculae indicating that it is an outgrowth of the trabeculae, probably by appositional new bone onto the pre-existing trabeculae. This is a solitary bone island (also known as solitary osteoma). This degree of intimate detail provides a complete evaluation of the bony structure and of the changes brought about by disease throughout the femoral head.

B. Case Report 2

In a 39-yr-old female, the femoral head was replaced with a total hip arthroplasty because of pain and limited function resulting from congenital dysplasia of the hip. Note the distortion and deformity of the outline, and the lack of organization of the trabecular pattern into a weight-bearing band such as the calcarine radiation from calcar to weight-bearing zone (Fig. 2). At the top of the articular surface, the soft-tissue shadow is that of the ligamentum teres, which has some mineralized tissue at its tip, from its acetabular attachment.

C. Case Report 3

This femoral head in a 77-yr-old female was replaced with a total hip arthroplasty because of the clinical diagnosis of degenerative arthritis (Fig. 3). Examination revealed the presence of a sequestered fragment of bone in the weight-bearing area. This was shown to overlie a zone of lucency, in which there appeared to have been resorption of trabeculae. Below this, there was increased density in a linear band that appeared to encircle the area of lucency. Note that the fragment is free-floating, and has at least one of its corners raised above the adjacent surface in the upper region of the femoral head. This is in keeping with the fact that the floating fragment of bone is supported by spongy, fibrous, or fibrocartilaginous tissue that was compressed by apposition to the acetabulum, while the femoral head was weight-bearing. Once acetabular pressure was removed, the floating fragment was pushed up by the elasticity of the subjacent soft tissues seen in the lucent zone on the X-ray.

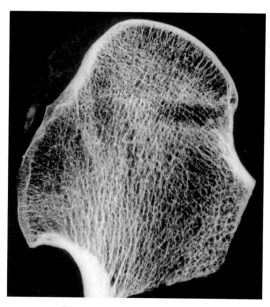

Figure 2. *See* case report 2.

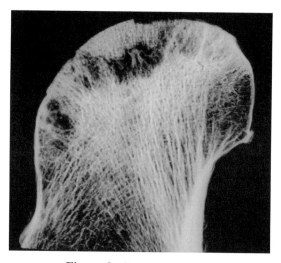

Figure 3. *See* case report 3.

The contrast between the sclerosis in the subjacent bone and the lack of modification of trabecular pattern in the free-floating fragments supports the diagnosis of avascular necrosis. The fact that the degenerative changes along the current joint surface are continuous between the free-floating fragment and the adjacent bone superolaterally lead to the conclusion that a subchondral cyst had undermined the overlying bone, which collapsed and became sequestered and avascular. This is a recently recognized association of osteoarthritis. Only through careful examination of the entire femoral head can this be identified. The fine-detail radiograph is particularly helpful in identifying such changes.

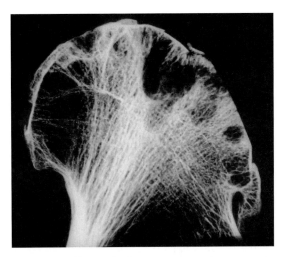

Figure 4. *See* case report 4.

D. Case Report 4

This femoral head in a 85-yr-old female was replaced with a total hip arthroplasty because of a clinical diagnosis of degenerative arthritis (osteoarthritis) (Fig. 4). There is erosion of the articular surface, consistent with a degenerative process. However, there are partly collapsed and free-floating fragments of the degenerated articular surface overlying the subchondral cyst, with a rounded outline sitting immediately under. Note the severe decrease in the trabeculae of the spongiosa inferomedially (to the left in figure). The coarseness of the trabeculae in the calcarine trabecular radiation reflects an overall decrease in the amount of bone present. This patient was osteopenic, and the degenerative arthritis was a concurrent process. The collapse of the osteochondral fragment overlying the subchondral cyst into the lucency representing the subchondral cyst is of particular interest. Note the good preservation of the subchondral bone plate with a smooth, linear outer surface and granular eroded trabeculae on the deep surface. The smoothness of the outer surface of the plate contrasts with the roughness of the outline of the adjacent articular surface. This suggests that this fragment collapsed early in the development of the degenerative arthritis. It became localized within the subchondral cyst and protected from the functional stresses of the adjacent articular surface. Grossly as well as microscopically, this was a fragment of articular cartilage with its intact subchondral bone plate. This collapsed and well-preserved articular osteochondral fragment contrasts with the surrounding degenerative changes, and is regarded as antedating the osteoarthritic changes seen in the remainder of the joint surface. As such, it has undergone post-collapse avascular necrosis. The obvious osteopenia of the bone in the femoral head may also have contributed to the collapse of this segment of the articular surface once the subchondral "cyst" was established early in the evolution of the osteoarthritic process.

F. Case Report 5

In a 79-yr-old male, this femoral head was replaced with a total hip arthroplasty with a clinical diagnosis of degenerative arthritis (osteoarthritis) secondary to avascular necrosis

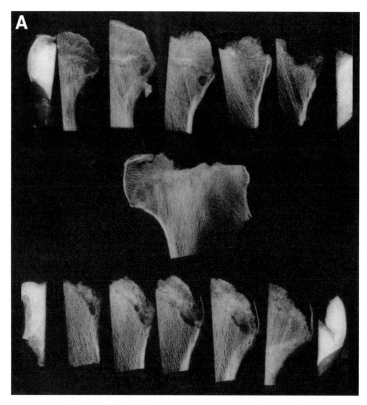

Figure 5. (A) *See* case report 5. *(Continued)*

(Fig. 5A). The upper series of sagittal sections from the anterior part of the femoral head show only focal remnants of the necrotic bone (section just to the right of center in the photograph). The coronal section in the center shows the extent of the erosive destruction of the necrotic portion of the femoral head with collapse of the osteochondral tissues, which probably remained viable but were poorly supported once the avascular portion of the femoral head was lost. In the lower series of sagittal sections from the posterior portion of the femoral head, there is a greater bolus of necrotic bone. Note that the three sections from center to the right in the figure show a small remnant of the osteochondral flap. The tip of the flap is free-floating, and the base of it is attached to the underlying femoral head.

In Fig. 5B, the trabeculae of the femoral head that reach the surface are sharply truncated and enveloped in appositional bone, making them look granular and making the overall pattern into a mildly sclerotic surface. Note the collapse of the osteochondral flap at the tip of the inferomedial portion of articular surface remaining (to the left of the figure). The abrupt disruption of the substance of the femoral head at the current free surface suggests a rapid destruction of a massive area of necrosis, with rounding off by abrasion occurring only at the superolateral border of the distorted articular surface (to the right in the figure). The rapid progression of the destructive process leaves little opportunity for reaction or repair on the part of the viable bone. When there is a large avascular zone, one expects a higher probability that the avascular bone will collapse

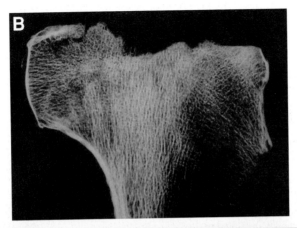

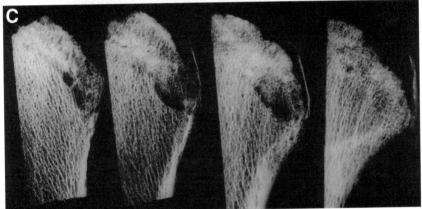

Figure 5. *(Continued)* (B, C) *See* case report 5.

and will be mechanically abraded, converting it into fragmented joint detritus that will precipitate out into the dependent zones of the synovium of the joint.

In Fig. 5C, note the osteochondral flap present to the right of the sections in the illustration. Where the osteochondral flap retains continuity with the subjacent bone, this acts as a hinge, allowing the osteochondral flap to pivot on this site. With function, a "wedge" of joint fluid and detritus is pushed under the flap and protrudes into the bone. As a result, one sees very active osteoclastic resorption of the bone associated with large numbers of histiocytes, including multinucleated giant cells. This is under the fluffy or cloudlike density in the adjacent spongiosa as a result of new bone formation on and between the existing trabeculae.

F. Case Report 6

In a 71-yr-old male, the femoral head was replaced with a total hip arthroplasty, with a diagnosis of avascular necrosis originally treated with vascularized fibular graft (Fig. 6). This fine-detail radiograph shows the effect of mechanical abrasion and loss of congruity of the joint with impingement of the altered femoral head surface onto the lip of the acetabulum. As a result, there is an indentation within the substance of the femoral head. The

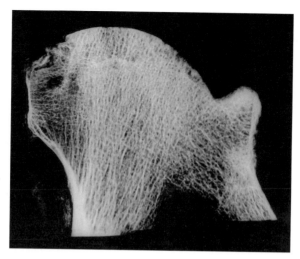

Figure 6. *See* case report 6.

smooth rounding off of the contour of the current articulating surface is the result of both new bone formation between the pre-existing trabeculae and impaction of joint detritus. Inferomedially (to the left of the illustration), there is a small remnant of the osteochondral flap from the original joint surface. It has collapsed into an erosive cavity in an area where there is patchy loss of trabeculae that is indicative of active resorptive activity. The granular shadows on the outside of the bone adjacent to the dense cortex representing calcar identify the presence of joint detritus within synovium. Some granular radio-densities can also be visualized at the margin of the original articular surface (to the left in the illustration), probably representing calcification or ossification within remnants of the articular cartilage. Please note that the smoothness of the so-called eburnated, exposed trabecular bone is interrupted by small lucencies representing foci of fibrous or fibrocartilaginous tissue that protrude onto the surface from the subjacent bone marrow. The granular filling-in of the intertrabecular space produces the solid-appearing bone, which, as one looks at the free surface, appears eburnated and ivory-like. Note the cloudlike increased density that encases the trabeculae near the articular surface. This extends for a short distance to a point where the trabeculae again become individual and are clear in outline. To the right of the photograph (superolateral cortex), note the small tufts of mineralized bone that protrude from the periosteal surface and the localized area of increased density within the subjacent trabeculae. This is part of a reactive process leading to new bone formation as part of abnormal stresses being applied by the acetabular lip onto the "new" joint margin.

G. Case Report 7

This 49-yr-old female patient had a long history of steroid therapy and 5 yr previously was found to have avascular necrosis. She underwent vascularized fibular graft, which only temporarily resolved her symptoms. With persistence of pain and loss of function, she was converted to a total hip arthroplasty. The overview of fine-detail radiograph of the sectioned femoral head shows various aspects of her original disease and of the attempted surgical repair (Fig. 7A). In the weight-bearing zone, the osteochondral tissues have collapsed. They are outlined by a margin of fragmented bone that produces a concavity into which the osteochondral flap has collapsed. Note the massive increased density present within the femoral head, adjacent to the fibular graft. In the coronal section, there is a very large, irregular area of sclerosis to the right of the coronal sections (inferomedial to the implant in the femoral head). In addition, there is a shell of sclerotic new bone outlining the graft. Note that there is a suggestion of lucency outlining the margin of the graft from the surrounding sclerotic bone reaction. The sagittal sections in the posterior part of the femoral head (inferior part of illustration) show extensive fragmentation and collapse right at the tip of the increased density at the end of the fibular graft. The anterior sagittal sections (upper part of illustration) show the collapse of the osteochondral flap, the irregular erosions along the bone under the osteochondral flap and metallic remnants of instrumentation from the vascular pedicle of the fibular graft. One also sees to greater advantage the lucent band of fibrous tissue that separates the graft from the surrounding host bone.

Fig. 7B shows that the tip of the implant has indeed been incorporated by a massive amount of new bone, which has overwhelmed the pre-existing trabeculae. However, note that the two masses of dense bone extending on either side of the tip of the graft have not protected the osteochondral flap from collapse. One can see coarse trabeculations reflecting new bone formation between the graft and the osteochondral flap in the upper right portion of the femoral head, adjacent to the right inside of the osteochondral flap. The linear lucency outlining the graft reflects the presence of a layer of fibrous tissue between the centrally placed graft that appears as dense cortical bone, and the appositional envelope of reactive bone from the host site in the femoral neck and head.

Fig. 7C shows a plastic-embedded undecalcified ground section of the central sagittal section of the anterior half of the femoral head. This section is approx 20 μm thick. The tip of the graft is on the right. Note the smoothness of the contour of the graft, its continuity at the upper region with the reactive bone, and its separation from the surrounding osseous shell by a band of lucency, where the metallic instrumentation remnants from the pedicle of the vascularized fibular graft are located. Note how little new bone exists in the upper left end of the graft toward the area of the collapsed osteochondral flap. The lucent areas between the osseous fragments in the upper weight-bearing zone were areas of gelatinous, fibrous granulation tissue. The scalloping and erosions seen in the sclerotic bone are indicative of osteoclastic resorption. Note the linear vascular markings within the sclerotic bone, which are much wider in the lower part of the illustration, where the fibular graft is being resorbed by the envelope of fibrous tissue. Note how the various metallic fragments of the pedicle are free within the fibrous tissue or have been incorporated in the reactive zone of the host bone.

Fig. 7D shows a cross-section of the neck at the base of the resected femoral head at the neck. The vascularized fibular graft occupies the center of the cross-section. The sclerotic portion of cortex in the lower right represents the medial cortex or calcar. The roughness in the upper zone represents muscle insertion onto the cortical outline. The fibular graft is the central circle of bone. It appears to be attached on the right side by incorporation and fusion to the host bone. The remaining surface is isolated from the surrounding host bone by a radiolucent wall of intervening fibrous tissue, in part representing the vascular pedicle. Note the abundance of new bone present in the area adjacent to the point of contact of the fibular graft with the host bone and the less prominent bone formation in most of the remainder of the circumference of the shell encircling the graft (where it is enveloped by

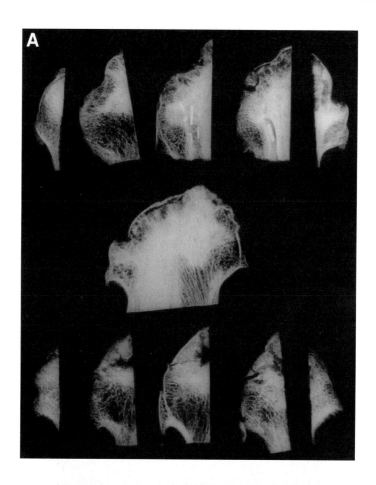

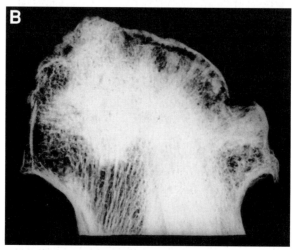

Figure 7. *See* case report 7. *(Continued)*

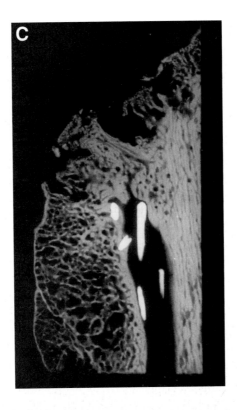

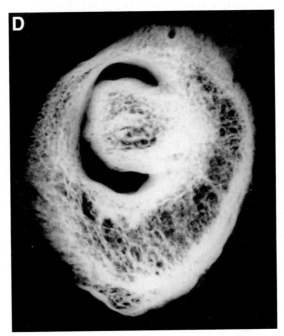

Figure 7. *(Continued)* (C, D) *See* case report 7.

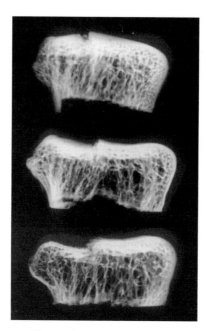

Figure 8. *See* case report 8.

the fibrous tissue). This pattern of partial incorporation denotes the effect on healing by biomechanical stresses, by the load applied to the graft and the effect of vascularization. This cross-section shows that although there is extensive new bone formation, the fibular graft is not well-incorporated. It has remained intact and partly sequestered by the host bone. In fact, it has acted as a strut within its implantation bed. Functionally, the sclerotic reaction with large amounts of bone distally in the femoral head supports small, localized areas of the articular surface, but in this case, there is little evidence of actual support for the articular surface, which has become an osteochondral flap and has collapsed despite of the subjacent reactive sclerosis.

H. Case Report 8

This radial head was removed because of painful arthritis (Fig. 8). Examination of these cross-sections by fine-detail radiograph demonstrated a step in the subchondral bone. The altered trabecular pattern below this helped to support the interpretation that this was an old fracture and that the arthritis was a secondary process superimposed on an old fracture. (No history of injury could be elicited from the patient).

REFERENCES

1. Amling M, Posl M, Ritzel H, et al: Architecture and distribution of cancellous bone yield vertebral fracture clues. A histomorphometric analysis of the complete spinal column from 40 autopsy specimens. *Arch Orthop Trauma Surg* 115:262–269, 1996.

2. Bogoch ER, Moran E, Crowe S, et al: Arthritis not immobilization causes bone loss in the carrageenan injection model of inflammatory arthritis. *J Orthop Res* 13:777–782, 1995.
3. Cameron HU, Fornasier VL: Trabecular stress fractures. *Clin Orthop* 111:266–268, 1975.
4. Chappard D, Legrand E, Audran M, et al: Histomorphometric measurement of the architecture of the trabecular bone in osteoporosis: comparative study of several methods. *Morphologie* 83:17–20, 1999.
5. Delichatsios HK, Lane JM, Rivlin RS: Bone histomorphometry in men with spinal osteoporosis. *Calcif Tissue Int* 56:359–363, 1995.
6. Fornasier VL: Fine detail radiography in the examination of tissue. *Hum Pathol* 6:623–631, 1975.
7. Fornasier VL, Villaghy MI: The results of bone biopsy with a new instrument. *Am J Clin Pathol* 60:570–573, 1973.
8. Fornasier VL, Cameron HU: Techniques of closed bone biopsy. *CRC Crit Rev Clin Lab Sci* 6:145–155, 1975.
9. Fornasier VL, Stapleton K, Williams CC: Histological changes in Paget's disease treated with calcitonin. *Hum Pathol* 9:455–461, 1978.
10. Fornasier VL, Czitrom AA: Collapsed vertebrae: a review of 659 autopsies. *Clin Orthop* 131:261–226, 1978.
11. Fornasier VL, Rabinovich S: A current look at hyperparathyroidism by the pathologist. *Modern Med Canada* 35:29–32, 1980.
12. Harris DJ, Fornasier VL: An ivory vertebra: monostotic Paget's disease of bone. *Clin Orthop* 136:173–175, 1978.
13. Harrison JE, Murray TM, Bayley TA, et al: Effect of estrogen and fluoride on bone. In: Martini L, Gordon GS, Shara F, eds: *Steroid Modulation of Neuroendocrine Function, Steroids and Bone Metabolism.* Elsevier, Amsterdam, The Netherlands, 1984:211.
14. Harrison JE, Bayley TA, Josse RG, et al: The relationship between fluoride effects from bone histology and of bone mass in patients with post-menopausal osteoporosis. *Bone Miner* 1:321–333, 1986.
15. Hsu AC, Kooh SW, Fraser D, et al: Renal osteodystrophy in children with chronic renal failure: an unexpected common and incapacitating complication. *Pediatrics* 70:742–750, 1982.
16. McCarthy JT, Dayton JM, Fitzpatrick LA, et al: The importance of bone biopsy in managing renal osteodystrophy. *Adv Ren Replace Ther* 2:148–159, 1995.
17. Johnell O, O'Neill T, Felsenberg D, et al: Anthropometric measurements and vertebral deformities, European Vertebral Study Group. *Am J Epidemiol* 146:287–293, 1997.
18. Legrand E, Chappard D, Pascaretti C, et al: Trabecular bone microarchitecture, bone mineral density, and vertebral fractures in male osteoporosis. *J Bone Miner Res* 15:13–19, 2000.
19. Legrand E, Chappard D, Pascaretti C, et al: Trabecular bone microarchitecture and male osteoporosis. *Morphologie* 83:35–40, 1999.
20. McCarthy EF: The pathology of transient regional osteoporosis. *Iowa Orthop J* 18:35–42, 1998.
21. Mirra JM, Brien EW, Tehranzadeh J: Paget's disease of bone: review with emphasis on radiologic features. Part 1. *Skeletal Radiol* 24:163–171, 1995.
22. O'Flaherty EJ: Modeling normal aging bone loss, with consideration of bone loss in osteoporosis. *Toxicol Sci* 55:171–188, 2000.
23. Ogilvie-Harris DJ, Fornasier VL: Pathological fractures of the hand in Paget's disease. *Clin Orthop* 143:168–170, 1979.
24. Ritzel H, Amling M, Posl M, et al: The thickness of human vertebral cortical bone and its changes in aging and osteoporosis: a histomorphometric analysis of the complete spinal column from thirty-seven autopsy specimens. *J Bone Miner Res* 12:89–95, 1997.
25. Urovitz EPM, Fornasier VL, Risen MI: Etiological factors in the pathogenesis of femoral trabecular fatigue fractures. *Clin Orthop* 127:275–280, 1977.

38

Microangiography, Macrosectioning, and Preparation for Contact Radiography

Yebin Jiang,[1] Yunzhao Wang,[2] Dianmin Xue,[2] and Yuming Yin[3]

[1]Osteoporosis and Arthritis Research Group, Department of Radiology, University of California, San Francisco, CA, USA
[2]Department of Radiologic Pathology, Beijing Institute of Traumatology and Orthopaedics, Beijing Ji Shui Tan Hospital, Beijing, P.R. China
[3]Department of Radiology, Washington University School of Medicine, St. Louis, MO, USA

I. INTRODUCTION

Musculoskeletal microangiography, histopathological macrosection, and contact microradiography are widely used for investigation of the microvasculature and macro- and microstructure of bone, cartilage, and muscles. The usefulness of these techniques has been documented in the literature of orthopedic research as well as in the literature of radiology studying radiologic-pathologic correlations, histopathologic characteristics, and explanations of radiologic manifestations.

These techniques are useful for the investigation of cortical and trabecular bone modeling and remodeling, and may find application in the study of skeletal developmental embryology, angiogenesis and osteogenesis (Fig. 1–4), bone tumors, fracture healing, metabolic bone diseases (Fig. 5), endemic bone and joint diseases, and arthritis.

II. MICROANGIOGRAPHY

There are several approaches to microangiography. One injects a contrast medium, such as barium sulfate, into the microvasculature, followed by radiography. Another approach is to stain the microvasulature using, for example, Chinese ink, and to examine the microvasculature histologically. These methods can be used in surgical specimens, dead embryos or fetuses, and various animal models.[1–4] Specimens should be fresh, so that the contrast media or staining materials can be successfully injected into the microvasculature.

A. Contrast Media Injection

Barium sulfate is the most commonly used media for microangiography. It shows very high contrast on radiographs.

From: *Handbook of Histology Methods for Bone and Cartilage*
Edited by: Y. H. An and K. L. Martin © Humana Press Inc., Totowa, NJ

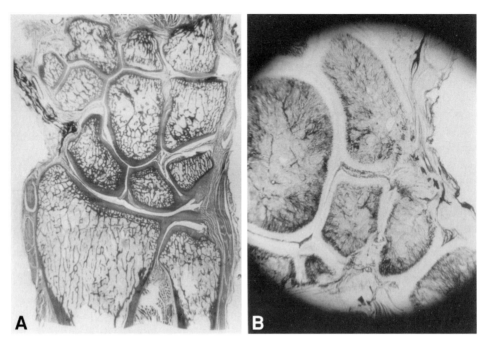

Figure 1. (A) Celloidin-embedded decalcified macrosection of the carpal bones and distal radius and distal ulna from an adult human cadaver (H&E stain). (B) Corresponding microvasculature with Chinese ink injection of the carpal bone.

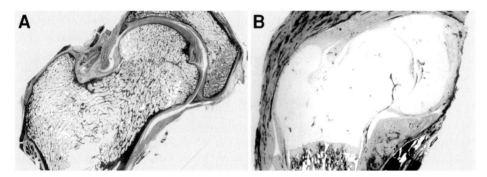

Figure 2. Celloidin-embedded decalcified macrosection of the hip from (A) an adult human cadaver or (B) a dead fetus (H&E stain).

Method: Commercially available barium sulfate that is commonly employed for radiological gastrointestinal examination can be used. Add 50 g of barium sulfate to 100 mL saline, and stir well until it becomes a homogenous suspension. Inject the suspension into a main artery through a catheter.

For bone microangiography, contact radiographs can be taken after injection of the contrast media, with or without decalcification. Higher contrast and more detailed structure of the microvasculature can be observed with decalcification of the bone specimen.

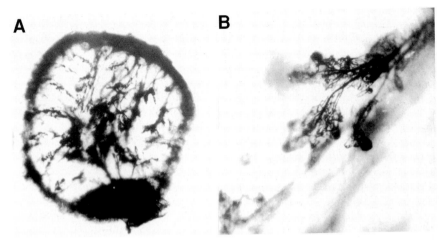

Figure 3. Celloidin-embedded macrosection with Chinese ink injection of the cartilage in the epiphysis of a fetus shows microvascular structure. Low- (A) and high- (B) power views.

Advantage: This method is relatively easy, and the procedures are clean compared to ink injection. Both bone tissue and microvasculature can be observed on undecalcified radiographs.

Disadvantage: The microvascular structure cannot be appreciated on histological sections because barium sulfate does not stain the structure. In addition, during the injection procedure, there is some resistance of the vessels to injecting the barium sulfate suspension.

B. Chinese Ink Injection

Chinese ink is a good staining agent for microangiography, because it stays firmly in the microvasculature, and will not influence histopathological observation of the structure of other cells in bones, joints, or muscles.

Method: Commercially available Chinese ink used for calligraphy and painting can be injected into a main artery through a catheter. The specimen is then processed for histological section for observation of microvasculature.

Advantage: Chinese ink is easy to inject, and provides very good staining for microvasculature. It is not expensive and is widely available, as it is extensively used in Chinese calligraphy and Chinese painting, and is waterproof in these applications.

Disadvantage: Microvasculature cannot be observed on radiography because, unlike barium sulfate, Chinese ink is not radiopaque.

C. Injection with a Mixture of Barium Sulfate and Chinese Ink

Mix equal amounts of the barium sulfate suspension and Chinese ink, stir very well, and inject the mixture into a main artery through a catheter. The specimen is radiographed, and then sectioned for histological examination.

Such an injection has advantages over the two techniques applied separately, as microvasculature can be examined on both histological section and microradiography.

D. Selecting an Artery for Injection

For surgical specimens such as amputated extremities, the main artery supplying the specimen should be found immediately and marked with a suture to avoid difficulty in locating the artery later following shrinkage into other soft tissues.

In animal studies, euthanasia should be immediately followed by injection of barium sulfate suspension, Chinese ink, or a combination of these through catheterization into the main artery—e.g., the right iliac artery for right lower extremity.

For studying the whole dead embryo or fetus, the contrast or stain agent should be injected through the umbilical artery.

E. Amount of Contrast Media or Chinese Ink to Be Injected

When effusion of the contrast media or Chinese ink can be observed through the skin, the injection can be stopped as soon as the contrast and/or staining agents have filled the microvasculature. To test whether the medium has diffused thoroughly, make a small cut in a distal phalanx: if drops of the contrast and/or staining agents emerge from the bone-marrow cavity the injection has been successful.

III. SPECIMEN PREPARATION

A. Fixing Specimens

Before fixing the specimen, it is useful to take a contact radiograph of the specimen to ascertain the structure and location of joint components.

The specimen can then be dissected, and placed in a container with 10% neutral buffered formalin (NBF). Small samples, such as rat bones, can be fixed in 24 h. Large specimens, such as whole adult human lower extremities, take about 2 wk to fix completely. Adding formalin to the contrast and/or staining agents and injecting them together will shorten the fixing duration by one-half, but will cause the tissue to contract, thus increasing resistance to injection.

B. Cutting, Slabbing, and Radiography

The fixed specimen can be further reduced by cutting and slabbing, using a band saw for big specimens or a low-speed metallurgical saw (Isomet saw) for smaller specimens. Slabs should be no more than 1 cm thick, and small specimens can be cut into thinner slabs. The thinner the specimen, the easier it is for graded alcohol or acetone to dehydrate the specimen and for embedding materials to infiltrate.

If the specimen is not well-fixed, the slabs can be further fixed with 10% NBF.

After cutting and slabbing the specimen, it is useful to take a contact radiograph of the slab specimen to examine its fine radiologic structure.

C. Decalcification

If the purpose of the investigation is to study cellular activities, especially those of the cell structure embedded in calcified bone matrix, it is important to clearly stain the cells after removing the calcium. An acid solution is commonly used to remove the calcium. Strong acid, such as nitric acid, removes the calcium quickly, but can easily destroy the bone matrix and cellular structure and is thus not recommended. The most commonly used acid is a mixture of 30% formic acid with 10% formalin. The formalin protects the cellular structure from damage by the acid. The volume of the acid solution should be 10 times the volume of the specimen, and should completely cover the specimen.

To check the progress of decalcification, insert a needle into the bone samples. If there is no resistance, or no more than in the soft tissue, decalcification is complete. To confirm the success of decalcification, a radiograph can verify that no calcium is present. If decalcification is incomplete, it will be very difficult to cut the specimen after it is embedded in paraffin or celloidin. The calcium can damage a cutting knife unless it is diamond- or tungsten carbide-tipped.

Decalcification can be accelerated, especially for large specimens from adult humans, by electrolysis. However, the temperature must be carefully monitored because it is easily raised, and this can destroy a specimen.

After fixing and/or decalcification, the slabs should be washed with continuously running tap water for about 3 d to clear the formalin and/or acid and allow better staining of cells and matrix.

D. Dehydrating, Trimming, and Defatting

After washing out the fixing formalin and/or decalcification acid, the slab should be dehydrated gradually with 80%, 95%, and 100% ethanol for 4 h to 2 d at each concentration, depending on the size of the specimen. The bigger and thicker the specimen, the longer it will take to dehydrate. Immediately after the 80% ethanol, the specimen should be trimmed, unnecessary tissues should be cut away, and the thickness minimized. A sharp knife should be used, to avoid deforming the tissue. The 100% ethanol should be repeated to ensure complete dehydration.

The specimen should then be defatted with two changes of acetone, for one-half to 2 d each, according to the thickness and size of the specimen.

IV. CELLOIDIN-EMBEDDED SPECIMENS

A. Characteristics of Celloidin

Celloidin can be dissolved in a mixture of equal amounts of ethanol and ether, in acetone and in clove oil. The mixture is highly volatile. The container should be closed and sealed. A celloidin block has a hardness similar to decalcified bone tissue and ligaments, and provides good tenacity. It does not usually break, and there is little visual distortion. The section can be stained without removing the celloidin. It is superb for thick-slice macrosections of microvasculature injected with Chinese ink. The hardness of the block can be adjusted by exposure to different concentrations of ethanol: immersion in 70% ethanol will increase hardness, in 85% ethanol will decrease hardness, and in 80% ethanol, hardness will be unchanged.

B. Infiltration and Embedding

The dehydrated specimen is infiltrated gradually with increasing concentrations of celloidin solution—i.e., 2%, 4%, 6%, 8%, 10%, 12%, for a few days to 1 wk in each according to the thickness and size of the specimen.

Place the well-infiltrated specimen in a glass dish filled with 15–20% celloidin solution. Place it gently to avoid air bubbles. The side that will be sectioned first should be face down. Cover the dish, but do not seal it so that the solution will slowly volatilize.

When the periphery of the block becomes solid and as hard as rubber, separate its edge from the dish with a knife, and fill the dish with 80% ethanol for 3–5 d to make the block homogeneously hard as rubber. Trim the block, leaving a celloidin margin about 2–3 mm thick around the specimen. Store the block in 80% ethanol.

C. Specimen Holder

Immerse a dry wood specimen holder in a solution of equal volumes of ethanol and ether for 5–10 min. Meanwhile, after clearing the other side (opposite sectioning side) of the block, place it in this solution for 1–3 min to make it soft and sticky. Put some 15–20% celloidin solution on one side of the wood specimen holder, and immediately place the soft and sticky side of the block onto the wood specimen holder. Gently press the block to eliminate air bubbles between the specimen holder and the block so that they adhere firmly to each other. Place the side of the block that will be sectioned into a glass dish with 80% ethanol to avoid further hardening of the block. Do not let the 80% ethanol touch the junction between the block and the wood specimen holder, or they may come apart. Cover the dish.

D. Sectioning

Fix the specimen holder on a microtome, and set the angle between the cutting surface of the knife and sectioning surface of the specimen at 45 degrees. Trim away the surface celloidin. When approaching the tissue, use a small brush to moisten the knife and specimen with 80% ethanol before each pass of the knife to reduce friction and contraction of the celloidin, which will lead to variations in the thickness of the slices. Place the slice in a glass dish filled with 80% ethanol.

For microvasculature, a thickness of 200 μm should be used. For histological observation, 5–20 μm thickness should be used. A few slices should be set aside for different staining methods such as hematoxylin and eosin (H&E), Masson's trichrome, and van Gieson's.

The microtome used can be manual or automatic, sliding or rotating. For large samples, a heavy-duty motor-driven sliding microtome is preferred (Fig. 6).

E. Mounting Microvascular Slices

The 200-μm slice for examining microvasculature needs no further staining, and is ready for mounting. Handling the slice with tweezers, dehydrate it in graded ethanols at 80%, 95%, and 100%, for 5–10 min at each concentration. Dehydrate further in two changes of absolute ethanol. Clear the slice in two changes of xylene, for 3–5 min each. Leaving the slice in the xylene too long will lead to deformities and hardening of the section, making it difficult to mount. An ample amount of Permount (Fisher Scientific) should be put on a glass slide, the section placed on top of the Permount, and a few drops of Permount put on top of the section. Use a few drops of xylene to eliminate air bubbles in the Permount, and cover slip with a thick glass. Extra care should be taken to prevent and remove air bubbles using extra drops of Permount and xylene afterward.

F. Staining

There are many staining methods, but the basic procedures are similar. Only the H&E staining procedures are presented here. After washing the 5–20 μm slices in distilled water to remove the alcohol, put them in hematoxylin solution for 20–30 min, then into

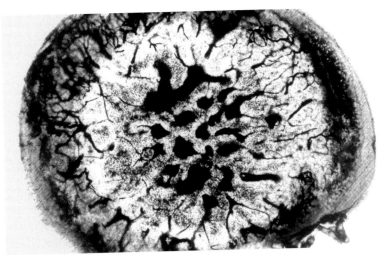

Figure 4. Microphotograph of cross-section of the femoral neck of an adult rat showing the microvascularity. Undecalcified 25-μm-thick sections with vascular microinjection of Chinese ink and Villanueva bone stain. Magnification ×40.

regular tap water until the celloidin margin around the specimen becomes dark blue. Place the slices into diluted HCl solution (1%) until the dark blue color in the celloidin margin is gone, and return them to tap water. Check a slice under a microscope to ascertain that the staining is satisfactory, then rinse in distilled water, place them in the eosin solution for 1 min, and dehydrate in graded ethanols. Place a single slice flat, with no buckling, on paper for support and transfer to two changes of absolute ethanol, clear in two changes of xylene, place on a glass slide, and finally cover slip with Permount. Take care to avoid air bubbles.

V. OTHER EMBEDDING MATERIALS

Paraffin can be used to embed large specimens for macrosectioning after decalcification. The technique is similar to microsectioning. The main difference is that a automatic sliding microtome should be used, freeing both hands to handle the specimen. Before sectioning, the embedded block should be cooled to harden the paraffin to the hardness of the decalcified specimen. Between sections and after trimming the block, ice should be placed on the surface to cool it again. Staining and mounting are the same as in microsectioning.

Paraffin should not be used for microvasculature studies because it is not strong enough to support thicker slices.

Methyl methacrylate (MMA) can be used for thicker microvasculature slices with or without decalcification (Fig. 4, 5). MMA is hard and difficult to cut with a microtome. The block should be cut using a saw, such as low-speed Isomet saw. The slice can then be ground to 200 μm for study directly under the microscope without mounting. Undecalcified sections can be ground to 30 μm for studying dynamic bone mineralization after double-labeling using dynamic bone histomorphometry, and then microradiographed for

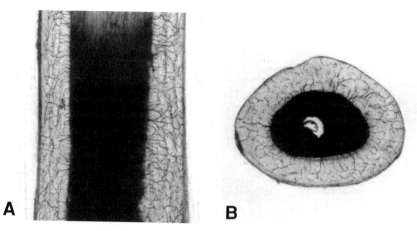

Figure 5. Microphotographs of the central coronal section (A) and cross-section of the distal femoral diaphysis (B) in an adult rat show that vascularity in the inner two-thirds of the cortex is radially oriented from the medullary canal and some short longitudinal channels are present in the outer one-third of the cortex. Undecalcified 200-μm-thick sections with vascular microinjection of Chinese ink and Villanueva bone stain. Magnification ×10.

bone microstructure and mineralization mapping within single trabeculae. A heavy-duty microtome can used to produce thin sections from decalcified or undecalcified MMA-embedded specimens (Fig. 6). Since thin-slice cutting and staining of macro- and microsections are very similar, refer to the chapter on microsectioning (*see* Chapter 13).

VI. MICROVASCULAR QUANTIFICATION

The microvascular macrosection can be digitized using a microscope coupled to a camera and computer. National Institutes of Health (NIH) imaging software or image-analysis software can be used. Each image must be corrected for background variations. For structural analysis, gray-scale images with a range of values must be segmented into binary images with only two values—white and black—representing vasculature and non-vasculature. The chosen threshold should give satisfactory segmentation, as determined by visual assessment. Total tissue area, microvascular area, and perimeter can be measured directly, and percentage microvascular area, microvascular number, thickness, and separation can be calculated according to node or the parallel-plate model assumptions used in bone histomorphometry.[2,5,8] Measurements of vascular connectivity such as the number of microvascular nodes, free ends, and branches can be obtained from a skeletonized trabecular network generated by using thinning algorithms.[6,7]

The three-dimensional (3D) structure of the microvasculature can also be obtained and directly quantified. If Chinese ink has been used, consecutive sections should be obtained with each slice digitized to generate 3D images, following any necessary image processing such as image registration. 3D images can also be obtained by sequentially imaging the surface of the block at regular increments as it is being ground to the specified thickness. Micro-CT can be used to generate 3D microvasculature from slices injected with barium sulfate.

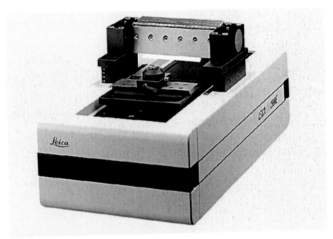

Figure 6. A heavy-duty, sliding automatic microtome (Polycut, Leica, Wetzlar, Germany) can free both hands to handle the sectioning procedures, for both macro- and micro-sectioning undecalcified or decalcified specimens embedded in paraffin, celloidin, or MMA.

Image processing algorithms, free from the model assumptions used in two-dimensional (2D) bone histomorphometry, can be used to segment and directly quantify 3D microvasculature, similar to assessment of 3D trabecular bone structure.[6] Vascular thickness is determined by filling maximal spheres in the structure with the distance transformation, then calculating the average thickness of all vascular voxels. Vascular separation is calculated with the same procedure, but the voxels representing nonvascular parts are filled with maximal spheres. Separation is the thickness of the nonvascular cavities. Vascular number is taken as the inverse of the mean distance between the mid-axes of the observed structure.

VII. SUMMARY

In practice, microangiography, histopathological macrosectioning and contact microradiography are tedious and labor-intensive, but quite straightforward. Creative but careful adherence to procedures will yield rewarding results. Whether for qualitative or quantitative assessment, these techniques have many interesting and useful applications in musculoskeletal research.

REFERENCES

1. Cheng X, Wang Y, Qu H, et al.: Ossification processes and perichondral ossification groove of Ranvier: a morphological study in developing human calcaneus and talus. *Foot Ankle Int* 16:7–10, 1995.
2. Jiang Y: *Radiology and Histology in the Assessment of Bone Quality.* Peeters, Leuven, Belgium, 1995:15–129.
3. Jiang Y, Wang Y, Zhao J, et al: Bone remodeling in hypervitaminosis D_3: Radiologic-microangiographic-pathologic correlations. *Invest Radiol* 26:213–219, 1991.
4. Jiang Y, Wang Y, Zhao J, et al: Metastatic calcification within bone, the main cause of osteosclerosis in hypervitaminosis D_3: Radiologic-pathologic correlations. *Invest Radiol* 25:1188–1196, 1990.

5. Jiang Y, Zhao J: Histomorphometry. In: Liu ZH, ed: *Osteoporosis.* Science Publication House, Beijing, China, 1998:443–456.
6. Jiang Y, Zhao J, White DL, et al: Micro CT and micro MR imaging of 3D architecture of animal skeleton. *J Musculoskel Neuron Interact* 1:45–51, 2000.
7. Korstjens CM, Geraets WG, van Ginkel FC, et al: Longitudinal analysis of radiographic trabecular pattern by image processing. *Bone* 17:527–532, 1995.
8. Parfitt AM, Drezner MK, Glorieux FH, et al: Bone histomophometry: standardization of nomenclature, symbols, and units. *J Bone Miner Res* 2:595–610, 1987.

VIII Recognizing and Avoiding Artifacts

39

Recognizing and Interpreting Histology Artifacts in Hard-Tissue Research

Thomas W. Bauer

Departments of Pathology and Orthopaedic Surgery, The Cleveland Clinic Foundation,
Cleveland, OH, USA

I. INTRODUCTION

An impressive spectrum of high-technology tools is now available to study the safety and efficacy of new materials and devices. Magnetic resonance and CT scanning along with transmission and scanning electron microscopy, confocal microscopy, and atomic force microscopy are only a few of the impressive tools now available and useful in biomedical materials research. In the face of such technological advances, it is surprising to some that the foundation upon which all other morphological studies are derived remains basic light microscopy. Tissues are sampled, fixed, dehydrated, embedded in paraffin wax, sectioned, stained, and viewed with an optical microscope using transmitted light in a manner that has changed little in more than a century.[4,7] Indeed, basic light microscopy of paraffin-embedded tissue, especially when interpreted in conjunction with other clinical findings, continues to be the most cost-effective method to diagnose the entire spectrum of inflammatory and neoplastic conditions, and forms a cornerstone for testing the biocompatibility of new materials.

Despite a century of use, routine tissue processing is far from perfect. Every microscope slide contains artifacts. Most experienced pathologists easily recognize and dismiss these artifacts, but some investigators who are involved in the evaluation of orthopedic biomaterials do not have extensive experience interpreting microscope slides, and artifacts misinterpreted as significant findings are relatively common in the published biomedical materials literature as well as in presentations and posters exhibited at major meetings. The purpose of this chapter is to describe and illustrate a few common histologic artifacts, and to draw attention to other aspects of specimen preparation and experimental design that may be helpful in the study of tissues around retrieved human devices as well as in preclinical animal studies.

II. ROUTINE, DECALCIFIED, PARAFFIN-EMBEDDED HISTOLOGY

The methods of routine histologic tissue processing include sampling, fixation, decalcification if necessary, dehydration, embedding, sectioning, staining, and interpretation. There are opportunities for artifacts at each of these steps.

From: *Handbook of Histology Methods for Bone and Cartilage*
Edited by: Y. H. An and K. L. Martin © Humana Press Inc., Totowa, NJ

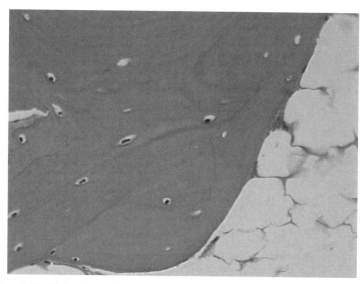

Figure 1. Decalcified histology of normal cancellous bone. Note that most, but not necessarily all, lacunae contain visible osteocytes.

A. *Obtaining the Sample*

Once a specimen has been obtained, it should be placed promptly into a suitable fixative. Although this seems obvious, there are countless examples of expensive preclinical studies that are essentially worthless because of unsatisfactory tissue handling. For example, it is common for investigators to do mechanical testing and histology on the same samples. Mechanical testing will inevitably compromise histology, even if that testing is not carried to mechanical failure, simply because of the delay in fixation that inevitably results from the mechanical testing. Delayed fixation causes air-dry artifacts as well as autolysis. If histology is given high priority for a given study, then samples should be dedicated to histology without mechanical testing, and should be placed into an appropriate volume of fixative within minutes of the time they are obtained. These samples should not be placed in saline, refrigerated, or frozen. Although the histology of frozen tissue is not worthless, it is not as useful as histology of well-fixed tissues (Figs. 1,2).

Specimens for histology should be handled gently at the time of sampling. Some types of cells are especially fragile, and are easily crushed. The resulting crush artifact seen on microscope slides is uninterpretable. Forceps should also be used with care in transferring tissue into fixative or other containers. Sometimes a small piece of tissue from one specimen can adhere to the tip of the forceps and be accidentally transferred to the container for a different specimen. This "carry-over" will be embedded and will appear in each histologic section. Although rarely a problem in biomedical materials research, this type of error has critical consequences when dealing with human biopsy specimens. Either fresh instruments should be used with each case, or at a minimum, forceps should be rinsed and cleaned before handling tissues from different cases.

The use of thermal cutting tools is common in surgery. Although these instruments have some advantages with respect to patient care, the heat causes thermal damage to adjacent tissues that can compromise slide interpretation.[1] Power drills also generate considerable

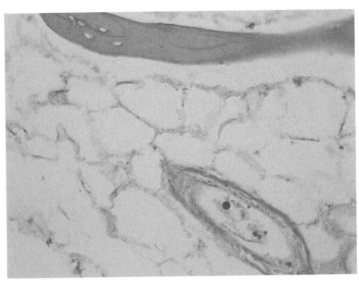

Figure 2. Decalcified histology of a specimen that was not placed promptly in fixative. Cells have lysed, and cell membranes are not distinct. This autolysis artifact should not be misinterpreted as necrosis or as bone-marrow edema.

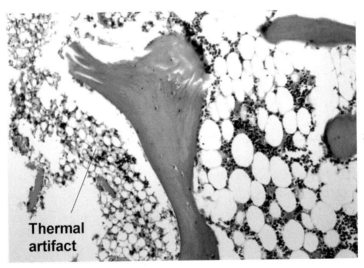

Figure 3. A power drill was used to obtain this core biopsy of a femoral head. The thermal artifact from the drill induces a "microvesicular" change to the marrow fat that should not be misinterpreted as early ischemic necrosis.

heat, and the thermal damage to bone and marrow fat can resemble the "microvesicular" appearance of early ischemic necrosis (Fig. 3).

B. Fixation

A common cause of poor-quality histology is inadequate fixation. Although 70% ethanol is satisfactory for some types of specimens, the most useful tissue fixative in general continues to be 10% neutral buffered formalin (NBF). Formalin penetrates tissues fairly well, and fixes tissues well enough to be suitable for transmission electron microscopy (TEM) as well as light microscopy, but good formalin fixation requires an adequate volume of fixative. The reaction product of the chemical reaction between formalin and tissue is water,[5] so if insufficient formalin surrounds a tissue specimen, the concentration of formalin decreases with time. The most common error in tissue processing is to put too large a piece of tissue into a small volume of fixative. Most protocols recommend a ratio of 10–20 volumes of fixative per volume of tissue.[3] We recommend using a saw to trim bone samples to a thickness of 2–5 mm prior to fixation. The use of a saw may impact small particles of bone (bone dust) into adjacent cancellous bone (Fig. 4). To minimize this artifact, bone specimens can be gently brushed under running water before being placed into fixative.

Tissue that has been formalin-fixed inevitably undergoes some shrinkage. The amount of volumetric shrinkage varies, but has been estimated to be about 10%. Some types of cells and tissues show more shrinkage than others, resulting in the appearance of empty spaces on microscope slides. For example, even well-fixed and processed cancellous bone will contain osteocytes that have shrunk within their lacunae (Fig. 1), creating the appearance of empty spaces surrounding pyknotic nuclei. The osteocyte lacunae in Fig. 1 measure about 17 μm in diameter, and the visible cells measure about 7 μm, creating an apparent space of several micrometers around each osteocyte nucleus. Based on these dimensions, we would expect to see some lacunae that appear to be empty simply based on the stereology of cutting 5-μm sections through lacunae with the contents previously described. This is one reason why the diagnosis of osteonecrosis requires more than simply noting the presence of occasional empty osteocyte lacunae.

Another artifact that can be misinterpreted as orthopedic wear debris is formalin pigment (Fig. 5). When acidic formalin reacts with hemoglobin, a brown pigment forms and precipitates onto the section, yielding a histologic appearance similar to hemosiderin or particles of wear debris. Formalin pigment precipitation is minimized by using formalin that has been buffered to nearly neutral pH.[6]

C. Improper Decalcification

Bone can be processed without decalcification, embedded in plastic, and either hand-ground or cut with a special microtome to provide excellent quality sections, but for most purposes decalcified sections still provide the most cost-effective way to evaluate ossified tissues. A number of different reagents are available to demineralize bone, but preparing "decals" of consistently good quality is a problem for many laboratories. Under-decalcified tissues chip or shatter when subjected to sectioning, and cells may be completely dissolved by over-decalcification in strong acids (Fig. 6). Cytolysis by over-decalcification is another reason why empty lacunae are not by themselves diagnostic of ischemic osteonecrosis. Although some investigators place large segments of bone into decalcifying solution for a prolonged period, we recommend trimming the sample with a saw before fixation and decalcification. It is necessary to use an adequate volume of decalcification solution, and using a magnetic stirrer to gently but constantly oscillate the solution may help yield uniform decalcification. Several different methods can be used to determine when sufficient decalcification has occurred. For

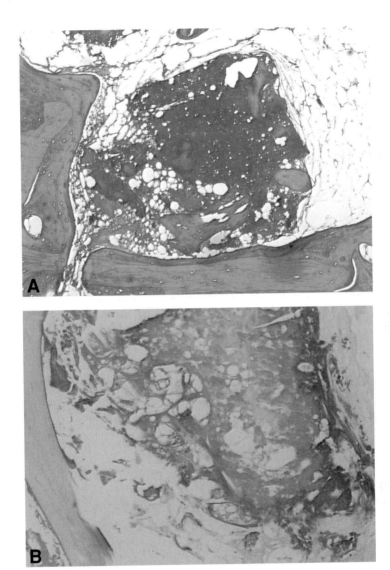

Figure 4. Bone dust can be impacted into cancellous bone when a specimen is cut with a band saw prior to fixation (A). This artifact should not be misinterpreted as the dystrophic calcium commonly seen in a bone infarct (B).

example, the specimen can be physically examined, the calcium content in the solution can be measured, or the tissue can be radiographed.

D. Inadequate Dehydration or Embedding

Tissue that is too rapidly processed through dehydration alcohols is very difficult to cut and has poor cellular preservation. The resulting block is brittle, and tends to chatter or shred when sectioned. Sometimes the specimen can be salvaged by rehydration followed by careful dehydration and re-embedding, but the final quality is still compromised, often because the tissue was inadequately fixed in the first place.

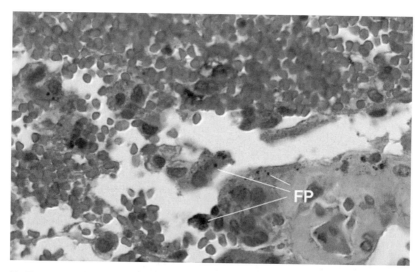

Figure 5. Formalin pigment (FP) may precipitate if the fixative pH is too low. This is especially common in areas of hemorrhage, and should not be misinterpreted as orthopedic wear debris. The pigment seems to adhere to macrophages and giant cells, making the distinction even more important.

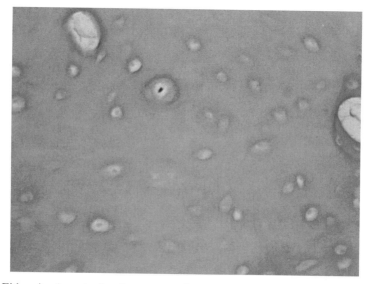

Figure 6. Either inadequate fixation or overdecalcification can destroy osteocytes. Empty lacunae are a common artifact, and should not be misinterpreted as diagnostic of osteonecrosis.

E. Sectioning Artifacts

Well-processed and embedded tissues are relatively easy to cut with a microtome. Simple cutting artifacts such as knife marks can be corrected by recuts with a suitable microtome blade. Unfortunately, most histologic artifacts in decalcified tissues are not based on errors in sectioning, but rather on inadequate fixation or tissue processing, so that deeper

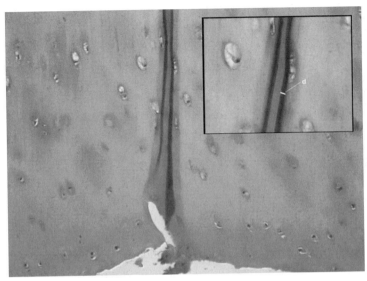

Figure 7. Some artifacts can be useful. Most sections contain folds, and by focusing on the edge of the fold, the thickness of the section can be visualized and, if necessary, measured (d).

sections from the same block are unlikely to show much improvement. Nevertheless, it is important to recognize sectioning artifacts, especially if histomorphometry will be used to quantify aspects of morphology. Sometimes trabeculae of cancellous bone are lifted out of the section, leaving behind apparent spaces. These spaces can be misinterpreted as vascular channels, and can be especially important if they are not recognized during a study in which different tissue compartments are being quantified with the use of histomorphometry.

One type of sectioning artifact can be an asset. Experimental studies often use morphometry to quantify histologic findings in sections from different experimental groups. An underlying assumption of all histomorphometry is that sections are of uniform thickness. In fact, minor differences in section thickness are common, and major differences in section thickness can have profound effects on the results of morphometry. Almost all histologic sections contain folds. By carefully focusing on the edge of the fold, the thickness of the section can be visualized and measured if necessary, thereby documenting the thickness in that part of the microscope slide (Fig. 7). Measuring multiple folds can provide information about thickness variability within an individual section as well as among sections of each experimental group.

Once a section has been cut with a microtome, it is floated on a water bath and then transferred to a microscope slide. In a busy laboratory, a histotechnologist may cut many blocks from different specimens, and occasionally a fragment from one sample is accidentally picked up along with the intended section from another specimen. This "pick-up" can be recognized and distinguished from a "carry-over" as a piece of tissue adjacent to one tissue section, but not present in serial sections of that block.

F. Staining

The frequency and importance of staining artifacts depend largely on the type of stain that is used. A common artifact is the presence of precipitated stain pigment such as hematoxylin or toluidine blue. Small grains of hematoxylin pigment can be misinterpreted as orthopedic wear debris. One clue to help recognize this stain artifact is the distribution of the pigment over all of the tissue and on the microscope slide away from the tissue.

Special histochemical or immunohistochemical stains can be used to identify specific cells or extracellular substances in microscope slides. It is beyond the scope of this chapter to describe potential artifacts related to these types of stains, but investigators who interpret special stains must be aware of the types of positive and negative controls required for documenting stain specificity.

Another artifact related to staining is the presence of stained keratinocytes derived from the hands of the histotechnologist. These cells can be found on most routinely processed slides, but usually are of no consequence and are easily dismissed by experienced pathologists.

It is appropriate to wear disposable gloves when handling tissues, and some histotechnologists wear gloves while preparing microscope slides. Although most gloves are now free of talc, other types of glove powder are birefringent, and can contaminate microscope slides. If not recognized, glove powder can be misinterpreted as particles of polarizable foreign debris.[2] Although this is not a common problem in routinely processed tissues, glove powder can often be visualized on frozen sections viewed with the use of polarized light.

III. FROZEN SECTIONS

The interpretation of histologic sections obtained from frozen tissue is not necessary for the evaluation of many orthopedic biomaterials, but still has an important place in the field of orthopedic pathology in general. For example, the interpretation of frozen sections can be helpful in determining the presence or absence of infection at the time of revision arthroplasty, and frozen sections play an important role in the diagnosis and staging of tumors. In addition, despite the principles described above, some investigators still insist upon mechanically testing orthopedic specimens prior to histology, and choose to preserve the specimens by freezing rather than by using fixative solutions. Finally, some proteins and other antigens are best identified with the use of immunohistochemical and other staining techniques that require the use of frozen tissue. Therefore, recognizing artifacts related to frozen tissue may be a necessary aspect of biomaterials research.

If tissue is to be frozen, the histologic features are best preserved by very rapid freezing to a low temperature. This is best achieved by covering a small tissue sample with an appropriate commercial embedding medium, such as OCT compound (Tissue Tek, Torrance, CA), immersing the tissue in liquid nitrogen, and obtaining a frozen section with the use of a cryostat. Although artifacts related to freezing and subsequent thawing are inevitable, the artifacts are not as severe as when a specimen is simply placed in a conventional freezer.

Under optimal conditions frozen sections obtained as described here yield relatively good morphology. However, it should be recognized that red blood cells and the granules within neutrophils are lysed by freezing, so their presence must be determined by other clues at the time of slide interpretation (such as the distinctive shape of the nucleus in the case of neutrophils). Slow freezing produces ice crystals that can drastically distort the tissue, and slow thawing encourages autolysis.

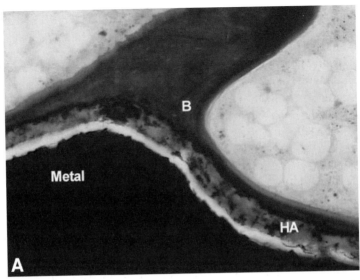

Figure 8. There are no empty spaces in vivo. Blood, serum, or cells make their way into all potential spaces. In (A), an artifact in which a hydroxyapatite coating (HA) has separated from the metal substrate during slide preparation is illustrated. This should not be interpreted as coating delamination in vivo. *(Figure continues)*

IV. UNDECALCIFIED HISTOLOGY

Routine histology with decalcification of bone is the most cost-effective way to process many orthopedic specimens, but if the experimental design requires the recognition of unmineralized bone (osteoid), or if it is desirable to evaluate the interface between bone and a synthetic biomaterial, undecalcified sections may be necessary. Undecalcified sections share many of the histologic artifacts described in Section III, and because these sections are often subjected to histomorphometry, it is especially important to recognize these artifacts. Several different techniques for preparing microscope slides of bone and implants are described elsewhere in this volume. Regardless of the methods of embedding and sectioning, it is difficult to consistently make perfect sections of hard tissues, and these microscope slides often contain artifacts, the most common of which relate to debris from the implant itself or from grit used to sand the sections. Whether cut with a saw or ground by hand, debris often becomes embedded in the section. It is sometimes not possible to definitively distinguish orthopedic wear debris from debris produced during section preparation. One approach is to study the nature of the cells around the particles. Particles that are within macrophages or giant cells are most likely not artifacts, whereas particles that are distributed across the tissue section without respect to background are more likely artifacts related to slide preparation. Similarly, empty spaces between bone and an implant or between an implant coating and its substrate are artifacts of section preparation. There are no "empty" spaces in vivo. If a coating delaminates in vivo, then something (e.g., serum, blood, or cells) will occupy the space between the delaminated coating and the substrate (Fig. 8). An empty space in a microscope slide is an artifact.

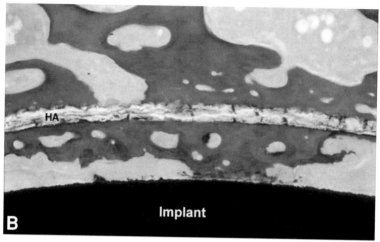

Figure 8. *(Continued)* (B) If the coating delaminated in vivo, cells, fluid, or extracellular matrix would be present between the coating and the substrate.

V. CONCLUSIONS

Despite many technological advances, simple light microscopy remains an indispensable part of biomedical materials research and patient care. No microscope slide is perfect, so it is necessary to recognize histologic artifacts and to interpret them appropriately. Commonly misinterpreted artifacts include contaminants misinterpreted as particles of wear debris, empty osteocyte lacunae mistakenly interpreted as diagnostic of osteonecrosis, and the mis-interpretation of empty spaces in microscope slides as representative of delamination or implant failure in vivo. Once artifacts are recognized, they can be dismissed, and other aspects of the microscope slide can be interpreted in the appropriate context.

Acknowledgement: The author would like to express his appreciation to the many his-totechnologists at the Cleveland Clinic Foundation who consistently strive to produce good quality "decals," especially Ms. Pavlina Pavlosky and Ms. Diane Mahovlic.

REFERENCES

1. Bauer TW, McCarthy JJ, Stulberg BN: Osteonecrosis of the femoral head: Histologic diagnosis and findings after core biopsy. In: Urbaniak JR, Jones JP, eds: *Osteonecrosis: Etiology, Diagnosis and Treatment.* AAOS Publishing, Chicago, IL, 1998:73–79.
2. Bauer TW: Identification of orthopaedic wear debris. *J Bone Joint Surg [Am]* 78:479–483, 1996.
3. DeLellis RA, Faller GT. Cell and tissue staining methods. In: Silverberg SG, Frable WJ, DeLellis RA, eds: *Principles and Practice of Surgical Pathology and Cytopathology, 3rd ed.* Churchill Livingstone, New York, NY, 1997:43–62.
4. Grehn J: *Leitz Microscopes for 125 Years.* Ernst Leitz Wetzlar GmbH, Rockleigh, NJ, 1977:6–10.
5. Pearse AGE: The chemistry of fixation. In: Pearse AGE, ed: *Histochemistry. Theoretical and Applied.* Little Brown and Co., Boston, MA, 1953:11–20.
6. Sheehan DC, Hrapchak BB: *Theory and Practice of Histotechnology.* Battelle Press, Columbus, OH, 1980:214–215.
7. Wright Jr., JR: The development of the frozen section technique, the evolution of surgical biopsy, and the origins of surgical pathology. *Bull Hist Med* 59:295–326, 1985.

INDEX

t: table
f: figure